Telemedicine, Telehealth and Telepresence

Rifat Latifi • Charles R. Doarn
Ronald C. Merrell
Editors

Telemedicine, Telehealth and Telepresence

Principles, Strategies, Applications, and New Directions

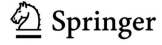

Editors
Rifat Latifi
Department of Surgery
Westchester Medical Center and New York
Medical College
Valhalla, NY
USA

Charles R. Doarn
Department of Environmental and Public
Health Sciences
University of Cincinnati
Cincinnati, OH
USA

Ronald C. Merrell
Virginia Commonwealth University
Mentone, AL
USA

ISBN 978-3-030-56916-7   ISBN 978-3-030-56917-4   (eBook)
https://doi.org/10.1007/978-3-030-56917-4

© Springer Nature Switzerland AG 2021, corrected publication 2021
Chapters 1, 6, 12 and 17 are licensed under the terms of the Creative Commons Attribution 4.0 International License (http://creativecommons.org/licenses/by/4.0/). For further details see license information in the chapters.

This work is subject to copyright. All rights are reserved by the Publisher, whether the whole or part of the material is concerned, specifically the rights of translation, reprinting, reuse of illustrations, recitation, broadcasting, reproduction on microfilms or in any other physical way, and transmission or information storage and retrieval, electronic adaptation, computer software, or by similar or dissimilar methodology now known or hereafter developed.

The use of general descriptive names, registered names, trademarks, service marks, etc. in this publication does not imply, even in the absence of a specific statement, that such names are exempt from the relevant protective laws and regulations and therefore free for general use.

The publisher, the authors and the editors are safe to assume that the advice and information in this book are believed to be true and accurate at the date of publication. Neither the publisher nor the authors or the editors give a warranty, expressed or implied, with respect to the material contained herein or for any errors or omissions that may have been made. The publisher remains neutral with regard to jurisdictional claims in published maps and institutional affiliations.

This Springer imprint is published by the registered company Springer Nature Switzerland AG
The registered company address is: Gewerbestrasse 11, 6330 Cham, Switzerland

Foreword

Few would argue the benefits of telemedicine to the patient, society, the community, the healthcare system, healthcare professionals, and funders. Despite the obvious, the uptake of telemedicine over the last three decades has remained slow, nascent in some parts of the developed world and a dream of unmet potential in the developing world. It is too often inhibited by bureaucracy, regulation, fear of change, lack of awareness, and ignorance. This is particularly unfortunate for the developing world in which I work, where the unmet healthcare burden is greatest. Increasing general awareness and knowledge of telemedicine in all settings is imperative.

The book's editors, Ron Merrell, Chuck Doarn, and Rifat Latifi, have impeccable telemedicine credentials and are acknowledged leaders in the field, having been at the coalface for many years. Ron and Chuck, have been the co-editors of the prestigious *Journal of Telemedicine* and *eHealth*. Rifat is respected internationally for his implementation of telemedicine in Kosova and Cabo Verde among others. All are Fellows of the American Telemedicine Association. They have assembled 66 experts from several countries to author the 28 chapters of this book which cover a wide range of issues. These are divided into Principles of Telemedicine and Telehealth, Strategies for Building Sustainable Telemedicine and Telehealth Programs, Outcomes Based Evidence Clinical Applications of Telemedicine, and the Next Generation of Telemedicine and Telepresence.

Rogers' Diffusion of Technology Curve describes the growing number of users of new technology as the innovators, the early adopters, the early majority, the late majority, and finally the laggards—or perhaps the Luddites. Telemedicine in many parts of the developed world has been at the stages of the early adopters, and in some disciplines, the early majority. The developing world lags at the innovator stage.

To paraphrase the 1956 Dinah Washington song, "What a difference a virus makes." The COVID-19 Pandemic has changed this. Telemedicine is alive and well. Through necessity, many have been obliged to adopt it for their own and their patients' safety. The majority are now using information technology in some form to provide care over distance, and in many countries in the developing world telemedicine is leapfrogging from the innovators to the early majority. Health professionals have discovered telemedicine, and many believe they are innovators because they have changed and adopted it. The need for the evidence behind what they are now doing in their daily telemedicine practice and advice on how to improve what they are doing has been of little importance to them—until now. They need this information.

This book meets that need and will serve those who read it well, as they embrace the culture of telemedicine and draw upon the hard-earned experience and battle scars of the many authors. The surge in telemedicine and its widespread incursion into daily practice will not go away when a vaccine is found. As Benjamin Franklin said, "Out of adversity comes opportunity." The timing of this book is serendipitous and its content welcomed.

Maurice Mars, MBChB, MD,
University of KwaZulu-Natal
Durban, South Africa

Preface

In late 2019 and early 2020, a Coronavirus 2019 (COVID-19) began to affect the entire world. As of June 1, 2020, over 6.3 million (and counting) people worldwide have been affected by COVID-19, with over 376,000 deaths in nearly every country. This pandemic sickens our hearts and minds as we individually are affected and we seem helpless to respond. As practitioners and researchers, we each have our own stories and some have even been sickened by the virus. Returning back to a new normal, whether the operating room, the hospital, or the office after working from home for a few weeks, while recuperating from COVID-19 has been such a treat. Our daily schedule is fuller than ever with virtual meetings using Zoom or Webex as well as normal face-to-face meetings with social distancing ever present in our minds. Yes, the world has changed rapidly and significantly. The old ways may be gone forever. Medical and surgical practice have changed not only from a response to patients with COVID-19 but how world health community has embraced telemedicine and telehealth. Is this a new world order for healthcare?

The pandemic caused by COVID-19 brought to light something that we, the telemedicine and telehealth enthusiasts, have been fighting toward for decades. We knew all along that telemedicine and telehealth can be an excellent model to care of the sick and injured in just about every discipline. Today, a search on PubMed for "COVID-19 and telemedicine or telehealth" results in over 500 manuscripts published for a disease that is less than 6 months old. There is no precedent for this in any field of medicine. These papers are from every aspect of medicine and surgery. Finally telemedicine at center stage [1].

Have you thought, as a surgeon, medical doctor, or any healthcare practitioner, how do we make a diagnosis and how do we create a plan for treatment? We teach our students that history and physical exam are the most important. The diagnosis is confirmed by studies. Yes, we still teach that. After all, most patients have some sort of diagnostic test, including radiologic (usually CT scan, MRI, PET scan, etc.) and other laboratory tests. Gone are the days when we made a diagnosis by examining the patient alone, unless the patient has a clear-cut surgical problem (peritonitis) and needs emergency surgery.

So what is the value of seeing a doctor in his/her office? If the medical and surgical history can be taken via interview across telehealth/telemedicine platform, if the laboratory and radiologic studies are accessible from anywhere in the world through sophisticated software, abundant and present in every laptop or other mobile devices, the question comes down to "why do we need to have a patient travel often for hours, interrupt their life and work, and come to see us in our fancy and expensive offices?" We can obtain the patient's temperature and weight as well as measure blood pressure, pulse, respiratory volume, and other basic medical information virtually while the patient remains in the comfort of their home, office, or where ever they are. Pre-operative and post-operative care can also be accomplished in the same manner so the patient does not have to come to the office.

Integrating telemedicine and telehealth into the healthcare system permits the following: patient safety and elimination of all the inconveniences the patient experiences, including interrupting their day, travel by car or other modality to the doctor's office, spending time parking (oftentimes they have to pay for parking), waiting in the waiting room with other sick patients, and eventually be seen by the provider. This process is long, arduous, and in many cases not necessary. Most clinical encounters can be done virtually using telemedicine and telehealth.

Telemedicine and telehealth have consistently been shown to be effective in regular medical and surgical practice, primary care, and second opinion to extreme conditions, such as crises, disasters, remote areas, or limited-resource locations. All of these are carefully documented in this book. Each chapter is written with the patient and the healthcare system in mind. Patients and the public at large want telemedicine, and so do hospitals and most doctors. While many of us have known the benefits that telemedicine and telehealth offer, convincing the majority of our colleagues has been a struggle, at least until COVID-19 became a threat to humanity [1].

The biggest advantage of telemedicine and telehealth in the current crisis is their ability to continue providing health services at a physical distance. In the USA, the majority of healthcare institutions use some form of telemedicine or telehealth thanks to significant advances in telecommunications including and not limited to improved high-resolution imaging and greater access to broadband. Although nascent technologies, infrastructure, and legislation are increasingly discussed and improved, they remain today at an early stage of integration and diffusion in the current healthcare system. While, we truly believe that telemedicine and telehealth are finally at the center stage, there are challenges to continue with this momentum [1]. The most important challenges the widespread diffusion of telemedicine is facing are: lack of standardized approach and guidelines describing the uniform criteria as to when telemedicine should be a part of the care; absence of clarity on the ways and mechanisms of reimbursement; licensure issues when telemedical care has to cross state lines; compliance with the Health Insurance Portability and Accountability Act (HIPAA) privacy and security rules; and liability and malpractice insurance issues. In addition, technology failures and human factors are also to be considered, but with recent advances, the integration of technology with human factors has become almost seamless. Moreover, with a perfect integration of telemedicine and telehealth in the care of chronic diseases, care continuity questions may arise. The aforementioned factors are probably the reason why telemedicine needs to be integrated into the current healthcare system. COVID-19 has changed this. Imagine, you wake up and the doctor comes to your home or your office virtually. If you have to wait, you are still working or enjoying your day wait ever you are doing. Now, that is a great day in healthcare.

The new world order caused by the COVID-19 virus, associated with severe acute respiratory syndrome, multiple organ failure, and very high mortality, has brought about one major change. Suddenly, the medical community, and those who finance the healthcare sector, realized that telemedicine and telepresence are applicable, desirable, acceptable, and much sought after by our patients and we can manage just about every disease and condition [1]. Although, by and large, telemedicine and telehealth have faced challenges and perhaps some resistance, despite their great potential, it has become evident that they can provide rapid, safe, and high-quality care remotely during this pandemic, the largest one since 1918. Perhaps one benefit of suffering through the COVID-19 pandemic will be the establishment of a new virtual medical world order, and that telemedicine has taken its deserving place in healthcare: prime time and a center stage. Let's call this period the rebirth of telemedicine.

We hope you find this text a worthy reference.

Reference

1. Latifi R, Doarn CR. Perspective on COVID-19: finally, telemedicine at center stage. Telemed J E Health. 2020;26(9):1106–9.

Valhalla, NY, USA	Rifat Latifi
Cincinnati, OH, USA	Charles R. Doarn
Mentone, AL, USA	Ronald C. Merrell
June 1, 2020	

The original version of the book was revised: Chapters 1, 6, 12 and 17 were originally published non-open access. They have been converted to open access under a CC BY 4.0 license and the Copyright is now with "The Author(s)". The correction to the book is available at https://doi.org/10.1007/978-3-030-56917-4_30

Acknowledgement

We would like to thank all the authors and co-authors for their selflessness and major contributions to this book. In addition to their efforts, we would like to thank the Springer team for both their patience and professionalism. Special thank you to Geena George, MPH, a Research Coordinator in the Clinical Research Unit, Department of Surgery, at Westchester Medical Center in Valhalla, NY. Without her help, this book would have never been finished.

Contents

Part I Principles of Telemedicine and Telehealth

1 First Trainees: The Golden Anniversary of the Early History of Telemedicine Education at the Massachusetts General Hospital and Harvard (1968–1970) 3
Ronald S. Weinstein, Michael J. Holcomb, Elizabeth A. Krupinski, and Rifat Latifi

2 Initiate-Build-Operate-Transfer (IBOT) Strategy Twenty Years Later: Tales from the Balkans and Africa. 19
Rifat Latifi

3 Clinical Telemedicine Practice: From Ad Hoc Medicine to Modus Operandi. 43
Rifat Latifi

4 Incorporation of Telemedicine in Disaster Management: Beyond the Era of the COVID-19 Pandemic 51
Rifat Latifi and Charles R. Doarn

5 Telemedicine and Health Information Exchange: An Opportunity for Integration. 63
Dale C. Alverson

6 Telehealth Dissemination and Implementation (D&I) Research: Analysis of the PCORI Telehealth-Related Research Portfolio. 77
Ronald S. Weinstein, Robert S. Krouse, Michael J. Holcomb, Camryn Payne, Kristine A. Erps, Elizabeth A. Krupinski, and Rifat Latifi

7 Standards and Guidelines in Teleheatlh: Creating a Compliance and Evidence-Based Telehealth Practice 97
Nina M. Antoniotti

8 Federal and State Policies on Telehealth Reimbursement. 115
Jordana Bernard and Mei Wa Kwong

| 9 | Legal and Regulatory Implications of Telemedicine 129
Geena George and Brandon E. Heitmann |
|---|---|
| 10 | Business Aspects of Telemedicine 141
Nina M. Antoniotti |
| 11 | Advancing Telehealth to Improve Access to Health
in Rural America. 157
Charles R. Doarn |

Part II Strategies for Building Sustainable Telemedicine and Telehealth Programs

| 12 | Innovative Governance Model for a Sustainable
State-Wide University-Based Telemedicine Program 171
Ronald S. Weinstein, Nandini Sodhi, Gail P. Barker, Michael
J. Holcomb, Kristine A. Erps, Angelette Holtrust, Rifat Latifi,
and Elizabeth A. Krupinski |
|---|---|
| 13 | Telehealth Patient Portal: Opportunities and Reality 189
Ronald C. Merrell |
| 14 | Technology Enabled Remote Healthcare in Public Private
Partnership Mode: A Story from India. 197
K. Ganapathy and Sangita Reddy |
| 15 | International and Global Telemedicine: Making It Work. 235
Dale C. Alverson |
| 16 | Technological Advances Making Telemedicine and Telepresence
Possible. 257
Charles R. Doarn |

Part III Outcomes Based Evidence Clinical Applications of Telemedicine

| 17 | Survey of the Direct-to-Hospital (DTH) Telemedicine
and Telehealth Service Industry (2014–2018). 275
Ronald S. Weinstein, Nicholas Rolig, Nancy Rowe,
Gail P. Barker, Kristine A. Erps, Michael J. Holcomb,
Rifat Latifi, and Elizabeth A. Krupinski |
|---|---|
| 18 | Telemedicine for Trauma and Emergency Care Management. 293
Rifat Latifi |
| 19 | Telemedicine for Burn Care: The Commonsense Telemedicine 307
Dylan Stewart, Joseph R. Turkowski, and Rifat Latifi |

20	**Telemedicine for Intensive Care**	321
	Rifat Latifi and Kalterina Osmani	
21	**Telehealth in Pediatric Care**.................................	333
	Jennifer L. Rosenthal, Jamie L. Mouzoon, and James P. Marcin	
22	**Overview of Child Telebehavioral Interventions Using Real-Time Videoconferencing**............................	347
	Alexandra D. Monzon, E. Zhang, Arwen M. Marker, and Eve-Lynn Nelson	
23	**Telemedicine for Psychiatry and Mental Health**	365
	Matthew Garofalo, Sarah Vaithilingam, and Stephen Ferrando	
24	**Telecardiology**	379
	Milena Soriano Marcolino, Maria Beatriz Moreira Alkmim, Maira Viana Rego Souza e Silva, Renato Minelli Figueira, Raissa Eda de Resende, Letícia Baião Silva, and Antonio Luiz Ribeiro	
25	**Telestroke and Teleneurology**.................................	401
	Benzion Blech and Bart M. Demaerschalk	
26	**Telemedicine for Prisons and Jail Population: A Solution to Increase Access to Care**..........................	419
	Rifat Latifi, Kalterina Osmani, Peter Kilcommons, and Ronald S. Weinstein	

Part IV The Next Generation of Telemedicine and Telepresence

27	**Surgical Telementoring and Teleproctoring**......................	431
	Rifat Latifi, Xiang Da Dong, Ziad Abouezzi, Ashutosh Kaul, Akia Caine, Roberto Bergamaschi, Aram Rojas, Igor A. Laskowski, Donna C. Koo, Tracey L. Weigel, Kaveh Alizadeh, Nikhil Gopal, Akhil Saji, Ashley Dixon, Bertie Zhang, John Phillips, Jared B. Cooper, and Chirag D. Gandhi	
28	**The Promise and Hurdles of Telemedicine in Diabetes Foot Care Delivery**	455
	Bijan Najafi, Mark Swerdlow, Grant A. Murphy, and David G. Armstrong	
29	**Telemedicine in Austere Conditions**	471
	Charles R. Doarn	
Correction to: Telemedicine, Telehealth and Telepresence		C1
	Rifat Latifi, Charles R. Doarn, and Ronald C. Merrell	

Index... 485

Contributors

Ziad Abouezzi Department of Surgery, Westchester Medical Center, Valhalla, NY, USA
New York Medical College, School of Medicine, Valhalla, NY, USA

Kaveh Alizadeh Department of Surgery, Westchester Medical Center, Valhalla, NY, USA
New York Medical College, School of Medicine, Valhalla, NY, USA

Maria Beatriz Moreira Alkmim Telehealth Center, University Hospital, Universidade Federal de Minas Gerais; Telehealth Network of Minas Gerais, Belo Horizonte, Brazil

Dale C. Alverson Health Sciences Center, University of New Mexico, Albuquerque, NM, USA

Nina M. Antoniotti Interoperability and Patient Engagement, St. Jude Children's Research Hospital, Edgar, WI, USA

David G. Armstrong Southwestern Academic Limb Salvage Alliance (SALSA), Department of Surgery, Keck School of Medicine of University of Southern California, Los Angeles, CA, USA

Gail P. Barker Arizona Telemedicine Program, The University of Arizona's College of Medicine, Tucson, AZ, USA

Roberto Bergamaschi Department of Surgery, Westchester Medical Center, Valhalla, NY, USA
New York Medical College, School of Medicine, Valhalla, NY, USA

Jordana Bernard InTouch Health, North Potomac, MD, USA

Benzion Blech Mayo Clinic College of Medicine and Science, Phoenix, AZ, USA

Akia Caine Department of Surgery, Westchester Medical Center, Valhalla, NY, USA
New York Medical College, School of Medicine, Valhalla, NY, USA

Jared B. Cooper New York Medical College, School of Medicine, Valhalla, NY, USA
Department of Neurosurgery, Westchester Medical Center, Valhalla, NY, USA

Bart M. Demaerschalk Medical Director of Center for Connected Care, Cerebrovascular Diseases Division, Mayo Clinic College of Medicine and Science, Phoenix, AZ, USA

Ashley Dixon New York Medical College, School of Medicine, Valhalla, NY, USA
Department of Urology, Westchester Medical Center, Valhalla, NY, USA

Charles R. Doarn Department of Environmental and Public Health Sciences, College of Medicine, University of Cincinnati, Cincinnati, OH, USA

Xiang Da Dong Department of Surgery, Westchester Medical Center, Valhalla, NY, USA
New York Medical College, School of Medicine, Valhalla, NY, USA

Kristine A. Erps Arizona Telemedicine Program, The University of Arizona's College of Medicine, Tucson, AZ, USA

Stephen Ferrando Department of Psychiatry, Westchester Medical Center Health System, New York Medical College, Valhalla, NY, USA

Renato Minelli Figueira Telehealth Center, University Hospital, Universidade Federal de Minas Gerais; Telehealth Network of Minas Gerais, Belo Horizonte, Brazil

K. Ganapathy Apollo Telemedicine Networking Foundation, Chennai, Tamil Nadu, India

Chirag D. Gandhi New York Medical College, School of Medicine, Valhalla, NY, USA
Department of Neurosurgery, Westchester Medical Center, Valhalla, NY, USA

Matthew Garofalo Department of Psychiatry, Westchester Medical Center Health System, New York Medical College, Valhalla, NY, USA

Geena George Department of Surgery, Clinical Research Unit, Westchester Medical Center, Valhalla, NY, USA

Nikhil Gopal New York Medical College, School of Medicine, Valhalla, NY, USA
Department of Urology, Westchester Medical Center, Valhalla, NY, USA

Brandon E. Heitmann Fitzpatrick & Hunt, Pagano, Aubert, LLP, New York, NY, USA

Michael J. Holcomb Arizona Telemedicine Program, The University of Arizona's College of Medicine, Tucson, AZ, USA

Angelette Holtrust Arizona Telemedicine Program, The University of Arizona's College of Medicine, Tucson, AZ, USA

Ashutosh Kaul Department of Surgery, Westchester Medical Center, Valhalla, NY, USA
New York Medical College, School of Medicine, Valhalla, NY, USA

Peter Kilcommons MedWeb, San Francisco, CA, USA

Donna C. Koo Department of Surgery, Westchester Medical Center, Valhalla, NY, USA

New York Medical College, School of Medicine, Valhalla, NY, USA

Robert S. Krouse University of Pennsylvania, Philadelphia, PA, USA

Elizabeth A. Krupinski Emory University, Atlanta, GA, USA

Mei Wa Kwong Center for Connected Health Policy, Sacramento, CA, USA

Igor A. Laskowski Department of Surgery, Westchester Medical Center, Valhalla, NY, USA

New York Medical College, School of Medicine, Valhalla, NY, USA

Rifat Latifi Department of Surgery, Westchester Medical Center Health, Valhalla, NY, USA

New York Medical College, School of Medicine, Valhalla, NY, USA

James P. Marcin Department of Pediatrics, UC Davis Health, Sacramento, CA, USA

Milena Soriano Marcolino Telehealth Center, University Hospital, Universidade Federal de Minas Gerais; Telehealth Network of Minas Gerais, Belo Horizonte, Brazil

Arwen M. Marker Clinical Child Psychology, University of Kansas, Lawrence, KS, USA

Ronald C. Merrell Virginia Commonwealth University, Mentone, AL, USA

Alexandra D. Monzon Clinical Child Psychology, University of Kansas, Lawrence, KS, USA

Jamie L. Mouzoon Department of Pediatrics, UC Davis Health, Sacramento, CA, USA

Grant A. Murphy Southwestern Academic Limb Salvage Alliance (SALSA), Department of Surgery, Keck School of Medicine of University of Southern California, Los Angeles, CA, USA

Bijan Najafi Interdisciplinary Consortium for Advanced Motion Performance (iCAMP), Division of Vascular Surgery and Endovascular Therapy, Michael E. DeBakey Department of Surgery, Baylor College of Medicine, Houston, TX, USA

Eve-Lynn Nelson Pediatrics, University of Kansas Medical Center, Kansas, KS, USA

Kalterina Osmani Department of Medicine, Westchester Medical Center, Valhalla, NY, USA

Camryn Payne Arizona Telemedicine Program, The University of Arizona's College of Medicine, Tucson, AZ, USA

John Phillips New York Medical College, School of Medicine, Valhalla, NY, USA

Department of Urology, Westchester Medical Center, Valhalla, NY, USA

Sangita Reddy Apollo Hospitals Group, Hyderabad, Telangana, India

Raissa Eda de Resende Telehealth Center, University Hospital, Universidade Federal de Minas Gerais; Telehealth Network of Minas Gerais, Belo Horizonte, Brazil

Antonio Luiz Ribeiro Telehealth Center, University Hospital, Universidade Federal de Minas Gerais; Telehealth Network of Minas Gerais, Belo Horizonte, Brazil

Aram Rojas Department of Surgery, Westchester Medical Center, Valhalla, NY, USA

New York Medical College, School of Medicine, Valhalla, NY, USA

Nicholas Rolig Arizona Telemedicine Program, The University of Arizona's College of Medicine, Tucson, AZ, USA

Jennifer L. Rosenthal Department of Pediatrics, University of California Davis, Sacramento, CA, USA

Nancy Rowe Arizona Telemedicine Program, The University of Arizona's College of Medicine, Tucson, AZ, USA

Akhil Saji New York Medical College, School of Medicine, Valhalla, NY, USA

Department of Urology, Westchester Medical Center, Valhalla, NY, USA

Letícia Baião Silva Telehealth Center, University Hospital, Universidade Federal de Minas Gerais; Telehealth Network of Minas Gerais, Belo Horizonte, Brazil

Nandini Sodhi Arizona Telemedicine Program, The University of Arizona's College of Medicine, Tucson, AZ, USA

Maira Viana Rego Souza e Silva Telehealth Center, University Hospital, Universidade Federal de Minas Gerais; Telehealth Network of Minas Gerais, Belo Horizonte, Brazil

Dylan Stewart Westchester Medical Center and Maria Fareri Children's Hospital, Valhalla, NY, USA

New York Medical College, School of Medicine, Valhalla, NY, USA

Mark Swerdlow Southwestern Academic Limb Salvage Alliance (SALSA), Department of Surgery, Keck School of Medicine of University of Southern California, Los Angeles, CA, USA

Joseph R. Turkowski Department of Surgery, Westchester Medical Center Health, Valhalla, NY, USA

Sarah Vaithilingam Department of Psychiatry, Westchester Medical Center Health System, New York Medical College, Valhalla, NY, USA

Tracey L. Weigel Department of Surgery, Westchester Medical Center, Valhalla, NY, USA

New York Medical College, School of Medicine, Valhalla, NY, USA

Ronald S. Weinstein Arizona Telemedicine Program, College of Medicine, The University of Arizona's, Tucson, AZ, USA

E. Zhang Pediatrics, University of Kansas Medical Center, Kansas City, KS, USA

Bertie Zhang New York Medical College, School of Medicine, Valhalla, NY, USA
Department of Urology, Westchester Medical Center, Valhalla, NY, USA

Part I
Principles of Telemedicine and Telehealth

First Trainees: The Golden Anniversary of the Early History of Telemedicine Education at the Massachusetts General Hospital and Harvard (1968–1970)

Ronald S. Weinstein, Michael J. Holcomb, Elizabeth A. Krupinski, and Rifat Latifi

Recently, interest in creating curriculum in telemedicine for medical students, and in telehealth for nurses and most other health professionals, has spiked because of the healthcare industry's rapid shift to providing care via telemedicine as a means of infection control due to the Covid-19 pandemic [1, 2]. This commentary describes the initial medical student and resident training in telemedicine at the Massachusetts General Hospital (MGH) a half century ago.

John H. Knowles, MD, a Unique Academic Medicine Leader

John H. Knowles, MD, was an MGH-trained cardiopulmonary internist and the MGH General Director who was a principal architect for the Logan International Airport MGH Medical Station multi-specialty telemedicine program (LIA-MGH-TP). He also touched the lives of both Michael Crichton and Ronald S. Weinstein, MD, two of the initial trainees in LIA-MGH-TP. Crichton was a Harvard Medical School (HMS) fourth year medical student, in 1969, and Weinstein was a third year MGH pathology resident a year earlier, in 1968, when each of them, separately, encountered telemedicine for the first time, unknowingly to become recognized as "pioneers in telemedicine training" a half century later.

The original version of this chapter was revised. The correction to this chapter is available at https://doi.org/10.1007/978-3-030-56917-4_30.

R. S. Weinstein (✉) · M. J. Holcomb
Arizona Telemedicine Program, The University of Arizona's College of Medicine, Tucson, AZ, USA
e-mail: rweinstein@telemedicine.arizona.edu

E. A. Krupinski
Department of Radiology, Emory University, Atlanta, GA, USA

R. Latifi
Department of Surgery, New York Medical College, School of Medicine and Westchester Medical Center Health, Valhalla, NY, USA
e-mail: Rifat.Latifi@wmchealth.org ; Rifat_Latifi@nymc.edu

© The Author(s) 2021, corrected publication 2021
R. Latifi et al. (eds.), *Telemedicine, Telehealth and Telepresence*,
https://doi.org/10.1007/978-3-030-56917-4_1

When John H. Knowles had enrolled in Harvard College, in the mid-1940s, he focused his attention on extracurricular campus activities including sports and college theater where he was a Hasty Pudding Club's Theater student performer. Knowles' fun-loving college years in Cambridge, and Scollay Square entertainment in Boston, caught up with him when ten medical schools rejected him for admission [3]. Fortunately for Knowles, and the academic medicine community as well, a curious dean at Washington University in St. Louis, Missouri took a chance on Knowles and admitted him into their freshman class. Knowles rose to the occasion and ended up graduating first in his class. He landed what was then the top prize for a medical student anywhere in the United States, an internship in medicine at the MGH.

When Knowles arrived at the MGH as an intern, in 1951, he was riding high on his widely admired Harvard reputation as a nine-varsity letter, three-sport, Harvard College athlete with a high profile on campus as a Hasty Pudding Club's Theater performer. Everyone knew about his miraculous academic turnaround at a highly ranked medical school in the mid-west. Knowles seemed comfortable with his celebrity status and was accustomed to being in the limelight.

Knowles more than lived up to his advanced billing. In addition to his talents as a physician, and his popularity throughout the MGH organization, he was strongly committed to community outreach. That combination resonated with the MGH power brokers in Boston's financial district and the wealthy MGH trustees. They were looking for a new kind of leader for the MGH, somebody who could help transform their stodgy, but beloved, inward-looking Ivy League-minded institution into an outward-looking community leader in healthcare.

Changes in the US healthcare industry, in the mid-1960s, also favored Knowles's emergence as a national leader. His interest in community outreach became relevant to the US healthcare policy agenda. It is noteworthy that the passage of Medicare and Medicaid legislation in 1965 was a game changer for the US university hospital industry. Nineteenth century-style charity wards were eliminated, with their patients being transferred into revenue-generating beds elsewhere in the hospital. Almost overnight, community engagement became a hot topic as a new potential source of revenue for hospitals. The seeds were sowed for the creation of a new wave of community health centers, in urban areas. Knowles had positioned himself to be a leader in that arena [4–6]. It was in that setting that telemedicine popped up on the radar screen in Boston, with Knowles cheering it on as one of its greatest advocates.

The First MGH Telemedicine Trainees

Historically, Michael Crichton was the first HMS student to take a clinical rotation in the pioneering LIA-MGH-TP, in 1969. He is the only HMS student known to have published a chapter in a book about that medical student experience. His book, *Five Patients. The Hospital Explained*, provides an interesting picture of various aspects of academic medicine at the time multi-specialty telemedicine appeared on the scene in Boston, Massachusetts, in 1968 [7]. With respect to his subsequent career, Crichton ultimately chose not to obtain a medical license, or practice medicine, but he followed the latest medical research advances throughout his career. Crichton wrote his first best-selling novel, *Andromeda Strain,* as an HMS student. He followed this up with his novel and movie *Jurassic Park*.

The first resident-trainee of LIA-MGH-TP was Ronald S. Weinstein, M.D., a coauthor of this article. Weinstein is 81 years old and still works full time as the Founding Director of the national award-winning Arizona Telemedicine Program, in Tucson, Arizona. Weinstein is President Emeritus of the American Telemedicine Association. He is a pathologist who had his fellowship training at the MGH and Harvard in cancer biology research. He spent much of his research career studying cancer cell invasion and metastasis and, later, mechanisms of cancer multi-drug resistance [8, 9]. Weinstein has been recognized as the "father of telepathology," a subspecialty of telemedicine. He invented, patented, and commercialized robotic telepathology and introduced the term "telepathology" into the English language [10, 11].

John H. Knowles, MD, as a Mentor

In 1962, John H. Knowles, MD, at age 35, became the youngest General Director in the history of the 150-year-old MGH [6] (Fig. 1.1). A high-energy individual, Knowles was actively involved in HMS training programs at multiple levels. As MGH Hospital General Director, Knowles personally took ward service call a week each month. Weinstein recalls Knowles participating in the weekly medicine

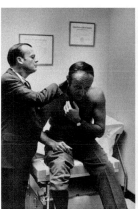
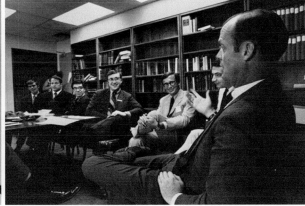

Fig. 1.1 (Left) Dr. John H. Knowles examining a patient. A highly competitive college athlete, Knowles had been a standout three-sport Harvard varsity letterman, in baseball, hockey, and squash. (Photo credit: Leonard McCombe/The Life Picture Collection/Getty Images). (Right) MGH General Director John Knowles meeting with a group of visitors at the MGH. He was "extraordinarily articulate, elegant in thought, scrupulous and respectful of language" [4]. Knowles was the administrator behind the establishment of the Logan International Airport MGH Medical Station telemedicine program. The MGH Medical Station was an integral component of Knowles MGH community outreach program for Boston. (Photo credit: Leonard McCombe/The Life Picture Collection/Getty Images)

morbidity and mortality (M&M) meetings in the Bulfinch Building. Knowles took pathology residents presenting their autopsy case results through their paces.

Knowles could discuss complicated medical cases on the fly, thinking out loud, using brilliant reasoning, presenting his summaries and conclusions in verbal paragraphs, always with theatrical flair. At the end of each commentary, he would stand with that endearing smile on his face, and methodically nod with raised eyebrows, individually, to each of the tenured Harvard professors in the conference room. In other settings, Knowles strongly encouraged MGH trainees, such as Weinstein, to step up into leadership positions that "would make a difference in the world" [4–6]. A decade later, still at the relatively young age of 45, Knowles was named President of the Rockefeller Foundation in New York City. This provided Knowles with a platform on which to continue his work on US healthcare delivery system reform and community outreach.

Origins Logan International Airport MGH Medical Station Telemedicine Program

On October 4, 1960, an Eastern Air Lines, Lockheed Electra L-188 prop-jet commercial airliner crashed immediately after takeoff from runway 9 the Logan International Airport, in Boston. The airplane struck a flock of starlings at an altitude of approximately 120 feet and crashed into Winthrop Harbor, an extension of Boston harbor. Dozens of passengers were killed. While many on board were killed instantly in the crash, there were also survivors with critical injuries that subsequently died without medical care. Getting emergency medical personnel out to Logan International Airport (LIA) was a logistical nightmare as the only ground transportation access was through the Callahan Tunnel, the single gateway to and from downtown Boston. Telemedicine emerged as a practical solution [12–14]. Knowles was a strong proponent from the start, although the idea for it was not his own. That came from his clinical counterpart, the cardiopulmonary internist, Kenneth T. Bird, MD.

In 1962, the same year Knowles became MGH General Director, Ronald S. Weinstein, a second-year medical student at Tufts Medical School (TMS) across town, accepted a one-year post-Sophomore fellowship in biophysics and electron microscopy in the MGH Department of Neurosurgery, which housed the Mixter Laboratory for Electron Microscopy, headed by Stanley Bullivant, PhD, a pioneer in a new field, freeze-fracture electron microscopy. Three years later, Weinstein was awarded a pathology residency at the MGH, becoming the first TMS graduate accepted into any MGH residency program. Knowles, and the MGH Chair of Neurosurgery, William H. Sweet, MD, encouraged Weinstein to apply for a National Institutes of Health (NIH) grant as a Principal Investigator on a Program Project grant. Knowles personally signed the request letter for an NIH waiver allowing the award [15–17]. Knowles liked Weinstein's career trajectory. He proudly acknowledged Weinstein's accomplishments as a success story for community outreach since Weinstein had been recruited to MGH from Tufts Medical School, across town.

On January 3, 1963, the Logan International Airport MGH Medical Station, a cooperative venture between MGH and the Massachusetts Port Authority, orchestrated by Knowles, opened to patients with Dr. Kenneth T. Bird as its medical director. Within a few years, the clinic was seeing 100 patients a day. The creation of a Logan International Airport telemedicine service was Bird's idea [12]. He was tired of driving back and forth between the MGH and the Logan Airport. Telemedicine stood out as a potential solution, and Knowles provided resources to support the effort. John Knowles saw telemedicine from a larger perspective. For him, it was a success in the development of his MGH community outreach programs. While Knowles would never detract from the originality and importance of Bird's contributions, nor fail to give Bird full credit for his innovations and achievements in LIA-MGH-TP, nevertheless LIA-MGH-TP was recognized as one of Knowles' signature achievements as well [14] (Fig. 1.2). Dr. Bird coined the term "telemedicine" [12].

To create the MGH telemedicine program, LIA was linked to the MGH, 2.7 miles away, over a private bidirectional microwave telecommunication linkage [13]. At that time, NASA (National Aeronautics and Space Administration) was exploring

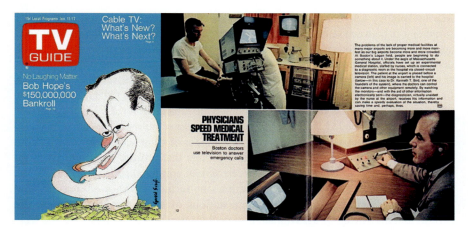

Fig. 1.2 Telemedicine (initially called "Telediagnosis" at the MGH) was featured in the January 11, 1969, issue of the popular magazine "TV Guide," nine months after the Logan International Airport-MGH Medical Station telediagnosis program became operational, on April 8, 1968. (Left) Cover of January 1969 TV Guide featuring the 65th birthday of the comedian Bob Hope. Hope died at age 100 in 2003. (Right—two-page spread in this issue of TV Guide). (Upper photo) A dermatology patient at the walk-in Logan International Airport MGH Medical Station "Telediagnosis clinic" is being examined remotely by television. (Lower photo) Kenneth T. Bird, MD, at the MGH, is examining the dark irregular purple skin lesion on the patient's left foot, using the robotically controlled-TV camera out at the Logan Airport. The patient's left leg is covered with a light-colored drape (Upper photo). Dr. Bird, looking straight ahead, is viewing the skin lesion on a black-and-white TV monitor. (not shown). He is adjusting the TV image magnification and focus of the patient's foot lesion by manipulating a TV control panel with his right hand. Dr. Bird uses ear buds to listen to heart and breath sounds coming from an electronic stethoscope (not shown)

terrestrial applications for technologies developed to care for astronauts in space [18, 19]. The health of astronauts was constantly in the news. Many doctors and nurses knew what an electronic stethoscope was and believed that it might even outperform the traditional stethoscope. The MGH was following NASA's lead in its implementations of electronic devices for remote patient care. As a frame of reference, the first lunar landing took place just a few months after Crichton graduated from HMS in 1969. The LIA-MGH-TP program was 4 years in the planning [12].

Crichton's and Weinstein's Involvements with Telemedicine as MGH Trainees

Crichton was a fourth year Harvard medical student when he rotated through the Medical Station telemedicine service (initially referred to as a "Tele-diagnostic Service"), in 1969.

In 1968, Weinstein had his first involvement with remote television microscopy. His background in biologic research and medical imaging was unusual for a medical student. He first became involved with high-resolution electron microscopy in 1960, when he was Head Chemist in the Department of Research Services, at the Woods Hole Marine Biology Laboratory (MBL), in Woods Hole, Massachusetts [20]. This was a summer job, between semesters, first at Albany Medical College, in Albany, New York, and then at Tufts Medical School, in Boston, where Weinstein became a transfer student. His assignment as an MGH post-sophomore fellow in electron microscopy was to redesign the equipment used for preparing biological specimens for high-resolution freeze-fracture specimen electron microscopy [21]. The goal was to take the resolution of freeze-fracture electron microscopy down to the molecular level.

Weinstein succeeded well beyond anybody's expectations. Use of his "Type II Freeze-Fracture Device" provided exquisite images of what became known as "connexin complexes" and their hydrophilic channels that are the structural basis for electronic and metabolic coupling between human epithelial cells [16, 17, 22]. He, and a collaborator, N. Scott McNutt, went a step further and showed that deficiencies in these complexes are early manifestations of malignant transformation in certain human cancers [23]. Weinstein's special interests in medical imaging were well known in the MGH Department of Pathology and at Harvard Medical School. This interest led directly to his involvement with the LIA-MGH-TP [15].

In 1967 prior to the opening of the LIA-MGH-TP clinic, a Harvard Medical School Professor and staff pathologist at the MGH, Robert E. Scully, MD, became involved in testing television microscopy equipment to determine its suitability for doing remote clinical microscopy (e.g., light microscopic examination of blood smears and urine sediments using television). Scully kept Weinstein in the loop. (Fig. 1.4) First, Scully examined the need for color television as compared with black-and-white television. He demonstrated nearly 100% diagnostic accuracy using standard black-and-white television [25]. This was not surprising since television microscopy (later called "video microscopy") had been used for biological research starting in 1955. When Weinstein was Head Chemist at the MBL, during

1 First Trainees: The Golden Anniversary of the Early History of Telemedicine…   9

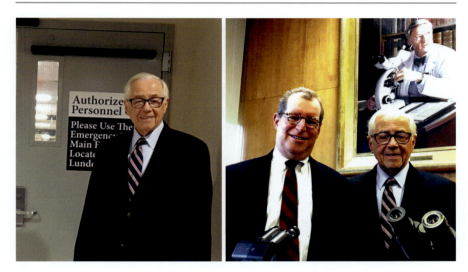

Fig. 1.3 (Left photo) Dr. Weinstein's 2018 visit to the MGH, marking the 50th anniversary of his original participation in television microscopy cases coming in from the Logan International Airport. MGH's White Building's first floor main hallway entrance into the Emergency Ward. The MGH Tele-diagnostic suite was on the first floor, in an alcove off the Emergency Ward. (Right photo) Marking the 50th anniversary of television microscopy in the Pathology Department at the MGH. Dr. David Louis, Castleman Chair of Pathology (left), is with Dr. Weinstein in the MGH Pathology Department Library (April 27, 2018). Dr. Castleman, for whom the Chair is named, is present in Fig. 1.4. (Fig. 1.4, front row). Dr. Robert B. Colvin, a former Castleman Chair of Pathology, is pictured in the oil painting on the wall. In the 1968 MGH Pathology Department annual photo (Fig. 1.4, taken 50 years previously, in 1968), Dr. Colvin was an MGH pathology trainee (Fig. 1.4, last row, second from the left). (Reproduced with permission from [20])

his summer breaks in medical school, he had frequently visited laboratories where video light microscopy experiments were underway and discussed the technology with senior investigators. Based on his survey of the field, Weinstein was able to reassure Dr. Scully that doing routine black-and-white television microscopy as a substitute to traditional hands-on light microscopy worked well and had little risk.

One day in 1968, while Weinstein was signing out surgical pathology cases with Dr. Scully, Dr. Scully invited him to lunch and said the reward would be "something special." Following lunch in the MGH staff cafeteria, they walked over to the telemedicine suite on the first floor of the White Building (Figs. 1.2 and 1.3). Once there, Dr. Scully telephoned the nurse-manager at the MGH Walk-In Clinic at Logan Airport. He reviewed the clinical history of the first patient with Weinstein and then asked the nurse to place the blood smear of Case #1 on the stage of the television light microscope out at the airport. An image of the blood smear popped up on the television monitor in their darkened room. (Fig. 1.5) Dr. Scully instructed the nurse on where to move the slide on the microscope stage, how fast to move it, and where to stop and focus. Several times Scully said "higher" or "lower" to instruct the nurse on bringing the blood sample on the glass slide into optimal focus. After examining a Wright Stain stained blood smear for several minutes, Scully asked Weinstein for

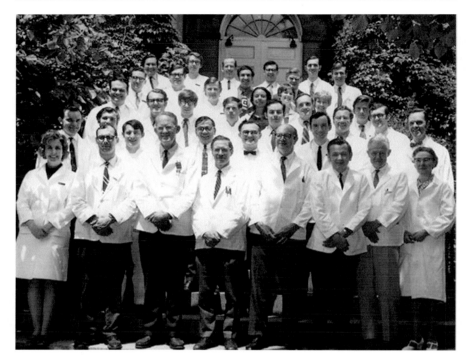

Fig. 1.4 1968 MGH Department of Pathology on the steps of the historic Bulfinch Building, a National Historic Landmark. Robert E. Scully, MD, is in the front row, 3rd from the right. Dr. Weinstein is in the 3rd row, 3rd from the right, standing behind Dr. Scully. Benjamin Castleman, MD, Chair of the MGH Department of Pathology, is in the front row, 4th from the right, standing next to Dr. Scully. Robert B. Colvin, MD, a future Castleman Chair, is in the last row, 2nd from the left. In his long career at the MGH, Dr. Castleman trained 15 future pathology department chairs and produced over 2000 professional publications, a nearly unimaginable number today. (Reproduced with permission from [24])

a diagnosis. Weinstein and Scully agreed on the diagnosis of "hypochromic microcytic anemia" which Scully then reported to the nurse over the telephone. They went through the same routine for Case #2, which turned out to be a "normal" blood smear. Dr. Scully said, "Well, Ronnie, we just made history." They agreed that the process had been straightforward, easy to do, that color television was not required, and the black-and-white television images were surprisingly good.

Crichton's Medical Student Book *"Five Patients. The Hospital Explained"*

Michael Crichton's student involvement with telemedicine education and training was much more extensive than Weinstein's. Crichton's experience was the subject of a chapter in *"Five Patients. The Hospital Explained,"* a book he completed writing just months before his graduation from HMS and published in 1970 [7].

1 First Trainees: The Golden Anniversary of the Early History of Telemedicine... 11

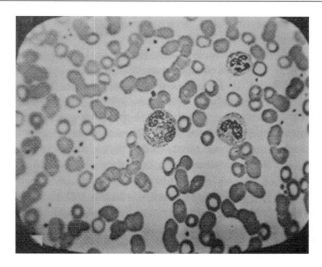

Fig. 1.5 Example of a television microscopy (video microscopy) image of a Wright Stain blood smear, originating at the Logan International Airport MGH Medical Station, and viewed on a black-and-white television screen at the MGH. (Photo credit: Raymond LH, Murphy, JR, "Telediagnosis: A new Community Health Resource: Observations on the Feasibility of Telediagnosis Based on 1000 Patient Transactions." American Journal of Public Health, February 1974; 64(2): 113 to 119, Figure 2, American Public Health Association [26])

While completing *"Five Patients,"* Crichton had discussions with Dr. Knowles about his experiences on the MGH telemedicine service, and their potential implications for healthcare in the future. Knowles' opinions and concerns show up in the text as sage observations by a learned mentor. Knowles also enriched Crichton's telemedicine experience by connecting him with senior MGH staff and with eminent professors at the Massachusetts Institute of Technology (MIT), a virtual temple for research on medical computer applications as well as leading edge research on Artificial Intelligence (AI).

Crichton's book *"Five Patients: The Hospital Explained"* is somewhat of a time capsule of what academic medicine was like a half century ago. On the one hand, Crichton was intrigued by the technologies of healthcare and the complexity of healthcare delivery, but on the other hand, hospital deficiencies were sobering to him, and the ambiguities of medical diagnostics and frustrations of the medical staff over uncertainties that permeate many aspects patient care, even in a world-class hospital, discouraged Crichton from taking the final step into medical practice (Fig. 1.6) . He did not apply for a medical license. Still, Crichton never lost his interest in medical sciences and emerging technologies, and he stayed current with advances in medical research for the rest of his life [27].

The "five patients" in Crichton's book were five actual cases of men and women in immediate need of medical help rushed to the MGH [7]. Crichton uses these cases to explain how hospital practice was changing in the age of science-technology explosion. Crichton used one of his cases to discuss the patient-experience using

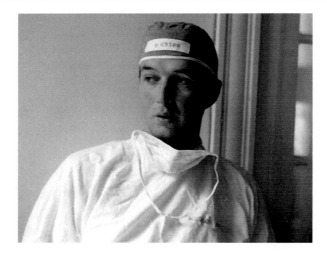

Fig. 1.6 Michael Crichton, dressed in surgical scrubs, during a Harvard Medical School (HMS) clinical rotation, in 1968. Crichton, a student of English literature, had a playful sense of humor regarding his own towering height. Here, the 6' 9" Crichton is dressed to recognize Sir Jeffrey Hudson (see surgical cap label), a storied member of the Seventeenth Century court of the English queen Henrietta Maria of France with height challenges. Crichton also wrote a medical mystery, "A Case of Need," for which he received an Edgar Award in 1968, using the pseudonym Jeffery Hudson. He wrote a collection ("The Med School Years Collection") of 8 paperback thrillers in medical school using the pseudonym John Lange. (This Figure is reproduced from http://www.michaelcrichton.com/doctor/, with permission from Taylor Crichton. Ronald S. Weinstein, M.D. was a Teaching Fellow at HMS, while an MGH pathology resident and laboratory director, and taught pathology to Michael Crichton's HMS class)

videoconferencing with a doctor on the other end. He discusses the limitations of the technology, and he considers advances in developing next-generation technologies for patient care, including decision support systems and Artificial Intelligence (AI). Crichton realized that computer programs could offer extraordinary possibilities: any community in the country, "or even a doctor's office could plug into the MGH program and let the computer monitor the patient and direct therapy" [28]. This sounds modern even today.

Crichton's Telemedicine Patient Workup

The telemedicine patient Crichton assisted in working up, as a senior medical student, was Mrs. Sylvia Thompson, a 56-year-old mother of three who began to experience severe, but not persistent chest pain over Ohio on a flight from Los Angeles to Boston. After the plane landed, she was directed to the Logan Airport MGH Medical Station near the Eastern Airlines terminal. After explaining her problem to the secretary, she was led to the telecommunications-equipped clinical examination room (Fig. 1.2). After a brief orientation by the nurse, Dr. Raymond Murphy, at the

MGH, popped up on the TV screen. He had gotten in on the ground floor of this new industry [26]. Off-camera was Michael Crichton watching the proceedings and taking notes [7].

After the Logan Airport Medical Station nurse gave a brief history and her physical findings, blood pressure 120/80, pulse 78, temperature 101.4, Dr. Murphy said, "How do you do, Mrs. Thompson." The nurse told a slightly flustered Mrs. Thompson, "Just talk to him," which she did. Dr. Murphy said, "I'm at the Massachusetts General Hospital. When was your first pain?" He then took a complete history.

This was followed by a physical examination, including a stethoscope examination of the patient's heart and lungs. The airport nurse, following verbal instructions from Dr. Murphy, at the MGH, placed the small electronic stethoscope bell on the patient, while Dr. Murphy listened to the patient's heart and lung sounds live through earbuds. After wheeling the remote controlled "portable" camera over to Mrs. Thompson, Dr. Murphy examined the patients' abdomen and face simultaneously on two separate monitors. The nurse took an ECG and transmitted an image of the ECG paper strip to Dr. Murphy who looked at it on a TV monitor.

While the examination was proceeding, another nurse was preparing samples of Mrs. Thompson's blood and urine in a laboratory down the hall. The nurse placed the samples on glass slides under a microscope attached to a black-and-white RCA TV camera. She and Dr. Murphy could view the images simultaneously as described earlier. The patient had a white count of 18,000.

Back in the examination room, Dr. Murphy said, "Mrs. Thompson, it looks like you have pneumonia. We'd like to have you come into the hospital (MGH) for x-rays and further evaluation." Although the telemedicine-enabled clinic had a television microscope for use for "clinical microscopy" from the beginning, teleradiology was still being evaluated and was not ready for implementation. Afterward, Mrs. Thompson said: "My goodness. It was just like the real thing."

When Mrs. Thompson set off for the MGH miles away, Dr. Murphy discussed her case, and the television link-up with Crichton. Dr. Murphy said, "It's interesting that patients accept it quite well." In retrospect, looking back 50 years, both the patient's perception of the encounter and Dr. Murphy's observations were very instructive. Today, we know that telemedicine is often convenient, efficient, easy to do, and generates a high level of both patient confidence and provider satisfaction. Why was telemedicine not widely adopted a half century ago? The answer turns out to be regulatory inertia, including the legal process that had imposed "deadweight costs" and impeded progress. Another huge barrier was reimbursement. A half century later, the Covid-19 pandemic has served as an innovation accelerator. Following Presidential and Governors' Executive Orders mandating social distancing and stay-at-home orders, and the waiving of burdensome restrictions on payment and urban, home, and nursing home telemedicine in general, telemedicine usage in the United States and the world took off. Tens of thousands of medical practices implemented telemedicine. Telemedicine cases soared 5000–8000%, or more, within months. Characterizations of telemedicine were in line with those of the pioneers. To patients, "It was just like the real thing." Providers were impressed that "patients accept it quite well." In Microsoft's ads for their Teams" products, the announcer says, "Telemedicine is here to stay."

Telemedicine and the Study of Innovations

While Crichton was on his telemedicine "rotation," he also became interested in the use of computer-based patient history taking. At that time, 15% of patients examined by Telediagnosis had their medical history taken by computer before they saw the tele-physician. Crichton was impressed with the remarkable ease with which patients accepted it. For the interview, the patient sat in front of a tele-type computer that asked questions, and they punched "yes" or "no" responses. "Yes" answers generated more questions. At the end of the interview, the computer produced a medical summary. Unlike the questions, the summary used medical terminology. The process took roughly 30 minutes.

Crichton simulated a computer interview in *"Five Patients."* He presented the computer with the same presenting complaint as that of Mrs. Thompson: chest pain. He then attempted to confuse it by feeding suggestive information, namely a family history of coronary artery disease and that the patient was taking digitalis. In later questions, the machine was fed a straightforward history for the type of chest pain most common in medical students—that of pain of psychogenic, or musculoskeletal, origin. At the conclusion, the computer printed out a summary.

Crichton noted that the computer program drew no conclusions about diagnosis: it only summarized answers to its own questions, and it did not cross-check itself. He also noted that there were more sophisticated programs available at the time and expands on the research taking place in the MGH Computer Science Laboratory [7]. Dr. Jerome Grossman said, "computers in the future will help with a doctor's critical decision, if a patient needs to see the doctor at all." In 1969, Grossman predicted that, "In the near future, when the home computer and the television set is practical, you're going to be able to plug right into the hospital computer without even leaving your home." It turns out that it took decades to have electronic health records with patient portals enabling patients' immediate access to their own records. Kathleen Dwyer, in Dr. G. Octo Barnett's Laboratory of Computer Science at the MGH, noted "there's no theoretical reason why you couldn't build a program to carry out some of the functions of a doctor…." In other words, the roles of physicians as diagnosticians may be endangered, but not eliminated completely [28].

In *Five Patients*, Crichton then discusses the broader implications of what he had observed on his two-week rotation and, in doing so, reveals his own remarkable level of sophistication in thinking about innovation and technology. There are echoes of John Knowles' voice in this conversation. First, Crichton acknowledges that it is the role of university medical centers to lead in the development of technology, and then disseminate it out into the community. He foresees that hospital physicians may some day direct the diagnosis and therapy of patients who never enter the hospital. In his day, neither television nor computers had much impact on hospital practices. They do today, in many parts of the hospital.

We are beginning to see the early fragmentation of the late twentieth-century and early twenty-first-century "big box" hospitals with the physical diffusion of some component parts out into the community. An example might be the loss of hospitals, and free-standing imaging centers, of their near monopolies of large diagnostic imaging equipment. For example, in a growing number of metropolitan areas, computed tomography (CT) scanners are being taken to patients' homes in specialized vans equipped for remote diagnosis by tele-physicians located at virtual hospitals or in HIPAA-compliant home offices. Nearly a dozen metropolitan areas in the United States already offer such direct-to-patient tele-stroke services. A prospective patient dials "911" and describes physical findings suggestive of an impending stroke. The message goes to a call center that dispatches a van, equipped with an on-board CT scanner, directly to the patient's home. The patient is placed in the head scanner. A medic performs the CT scan, which is transmitted, typically via cellular data networks, directly to an on-call tele-vascular neurologist or neuroradiologist. CT images are immediately interpreted, and a vascular tele-neurologist carries out the complimentary physical examination via telemedicine, often rendering the diagnosis from the display on a smartphone. A diagnosis of ischemic stroke results in the immediate intravascular infusion of tPA, the "clot busting" drug, averting a potentially life-threatening stroke. "Door-to-needle" times have been reduced to under 30 minutes for thousands of impending stroke cases. Barrow Neurological Institute, in Phoenix, Arizona, offers this service 24/7 [29].

What Will Harvard Medical School Teach Students in Their Telemedicine Courses?

Recently, HMS proudly announced they are introducing telemedicine into curriculum at multiple points. That is good news for the telemedicine industry, but not necessarily good for traditional medical practices (i.e., pre-Covid-19) [1, 30].

Harvard Medical School's adoption of a telemedicine-centric curriculum was done on-the-fly, apparently with an "all hands-on deck" sense of urgency [1]. Of course, this is best viewed through the lens of Covid-19 pandemic. The Covid-19 pandemic has caused a sea change in the healthcare industry, affecting far more than telemedicine. Many medical practices have gone "virtual" in a matter of a few months. Anecdotal evidence indicates that the transformation from in-person office appointments to "virtual" visits has taken place at previously unimaginable rates. Earlier predictions of 36 million telemedicine cases for 2020 before the Covid-19 pandemic set in are now being increased to 1 billion or more telemedicine cases by the end of 2020 [31]. Adding telephony (telephone only cases) and text-messaging into the equation, these numbers become staggeringly large going forward.

The good news is that the transition from traditional bricks-and-mortar practices to virtual practices seemed reasonably straight forward. The rise of high-speed broadband Internet communications over the past 25 years, the widespread adoption of mobile smartphones by businesses and consumers, the availability of rapidly scalable cloud computing infrastructure and services, and, most recently, the accessibility of secure and reliable synchronous video communications and asynchronous messaging, all laid the groundwork necessary for the recent explosive growth in implementation and utilization of telemedicine by healthcare providers and the patients they serve throughout the United States and the world.

The Association of American Medical Colleges (AAMC), the leading voice for medical education in the United States, has recognized the importance of including telemedicine in medical school curriculum of US medical schools. What will the core competencies be? Are there lessons to be learned from earlier efforts to teach a telemedicine curriculum? What is missing in this conversation? [2, 30, 31].

It is likely that both Crichton and Weinstein would express their concerns over a loss of the in-person humanity, empathy, and caring in the current Zoom-based world, even though Crichton chose not to practice medicine and Weinstein became a pathologist, a field with minimal direct patient contact. Even they knew that body language matters, and environment affects behavior. Although they went separate ways following their training, Weinstein into cancer research and academic department leadership, and Crichton into full-time writing and movie directing, each valued their professional relationships, their interpersonal interactions, and even their patient interactions in medical school. It could be that Zooming would not have been either of their preferred choices for people-to-people communication.

As Eric Topol, MD, a leading thinker in the Artificial Intelligence arena, and an outstanding practicing physician, has noted, "All of these humanistic interactions are difficult to digitize, which further highlight why doctors are irreplaceable by machines." He wisely concludes, "Machine medicine need not be our future" [32]. However, healthcare technologies do belong in the modern doctor's bag. Physicians will want to include telemedicine and other healthcare technologies as instruments in their medical tool kit, which they can utilize as needed to aid in the diagnosis and care of patients [33].

References

1. COVID-19 pandemic spurs creation of new, remote teaching methods at HMS. https://news.harvard.edu/gazette/story/2020/05/harvard-medical-school-uses-telemedicine-as-a-way-forward/. Last accessed 11 June 2020.
2. AMA encourages telemedicine training for medical students, residents. https://www.ama-assn.org/press-center/press-releases/ama-encourages-telemedicine-training-medical-students-residents. Last accessed 11 June 2020.
3. Schorow S. Inside the combat zone. The stripped-down story of Boston's Most notorious neighborhood. Guilford: Globe Pequot; 2017.
4. Castleman B, Crockett DC, Sutton SB, editors. The Massachusetts General Hospital. 1955–1980. Boston: Little Brown & Company; 1983. p. 17–25.
5. Knowles JH. The responsibility of the individual. Daedalus. 1977:57–80.
6. John H. Knowles, leading medical figure dies at age 52. https://www.nytimes.com/1979/03/07/archives/john-h-knowles-leading-medical-figure-dies-at-52-individual-can.html. Last accessed 7 June 2020.

7. Crichton M. Five patients: the hospital explained. New York: Alfred A. Knopf; 1970.
8. Weinstein RS, Jakate SM, Dominguez JM, Lebovitz MD, Koukoulis GK, Kuszak JR, Kluskens LF, Grogan TM, Saclarides TJ, Roninson IB, Coon JS. Relationship of the expression of the multidrug resistance gene product (P-glycoprotein) in human colon carcinoma to local tumor aggressiveness and lymph node metastasis. Cancer Res. 1991;51:2720–6.
9. Coon JS, Knudson W, Clodfelter K, Lu B, Weinstein RS. Solutol HS 15, nontoxic polyethylene esters of 12-hydroxystearic acid, reverses multi-drug resistance. Cancer Res. 1991;51:897–902.
10. Weinstein RS, Graham AR, Richter LC, Barker GP, Krupinski EA, Lopez AM, Erps KA, Bhattacharyya AK, Yagi Y, Gilbertson JR. Overview of telepathology, virtual microscopy, and whole slide imaging: prospects for the future. Hum Pathol. 2009;40:1057–69.
11. Weinstein RS, Holcomb MJ, Krupinski EA. Invention, and early history of telepathology (1985-2000). J Pathol Inform. 2019;10:1.
12. Next best thing to being there? https://nihrecord.nih.gov/2016/06/03/history-tv-tech-medicine-mined-21st-century-lessons. Last accessed 13 June 2020.
13. Bashshur RL, Shannon GW. History of telemedicine. Evolution, context, and transformation. New Rochelle: Mary Ann Liebert, Inc., Publishers; 2009. p. 165–72.
14. Bull W, Bull M. Something in the ether. A bicentennial history of Massachusetts General Hospital. 1811–2011. Beverly: Memoirs Unlimited; 2011. p. 281–7.
15. Louis D, Young RH. Keen minds to explore the dark continents of disease. A history of the pathology services at the Massachusetts General Hospital. Boston: Massachusetts General Hospital and Harvard Medical School; 2011. p. 255.
16. Weinstein RS, McNutt NS. Current concepts: cell junctions. N Engl J Med. 1972;286:521–4.
17. McNutt NS, Weinstein RS. Membrane ultrastructure at mammalian intercellular junctions. Prog Biophys Mol Biol. 1973;26:45–102.
18. Bashshur RL, Shannon GW. History of telemedicine. Evolution, context, and transformation. New Rochelle: Mary Ann Liebert, Inc., Publishers; 2009. p. 189–202.
19. Freiburger G, Holcomb M, Piper D. The STARPAHC collection: part of an archive of the history of telemedicine. J Telemed Telecare. 2007;13:221–3. https://doi.org/10.1258/135763307781458949.
20. Weinstein RS. On being a pathologist: a pathway to pathology practice; the added value of supplemental vocational training and mentoring in college and medical school. Hum Pathol. 2018;82:10–19.
21. Weinstein RS, McNutt NS. Heat-etching with a Bullivant type II simple freeze-cleave device. Proc Electron Micros Soc Am. 1970;28:106–7.
22. McNutt NS, Weinstein RS. The ultrastructure of the nexus: a correlated thin-section and freeze-cleave study. J Cell Biol. 1970;47:666–88.
23. McNutt NS, Weinstein RS. Carcinoma of the cervix: deficiency of nexus intercellular junctions. Science. 1969;165:597–9.
24. Weinstein RS, Holcomb MJ. Case Study: Congenital Toxoplasmosis Diagnosis and a Pair of Myers-Briggs Type Indicator® (MBTI®) Test Results for an Academic Pathologist. JSM Clic Pathol 2019;4:6.
25. Park B. Communications aspects of telemedicine. In: Bashshur RL, Armstrong PA, Youssef ZI, editors. Telemedicine. Explorations in the use of telecommunications in health care. Springfield, Illinois: Charles C. Thomas, Publisher; 1975. p. 54–86.
26. Murphy RL, Bird KT. Telediagnosis: a new community health resource: observations on the feasibility of telediagnosis—based on 1000 patient transactions. Am J Public Health. 1974;64:113–9. https://doi.org/10.2105/AJPH.64.2.113.
27. Steven T. Biography of Michael Crichton. The best little book, Hyperlink.
28. G. Octo Barnett. http://www.mghlcs.org/about/team/octobarnett. Last Accessed 7 June 2020.
29. Barrow Stroke Program Receives Top Honors. https://www.barrowneuro.org/in-the-news/stroke-program-honors/. Last Accessed 7 June 2020.

30. From bedside to webside: future doctors learn how to practice remotely. From bedside to webside: future doctors learn how to practice remotely. https://www.aamc.org/news-insights/bedside-webside-future-doctors-learn-how-practice-remotely. Last accessed June 11, 2020.
31. Coombs B. Telehealth visits are booming as doctors and patients embrace distancing amid the coronavirus crisis. https://www.cnbc.com/2020/04/03/telehealth-visits-could-top-1-billion-in-2020-amid-the-coronavirus-crisis.html. Last accessed 13 June 2020.
32. Topol E. Deep medicine: how artificial intelligence can make healthcare human again. New York: Basic Books; 2019.
33. Weinstein RS, Krupinski EA, Doarn CR. Clinical examination component of telemedicine, telehealth, mhealth and connected health medical practices. Med Clin N Am. 2018;102:533-44.

Open Access This chapter is licensed under the terms of the Creative Commons Attribution 4.0 International License (http://creativecommons.org/licenses/by/4.0/), which permits use, sharing, adaptation, distribution and reproduction in any medium or format, as long as you give appropriate credit to the original author(s) and the source, provide a link to the Creative Commons license and indicate if changes were made.

The images or other third party material in this chapter are included in the chapter's Creative Commons license, unless indicated otherwise in a credit line to the material. If material is not included in the chapter's Creative Commons license and your intended use is not permitted by statutory regulation or exceeds the permitted use, you will need to obtain permission directly from the copyright holder.

Initiate-Build-Operate-Transfer (IBOT) Strategy Twenty Years Later: Tales from the Balkans and Africa

2

Rifat Latifi

"Initiating, building, implementing and finally being able to see the result of 20 years of intensive work on telemedicine around the world, has been a great personal journey filled with joy, excitement, drama, an occasional disappointment, and many, many hours traversing the world from one corner to the other; away from my family, building bridges and friendships, laying down one brick building, a better healthcare system, a better future on each continent, expect Antarctica. And it was worth it. Every bit of it! What started as a desperation attempt to rebuild Kosova's destroyed healthcare, before and during the war of 1998/1999, the Telemedicine Project of Kosova (TPK) has been transformed into an establishment and dissemination of telemedicine everywhere, a passion, my second professional life, a part from surgery. Furthermore, it has been most enriching experience, an experience that I would not trade for anything in the world. Some would say it has been a destiny. This book is a further testament of the work that has been done over the last two decades, and it comes at the anniversary of 20 years of telemedicine in Kosova, 25 years of Arizona Telemedicine, and 50 years of telemedicine at Harvard University. Now we have much to celebrate and thank many people from many countries have contributed to this in one way or another."

Introduction

Establishing sustainable telemedicine has become a goal of many countries around the world, and most recently, with the COVID-19 pandemic, telemedicine has gained substantial traction. Despite the fact that World Health Organization (WHO)

R. Latifi (✉)
Department of Surgery, New York Medical College, School of Medicine and Westchester Medical Center Health, Valhalla, NY, USA

International Virtual e-Hospital Foundation, Arlington, VA, USA
e-mail: Rifat.Latifi@wmchealth.edu; Latifi@iveh.org

reports that at least 124 countries [1] in the world have some form of telehealth, and despite initiatives from a select few individuals and on occasion from various governments, often these initiatives never mature to become sustainable programs for daily clinical applications and a mainstream provider of clinical care. Telemedicine programs increase the access to care in all clinical disciplines everywhere. It is particularly true in remote areas and developing countries which lack specialists and other human capacities to provide healthcare. This is especially true in high-end clinical disciplines such as trauma, intensive care, neurosurgery, neurology, cardiology, and other disciplines. The telemedicine programs of Albania and the Republic of Cabo Verde are built based on the Initiate-Build-Operate-Transfer (IBOT) strategy formulated by the International Virtual e-Hospital Foundation (IVeH) and with support from the U.S. government agencies such as U.S. Agency for International Development (USAID) [2], Department of State, and United States European Command (EUCOM) [3], and the Slovenian government (Ministry of Foreign Affairs), among other partners. These two programs have been developed based on a model from telemedicine of Kosova [4].

The Birth of the Kosova Telemedicine Program and IBOT Concept

On June 10, 1999, the United Nations Security Council adopted Resolution 1244 authorizing civilian administration of Kosova in a partnership called the United Nations Interim Administration Mission in Kosova (UNMIK) to provide "…a framework for the resolution of the conflict in Kosova by authorizing the deployment of an international civilian and military presence that would provide an international transitional administration and security presence that would oversee the return of refugees and the withdrawal of military forces from Kosova." [5]

Civil administration was led by the UN, and humanitarian efforts were led by the Office of the United Nations High Commissioner for Refugees (UN-HCR). Reconstruction was the responsibility of the European Union with institution building by the Organization for Safety and Cooperation in Europe. Security was provided by North Atlantic Treaty Organization (NATO). A million refugees began returning home to a country devastated in terms of infrastructure and services. Large numbers of non-governmental organizations (NGOs) registered to assist in Kosova, and the initial assessment of the medical situation was grim. With the eruption and the internationalization of war and devastation, an exceptional and unprecedented example of disrupted medical care in this volatile region came to light. The government of Serbia had dismissed the entire Albanian medical staff from the University Clinical Center of Kosova (UCCK), and all other regional hospitals, and closed the only medical school, the Medical Faculty of University of Prishtina in Kosova a decade before. There was an obvious need for electronic information and distance learning because there was no medical library, information system, or facility for training. It was impossible to send Kosovar physicians for a rapid training out of the country. The situation invited electronic and telemedicine solutions with international cooperation, but this was 1999, and we could still smell the ashes. The only new things that were being built in Kosova were graves, endless sites of graves everywhere.

Following graduation from General Residency at Yale University (June 19, 1999), I left for Albania, where my parents and the rest of family that survived the killings by the Serbian government were refugees. July 1, 1999, I returned home to Kosova from Albania with a river of refugees who were returning back on buses, tractors, and all sort of trucks. The caravan of refugees that warm July night stretched for miles and miles in a dangerous and winding road that seems endless. They were returning to Kosova with hopes to find their homes, friends, and members of families, but instead most found nothing but destruction of their properties, death, and misery. I felt guilty returning to Kosova with refugees. This was their moment in history [6].

When I arrived in Kllodërnicë, Drenica, the village I grew up in, everything was destroyed. I learned that my uncle, aunt, many cousins, neighbors, and friends had all been killed, all shot at point blank range. I knew our house had been burned also. Our house in Kllodërnicë was burned the same day my wife Drita and I were closing on a new home in Richmond, Virginia. Ironic. I was hoping that at least some of thousands of books had survived the fire. I was wrong. Everything was gone: the books, the memories. Hope was the only survivor.... As I looked over the ravages of my old home, I became numb. There were no tears. There was nothing I could feel or do.

On July 2, 1999, at the gate of UCCK in Prishtina, a British soldier greeted me. He was a young man with boyish face, a machine gun in his hand, and a frightening look. I pulled out my American passport and told him that I used to work there, pointing at the Surgery Clinic. The soldier stood at attention and saluted me: *"Welcome Home, Sir."* I fought back my tears and saluted him. I have never forgotten his face. When I entered the emergency room, one of the senior surgeons recognized me and asked if I was on call that night. "No, I am not," I replied matter-of-factly, and we hugged each other. "It is good to see you alive," we said to each other. "I do not deserve to be on call now that there is peace. I was not here during the war thus; I cannot be on call tonight. I just came to find out who is still alive." I thought but never said a word. I think he understood me.

In early spring of 2000, as assistant professor of surgery at Virginia Commonwealth University, Dr. Ronald C. Merrell, then Chairman of the Department of Surgery, asked me to go to Toulouse, France, to participate in a telemedicine conference. This was my first telemedicine conference. I really enjoyed the conference and the City of Toulouse. I spent part of one evening at the Hemingway joint.

Most delegates knew each other, but I was new to this world. Professor Michael Nerlich, a trauma orthopedic surgeon from Regensburg University, Regensburg, Germany, during the dinner with Professor Charles Doarn, then working with Dr. Merrell, invited me to participate at the final conference of the G-8 meeting in Berlin, to take place on May 3–5, 2000.

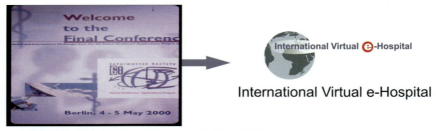

Berlin, May 4-5, 2000

R. Latifi: The Anatomy of War and Destruction of Kosova: An Alumnus Surgeon View on Reconstructing Health Care"

Fig. 2.1 The birthplace of the International Virtual e-Hospital and Initiate, Build, Operate, Transfer Strategy

The idea to establish and implement telemedicine in Kosova I presented for the first time at a G-8 Telemedicine meeting in Berlin on May 4, 2000 [7] (Fig. 2.1). I explained the dire state of postwar Kosova healthcare and suggested the creation of the IVeH as a way of change. This was my first international telemedicine presentation, and the auditorium was the right place to give this kind of futuristic talk as one needed for the Balkan's future. Speaker after speaker got up to offer me help, but they were unable to talk because they were in tears. It became clear that I had hit a cord, I had infused some new blood into this meeting, and I simply challenged the audience that if we were serious about offering help to developing countries and countries in disarray like Kosova, we should provide real structured help. This was the idea. I think the message came across clearly to everyone's mind and heart. I felt elated. Later in the evening reception held at the building of the German Parliament, the Minister of Health of Germany, Mrs. Anne Fisher, during the welcoming speech, said "I am very happy that today in Berlin you have created the International Virtual e-Hospital of Kosova." To the rest of the delegates present this appeared almost as if it was planned and orchestrated. No one but me knew that 28 hours ago this concept did not have a name. What became very clear to me was my life changed that very same morning in Berlin, Germany. Life that I would not change for anything.

By September 2003, I presented this concept and the results of establishing telemedicine of Kosova to 30 international conferences and meetings [6]. Over the next year, the idea was pursued appropriately by potential partners and sponsors. In October 2002, The First Intensive Balkan Telemedicine Seminar was held in Prishtina with some 400 participants from 21 countries (Fig. 2.2). Proceedings from this international telemedicine meeting were published by IOS Press as a book entitled *Establishing Telemedicine in Developing Countries: From Inception to Implementation* [8].

During this seminar, the newly acquired infrastructure permitted live demonstration from the medical campus of Virginia Commonwealth University in Richmond,

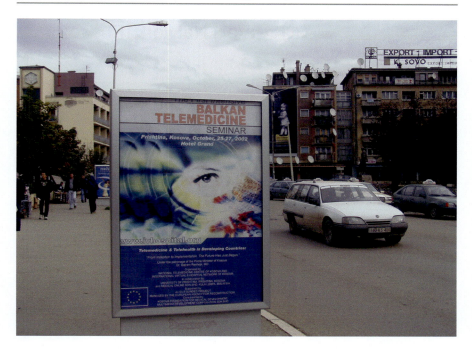

Fig. 2.2 The poster for the first telemedicine seminar in the Balkans, October 2002

including intraoperative distance learning demonstration. On December 10, 2002, the Telemedicine Center of Kosova (TCK) became operational (Fig. 2.3). The TCK was funded by a $1.5 million grant from the European Union through European Agency for Reconstruction [9]. The news of the first ever telemedicine conference in the Balkans held in Prishtina was widely publicized. Telemedicine was transforming healthcare and medical education around the world. In south-eastern Europe, Kosovo was at the forefront of this discipline. At the telemedicine conference, telemedicine practitioners from all over the world discussed how telemedicine can help transform healthcare. How to establish sustainable telemedicine programs; the clinical applications of telemedicine; and telemedicine's role in distance learning were all subjects for debate. The conference was funded by the EU via the European Agency for Reconstruction, as part of the EU's program to bring Kosovo's health system up to EU and world standards. At the opening ceremony, during the conference we were telepresent live with an operating theatre at Virginia Commonwealth University Hospital in Richmond to watch an operation taking place from thousands of miles away, high-quality sound and pictures allowed participants at the conference to see how that particular operation was being performed, and to hear the surgeon talking them through what he and his surgical team were

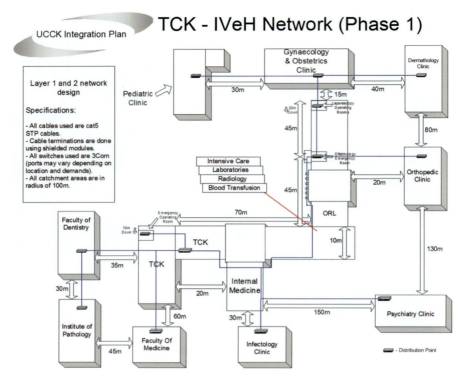

Fig. 2.3 The initial blueprint of Phase I, Telemedicine center of Kosova. 2020 TCK- Telemedicine Center of Kosova; IVeH- International Virtual e-Hospital

doing. At the opening ceremony, Kosovo's Prime Minister, Dr. Bajram Rexhepi (Fig. 2.4), a general surgeon, said: *"The development of the telemedicine project is an attempt to integrate medical institutions in Kosova with medical institutions of the world,"* he said. *"Furthermore, it will become a great tool and bridge for collaboration between doctors and nurses, narrowing the gap between developed countries and Kosova."*

The physical space was provided by the UCCK University Hospital. It was completed and inaugurated on December 10, 2002. Telecommunications connectivity was provided by Telecom of Kosova. There was lots of excitement about the telemedicine center in the country and its utility, but the greatest utility of the Center was not foreseen by many, that is the new telemedicine model that was being created.

The telemedicine program in Kosova, de facto was the seed for the IBOT concept, based upon the assessments done by the authors, medical volunteers in Kosova and the WHO findings, the objective was to design and implement the TCK as a

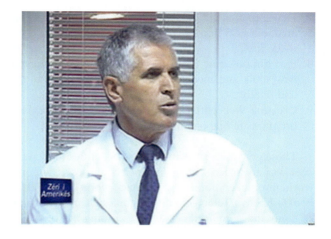

Fig. 2.4 At the opening ceremony, Kosovo's Prime Minister, Dr. Bajram Rexhepi. (Web Source: https://en.wikipedia.org/wiki/Bajram_Rexhepi)

sustainable and functional portal for information within and outside the region with a training center for telemedicine. The system would provide state-of-the-art medical education, consultation, and transmission of medical clinical data between the UCCK and the regional hospitals in Kosova, as well as between Kosova and the international medical community. In order to achieve the mission of reintegrating Kosova healthcare into healthcare community of the world, and to improve the desperate state of healthcare of Kosova [4], we set these intermediate goals for the program:

1. Establish advanced and sophisticated communication systems within the UCCK in Prishtina, and between UCCK in Prishtina and regional hospitals and health house centers in Kosova
2. Create human capacity to operate the telemedicine program and all its services (technological, educational, electronic library) independently from other local and/or international institutions
3. Establish the process whereby physicians and patients from Kosova use communications tools to peer hospitals and medical institutions abroad for consultations, academic discussion, and peer review of clinical scenarios
4. Provide medical students and Medical Faculty in Prishtina and its dentistry and pharmacy branches with electronic medical textbooks, scientific journals, and other teaching and didactic materials that are equal to that of peers of medical schools throughout Europe and the Western world
5. Advance and integrate telemedicine principles into the fabric of medical and surgical practice in the region
6. Incorporate telemedicine and medical informatics into the clinical curriculum of the Medical Faculty of University of Prishtina in Kosova

7. Develop, conduct, and support research protocols not only in the telemedicine area, but also in other clinical fields, in order to test and obtain evidence-based medicine
8. Perform outcome analyses of telemedicine applications in Kosova and develop new tools and means to provide telemedicine and virtual medical education, and finally
9. Create a Web portal and provide links to the existing Web-based educational programs in one organized step

These goals served as important modalities to increase access to care as the concept was advanced further in other countries. The concept was taught around the world through conferences, seminars, workshops, and peer review publications and books. Kosova Telemedicine Program became a subject of discussion and interest of many those countries that were coming out of the war, conflicts, and /or other disasters.

The two telemedicine programs subject of this chapter, Albania and Cabo Verde, while geographically different and on two separate continents, share many similarities. Both have remote sites and difficult terrain to traverse, and both are in rebuilding or transition phase of healthcare services. Moreover, the telemedicine program of each of these countries has been built based on the IBOT [9].

This ensures the final product (transfer to Ministry of Health) as an integral part of healthcare services. The telemedicine program of Cabo Verde was transferred to Ministry of Health in 2014, and the telemedicine program of Albania was transferred in 2017.

Initiate, Build, Operate, Transfer Strategy

The introduction of telemedicine and e-learning in Kosova in 2002 has been a pivotal step in advancing the quality and availability of medical services in a region whose infrastructure and resources have been decimated by wars, neglect, lack of funding, and poor management. The concept and establishment of the IVeH has significantly impacted telemedicine and e-health services in the Balkans and has served as an example for many. A comprehensive, four-pronged strategy, IBOT [9] (Fig. 2.5), has been useful approach in establishing telemedicine and e-health educational services in developing countries. IBOT includes assessment of healthcare needs of each country, but can be used for a region (as it was a case in the Hanoi region of Vietnam [10]), the development of a curriculum and education program, the establishment of a nationwide, regional, or healthcare system telemedicine network, and the integration of the telemedicine program into the healthcare infrastructure. The endpoint is the transfer of a sustainable telehealth program to the nation, region, or healthcare system involved. Once fully matured, the program will be transitioned to the national Ministry of Health, which ensures the sustainability and ownership of the program. The IBOT model has been effective in creating sustainable telemedicine and e-Health integrated programs in the Balkans and may be a

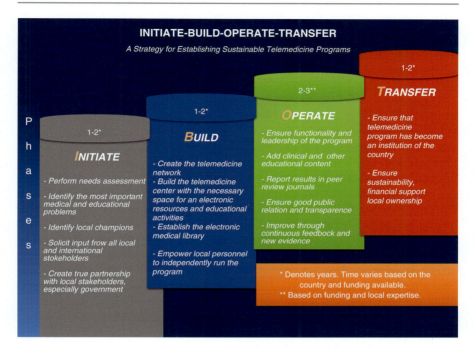

Fig. 2.5 A comprehensive, four-pronged strategy, "Initiate-Build-Operate-Transfer" (IBOT)

good model for establishing such programs in developing countries. The IBOT comprehensive four-pronged strategy, which ensures a step-by-step sustainable approach to rebuild the healthcare system using telemedicine and advanced technologies, has been reported elsewhere [11].

Initiating Phase: Assess the Local Context and Collaborate

This first phase in the IBOT strategy is structured to provide the nation's leadership with a broader understanding of telemedicine and the necessity of establishing such a program. The first set of questions that need to be answered is what is the level of need for a telemedicine program in the country or region, or institution and is the political leadership (or in case of institution or clinical department, is there a clinical appetite for it) willing and able to support such a program. In other words, are local officials, physicians, and/or the Ministry of Health willing to support and endorse the program?

Once you have these questions answered positively, then the next issue to address is does the nation or region, or institution have the technical infrastructure in place to support the program, or are they willing to support establishment of such structure? Other questions that need to be addressed are as follows: Are the people of the country or region or the institution interested in receiving training in telemedicine and, in the future, independently running the program, and what types of clinical services and educational programs are needed? However, the overarching question of this assessment process is: Once established, usually by external donors, will the telemedicine program be sustainable? This becomes acutely important in countries with political instability and frequent changes of political leadership.

If suitable answers are determined for these questions, then the IVeH will identify partners (local and international) and proceed in collaboration with, and/or on behalf of, the country. Once financial support for the project has been secured, massive intensive telemedicine and e-Health training on such topics as telecommunication, clinical applications, and services that may be implemented through telemedicine, data security, virtual educational programs, planning and implementing electronic libraries, and related business and financial issues is undertaken. Bringing together the relevant local stakeholders, including key politicians and other government officials, these prestigious and informative seminars, conducted by world-renowned telemedicine experts, demonstrate how different governmental agencies and universities can collaborate to provide care to patients and support to clinicians. Most of these seminars share the same basic content and usually are conducted by more than one group of experts, but training is tailored to the unique medical needs of a specific country or region. The seminars have served as galvanizing events, enabling a large number of health professionals to develop new capabilities. Physicians, nurses, students, information technology personnel, hospital administrators, government officials, politicians, and numerous others have actively participated in these presentations.

Building Phase and Creation of a Robust Infrastructure

The details of the building phase are based on the initial technical assessment and on the goals of the project. The four main steps of this phase are as follows: (1) building the network; (2) developing the main physical telemedicine center with the necessary space for an electronic auditorium, training areas, servers, administrative offices, and, ideally, additional resource or educational rooms; (3) establishing the electronic medical library. This is particularly essential for low- and middle-income countries (LIC and MICC) that do not have readily access to electronic libraries and research data and other resources, and produce training and educational opportunities so that local personnel can independently run the program and effectively offer clinical and educational services in the future.

The backbone of any telemedicine program is its network infrastructure and available bandwidth with optimal configuration and hardware. In each country, we require the establishment of a virtual private network that connects the national telemedicine center (usually based at the country's university clinical center or main hospitals) with regional telemedicine centers (RTCs) based at major hospitals in the area. This connectivity is based on fiber-optic lines provided by local telecommunications company or on some other form of Internet communications technology, including 3G, 4G, and now 5G. Regardless of what type of connection is established, it should be dedicated, secure, and compliant with the Health Insurance Portability and Accountability Act (HIPAA) privacy rules, due to the fact that most of the funding has come from various organizations in the USA. It also needs to be managed locally.

For the IVeH's current programs, communications have been supported by a Polycom VSX 7000 view station for point-to-point and multipoint communications via a Polycom MGC-25 Multiconference Unit or via some other product or technology, but there has been tremendous progress in technology with major trend toward mobile devices. All communications should be capable of recording and streaming live on the Internet for educational purposes. In addition, our telemedicine program should use a redundant technological system for educational programs, the electronic library, and teleconsultations. Each emergency room of every hospital involved in the program should have telemedicine capability and should be independent of the electronic library and of the educational videoconferencing system. More recently a number of software programs have made possible telehealth visits from any computer or mobile device.

In addition, a physical space that will serve as the main center of operations must be established. It is from this site that content will be dispersed and communication among the regional centers will be coordinated. This control center should house an electronic auditorium, training areas, servers, and administrative offices. Additional resource or educational rooms, such as simulation laboratories and smaller video-enabled conference rooms, provide additional flexibility and are highly advisable and encouraged. Such amenities add a special character and depth to the center, empowering leaders to undertake new, smaller-scale projects. Sophisticated computerized classrooms will facilitate the diffusion of the latest information to medical personnel. The main center should be connected to the local institution's operating rooms and other auditoriums and classrooms, fostering integration of telemedicine into overall medical operations and thus avoiding the perception of the telemedicine center as an isolated place within the institution and the country.

Because universities and medical schools in developing countries cannot afford subscriptions to expensive medical scientific journals, they rely on written manuscripts from professors and other faculty members. Yet, the cost of even those print materials often is prohibitive. Creation of an electronic medical library, using the WHO's Health Internetwork Access to Research Initiative (HINARI) and other open resources, has been extremely beneficial in supporting the cognitive needs of the medical community. Since the inception of the Telemedicine Program of Kosova (TMPK), the telemedicine center has become an arm of the medical faculty and University of Prishtina, where thousands of continuing medical education (CME), international teleconsultations, videoconferences, lectures, and seminars are being held, contributing this way significantly to healthcare system by advancing the knowledge of medical and nursing staff and exposing medical and other healthcare-related students to new advances in medicine. Hundreds of thousands of individuals have visited the TCK e-library. TMPK has been an efficient mechanism for CME and a sustainable model for rebuilding the medical system. TMPK has been successful in offering physicians, nurses, and other medical professionals access to the electronic information. The library benefits all healthcare workers, medical students, residents, other trainees, and, ultimately, patients.

Established in 2002, HINARI is a cooperative program comprising WHO, publishers, and various national medical libraries. This program provides online access to 7000 biomedical journals, and offers robust search engine functionality. Physicians, nurses, students, and other library users have constant, password-protected access to HINARI, even from their homes. Each telemedicine center can modify access to library materials as it deems appropriate. Conveniently offering remote access to the latest evidence-based medicine, the electronic library is one of the most important segments of an integrated telemedicine and e-health educational program for developing countries.

The Operating Phase: Build the Human Capacities and Protocols of Operations

The operating phase is likely the most challenging phase of the IBOT strategy and is conducted concomitantly with the building phase. As the capacity-building phase, this part of the process focuses on creating telemedicine experts, clinical ambassadors, and physician and nursing champions. In developing countries, new institutions or new concepts are sometimes met with hesitation from those who will benefit the most—medical professionals. Without healthcare professionals on board who are able and willing to lead the program, it cannot be sustained. Therefore, for the first two to three years of each telemedicine program that is launched, special attention to training and educating staff who can independently run the program—including technical, educational, library, clinical, research, development, financial, and managerial staff—should be paid. This all-inclusive concept is of the utmost importance. No matter what their area of specialization, all staff members are the future leaders of the program. Building clinical protocols of operations is a must during early stage of this phase.

Transferring Phase: Turn the Program Over to a Local Institution

Ideally, in this fourth and final phase of IBOT, the completed telemedicine program is transferred to the local public institution that it primarily serves. The Ministry of Health of that country becomes the official "owner" of the telemedicine center and equipment. Institutionalization of telemedicine is vital for sustainability; it must become an integral, long-term part of standard protocols and procedures and part of national, regional, or institutional budget.

IVeH has found that full incorporation of the four-phase implementation process is dependent on the following elements: flexibility in the architectural design of the

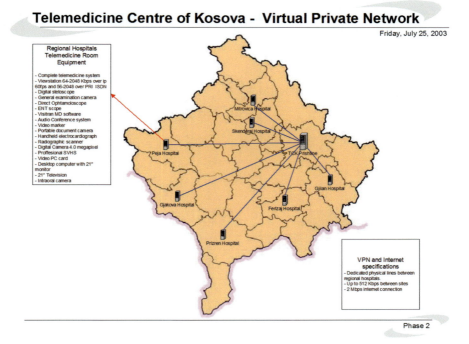

Fig. 2.6 Telemedicine Network of Kosova

network and infrastructure; multidisciplinary and functional interoperability of well-trained, actively participating individuals and teams; delivery of effective consultative clinical services; locally relevant, structured educational content through discipline-specific seminars and leadership courses; professional dedication; strategic flexibility; continuous advocacy; and development of specific indicators that go beyond creating a program or center [12].

Two Examples of Successful Implementation of IBOT Strategy

Using the IBOT strategy, the IVeH has now established and managed the telemedicine program in Kosova (2002–2007) and in Albania (2008–2016), and Cabo Verde telemedicine program (2010–2012). Each of those programs consists of a national telemedicine center in the nation's capital, Prishtina (Kosova) (Fig. 2.6), Tirana (Albania) (Fig. 2.7), and Praia (Cabo Verde) (Fig. 2.8). In this chapter, I will review the Albanian and Cabo Verdean telemedicine programs. As in the case of Kosova, programs in Albania and Cabo Verde started with intensive telemedicine seminars (Figs. 2.9 and 2.10).

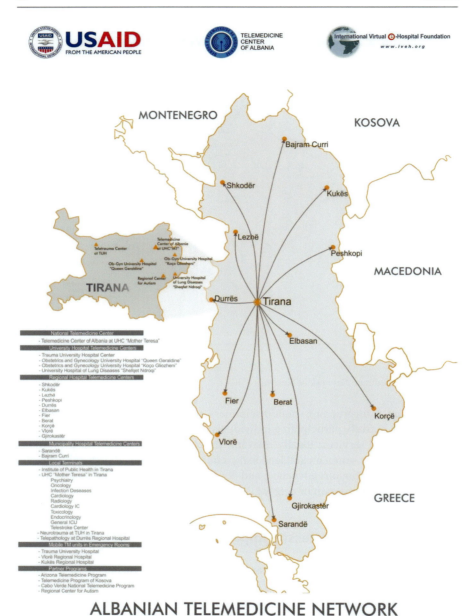

Fig. 2.7 Telemedicine Network of Albania

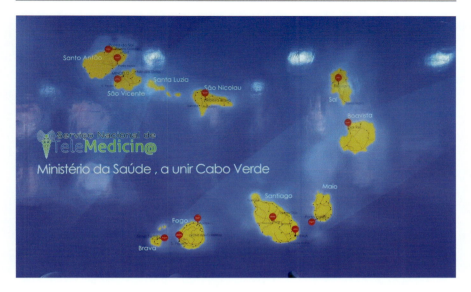

Fig. 2.8 Telemedicine Network of Cabo Verde

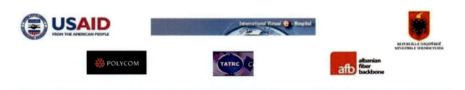

Fig. 2.9 Poster for telemedicine-intensive seminar in Albania

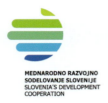
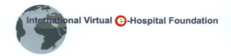

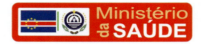

Fig. 2.10 Poster for telemedicine-intensive seminar in Cabo Verde

Albania Telemedicine Program

Albania, a South East European country with 2,938,275 population and 27,400 km² total land [4], has a robust telemedicine program that has previously been reported [3]. According to the WHO, physician density per 1000 population is 1.286 (2013), and the density of nursing and midwifery personnel per 1000 population is 5.161 (1994) [5]. Since then, the situation has changed dramatically in Albania, as hundreds, if not thousands, of physicians and nurses have been migrating to Western Europe, in dying need for new cadre of doctors and nurses. To this end, the provision of the overall high-quality healthcare services is still a major challenge [6–8], with infant mortality rate per 1000 live birth of 6.1 (2017) and maternal mortality ratio per 100,000 live births of 29 (2015), while health expenditure is 5.88% of the GDP (2014). As in most LIC and MICC, there are a number of regional hospitals in Albania, but the majority of specialists live and work in Tirana, leaving rural Albania devoid of medical services. For example, there are only two hospitals with neurosurgery services (one of them serves as the only trauma center in the country), and both are in Tirana. Emergency and trauma services around the country have serious challenges [6, 7].

The Integrated Telemedicine and e-Health program in Albania (ITeHP-Albania) was established by the IVeH in a collaborative effort with the USAID)/Albania, the U.S. Army Corps of Engineers, the government of Albania (Ministry of Health and Social Affairs [MOHSA]), and the University of Arizona, while the author was on faculty there. This program was developed based on previous telemedicine models implemented in Kosova. In the first paper on telemedicine of Albania [13], we described a successful model of a multi-partnership collaborative approach among two agencies of the U.S. Government (the USAID and the U.S. Department of Defense through the U.S. military [U.S. Army Corps of Engineers] of the EUCOM), the Government of Albania led by Dr. Salih Berisha, Prime Minister, a cardiologist (Fig. 2.11). The IVeH designed, led, and implemented the telemedicine program as a tool to assist in rebuilding the medical system and the healthcare system of Albania. The program in Albania has matured into the "Integrated Telemedicine and e-Health in Albania," which has been incorporated into the strategy of healthcare reforms supported by the Ministry of Health of Albania, and has been operational from inception in 2009 and has grown into a large telemedicine network (Fig. 2.5).

In the prospective descriptive analysis of the processes of establishing a telemedicine program in Albania, based on the comprehensive IBOT strategy, we divided the study period into three timeframe periods: (1) September 2007–December 2009, the initiation phase; (2) January 2009–September 2011, the building phase; and (3) October 2011–June 2014, the operating phase. We compared the progress of implementation of IBOT in Albania with the previously published prediction of length and timeframe required for each phase of IBOT [13]. Data on number of telemedicine centers established, including physical rehabilitation of the premises, number of clinical telemedicine programs initiated, number of teleconsultations performed, the electronic library (e-library) based on the WHO's Health InterNetwork Access Research Initiative, and the number of participants and the types of CME sessions as part of the virtual educational programs, were analyzed. Moreover, data on other innovative programs such as telestroke, teletrauma, teleautism, telediabetes, and telenursing programs and development of software

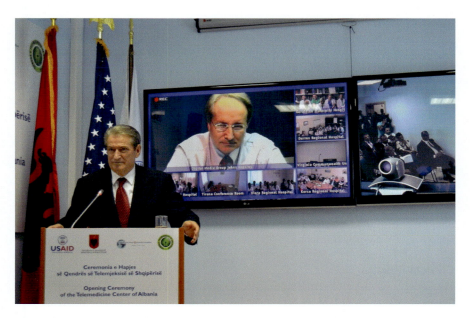

Fig. 2.11 Inauguration of Telemedicine in Albania by Prime Minister Dr. Salih Berisha, the strongest supporter of telemedicine in the Balkans, 2011; In the background Dr. Rifat Latifi participating virtually

programs to aid telemedicine programs were gathered between October 2011 and June 2014 and are presented as part of the implementation of the telemedicine program in Albania. During the study period (September 2007–June 2014), we reported that the National Telemedicine Center of Albania in Tirana and 12 regional telemedicine centers were established. The necessary policies and procedures to support the activities of this program were also completed. IVeH's four pillars, which include (1) a nationwide telemedicine network, (2) clinical programs, (3) educational programs, and (4) the e-library, have been completed.

Moreover, in that paper we reported four software applications' developments: (1) telestroke software, the beta version of a Web-based patient form and the Digital Imaging and Communications in Medicine viewer to support the activity of the telestroke program; (2) teleradiology software, a modified version of the telestroke software that provides the possibility to download the images for viewing and diagnosis, but also online viewing for the purpose of quick second-opinion provision; (3) telediabetes software, a Web-based blog-like program by means of which recently diagnosed diabetes patients can interact with experts of the Albanian Diabetes Association; and (4) the software that captures and stores research data for the Neurosurgery Service of the "Mother Theresa" University Hospital Center.

During this period, we added more clinical content including teletrauma, teleophthalmology, telecardiology, and telenursing that have also been developed and are in use. The virtual educational programs consisting of both national and international components have been active since January 2012. In addition, there were one to three weekly lectures organized by the Telemedicine Center of Kosova and the biweekly lecture series of the Albanian Association of Nurses, as well as many other training programs.

We described somewhat of a slow progression the clinical telemedicine program experienced initially, but with time things improved. Overall, the results of our study of establishment and implementation of telemedicine of Albania are compatible with the previously reported timeframe of IBOT implementation. With collaboration among U.S. governmental agencies working in Albania, Albanian governmental institutions, and IVeH, a medical system that was in need of major reform was revitalized using telemedicine and advanced technologies through the principles of the IBOT approach.

Today, telemedicine program in Albania serves the entire country with a total of 36 active telemedicine centers and telemedicine clinical portals/units. Out of these, 19 centers provide teleconsultations, and 11 regional hospitals and 3 municipal hospitals refer the patients. There are three mobile units to complete telemedicine network in Albania. In January 2017, the program was transferred to MOHSA as an integral part of the National Center of Biomedical Engineering (NCBE) and is fully supported by the government.

Clinical Results

Previously, we have reported telemedicine results in Albania [14]. Recently [15], however, we analyzed 2842 patients who were managed using telemedicine program in all clinical disciplines. We excluded 118 patients—90 teleautism patients and 28 patients with missing data (unknown clinical discipline and unknown or no action taken during the consult). Ultimately, 2724 patients remained for analysis. The most frequently consulting clinical disciplines were radiology (39.0%), neurotrauma (27.2%), and stroke (16.7%). The difference in transfer status was statistically significant ($p < 0.001$) for radiology, neurotrauma, stroke, pneumatology, psychiatry, nephrology, and surgery. Elderly (the age group 70–79) had higher rate of transfer rate. While the rate of transfer patients increased from 2014 through 2017, overall there is a smaller size of transferred patients to a tertiary center in each year. The rate of transfer patients decreased in 2018 patients.

Overall, transfer neurotrauma patients were slightly older (42.5 vs. 44.8, $p = 0.215$), but there was no statistical difference. However, the difference was statistically significant in the stratum of patients 80 years of age ($p = 0.021$). Similar to overall clinical disciplines, only a smaller portion of neurotrauma patients were transferred to a tertiary center each year (as follows: 23.8–35.9%). The two centers that requested most consults for neurotrauma were Vlora Regional Hospital (51.8%) and Korca Regional Hospital (32.9%). All the teleneurotrauma consults (100%) were provided by University Hospital of Trauma in Tirana. The transfer rate in Vlora Regional Hospital was 22.7%, and in Korca Regional Hospital it was 46%. Most successful clinical program has been neurotrauma [16].

Telemedicine in Cabo Verde

The telemedicine program in Cabo Verde, a nation of 10 islands of West Africa, started in 2012 as a 10-center program, which later progressed to 14 centers. The population of Cabo Verde is 560,084, and the total land is 4030 km^2. According to the WHO, the density of physicians is 0.788 per 1000 population (2015). The nursing and midwifery personnel density is 1.256 per 1000 population (2015). Economically, 4.8% of the GDP goes toward health (2014). The infant mortality rate is 10.4 deaths per 1000 live births (2017), whereas the maternal mortality rate is 42 deaths per 100,000 live births (2015) [17].

There is no medical school, and all doctors are graduates from other countries such as Portugal, Brazil, Russia, China, and Cuba among others [11]. Santiago and Sao Vicente islands are the most populated islands. The majority of physicians are concentrated in Santiago, and nurses are mostly concentrated in Sao Vicente [18].

Cabo Verde has proven a great success story of telemedicine in Africa [17–20]. Although Cabo Verde has had a long history of telemedicine for pediatric cardiology [19], in 2014, we reported the first establishment of nation-wide telemedicine in Cabo Verde [17]. The Minister of Health of Cabo Verde, Dr. Maria Cristina Fontes Lima (Fig. 2.12), was an incredible supporter of the program. Over a 26-month period (November 2011–December 2013), the program implemented: (1) capacity building; (2) network development and deployment of equipment; (3) implementation of clinical telemedicine; (4) implementation of activities related to continuing medical education, delivered from within the country and from abroad; and (5) establishment and use of the electronic virtual library.

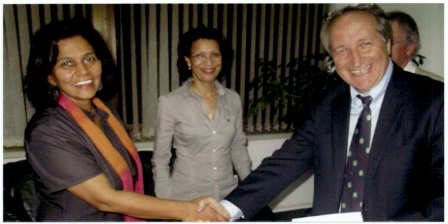

Dr. Latifi during a meeting with the Minister of Health of The Republic of Cabo Verde, Dr. Maria Cristina Fontes Lima.

Fig. 2.12 The Minister of Health of Cabo Verde, Dr. Maria Cristina Fontes Lima

Most recently we reported the follow-up study on Cabo Verde telemedicine [21] and updated the clinical results and expansion of the telemedicine program from 10 centers to 14 telemedicine centers in 9 populated islands (Fig. 2.7).

During the period 2014 to 2019, there were a total of 2442 telemedicine consultations performed, however. A total of 404 consultations had incomplete data and were excluded. The patients ranged from infancy to the elderly. Overall, the median age was 35 years. There were more female than male (54.9% vs. 45.9%). Telemedicine consultations have grown steadily. For example, in 2014, 128 patients, while in 2018, 796 patients were seen, from all islands; however, Fogo (22.0%) and Santo Antão (16.2%) requested the highest number of teleconsultations. Hospital Dr. Agostinho Neto (HAN) received the majority (81.0%) of the telemedicine consults. Overall, the transfer rate was 34.3%. The most common clinical disciplines using telemedicine were neurology, cardiology, orthopedic surgery, general surgery, endocrinology, otolaryngology, urology, and dermatology.

The most active specialty was neurology (29.5%), and 12.4% (89/720) of neurology patients were transferred. Cardiology comprised the greatest portion of transfer patients (17.6%), and it was statistically significant. In 2018, a statistically significant increased rate of transfer was seen in otolaryngology, surgery, and cardiology. Among surgical specialties, orthopedic surgery demonstrated a non-significant pattern of transfer in all years of the study except 2015.

As expected, there is similar transfer rate in all the islands except Boa Vista, which showed an increase, while the island of Santo Antão showed significant decrease in transfer rate. Generally, however, Cabo Verde telemedicine program has continued to expand both in volume and centers since 2014. At the same time, a continuous decrease in the number of transfer cases has been demonstrated.

Telemedicine Champions

The question that has been raised over the last two decades is that what should the success of telemedicine program be attributed to? We examined the relationship between the clinical teleconsultations as an indicator of healthcare system needs and the contribution of local telemedicine champions based on data prospectively collected data between 2014 and 2018 from Albania and Cabo Verde [21]. For the purpose of this study, the telemedicine champion was defined as an individual, clinical discipline or hospital that contributed with at least 100 telemedicine consultations during the study periods. Individual telemedicine champion was defined as an individual physician from any clinical discipline or hospital receiving and responding to or requesting telemedicine consultation. Based on this definition, we developed the new concept of clinical discipline champion and hospital champion.

As reported above, there were a total of 2442 teleconsultations in Cabo Verde and 2724 teleconsultations in Albania during the study periods. These two telemedicine programs have similar clinical disciplines and with only small differences. In total, there were 173 physicians in Albania and 108 physicians in Cabo Verde from different specialties that performed or asked for telemedicine consultations.

Based on the 100-telemedicine consultation definition, radiology ($n = 1061$), neurotrauma ($n = 742$), and neurology or stroke ($n = 489$) were clinical discipline champions. On the other hand, in Cabo Verde, there were eight champion clinical disciplines including neurology ($n = 720$), cardiology ($n = 313$), orthopedics ($n = 190$), surgery ($n = 143$), endocrinology ($n = 141$), otolaryngology ($n = 139$), urology ($n = 139$), and dermatology ($n = 126$).

Using the 100-requesting teleconsultation as the indicator of local hospital champion, we identified the hospital champion in seven islands in Cabo Verde and four in Albania. The Cabo Verde hospital champions were in Fogo ($n = 537$), Santo Antao ($n = 396$), Boa vista ($n = 246$), Sal ($n = 241$), Sao Nicolau ($n = 231$), Brava ($n = 175$), and Maio ($n = 157$), while four requesting champion hospitals in Albania were Vlora ($n = 1249$), Korca ($n = 740$), Shkodra ($n = 222$), and Kukes ($n = 202$). Similarly, based on the indicator of 100 performing teleconsultations, in Cabo Verde, the receiving hospital champions were Hospital of Dr. Agostinho ($n = 1978$) and Hospital of Dr. Baptitsa de Sousa ($n = 464$). The receiving hospital champions in Albania were UHC Mother Teresa ($n = 1483$) and University Trauma Hospital ($n = 1119$). In Albania, there is a well-developed teleradiology (20 physicians, 4 champions), teleneurotrauma (7 physicians, 5 champions), and neurology/telestroke program (16 physicians and 2 champions).

In Cabo Verde, champion clinical disciplines were teleneurology (3 physicians, 2 champions), telecardiology (8 physicians, 1 champion), teleorthopedics (11 physicians, no champion), telesurgery (13 physicians, no champion), tele-endocrinology (3 physicians and 1 champion), teleotolaryngology (7 physicians, no champion), teleurology (3 physicians, no champion), and teledermatology (3 physicians and 1 champion).

Summary and the Road of Telemedicine Ahead?

Twenty years from the Berlin G8 conference, I continue to be as enthusiastic, optimistic, and determined that the future of the telemedicine will be as brighter as ever in the past. In conclusion, both programs have been running progressively. They have reduced the rate of unnecessary transfers, resulting in saved resources. Although they are in two different geographical locations and have different populations and cultures, they work well under the same system. This stems from the same platform that these two programs have been established on (IBOT) basis. Also, the key to success for these two programs is trying to assess the need, infrastructure, and resources as well as involving the host government and academic leaders from the beginning. In 2018, both countries improved their telemedicine program. There is still more room to grow, and these two programs can serve their host counties better.

Overall, telemedicine has made great strides, from both a research standpoint and an organizational standpoint. We do need, however, to harness new and innovative concepts, such as smartphone health apps, as long as they are clinically sound, secured, and deployable. We also need to further test their potential effectiveness as principal components of the existing infrastructure.

IVeH previously published data on the cost-effectiveness of the TMPK [9]. Yet clearly, more vigorous analyses of these programs are needed. We await research by other impartial investigators to demonstrate the strengths and weaknesses of the IBOT strategy in other parts of the world. It goes without saying that just like in any other surgical mission, the implementation of telemedicine programs in developing nations requires the involvement of people who are passionate about their work and are willing to make personal and professional sacrifices. The intellectual and emotional satisfaction resulting from working with these programs, however, is enormous and most fulfilling, particularly when one considers the sustainable potential impact on patient care in developing countries. Moreover, for those of us who have moved to the USA and made it our home, these programs make virtual return possible anytime, anywhere.

The IVeH has received three significant awards for its efforts to promote telemedicine and e-health. In June 2011, the Computerworld Honors Program awarded to the IVeH the prestigious twenty-first Century Achievement Award in the Health category [22]. The award recognizes the utility of the IBOT strategy and its successful implementation in Kosova and Albania. In December 2011, the Utilization Review Accreditation Commission and the Care Continuum Alliance awarded the 2011 International Health Promotion Award in the International Community Health category to the IVeH. Most recently, the IVeH and the seven telemedicine centers in Kosova received the 2011 Visual Communications User Application Healthcare Award at the Telepresence and Videoconferencing Editor's Choice Awards ceremony [23].

For the IBOT model that ensures the program's sustainability and has been successfully replicated in Albania and Cabo Verde, Africa, and for helping to establish telemedicine and e-health programs in underdeveloped countries, especially those recovering from conflict and in need of major rebuilding of their healthcare systems, the American College of Surgeon's Operation Giving Back awarded the 2015 International Surgical Volunteerism Award [24].

References

1. World Health Organization. Atlas of eHealth country profiles 2015: the use of eHealth in support of universal health coverage | based on the findings of the 2015 global survey on eHealth. WHO | Atlas of eHealth country profiles 2015 Web site. Published February 2016. Updated 2016. https://www.who.int/goe/publications/atlas_2015/en/. Last accessed 26 May 2020.
2. Pepi SA. USAID | from the American people. US Embassy Funds Renovation of Telemedicine Centers in Albanian Regional Hospitals Web site. Published May 13, 2014. Updated 2014. https://2012-2017.usaid.gov/albania/news-information/press-releases/us-embassy-funds-renovation-telemedicine-centers-albanian. Last accessed 26 May 2020.
3. Little V. US army corps of engineers. Albania telemedicine network fully connected Web site. Published October 24, 2015. Updated 2015. https://www.nau.usace.army.mil/Media/News-Stories/Article/625824/albania-telemedicine-network-fully-connected/. Last accessed 26 May 2020.
4. Latifi R, Muja S, Bekteshi F, Reinicke M. Use of information technology to improve quality of healthcare: Kosova's telemedicine project and international virtual e-hospital as an example. Stud Health Technol Inform. 2004;104:159–67.
5. United nations peacemaker. Security Council Resolution 1244. 1999. On the situation relating Kosovo Web site. Published June 10, 1999. Updated 1999. https://peacemaker.un.org/kosovo-resolution1244. Last accessed 26 May 2020.
6. Latifi R. Instead of a prologue establishing telemedicine in the Balkans from berlin to Prishtina via Mars -a personal journey. In: Latifi R, editor. Telemedicine in developing countries: from inception to implementation: IOS Press; 2004. p. 8–21. Last accessed 26 May 2020.
7. Latifi R. The anatomy of war and destruction of Kosova: an Alumni view on restructuring health care. Final Conference of G-8, Global Applications Health Project, Berlin, May 3–5, 2000.
8. Latifi R, editor. Establishing telemedicine in developing countries: from inception to implementation. IOS Press; 2004. Latifi R., ed. Last accessed 26 May 2020.
9. Latifi R, Merrell RC, Doarn CR, et al. "Initiate-build-operate-transfer"--a strategy for establishing sustainable telemedicine programs in developing countries: initial lessons from the Balkans. Telemed J E Health. 2009;15(10):956–69.
10. International Virtual e-Hospital www.iveh.org. Last accessed 26 May 2020.
11. Latifi R. Using telemedicine to strengthen medical systems in limited-resource countries. Bull Am Coll Surg. 2012;97(10):15–21.
12. Latifi R. "Initiate-build-operate-transfer" - a strategy for establishing sustainable telemedicine programs not only in the developing countries. Stud Health Technol Inform. 2011;165:3–10.
13. Latifi R, Dasho E, Shatri Z, et al. Telemedicine as an innovative model for rebuilding medical systems in developing countries through multipartnership collaboration: the case of Albania. Telemed J E Health. 2015;21(6):503–9.
14. Latifi R, Gunn JK, Bakiu E, et al. Access to specialized care through telemedicine in limited-resource country: initial 1,065 teleconsultations in Albania. Telemed J E Health. 2016;22(12):1024–31.

15. Latifi R, Parsikia A, Boci A, Doarn CR, Merrell RC. Increased access to care through telemedicine in Albania: an analysis of 2,724 patients. Telemed J E Health. 2020;26(2):164–75.
16. Olldashi F, Latifi R, Parsikia A, et al. Telemedicine for neurotrauma prevents unnecessary transfers: an update from a nationwide program in Albania and analysis of 590 patients. World Neurosurg. 2019;128:e340–6.
17. Azevedo V, Latifi R, Parsikia A, Latifi F, Azevedo A. Cabo Verde telemedicine program: an update report and analysis of 2,442 teleconsultations. Telemed J E Health. (In press).
18. Correia A, Azevedo V, LV LÃ£o. Implementation of telemedicine in Cape Verde: influencing factors. Acta Medica Port. 2017;30(4):255–62.
19. Castela E. Coimbra telemedicine service improves access to pediatric cardiology in Cape Verde. Acta Medica Port. 2017;30(4):253–4.
20. Latifi R, Dasho E, Merrell RC, et al. Cabo Verde telemedicine program: initial results of nationwide implementation. Telemed J E Health. 2014;20(11):1027–34.
21. Latifi R, Azevedo V, Boci A, Parsikia A, Latifi F, Merrell RC. Telemedicine consultation as an indicator of local telemedicine champions contributions, healthcare system needs or both - tales from two continents. Telemed J E Health. 2020. https://doi.org/10.1089/tmj.2019.0290. Online ahead of print.
22. The Computerworld Honors Program. Published June 2011. https://na.eventscloud.com/file_uploads/52b680fc313c6a4e7e1459f8bf7b6ce8_International_Virtual_e-Hospital_-_Balkan_Telemedicine_Program.pdf. Last accessed 26 May 2020.
23. Polycom. IVeH -Albania- Customer Success Story - Polycom, Inc.Web site. https://www.polycom.es/global/en/customer-stories/iveh-albania.html. Last accessed 26 May 2020.
24. American college of surgeons. 2015 International Volunteer Award: Rifat Latifi Web site. Updated 2015. https://www.facs.org/ogb/award-winners/international/latifi. Last accessed 26 May 2020.

Clinical Telemedicine Practice: From Ad Hoc Medicine to Modus Operandi

Rifat Latifi

Introduction

Clinical telemedicine has been adopted by several countries around the world, although it was expected that by now large-scale telemedicine expansion would have occurred. Successful telemedicine programs have been implemented and provide excellent examples for others [1–4]; however, the adoption of technology, programs, and systems has not happened as readily as expected, until this recent year. Of the successful programs that do exist, many have not spread to large-scale applications. These programs typically have champions who facilitate program funding with government and private sector connections, or who have successful granting, but importantly have clinicians who have embraced and adopted telemedicine. Despite the current growth and newer enthusiastic acceptance of telemedicine during COVID-19, when one considers the potential of telemedicine, this is all still on a smaller scale, and there is much room for improvement. We need to move from crisis mode to sustainable modus operandi on clinical applications of telemedicine [5].

There are a number of organizations that have produced their own guidelines on clinical telemedicine from WHO to ATA, ISTeH, and other subspecialty societies. The aim is to facilitate the successful implementation and incorporation of telemedicine by providing guidance for establishing programs and requiring member states to participate by developing local telemedicine efforts [4, 6, 7]. The benefits of clinical telemedicine are many, including remote monitoring, offering telehealth services to rural populations who may not normally receive adequate healthcare, providing expertise from a distance, cost savings, and educational purposes; however, with the many benefits that come with telemedicine, there are also many

R. Latifi (✉)
Department of Surgery, New York Medical College, School of Medicine and Westchester Medical Center Health, Valhalla, NY, USA
e-mail: Rifat.latifi@wmchealth.org; Rifat_Latifi@nymc.edu

barriers. The major barriers until now have been economic, legal, and some technical [5]. However, in response to COVID-19, the Center for Medicaid and Medicare Services has permitted patients to be seen via videoconferencing in their homes, without having to travel to a qualifying "originating site" for Medicare telehealth encounters. Furthermore, the Drug Enforcement Administration (DEA) approved an exception that allows prescriptions for controlled substances via telemedicine without a prior in-person evaluation. It is our hope that these guidelines will not be revoked once this pandemic has subsided. While this is very positive news for telemedicine overall, we will need to carefully document the benefits of telemedicine during this pandemic, in order to continue to pressure the policy makers to recognize that there is a need for continuous support and advancement of telemedicine services [5].

Hopefully, these examples, new support for telemedicine from the U.S. and other governments, along with other lessons from around the world that have been well documented will ensure continuation, expansion, and sustainability of the current enthusiasm for telemedicine across the world and in all clinical disciplines.

Telemedicine programs should be incorporated with, and be part of, local healthcare systems and the culture of individual organizations [8–10]. The objective of this chapter is to discuss current evidence of successful clinical telemedicine programs and to provide guidance on establishing and maintaining successful programs for others.

Telemedicine Modalities

Store and forward, and synchronous (real-time) methods are the most frequently used forms of telemedicine. Store and forward is typically used for the transmission of history, physical examination, and image-based diagnostic materials, such as in radiology [1–3]. In addition, real time is a common technique that involves live assistance with clinical conditions, while both patients and local healthcare providers are present. Moreover, telemedicine networks can be used for educational and telehealth consultations [11]. A third form of telemedicine, remote monitoring has been used extensively in emergency situations [12] and has gained wider acceptance as relevant technologies have become less expensive and more readily available. All three forms of telemedicine are beneficial in clinical telemedicine settings.

Clinical Telemedicine

Clinical telemedicine can be applied to every aspect of healthcare including primary care [13], cardiology [14], neurology [15], orthopedics and traumatology [16], psychiatry [17], home healthcare [18], rehabilitation [19], wound care [20], pathology [21], dermatology [22], oncology [23], and palliative care [24]. However, there is no clinical discipline in which telemedicine cannot be applied [25]. Radiology [26], on the other hand, is most commonly. Artificial intelligence is gaining momentum and will become part of the armamentarium and part of telemedicine. Other disciplines such as trauma, particularly neurotrauma, and intensive care will be addressed in separate chapters in this book.

In the last few years, many telemedicine applications have changed into mobile health and involve sensors, mobile apps, social media, and location-tracking technology that are used in disease diagnosis, prevention, and management [27]. These technologies include heart rate monitors, blood pressure monitors, and blood sugar monitors. Newer technologies are continually being developed for clinical telemedicine usage.

Clinical Telemedicine Guidelines

Many organization and association have designed their telemedicine guidelines. The American Telemedical Association has created a set of guideline to serve as standards for telemedicine practices in various clinical disciplines including stroke, mental health, burn, teleICU, pathology, and others [28–34]. The use of, and the need for, guidelines was also reviewed [35]. These guidelines and standards include clinical, administrative, and technical requirements for telemedicine networks that evolve with time and should be evidence based. A recent study revealed major weaknesses in current guidelines for electronic communication between patients and providers, and the guidelines appear to be based on minimal evidence and offer little guidance on how best to use electronic tools to communicate effectively [36].

The requirements include human resource management, privacy and confidentiality, federal, state, and other credentialing, regulatory agency requirements, fiscal management, ownership of patient records, patient rights and responsibilities, documentation protocols, network security, equipment use, and research protocols.

Policies and Protocols/Agreement Required

With each policy and protocol, all personnel, contractors, and members of a clinical medicine group will need to complete appropriate paperwork that includes security policies, personnel policies, and technical policies that ensure the confidentiality and integrity of data are maintained. Inclusion of local legal policies is necessary in these agreements.

Technical Requirements

The technology of clinical telemedicine has been advancing greatly in the last few years, from telemedicine towers to smart software and mobile devices. Technical requirements include high-quality network communications and often depend on the stage of the program. For mature programs, data communication networks can include local area networks (LAN), which interconnect hosts in small areas, such as a building; small office/home office networks (SOHO), which are similar to a LAN, but contain less hosts; metropolitan area network (MAN), which connects multiple sites; or a wide area network (WAN), which interconnects multiple sites over long distances. Other options that include plain old telephone service (POTS), which is an analog dial up telephone that provides voice and limited amounts of data between two points, are for the most part a thing of the past. With the rapid advancements in cellular technology, cellular/mobile broadband technology is becoming a viable form of telemedicine technology. Another form of connectivity is that of T-carrier lines. T-carrier lines are high-speed digital network transport services that support both voice and data transmission and link other organizations to provide services over large areas. Satellite connectivity is another connectivity option that is used widely across the world. Recent advances in satellite technology allow for portable satellite applications. Broadband global area network (BGAN) is one example of a portable satellite application. It uses a compact, portable satellite terminal that is easy to set up and use. Video conferencing can be used for educational purposes, consultation following surgery, surgical telementoring, trauma and emergency medicine situations, and discussions among multidisciplinary teams (see chapters 18, 27).

How to Perform Teleconsultations

Well-planned, structured, and integrated telemedicine consultation should become a part of regular clinical practice, and it is best if it is incorporated into clinical practice through integrated EMR, so it can be shared and viewed by other providers of healthcare systems participating in the care of the patient. Privacy and confidentiality should be a priority, as well as documentation. The teleconsultation office must be set up much like being in a regular office where patients are seen. Additionally, the patient should establish a secure and comfortable area from where they can contact the clinician.

Saving the Data

Data security and accessibility are essential to a successful telemedicine program [37]. Several protocols should be established for saving and using the data. These protocols include authentication, encryption, access control, integrity, confidentiality, auditing and accounting systems, and security policy. User control has to be established for every stage of access to the system. Encryption, or the scrambling transmission of data, should be carried out using a "behind the scenes" algorithm or program. A policy that is strictly adhered to, that incorporates effective procedures to maintain confidentiality, data integrity, and security, should be established.

Reporting the Data

When reporting the data, all rules regarding confidentiality and security of the data are paramount. This should be no different than any other data on EMR.

Summary

Clinical telemedicine has gained great popularity, particularly following the COVID-19 pandemic. Throughout the last few years, telemedicine has become more acceptable, even though in the past telemedicine has been ignored despite a great potential to provide rapid, safe, and high-quality care. Although a number of world enthusiastic surgeons and physicians have been teaching and practicing telemedicine around the world, only recently has telemedicine taken center stage. Specific clinical disciplines have been addressed in this book.

References

1. Latifi R. Establishing telemedicine in developing countries: from inception to implementation. Amsterdam: IOS Press; 2004. p. 159–67.
2. Latifi R. Telemedicine for trauma, emergencies, and disaster management. Norwood: Artech House Publishers; 2010.
3. Latifi R. Current principles and practices of telemedicine and e-health. Amsterdam: IOS Press; 2008.
4. World Health Organization. Atlas of eHealth country profiles 2015: the use of eHealth in support of universal health coverage. World Health Organization. https://www.who.int/goe/publications/atlas_2015/en/. Published December 15, 2016. Accessed 28 Apr 2020.
5. Latifi R, Doarn CR. Perspective on COVID-19: Finally, telemedicine at center stage [published online ahead of print, 2020 May 14]. Telemed J E Health. 2020; https://doi.org/10.1089/tmj.2020.0132. Published May 14, 2020.
6. Home page. https://www.who.int/data/gho/indicator-metadata-registry/imr-details/4782-.
7. Home page. https://www.isfteh.org. Accessed 5 May 2020.
8. Home page. The Arizona Telemedicine Program. https://telemedicine.arizona.edu. Accessed 5 May 2020.
9. Office of Telehealth & Telemedicine. Georgia Department of Public Health. https://dph.georgia.gov/office-telehealth-telemedicine. Accessed 5 May 2020.
10. Home page. http://dhss.alaska.gov/dph/HealthPlanning/Pages/telehealth/default.aspx. Accessed 5 May 2020.
11. Latifi R, Dasho E, Shatri Z, et al. Telemedicine as an innovative model for rebuilding medical systems in developing countries through multipartnership collaboration: the case of Albania. Telemed J E Health. 2015;21(6):503–9. https://doi.org/10.1089/tmj.2014.0138.
12. Latifi R, Weinstein RS, Porter JM, et al. Telemedicine and telepresence for trauma and emergency care management. Scand J Surg. 2007;96(4):281–9. https://doi.org/10.1177/145749690709600404.
13. Bashshur RL, Howell JD, Krupinski EA, et al. The empirical foundations of telemedicine interventions in primary care. Telemed J E Health. 2016;22(5):342–75. https://doi.org/10.1089/tmj.2016.0045.
14. Lopes MACQ, Oliveira GMM, Ribeiro ALP, et al. Guideline of the Brazilian Society of Cardiology on telemedicine in cardiology – 2019. Arq Bras Cardiol. 2019;113(5):1006–56. https://doi.org/10.5935/abc.20190205.

15. Bramanti A, Calabrò RS. Telemedicine in neurology: where are we going? Eur J Neurol. 2018;25(1):e6. https://doi.org/10.1111/ene.13477.
16. Prada C, Izquierdo N, Traipe R, et al. Results of a new telemedicine strategy in traumatology and orthopedics. Telemed J E Health. 2020;26:665–70. https://doi.org/10.1089/tmj.2019.0090.
17. Fortney JC, Pyne JM, Turner EE, et al. Telepsychiatry integration of mental health services into rural primary care settings. Int Rev Psychiatry. 2015;27(6):525–39. https://doi.org/10.3109/09540261.2015.1085838.
18. Michaud TL, Zhou J, McCarthy MA, et al. Costs of home-based telemedicine programs: a systematic review. Int J Technol Assess Health Care. 2018;34(4):410–8. https://doi.org/10.1017/S0266462318000454.
19. Galea MD. Telemedicine in rehabilitation. Phys Med Rehabil Clin N Am. 2019;30(2):473–83. https://doi.org/10.1016/j.pmr.2018.12.002.
20. Bianciardi Valassina MF, Bella S, Murgia F, et al. Telemedicine in pediatric wound care. Clin Ter. 2016;167(1):e21–3. https://doi.org/10.7417/T.2016.1915.
21. Griffin J, Treanor D. Digital pathology in clinical use: where are we now and what is holding us back? Histopathology. 2017;70(1):134–45. https://doi.org/10.1111/his.12993.
22. Trettel A, Eissing L, Augustin M. Telemedicine in dermatology: findings and experiences worldwide – a systematic literature review. J Eur Acad Dermatol Venereol. 2018;32(2):215–24. https://doi.org/10.1111/jdv.14341.
23. Fallahzadeh R, Rokni SA, Ghasemzadeh H, et al. Digital health for geriatric oncology. JCO Clin Cancer Inform. 2018;2:1–12. https://doi.org/10.1200/CCI.17.00133.
24. Worster B, Swartz K. Telemedicine and palliative care: an increasing role in supportive oncology. Curr Oncol Rep. 2017;19(6):37. https://doi.org/10.1007/s11912-017-0600-y.
25. Weinstein RS, Krupinski EA, Doarn CR. Clinical examination component of telemedicine, telehealth, mHealth, and connected health medical practices. Med Clin North Am. 2018;102(3):533–44. https://doi.org/10.1016/j.mcna.2018.01.002.
26. Bashshur RL, Krupinski EA, Thrall JH, et al. The empirical foundations of teleradiology and related applications: a review of the evidence. Telemed J E Health. 2016;22(11):868–98. https://doi.org/10.1089/tmj.2016.0149.
27. Sim I. Mobile devices and health. N Engl J Med. 2019;381(10):956–68. https://doi.org/10.1056/NEJMra1806949.
28. Demaerschalk BM, Berg J, Chong BW, et al. American Telemedicine Association: telestroke guidelines. Telemed J E Health. 2017;23(5):376–89. https://doi.org/10.1089/tmj.2017.0006.
29. Powers WJ, Rabinstein AA, Ackerson T, et al. Guidelines for the early management of patients with acute ischemic stroke: 2019 update to the 2018 guidelines for the early management of acute ischemic stroke: a guideline for healthcare professionals from the American Heart Association/American Stroke Association [published correction appears in Stroke. 2019;50(12):e440–e441]. Stroke. 2019;50(12):e344–418. https://doi.org/10.1161/STR.0000000000000211.
30. Myers K, Nelson EL, Rabinowitz T, et al. American Telemedicine Association practice guidelines for telemental health with children and adolescents. Telemed J E Health. 2017;23(10):779–804. https://doi.org/10.1089/tmj.2017.0177.
31. Theurer L, Bashshur R, Bernard J, et al. American Telemedicine Association guidelines for teleburn. Telemed J E Health. 2017;23(5):365–75. https://doi.org/10.1089/tmj.2016.0279.
32. Davis TM, Barden C, Dean S, et al. American Telemedicine Association guidelines for teleICU operations. Telemed J E Health. 2016;22(12):971–80. https://doi.org/10.1089/tmj.2016.0065.
33. Pantanowitz L, Dickinson K, Evans AJ, et al. American Telemedicine Association clinical guidelines for telepathology. J Pathol Inform. 2014;5(1):39. https://doi.org/10.4103/2153-3539.143329.
34. Richmond T, Peterson C, Cason J, et al. American Telemedicine Association's principles for delivering telerehabilitation services. Int J Telerehabil. 2017;9(2):63–8. https://doi.org/10.5195/ijt.2017.6232.

35. Krupinski EA, Antoniotti N, Bernard J. Utilization of the American Telemedicine Association's clinical practice guidelines. Telemed J E Health. 2013;19(11):846–51. https://doi.org/10.1089/tmj.2013.0027.
36. Lee JL, Matthias MS, Menachemi N, et al. A critical appraisal of guidelines for electronic communication between patients and clinicians: the need to modernize current recommendations. J Am Med Inform Assoc. 2018;25(4):413–8. https://doi.org/10.1093/jamia/ocx089.
37. Hadeed GJ, Holcomb M, Latifi R. Communication technologies: an overview of telemedicine connectivity. In: Latifi R, editor. Telemedicine for trauma, emergencies, and disaster management. Norwood: Artech House Publishers; 2011. p. 37–51.

Incorporation of Telemedicine in Disaster Management: Beyond the Era of the COVID-19 Pandemic

Rifat Latifi and Charles R. Doarn

At the time of writing this chapter, the COVID-19 pandemic has affected more than 2.5 million (and by the time it is published, this number may very well increase to many more millions with mortality in hundreds of thousands of patients worldwide), economy has suffered tremendously, unemployment has increased greatly, and life that we knew months ago has changed. We all long to return to a normal life, which we are not sure we treated as such, but now that we do not have it, we miss it.

Introduction

Numerous disasters have occurred over the past 15 years, but nothing has prepared us for a global pandemic from COVID-19. This highly infective virus has turned our world, impacting global health, commerce, education, and daily life. According to the International Disaster Database, there were 6973 disasters between the years 2000 and 2015 [1]. The numbers of disasters since 2015 have been fairly significant in death and destruction. The largest natural disaster in 2010 was an earthquake in Nepal in April where 8831 people were killed. Then, there were three heat waves through France, India, and Pakistan which killed 3275, 2248, and 1229 people, respectively. A landslide in October killed 627 people in Guatemala. A heat wave in Belgium killed 410 people. Floods in India killed 325 people in November and 293 people in July. An earthquake in Pakistan killed 280 people in October, and a flood in Malawi killed 278 people. In 2016, 1600 people were killed by Hurricane Matthew. An earthquake in

R. Latifi (✉)
Department of Surgery, New York Medical College, School of Medicine and Westchester Medical Center Health, Valhalla, NY, USA
e-mail: Rifat.Latifi@wmchealth.org; Rifat_Latifi@nymc.edu

C. R. Doarn
Department of Environmental and Public Health Sciences, University of Cincinnati College of Medicine, Cincinnati, OH, USA

© Springer Nature Switzerland AG 2021
R. Latifi et al. (eds.), *Telemedicine, Telehealth and Telepresence*,
https://doi.org/10.1007/978-3-030-56917-4_4

Taiwan killed 116 people. An earthquake in Italy killed 247 people. In 2017, flooding killed 1000 people in Sierra Leone; earthquakes in Mexico killed 460 people; Hurricane Maria killed 3057 people; an earthquake in Iran killed 500 people; a flood in China killed 144 people; a flood in Peru killed 150 people; an avalanche in Afghanistan killed 156 people; a landslide in the Congo killed 174 people; a flood in South Asia killed approximately 1200 people. In 2018, an earthquake and tsunami killed 2783 people in Indonesia; a flood in India killed 361 people; a flood in Nigeria killed 200 people; a heat wave in Pakistan killed 180 people. An earthquake in Papua New Guinea killed 145 people. In 2019, a heat wave in Japan killed 160 people; a cyclone in Africa killed 900 people; a cyclone in Mozambique killed 1000 people; and fires ravaged California and Australia. We have to remember that Ebola, on the other hand, had ravaged West Africa between 2014 and 2016, killing 11,325 people, and fight has still not ended, and the war is ongoing. The decade that we just left was bookended with the devastating earthquake in Haiti that killed over 230,000 people, and with wildfires consuming millions of acres across Australia.

When a little known viral infection in Wuhan, China, began in late 2019, no one would have predicted what COVID-19 could do to the entire world in a few short months. It has only been 100 years since the last global pandemic caused by a virus; the Spanish Influenza killed 500 million people or one third of the world's population. But our memory has faded and history seems to be reminding us of how unprepared we are for biological disasters.

Disasters present a worldwide problem that requires systematic, methodological preparation, and most of the time, response by multiple partners. The disaster management cycle includes preparation and simulation, mitigation, response, recovery, and post-disaster analysis. To effectively respond to major disaster crises and engage in management of disasters, a multi-national coordinated system is often required. Disasters always impact the healthcare sector of the population, and as such novel technologies and capabilities, including telemedicine, have been brought to bear.

Telemedicine technologies should be incorporated into these systems based on the effectiveness of mobile technologies and capabilities of providing remote expertise in crisis situations. Multiple organizations are engaged in testing the effectiveness of training, preparation, and simulated responses in order to better manage disaster response and recovery. One additional element to increase effective disaster management must be the creation of a telemedicine infrastructure prior to a disaster that can be incorporated into the management phases. This solution will assist in ultimately saving lives and reducing human consequences of disaster response.

However, in order to truly be effective during the pre-disaster period, telemedicine infrastructure needs to be established and not attempted only during the crisis. While there are many pressing issues that need to be normalized following a disaster such as water, electricity, transportation, and overall infrastructure, the first and foremost importance is saving the injured patients and getting survivors from the rubble, while you maintain services for other patients. Remember, during the disaster, people still can have medical events such as a heart attack, appendicitis, cholecystitis, bowel obstruction, cancer, etc., so medical and surgical teams need to be prepared.

Medical response is difficult to be coordinated, and often is risky for rescue teams. In this chapter, we deal mainly with the potential use of telemedicine in disaster management and will not dwell on medical management of disaster. Furthermore, this chapter provides an updated review of telemedicine programs that have been implemented and research that has been conducted while following the three-phase emergency management system and how the incorporation of telemedicine into disaster management phases can enhance emergency preparedness, response, and recovery.

Disaster Classifications

The *Emergency Events Database (EM-DAT)* was developed in 1988 with the aim to rationalize decision-making for disaster preparedness, while also providing an objective base for *vulnerability assessment and priority setting*. EM-DAT contains essential core data on the occurrence and effects of over *18,000 mass disasters* all over the world, running from *1900 to the present day* [1]. Disasters are broadly categorized as (1) natural, (2) man-made, (3) war and conflict related, and (4) land mines and unexploded devices or ordnance. Other sub-types of disaster include epidemics or pandemics, floods, volcanic activity, transportation problems, and many more. Interestingly, this EM-DAT does not include the new pandemic caused by COVID-19. The nature of the spread of the virus and its rapidly evolving morbidity and mortality in such short period and the resultant financial impact to the world's economy make this a biological disaster. The viral catastrophe, we can call this one. The public health experts would agree with us. Can we call this a biologic catastrophe? Not sure but on March 11, 2020, the World Health Organization (WHO) declared that COVID-19 was a pandemic. On April 15, 2020, the WHO reported 71,572 new cases, 1,914,916 confirmed cases, and 123,010 deaths with Europe and Americas most affected with 977,596 and 673,361 confirmed cases [2]. These are grossly underestimated cases for the rest of the world, as testing has been a major issue.

Disaster Management

Disaster management is a complex process that broadly includes three phases. Others have described this process as four phases of disaster management that include (1) mitigation, (2) preparedness, (3) response, and (4) recovery [3–5]. The use of telemedicine has been used in disaster response for several decades [6–20]. However, incorporation of telemedicine technology in disaster and emergency pre-planning and pre-response has been lacking [6]. Only recently, efforts to include telemedicine in disaster simulation have been reported [21–23]. Depending on the infrastructure and resources available in a particular country [6, 24], response to a disaster may involve multiple countries, but the effectiveness of these responses is determined by several factors, including medical documentation established prior to disaster [24]. This infrastructure should include an access to proper documentation from before the incident.

Can We Create 24/7 Mass Casualty Center That Will Deal with Local Disaster Management?

The rationale for establishing the idea and the concept to create 24/7/365 centers has been discussed over a number of decades. However, within the past several years such capability was develop and tested. The results of this multinational group of subject matter experts have been well documented [25, 26].

Globally, 5 billion people lack surgical care, resulting in one third of all deaths, with lost gross domestic product (GDP) exceeding 1 trillion (USD) by 2030; disasters (both natural and man-made) typically result in 100,000 or more deaths per year, many of which could be avoided with improved emergency care; mass casualty centers (MCC) would combine the trauma/stroke center model with integration of healthcare personnel, technology, and equipment to improve both daily and mass casualty care. The MCC would be practical and cost-effective mechanism to achieve the healthcare-related United Nations Sustainable Development Goals for 2030. Moreover, MCC will reduce the duplication of services across the military and civilian world.

Even in the middle of COVID-19 pandemic, military floating hospitals basically are empty, while public hospitals are inundated by patients (Fig. 4.1). Duplication of emergency services, especially civilian and military, often results in suboptimal, expensive care. The challenge to overcome the work between the various layers of agencies within same country is just as challenging between other countries. MCCs would integrate resources for both routine and emergency care—from prevention to acute care to rehabilitation. Integration of the various healthcare systems—governmental, non-governmental, and military—is key to avoid both duplication and gaps. Of course, these centers should be equipped with technology to provide seamless telemedicine services.

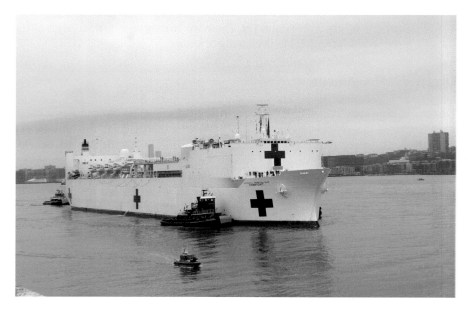

Fig. 4.1 US Navy Hospital Ship in NY, April 2020. (Source: U.S. Navy photo by Mass Communications Specialist 2nd Class Adelola Tinubu/Released) https://www.navy.mil/submit/display.asp?story_id=112806

Incorporation of Telemedicine in Each Phase of a Disaster

In order for telemedicine to be beneficial for any management, it should be part of the entire process, from preparation phase to recovery phase. In this section, we will address each of the disaster phases and how telemedicine can be helpful (Table 4.1).

Table 4.1 Phases of Emergency and Disaster Response and Telemedicine Solutions

The Three Phases of Emergency Management		Telemedicine Solutions
PHASE 1: BEFORE THE DISASTER (Mitigation and Preparation)	Includes any activities that prevent an emergency, reduce the chance of an emergency happening, or reduce the damaging effects of unavoidable emergencies. Incorporates plans or preparations made to save lives and to help response and rescue operations. Developing and establishing an operational telemedicine network	Multiple entity collaboration of communication, policy development, and implementation Standardization of practices across regions within the network Coordination of Pre-event training Standardization of pre-event telemedicine field kits Provide foundation for ensuring that adequate resources are in supply for event (satellite technology, telemedicine field kits, etc.) Scheduling of training is well-coordinated at a multi-national level rather than independently within each area, facilitates rapid and effective response
PHASE 2: DURING Response Responding safely to an emergency	Includes actions taken to save lives and prevent further property damage in an emergency situation. Response is putting your preparedness plans into action.	Situational awareness: Coordination of event response and outcomes at a multi-national level Facilitation of use of resources due to training and accessibility of resources Rapid advances in telemedicine technology that facilitate medical response to remote or disaster effected regions
PHASE 3: AFTER Recovery Recovering from an emergency	Includes actions taken to return to a normal or an even safer situation following an emergency.	Includes mitigation solutions in light of lessons learned during emergency: training, scheduling, reviewing coordination and communication successes and failures Usage of telemedicine technology to adapt resources to needs after a disaster

Reprinted from A multinational telemedicine systems for disaster response: opportunities and challenges, Vol. 130, C.R. Doarn, R. Latifi, C. Zoicas, Incorporation of Telemedicine in Disaster Management, 102, Copyright (Year), with permission from IOS Press
The publication is available at IOS Press through https://doi.org/10.3233/978-1-61499-728-3-99

Phase 1: Pre-Disaster

In order to use telemedicine pre-disaster, we believe that one has to have complete and functional infrastructure in place, with expertise to independently and professionally run the program. This program should be used continuously not only in non-disaster mode, that is for daily clinical activities, but in fact should simulate a disaster and practice again and again various scenarios and with various technologies to maintain competencies and a state of readiness. Moreover, it is imperative to maintain a strict and up to date research database and analyze the best outcomes of such exercises, preferably by independent assessment and evaluation teams, which should be shared with stakeholders and eventually reported in peer-review publications as appropriate. In expecting the disaster, there is work to be done that should involve multiple entities for collaboration in communication, policy development and implementation, and standardization of practices across regions within the network. This phase should also coordinate training and simulation, standardization of pre-event telemedicine field kits, communication capabilities, and a network of clinical expertise that are rapidly deployable so they can provide a rapid response.

Phase 2: During the Disaster

Setting up of telemedicine during the disaster may be challenging, especially if there was no infrastructure in place prior to the event, although the mobility of such technologies in recent years has improved significantly and their quick deployment has become much easier. Although the mobile, web-based solutions are easy to use, training and preparing human capacities to use mobile and other telemedicine solution should be part of preparedness [21–23].

Advances in global positioning system (GPS) have made it possible where wearable sensor nodes enable more efficient disaster response. Smart phones have been demonstrated to be a useful disaster and emergency response tool when situations do not allow for expert advice at the scene. For example, a lung ultrasound was performed by Crawford et al. [15] via a smart phone. Off-site experts were able to view real-time Point-of-Care Limited Ultrasound (PLUS) images that were displayed and transmitted via a smartphone. A portable ultrasound was interfaced to a laptop computer via an analog-to-digital converter. A new creative version of telemedicine for war and major conflicts has been created and reported using low-cost technology and Arabic-speaking intensivist from North America. Tele-ICU program was launched in December 2012 to manage the care of ICU patients in parts of Syria by using inexpensive, off-the-shelf video cameras, free social media applications, and a volunteer network of Arabic-speaking intensivists in North America and Europe [27]. Within 1 year, 90 patients per month in three ICUs were receiving tele-ICU services. At the end of 2015, a network of approximately 20 participating intensivists was providing clinical decision support 24 hours per day to 5 civilian ICUs in Syria. The volunteer clinicians manage patients at a distance of more than 6000 miles, separated by seven or eight time zones between North America and Syria. The program is implementing a cloud-based electronic medical record for physician documentation and a medication administration record for nurses.

Telemedicine During COVID-19

The new world order caused by COVID-19 has brought about many changes in our new world order. One of these changes is that almost overnight, the medical community realized that telemedicine and telepresence in fact are not only desirable, acceptable, and much sought after by patients and hospitals but by the entire community at large. Why risk your life by going to a busy academic hospital inundated by COVID-19 patients to simply see your doctor? Time for virtual visit has come; telemedicine after all is at the forefront. For more on the use of telemedicine in COVID-19 pandemic, see the first chapter of this book [28].

Phase 3: Post-Disaster

Telemedicine has great potential uses for large-scale man-made or natural disasters and emergencies that are characterized by unpredictability to place, time, and the number of injured people as well as their injury severity score, when other mode of transmission of information is not possible, or when the terrestrial infrastructure is lacking or has been destroyed. Recovery from disaster includes re-establishing infrastructure or revising infrastructure to more adequately meet the needs of disaster management. Disaster resilience is a term that is commonly used when assessing vulnerability of communities and ability to adapt after disaster [29, 30]. Lam et al. [30] suggest that vulnerability and adaptive capacity need to be assessed over time. Vulnerability is the latent relationship between exposure and damage. Adaptability is the latent relationship between damage and recovery. Both vulnerability and adaptability can fall under the third phase of disaster management because they represent a relationship that is intricately related throughout the disaster management process [31].

Telemedicine and telehealth technologies are particularly useful in managing disaster resilience and recovery. In conducting a review of literature on the subject of disaster recovery and benefits of telemedicine technology, very few articles describing the usefulness of technology during recovery were found [31]. The usefulness of telemedicine for disaster recovery during the Armenian Earthquake of 1988 [32, 33]. As stated eloquently, the disaster is usually unpredictable, and impersonal. So the only predictable element of disaster is its unpredictability [34], and we have to adapt to something that may not be able to be predicted.

Training and Simulation

Incorporating telemedicine in disaster management has not yet become an acceptable practice for most countries. As described in more detail [23], a Multinational Telemedicine System (MnTS) was tested during the NATO Consequence Management Field Exercise, "Ukraine 2015" [21]. This exercise was sponsored by Ukraine and its State Emergency Service [21, 22], and teams from four of the seven bordering countries of Ukraine participated. We demonstrated that an integrated system, including personnel, hardware, communication protocols, portable power generation, medical kits, and Web-based tools, was developed and successfully tested in the Euro-Atlantic Disaster Response Coordination Centre's Exercises Ukraine 2015. The field exercise tested and validated the MnTS and identified areas of improvement. The system and its evaluation provide additional information for establishing deployment capabilities.

The major difference between the Centre for Research on the Epidemiology of Disasters (CRED) programs and the NATO program is that the NATO MnTS explicitly tests simulation exercises in mock scenarios using telemedicine technology. These simulation exercises provide training for medical professionals and all levels of emergency staff within the trauma response network. The advantages of telemedicine technology need to be acknowledged when considering the most effective strategies for disaster management. We describe the multiple uses of telemedicine in disaster response [6]. Although the benefits are obvious, the adaptation of telemedicine technology has been slower in disaster response situations than would be expected. However, as described in Chaps. 5 and 7 of this book, NATO has incorporated telemedicine field kits, remote connectivity, and satellite and solar panels in their MnTS program. Demonstrated usefulness and efficiency of these systems was provided during the Ukraine 2015 multi-national disaster simulation exercise. Each of these telemedicine systems was set up in less than 25 minutes [21] (see Fig. 4.2).

The NATO Science for Peace and Security (SPS) Program also provided an example of how scientists and medical professionals can advance the disaster management processes by increasing the knowledge base for all parties involved in disaster. The SPS program not only focuses on the incorporation of scientific perspectives into developing solutions to global problems, but it also provides a multi-national collaborative aspect to developing these solutions. This collaborative spirit encourages a depth to problem-solving that is enhanced by multiple vantage points and knowledge bases.

In a recent publication, telemedicine was adopted into a simulation where 92 US Army Forward Surgical Team (FST) members participated in a high-fidelity mass casualty simulation at the Army Trauma Training Center (ATTC) [35]. However, only 10.9% of participants chose to use telemedicine, and those who used it believed it somewhat improved patient care, attainment of expert resources, decision-making, and adaptation, but not the timeliness of patient care. However, participants reported several barriers to using telemedicine in the mass casualty setting, including (1) confusion around team roles, (2) time constraints, and (3) difficultly using the mass casualty setting (e.g., due to noise and other conditions). Interestingly, the most common users were surgeons and nurses. It becomes clear that telemedicine was not integrated part of the simulation and still needs to have "Telemedicine Chief". Scheduling of training is well-coordinated at a multi-national level rather than independently within each area, and facilitates rapid and effective response.

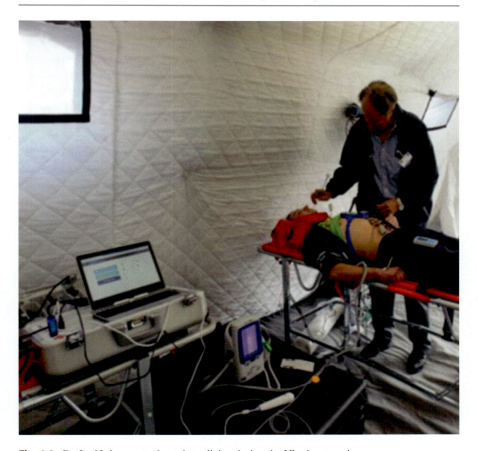

Fig. 4.2 Dr. Latifi demonstrating telemedicine during the Ukraine exercise

Administrative Requirements

Managing catastrophes like those described above takes creativity, but above all it requires technology and collaboration of wide variety of individuals, organizations, and systems. Apart from other intricacies and the peculiarities of such disasters such as managing a great number of authorities and organizations, there is a need for a high-level demand for Command, Control, and Communications (C3). The American Telemedicine Association has created guidelines of standards for telemedicine practices. These standards include administrative requirements for telemedicine networks [35]. These requirements include human resources management; privacy and confidentiality; federal, state, and other credentialing and regulatory agency requirements in the country where the telemedicine is practiced; fiscal management; ownership of patient records; patient rights and responsibilities; documentation protocols; network security; equipment use; and research protocols [35].

Conclusion

Disasters such as the COVID-19 pandemic pose a serious threat and challenge to the life of every individual and their daily activities, and overall to national and international infrastructure, economy, and well-being. Telemedicine, broadly speaking, can play a major role in the management of medical consequences of the disaster. But in order to have telemedicine and telehealth ready for the use during the disaster, we need to have telemedicine programs in place during the peace times. In addition, using telemedicine for local disaster management, we should establish programs that will incorporate telemedicine technology to solve disaster management problems as well as provide assistance in regional and multi-national collaborative environments to address problems posed by disaster scenarios.

References

1. Center for Research on the Epidemiology of Disaster (CRED). http://www.cred.be/. Last accessed 15 April 2020.
2. World Health Organization. http://who.int. Last accessed 15 April 2020.
3. Federal Emergency Management Agency. Phases of emergency management. Taken from www.training.fema.gov/emiweb/downloads/is10_unit3.doc. Last Accessed 5 Aug 2016.
4. Latifi R. Telemedicine-trauma-emergencies-disaster-management- https://www.amazon.com/ebook/dp. Last accessed 2020.
5. Doarn CR, Latifi R, Zoicas C, editors. A multinational telemedicine system for disaster response: opportunities and challenges, vol. 130. Amsterdam: NATO Publication/IOS Press; 2016.
6. Latifi R, Tilley EH. Telemedicine for disaster management: can it transform chaos into an organized, structured care from the distance? Am J Disaster Med. 2014;9(1):25–37.
7. Rolston DM, Meltzer JS. Telemedicine in the intensive care unit: its role in emergencies and disaster management. Crit Care Clin. 2015;31(2):239–55.
8. Ajami S, Lamoochi P. Use of telemedicine in disaster and remote places. J Educ Health Promot. 2014;3:26.
9. Murren-Boezem J, Solo-Josephson P, Zettler-Greeley CM. A pediatric telemedicine response to a natural disaster. Telemed J E Health. 2020;26(6):720–724.
10. Natenzon MY. New generation of mobile telemedicine units creates new possibilities for medical services to population in the remote and hard-to-access districts. Reveue internationale des services de sante des forces armees. 2012;85(4):60–69.
11. Stawicki SP, Howard JM, Pryor JP, Bahner DP, Whitmill ML, Dean AJ. Portable ultrasonography in mass casualty incidents: the CAVEAT examination. World J Orthop. 2010;1(1):10–9.
12. Hadeed G, Holcomb M, Latifi R. Communication technologies: an overview of telemedicine connectivity. In: Latifi, editor. Telemedicine for trauma, emergencies, and disaster management; 2011. p. 37–52.
13. Boniface KS, Shokoohi H, Smith ER, et al. Tele-ultrasound and paramedics: real-time remote physician guidance of focused assessment with sonography for trauma examination. Am J Emerg Med. 2011;29:477–81.
14. Crawford I, McBeth PB, Mitchelson C, et al. Telementorable, "just-in-time" lung ultrasound on an iPhone. J Emerg Trauma Shock. 2011;4:526–7.
15. Brown SW, Griswold WG, Demchak B, et al. Middleware for reliable mobile medical workflow support in disaster settings. AMIA Annu Symp Proc. 2006;2006:309–13.

16. Yang C, Yang J, Luo X, et al. Use of mobile phones in an emergency reporting system for infectious disease surveillance after the Sichuan earthquake in China. Bull World Health Organ. 2009;87(8):619–23.
17. Abdul Karim R, Zakara NF, Zulkifley MA, et al. Telepointer technology in telemedicine: a review. Biomed Eng Online. 2013:12–21.
18. Yuce M. Wireless technologies: potential use in emergencies and disasters. In: Latifi R, editor. Telemedicine for trauma, emergencies, and disaster management; 2010. p. 69–88.
19. MedWeb. https://www.medweb.com. Last accessed 19 April 2020.
20. Yu JN, Brock TK, Mecozzi DM, et al. Future connectivity for disaster and emergency point of care. Point Care. 2010;9(4):185–92.
21. Doarn CR, Hostiuc F, Zoicas C, Latifi R, Lester C. Development, structure, and organization of the MnTS. In: Doarn, Latifi, Hostiuc, Arafat, Zoicas, editors. Developing a multinational telemedicine system for emergency situations. Amsterdam: IOS Press.
22. Hosituc F, Latifi R, Poropatich R, Sokolovich N, Zoicas C, Doarn C. Validation of the MnTS in a simulated environment – Ukraine. In: Doarn, Latifi, Hostiuc, Arafat, Zoicas, editors. Developing a multinational telemedicine system for emergency situations. Amsterdam: IOS Press.
23. Doarn CR, Latifi R, Poropatich RK, Sokolovich N, Kosiak D, Hostiuc F, Zoicas C, Buciu A, Arafat R. Development and validation of telemedicine for disaster response: the North Atlantic Treaty Organization Multinational System. Telemed J E Health. 2018;24(9):657–68.
24. Aung E, Whittaker M. Preparing routine health information systems for immediate health responses to disasters. Health Policy Plan. 2013;28(5):495–507.
25. Aguilera S, Quintana L, Khan T, Garcia R, Shoman S, Caddell L, Latifi R, Park KB, Garcia P, Dempsey R, Rosenfeld JV, Scurlock C, Crisp N, Samad L, Smith M, Lippa L, Jooma R, Andrews RJ. Global health, global surgery and mass casualties: II. Mass casualty Centre resources, equipment and implementation. BMJ Glob Health. 2020;5(1):e001945.
26. Khan T, Quintana L, Aguilera S, Garcia R, Shoman H, Caddell L, Latifi R, Park KB, Garcia P, Dempsey R, Rosenfeld JV, Scurlock C, Crisp N, Samad L, Smith M, Lippa L, Jooma R, Andrews RJ. Global health, global surgery and mass casualties. I. Rationale for integrated mass casualty centres. BMJ Glob Health. 2019;4(6):e001943.
27. Moughrabieh A, Weinert C. Rapid deployment of international tele-intensive care unit services in War-Torn Syria. Ann Am Thorac Soc. 2016;13(2):165–72.
28. Hollander JE, Carr BG. Virtually perfect? telemedicine for covid-19. N Engl J Med. 2020;382(18):1679–81.
29. Miles SB, Green RA, Svekla W. Disaster risk reduction capacity assessment for precarious settlements in Guatemala City. Disasters. 2012;36(3):365–81.
30. Lam NS, Reams M, Li K, Li C, Mata LP. Measuring community resilience to coastal hazards along the Northern Gulf of Mexico. Nat Hazards Rev. 2016;17(1):pii: 04015013.
31. Uscher-Pines L, Fischer S, Chari R. The promise of direct-to-consumer Telehealth for disaster response and recovery. Prehosp Disaster Med. 2016;31(4):454–6.
32. Doarn CR, Merrell RC. Spacebridge to Armenia: a look back at its impact on telemedicine in disaster response. Telemed J E Health. 2011;17(7):546–52.
33. Nicogossian AE, Doarn CR. Armenia 1988 earthquake and telemedicine: lessons learned and forgotten. Telemed J E Health. 2011;17(9):741–5.
34. Andrews RJ, Quintana LM. Unpredictable, unpreventable and impersonal medicine: global disaster response in the 21st century. EPMA J. 2015;6(1):2.
35. Gregory M, Sonesh S, Hughes A, Marttos A, Schulman C, Salas E. Using telemedicine in mass casualty disasters. Disaster Med Public Health Prep. 2020:1–8. Ahead of print.

Telemedicine and Health Information Exchange: An Opportunity for Integration

Dale C. Alverson

Why Telemedicine and Health Information Exchange Should Work Together

Telemedicine is the provision of healthcare services over distance when the healthcare providers and/or their patients are at different locations and also encompasses several definitions [1]. Healthcare services offered via telemedicine can include case reviews, consultations, and direct patient care using synchronous videoconferencing, as well as asynchronous interpretation of forwarded images, such as x-rays, ultrasound, dermatology photos, ophthalmology retinal images, and pathology micrographs. In fact, images transmitted via telemedicine systems can also be classified as health information. Therefore, radiologic, pathology, retinal, or dermatologic images are often considered part of telemedicine as teleradiology, telepathology, teleophthalmology, or teledermatology but at the same time can be considered health information and be incorporated into an electronic medical record or as part of a health information exchange. Together and when integrated, Telemedicine and health information exchanges provide a means to better evaluate and manage a patient's care over distance, benefitting the patients, the local primary care providers, and the associated specialists, thus supporting the patient-centered medical home. These health information technologies both can use a spectrum of communication systems, such as the internet, wireless networks, microwave, cellular, and satellite, as well as the plain old telephone system and web-based portals along with a variety of devices for video-conferencing, including mobile phones and tablets with cameras and cloud-based audio-video platforms, blended into an improved platform for coordination and continuity of care.

D. C. Alverson (✉)
Health Sciences Center, University of New Mexico, Albuquerque, NM, USA
e-mail: dalverson@salud.unm.edu

© Springer Nature Switzerland AG 2021
R. Latifi et al. (eds.), *Telemedicine, Telehealth and Telepresence*,
https://doi.org/10.1007/978-3-030-56917-4_5

Just as when a patient is seen face-to-face in-person, when providing services via telemedicine, the healthcare professionals need access to the patient's protected health information (PHI) and need to document the patient encounter or consultation. However, particularly when using telemedicine between different locations and healthcare systems, the providers and the patients are often on different electronic health records (EHRs) that cannot easily share PHI. This makes the patient evaluation more difficult, at times incomplete, less efficient, and often leads to unnecessary duplication of tests and procedures [2, 3].

Having access to HIE during a telemedicine encounter, as when seeing patients in-person, can improve care coordination and continuity, and enhance the evaluation and treatment even when the patients and their providers are in different healthcare systems using different EHRs. Thus, telemedicine and the HIE become complementary as the HIE provides the appropriate, needed, and often critical health information at the right time and at the right place at the point of care [4]. Rather than viewing telemedicine and health information as separate, they are best applied in a complimentary manner to provide effective patient care (Figs. 5.1 and 5.2).

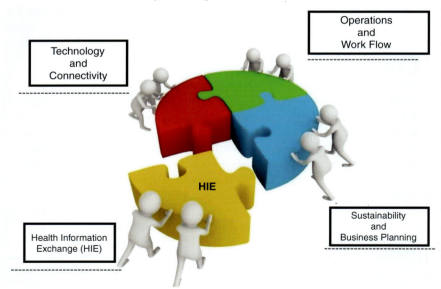

Fig. 5.1 HIE and telemedicine integration

Fig. 5.2 A health information exchange

What is a Health Information Exchange?

- Technology and services to make sure health information is available when and where it is needed.
- "Interoperability"- the ability of systems to exchange & use electronic health information from other systems without special effort on the part of the user.

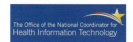

Creating Standards for Merging Health Information

With the appropriate secure interfaces, the health information exchange (HIE) can consolidate the patient's information into one set of documents from all the different EHRs allowing the telemedicine provider to have a much more comprehensive overview of the patient at the time of provision of care [5–7]. The HIE can display all of a patient's diagnoses, medications, allergies, immunizations, procedures, lab and radiology results, as well as other consultations and discharge summaries, as well as specific places of receiving healthcare services using admission, Discharge, and transfer (ADT) feeds, from other healthcare systems and their EHR into the HIE independent of the different EHRs or databases in which that information is housed [8–15]. A challenge is the provision of a standard data set from individual EHRs and different health systems that are needed to provide a more comprehensive and complete view of a patient's health information [16]. Therefore, an adequate interface with each EHR is necessary so those standard data sets can flow into the HIE. Efforts are underway and being developed to create a core date set of healthcare information that should be provided by each EHR such as the United States Core Data Set for Interoperability (USCDI) [17, 18] (Fig. 5.3).

Accomplishing those interfaces with a health system's EHR in a cost-effective manner can be another challenge. Furthermore, when developed and parsed appropriately, a user can more easily and effectively navigate that consolidated information when evaluating and managing a patient via telemedicine, as well as in-person. Although exchange of a Continuity of Care Document (CCD) [19, 20] or Consolidated-Clinical Document Architecture (C-CDA) [21] document is offered

Fig. 5.3 The core HIE data sets

Core HIE data

- Demographics
- Allergies
- Medications
- Immunizations
- Insurance
- Procedures
- Problem List
- Encounters (Visits) & Diagnoses

- Lab Data
- Radiology Data
- Clinical Notes

Note: Data available varies by organization

as a solution for health information exchange, they may be limited to interaction and document exchange between just two EHRs and may be more challenging to navigate since individual information is not generally parsed but combined into one large electronic document.

Health information merger from different data sets can be facilitated using other established common language platforms, such as SNOMED, RXNORM, and LOINC [22–24]. SNOMED is an international global standard for health terms [22]. As noted on their Web page, "LOINC is the international standard for identifying health measurements, observations, and documents. Reference labs, healthcare organizations, U.S. federal agencies, insurance companies, software vendors, in vitro diagnostic testing companies, and more than 85,900 registered users from 176 countries use LOINC to move data seamlessly between systems" [23]. As noted on their Web page, "RxNORM provides normalized names for clinical drugs and links its names to many of the drug vocabularies commonly used in pharmacy management and drug interaction software" [24].

As noted, even the sharing of images overlaps in the categories of health information and what was typically considered part of telemedicine. Furthermore, the integration of the HIE to support telemedicine can not only improve access and health outcomes, but also reduce costs. Telemedicine and HIE together can share similar secure networks and provide complimentary services to healthcare systems, their providers, and patients. The opportunities for collaboration between telemedicine programs and the HIE are significant and potentially synergistic during this unprecedented period of healthcare reform, and emergence of new innovative information and communication technologies. Specifically, state-wide or regional HIEs may wish to consider collaboration with the state or regional telehealth organizations in order to determine the best manner to integrate the two platforms.

A robust HIE can provide a rich data set for population health and community health assessment and data analysis providing insight as to a population health issues, needs, and a focus on effective interventions. Using the patients' Zip Codes

5 Telemedicine and Health Information Exchange: An Opportunity for Integration

and a relational database, geospatial information systems (GIS) can be combined with these data sets to provide a visualization of distribution of disease and impact of health programs addressing those health issues over time. That population health date combined with GIS can assist in focusing healthcare services where they are most needed (Fig. 5.4).

As opposed to an electronic health record (EHR) or health information exchange (HIE), Telemedicine provides direct patient care or support for their healthcare provider at the point of care. However, patient health information contained in their EHR or the HIE is a critical component of overall patient management, diagnosis, and treatment, whether provided via telemedicine or in-person. Thus, integrating both telemedicine and health information is becoming an important aspect of the use of these tools in new paradigms of healthcare during this remarkable period of health reform. An HIE can play an important role when providing telemedicine services to patients and their providers when the interactions are occurring between

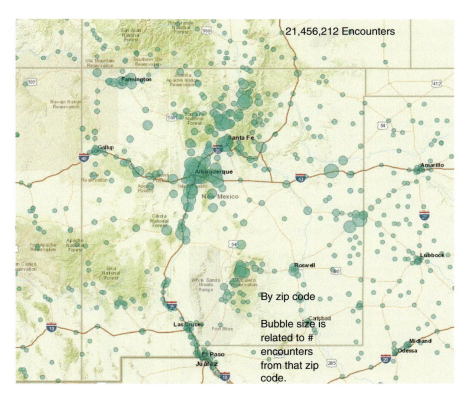

Fig. 5.4 Combing zip code date with patient healthcare information in the HIE

healthcare providers using different EHRs. Currently, the vast spectrum of certified EHRs cannot easily share the patient's health information but can be critical in the overall patient evaluation.

A survey of US households from the Practice Fusion GfK OmniWeb survey was conducted via omnibus April 17–18, 2010, using interviews conducted from among a nationally representative sample of 1035 adults age 18 or older [25]. That survey notes that patients see 18 different doctors in their lifetime. For patients >65 years old, they see 28 different doctors. A patient's health is dependent on equivalent of 200 pieces of paper in almost 19 different locations (Fig. 5.5).

Using interoperability standards, such as HL7 and Fast Healthcare Interoperability Resources (FHIR) [26–28], an HIE can consolidate health information from different EHRs and be made available during a telemedicine encounter. As noted in the HL7 webpage [24], "HL7, (Health Level Seven), is a standard for exchanging information between medical applications. This standard defines a format for the transmission of health-related information. Information sent using the HL7 standard is sent as a collection of one or more messages, each of which transmits one record or item of health-related information. Examples of HL7 messages include patient records, laboratory records and billing information." As an evolution of HL7, Fast Healthcare Interoperability Resources (FHIR) further facilitates interoperability of patient health information; "FHIR was developed by Health Level Seven International (HL7), a not-for-profit organization accredited by the American National Standards Institute that develops and provides frameworks and standards for the sharing, integration and retrieval of clinical health data and other electronic health information" [28].

Why use a Health Information Exchange?

- 18 different doctors in your lifetime

- >65 years old- 28 different doctors

- Your health is dependent on equivalent of 200 pieces of paper in almost 19 different locations.

Average values for the US from the Practice Fusion survey conducted via omnibus survey April 17- 18, 2010. The GfK OmniWeb survey is a weekly national web survey of US households. Interviews were conducted from among a nationally representative sample of 1,035 adults age 18 or older

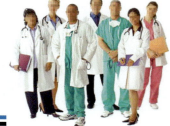

Fig. 5.5 Individual patient data

Creating a Nation-Wide HIE; Integrating Different HIEs

Ongoing efforts have been underway to create a nation-wide health information exchange as initially spearheaded by the Office of the National Coordinator (ONC) for Health Information Technology [29]. As noted on their Web page, "President George W. Bush created the position of National Coordinator on April 27, 2004. Congress later mandated ONC in the Health Information Technology for Economic and Clinical Health Act provisions of the American Recovery and Reinvestment Act of 2009, under the Obama Administration. The Office of the National Coordinator for Health Information Technology (ONC) has been at the forefront of the administration's health IT efforts and is a resource to the entire health system to support the adoption of health information technology and the promotion of nationwide health information exchange to improve healthcare. ONC is organizationally located within the Office of the Secretary for the U.S. Department of Health and Human Services (HHS). ONC is the principal federal entity charged with coordination of nationwide efforts to implement and use the most advanced health information technology and the electronic exchange of health information. The position of National Coordinator was created in 2004, through an Executive Order, and legislatively mandated in the Health Information Technology for Economic and Clinical Health Act (HITECH Act) of 2009" [29]. The first National Coordinator of Health Information Technology was David Brailer who laid the initial groundwork for a vision of the role electronic health records could play in the modernization of clinical digitization of healthcare. Since then ongoing efforts have been initiated to create a nation-wide health information exchange through different collaborations. The Sequoia Project is the independent, trusted advocate for nationwide health information exchange. In the public interest, we steward current programs, incubate new initiatives, and educate our community [30]. CommonWell Health Alliance [31] is a not-for-profit trade association devoted to the simple vision that health data should be available to individuals and caregivers regardless of where care occurs. Additionally, access to this data must be built into health IT at a reasonable cost for use by a broad range of healthcare providers and the people they serve. Currently, the "eHealth Exchange" [32], active in all 50 states, is the largest query-based, health information network in the country. It is the principal network that connects federal agencies and non-federal organizations, allowing them to work together to improve patient care and public health. Another organization called Strategic Health Information Exchange Collaborative (SHIEC) has been formed to facilitate sharing knowledge and finding solutions for HIE adoption, "SHIEC is a national collaborative representing health information exchanges (HIEs). The organization already represents 70+ HIEs, and these HIEs collectively cover more than 200 million people across the U.S., well over half of the American population" [33] (Fig. 5.6).

SHIEC has developed an effort called the Patient-Centered Data Home (PCDH) [34] currently centered in Utah's HIE, the Utah Health Information Network (UHIN). That platform allows exchange of patient encounters between different

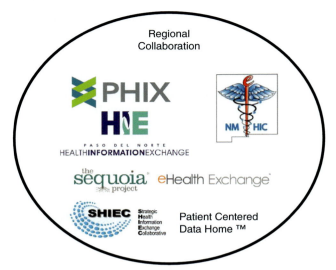

Integration of Data from NM and Western Texas (El Paso and Lubbock)
SHIEC PCDH would also allow connection with Utah, AZ, Western Colorado

Fig. 5.6 Regional HIE collaboration

states where patients may have received healthcare services, that is linking the "home" HIE with the "Away" HIE. For example, if a patient from Utah receives healthcare services in another participating state, such as Texas, that information is then shared within the UHIN and the Utah Providers are alerted about that encounter. Similarly, if a patient is seen in Utah, the UHIN shares that health information with the HIE in Texas and the Texas providers are alerted about that encounter. The patient's home HIE can be determined through Zip codes. Key to that exchange regarding specific patients is the sharing of each HIE's master patient Index (MPI) that allows the link to an individual patient with a high degree of specificity and sensitivity.

In addition, the telemedicine encounters need to be documented in the patient provider's EHR, as well as made accessible through the HIE, for future review and reference to enhance care coordination and continuity. Other approaches that allow the EHR user to take advantage of a related HIE is single sign-on where patient data in the HIE can be viewed in the EHR without additional effort of the user.

Often a state-wide or regional HIE offers Direct Secure Messaging (DSM) services. DSM is an electronic, standard-based, vendor-neutral, ONC-approved, mechanism for exchanging protected health information (PHI) between authenticated users. Therefore, it is a one-to-one efficient communication transaction of PHI but doesn't have the overall sharing of PHI between all HIE participants that is provided through access to an HIE. It provides an audit trail and confirmations and eliminates faxing, saving the cost of fax ink cartridges, paper, and support staff time. DSM requires access to the Internet but doesn't require an EHR. Furthermore, it can satisfy meaningful use for transitions of care requirements. DSM is used for referrals and other transitions of care, that is, summary of care records, billing and coding

Fig. 5.7 NMHIC consent model

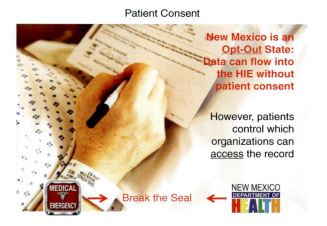

inquiries, sharing test results, coordination of care, for example, sharing care plans, and thus shared mailboxes aid care management teams.

HIEs can represent federated versus centralized database models or combination of those approaches.

In a federated model, PHI is stored in independent databases or repositories. Each healthcare organization or provider maintains ownership of and control over the health records; access to the health record is granted to users only when needed. Whereas, in a centralized model, health records are merged from participants in the HIE and stored in a single repository or database.

A combined model utilizes both centralized and decentralized platforms. Data exchange in an HIE can also be either pushed to the healthcare provider or pulled by the healthcare provider.

For example, a message or document, such as a lab result, is sent from one participant to another, this is called a "push" exchange. Whereas, when a provider searches for or queries a patient's health information, this is called a "pull" exchange. The types of data that can be exchanged not only include clinical information but also claim public health, quality, and reporting data.

Most HIEs require consent either as an "Opt-in" versus "Opt-out" approach. The "Opt-in" model requires patient consent to have their data provided into the HIE. The "Opt-out" doesn't require patient consent for their data to flow into the HIE but does usually require patient consent for users to view the data. Some HIEs provide a "break the seal" opportunities for providers to view the PHI in confirmed emergency situations without patient consent (Fig. 5.7).

Another exception precluding consent can be reportable health conditions being collected by public health agencies. To avoid inappropriate access to sensitive conditions within the patient's PHI, some HIEs can segregate data about those sensitive conditions such as mental health information, HIV/AIDS, sexually transmitted diseases, and certain genetic conditions. If not segregated, the patient is informed that HIE users may be able to view information about those sensitive conditions.

The New Mexico Health Information Collaborative (NMHIC) is an example of state-wide "Opt-out" HIE model (Figs. 5.8 and 5.9).

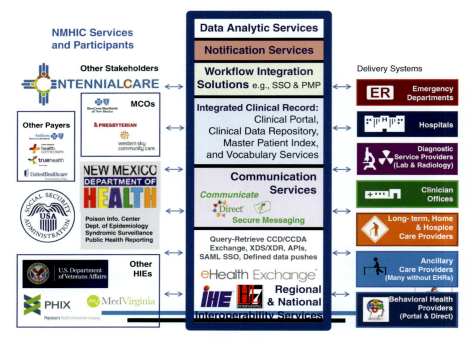

Fig. 5.8 New Mexico Health Information Collaborative (NMHIC) model

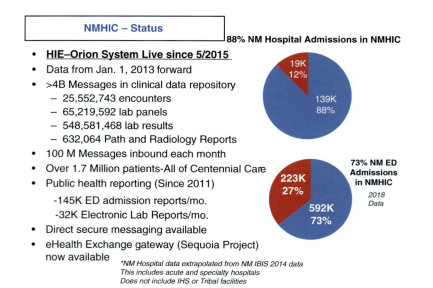

Fig. 5.9 NMHIC data acquisition as a state-wide HIE

5 Telemedicine and Health Information Exchange: An Opportunity for Integration

By New Mexico statute, patient data can flow into the HIE with patient consent.

Information within the NMHIC HIE is subject to Federal and State Privacy and Security Regulations which includes HIPAA, HITECH, and other regulations. Data in the HIE is encrypted at rest and in transit. Access is limited to authorized users only. NMHIC uses a spectrum of security systems, such as Insomnia Security that has done penetration testing on our NMHIC Orion environment and British Telecom America that has done an external HIPAA audit. Thus, security should meet industry standards such as SSAE16 (auditing), ISO 27001, and EHNAC.

Business model and sustainability approaches vary across HIEs. Some HIEs are subsidized by state agencies involved in health and human services, and others use a subscription model, where users contribute financial support for participation and use of the HIE based upon a return on investment and value added. Participating HIE users can include healthcare organizations, hospitals, clinics, private practices, individual providers, payers, and ancillary health service organizations, such as laboratories and radiologic imaging organizations (Fig. 5.10).

Social Determinants of Health (SDOH) are paying an important role in healthcare for a wide spectrum of patients. SDOH influence the capability of patients to comply with their healthcare management plans [35–37]. Many HIEs are now beginning to include exchange of SDOH so that healthcare providers and others managing care organizations can apply that additional information for more appropriate coordination of care and a more effective and realistic means to provide the desired care for individual patients.

Furthermore, rather than being in silos, efforts related to the meaningful use of EHRs and HIEs should be combined with the meaningful use of telemedicine in a collaborative manner in order to reach the goal of the Triple Aim [38], patient

Full Medical Record Interoperability in New Mexico

Value for NM
↑ Quality
↑ Safety
↓ Cost

References for Analysis:

The Business Case for interoperability and health Informaion Exchange HIMSS 8/2004 Gartner Study done for Arkansas extrapolated for New Maxico-AppendixD
http://www.himss.org/ResourceLibrary/genResourceDataIIPDF.as px?ItemNumber=32781

Similar results seen with financial analysis done by UNM Health Economist and a third party actuarial a nalysis for the NM Department of Health for the State Innovation Model project. Both showed a quick and significant return of investment.

Full value is only seen with full participation

Fig. 5.10 Making the business case

centeredness, improved health outcomes, and cost reduction, while enhancing the quality of care. Telemedicine can improve access to care but is best when combined with access to relevant patient health information and documentation. An HIE along with Telemedicine can also play an important role in transitions of care when patients are moving from one aspect to the healthcare system to another, such as from hospital to rehabilitation, to skilled nursing facilities, or home. Use of HIE and Telemedicine technologies can assist in avoidance of unnecessary rehospitalization or utilization of emergency department services. Organizations and individual experts involved in these initiatives should work together collaboratively to achieve these goals, providing the right care at the right place and at the right time.

Future

In the future, the goal of creating a nation-wide health information exchange can provide better care for patients who may receive services in different states, as well as provide healthcare support when traveling to other states and faced with an unexpected medical event.

An HIE can also play important role during a disaster when patients are disconnected from their primary care providers [39–41]. Outside healthcare providers in a disaster response facility who are seeing patients can access their health information and make more appropriate decisions about their healthcare management and provide continuity in their care and critical medications needed to provide adequate support.

Those same concepts apply to creating an international health information exchange where telemedicine can connect back to the patient's care team in their country of origin and where their care is primarily provided as well as overcome any potential language barriers. Integrating Telemedicine and HIE has the potential of enhancing healthcare worldwide as well as locally.

References

1. Bashshur R, Shannon G, Krupinski E, Grigsby J. Taxonomy of telemedicine. Telemed e-Health. 2011;17:484–94.
2. Saeed SA. Tower of babel problem in telehealth: addressing the health information exchange needs of the North Carolina Statewide Telepsychiatry Program (NC-STeP). Psychiatry Q. 2018;89(2):489–95. https://doi.org/10.1007/s11126-017-9551-6.
3. Ranganathan C, Balaji S. Key factors affecting the adoption of telemedicine by ambulatory clinics: insights from a statewide survey. Telemed J E Health. 2020;26:218–25. https://doi.org/10.1089/tmj.2018.0114.
4. Alverson DC. Health care in a perfect storm: a time for telemedicine and health information technology. In: Sikka N, Pion R, Tritle B, Weinstein R, editors. The thought leaders project. e-health, telemedicine, connected health-the next wave of medicine. Lexington: Bierbaum Publishing, LCC; 2012. p. 29–37.
5. Defining Health Information Exchange (HIE). https://searchhealthit.techtarget.com/definition/Health-information-exchange-HIE. Verified November 21 2019.

6. Prestigiacomo J. Telemedicine and health information exchange. 2013. https://www.hcinnovationgroup.com/interoperability-hie/infrastructure/article/13019394/telemedicine-as-the-backbone-to-hie. Verified November 19, 2019.
7. AHIMA Practice Brief. Telemedicine services and the health record (2013 update). (Updated May 2013). http://library.ahima.org/doc?oid=300269#.XdR9t25Fy6s.
8. Holmgren AJ, Adler-Milstein J. Health information exchange in US hospitals: the current landscape and a path to improved information sharing. J Hosp Med. 2017;12(3):193–8. https://doi.org/10.12788/jhm.2704.
9. Rudin RS, Motala A, Goldzweig CL, Shekelle PG. Usage and effect of health information exchange: a systematic review. Ann Intern Med. 2014;161(11):803–11. https://doi.org/10.7326/M14-0877.
10. Attallah N, Gashgari H, Al Muallem Y, Al Dogether M, Al Moammary E, Almeshari M, Househ M. A literature review on health information exchange (HIE). Stud Health Technol Inform. 2016;226:173–6.
11. Hersh WR, Totten AM, Eden KB, Devine B, Gorman P, Kassakian SZ, Woods SS, Daeges M, Pappas M, McDonagh MS. Outcomes from health information exchange: systematic review and future research needs. JMIR Med Inform. 2015;3(4):e39. https://doi.org/10.2196/medinform.5215.
12. Dobrow MJ, Bytautas JP, Tharmalingam S, Hagens S. Interoperable electronic health records and health information exchanges: systematic review. JMIR Med Inform. 2019;7(2):e12607. https://doi.org/10.2196/12607.
13. Sadoughi F, Nasiri S, Ahmadi H. The impact of health information exchange on healthcare quality and cost-effectiveness: a systematic literature review. Comput Methods Prog Biomed. 2018;161:209–32. https://doi.org/10.1016/j.cmpb.2018.04.023. Epub 2018 Apr 28.
14. Dendere R, Slade C, Burton-Jones A, Sullivan C, Staib A, Janda M. Patient portals facilitating engagement with inpatient electronic medical records: a systematic review. J Med Internet Res. 2019;21(4):e12779. https://doi.org/10.2196/12779.
15. Hoyle P. Health information is central to changes in healthcare: a clinician's view. Health Inf Manag. 2019;48(1):48–51. https://doi.org/10.1177/1833358317741354. Epub 2017 Nov 26.
16. Parker C, Weiner M, Reeves M. Health information exchanges--unfulfilled promise as a data source for clinical research. Int J Med Inform. 2016;87:1–9. https://doi.org/10.1016/j.ijmedinf.2015.12.005. Epub 2015 Dec 11.
17. U.S. Core Data for Interoperability (USCDI). https://www.healthit.gov/isa/us-core-data-interoperability-uscdi. Verified November 26, 2019.
18. Draft U.S. Core Data for Interoperability (USCDI) and Proposed Expansion Process. https://www.healthit.gov/sites/default/files/draft-uscdi.pdf. Verified November 26, 2019.
19. D'Amore JD, Sittig DF, Ness RB. How the continuity of care document can advance medical research and public health. Am J Public Health. 2012;102(5):e1–4. https://doi.org/10.2105/AJPH.2011.300640. PMC 3483927. PMID 22420795.
20. Ferranti JM, Musser RC, Kawamoto K, Hammond WE. The clinical document architecture and the continuity of care record: a critical analysis. J Am Med Inform Assoc. 2006;13(3):245–52.
21. C-CDA. https://www.healthit.gov/sites/default/files/ccda_and_meaningfulusecertification.pdf. Verified November 21 2019.
22. SNOMED. http://www.snomed.org/.
23. LOINC. https://loinc.org.
24. RXNORM. https://www.nlm.nih.gov/research/umls/rxnorm.
25. GfK OmniWeb Survey 2010: patients see 18.7 different doctors on average. https://www.fiercehealthcare.com/healthcare/survey-patients-see-18-7-different-doctors-average. Verified November 19 2019.
26. Health Language 7 (HL7). https://blog.interfaceware.com/hl7-overview/. Verified November 9, 2019.
27. Definition of Fast Healthcare Interoperability Resources (FHIR). https://www.fiercehealthcare.com/healthcare/survey-patients-see-18-7-different-doctors-average. Verified November 9, 2019.

28. FHIR. http://hl7.org/fhir/DSTU1/fhir-summary.pdf. Verified November 9, 2019.
29. HIE and Office of the National Coordinator (ONC). https://www.healthit.gov/topic/about-onc. Verified November 9, 2019.
30. Sequoia. https://sequoiaproject.org/. Verified November 9, 2019.
31. Common Well. https://www.commonwellalliance.org/.
32. eHealth Exchange. https://ehealthexchange.org/.
33. Strategic Health Information Exchange Collaborative (SHIEC). https://strategichie.com/about/.
34. SHIEC Patient Centered Data Home™ (PCDH). https://www.himss.org/resource-environmental-scan/shiec-patient-centered-data-hometm-pcdh.
35. Social Determinants of Health. https://www.healthypeople.gov/2020/topics-objectives/topic/social-determinants-of-health. Verified November 26, 2019.
36. CDC and Social Determinants of Health. https://www.cdc.gov/socialdeterminants/index.htm. Verified November 26, 2019.
37. WHO Social Determinants of Health. https://www.who.int/social_determinants/en/. Verified November 26, 2019.
38. The Triple Aim. http://www.ihi.org/engage/initiatives/TripleAim/Pages/default.aspx. Verified November 26, 2019.
39. Stevens L, Abbey R. HIE supports disaster preparedness and emergency services. May 14, 2014. https://www.healthit.gov/buzz-blog/health-information-exchange-2/hie-supports-disaster-preparedness-emergency-services. Verified November 26, 2019.
40. Southeast Regional HIT-HIE Collaboration final report: disaster preparedness must include HIE. https://www.healthdataanswers.net/disaster-preparedness-must-include-hie/. Verified November 26, 2019.
41. John Gregory J. Care delivery, March 12, 2018. Disasters bring unexpected use cases for HIE. https://www.healthexec.com/topics/care-delivery/disasters-bring-unexpected-use-cases-hie. Verified November 26, 2019.

Telehealth Dissemination and Implementation (D&I) Research: Analysis of the PCORI Telehealth-Related Research Portfolio

Ronald S. Weinstein, Robert S. Krouse, Michael J. Holcomb, Camryn Payne, Kristine A. Erps, Elizabeth A. Krupinski, and Rifat Latifi

Introduction

Improving outcomes through "patient-centered care" has emerged as an important focus of study in clinical practice and research over the past decade [1–8]. While the principles of patient-centered care and community-centered care are found in philosophical writings from ancient times, with the recent paradigm shift toward patient-centered care, physicians have begun to accept that the health and well-being of patients depends upon a collaborative effort between healthcare professionals, patients, and their communities [8–15].

As a result, the idea of active engagement of patients when critical healthcare decisions are being made (e.g., when patients arrive at a crossroads of medical options, where diverging paths have different and important consequences) is becoming increasingly acceptable and part of the standard of care. Of course, the preparedness of patients to fully accept that role and providers' willingness to promote active engagement is open to question [15]. More importantly, does the medical profession fully understand how unprepared patients and healthcare enterprises

---

The original version of this chapter was revised. The correction to this chapter is available at https://doi.org/10.1007/978-3-030-56917-4_30.

R. S. Weinstein (✉) · M. J. Holcomb · C. Payne · K. A. Erps
Arizona Telemedicine Program, The University of Arizona's College of Medicine, Tucson, AZ, USA
e-mail: rweinstein@telemedicine.arizona.edu

R. S. Krouse
University of Pennsylvania, Philadelphia, PA, USA

E. A. Krupinski
Department of Radiology, Emory University, Atlanta, GA, USA

R. Latifi
Department of Surgery, New York Medical College, School of Medicine and Westchester Medical Center Health, Valhalla, NY, USA

© The Author(s) 2021, corrected publication 2021
R. Latifi et al. (eds.), *Telemedicine, Telehealth and Telepresence*,
https://doi.org/10.1007/978-3-030-56917-4_6

are to "fully participate" in the decision-making processes? [16–19]. What strategies successfully enable patients and their caregivers to optimally provide self-care to manage chronic health conditions?

Questions related to population health literacy in the USA were barely on medical professions' radar screen prior to 2000 when news that more patients die each year from preventable medical errors than in car crashes shocked the nation [20–22]. While the magnitude of this problem remains controversial, there is a general awareness that the poor populational health literacy in the USA, and the relative absence of patient participation in clinical decision-making, may be contributing factors to the medical error problem [23–25]. Since the year 2000, beginning with the publication of the US Institute of Medicine's warnings concerning the possible presence of unacceptably high levels of preventable medical errors within the US healthcare system, not nearly enough has been done to improve patient healthcare education for our K-12 students, as well as future interprofessional team members [16–19]. The question of whether "the inclusion of sharp-eyed, medically savvy patients on their own personal interdisciplinary healthcare teams would make a difference" will likely need to be addressed through randomized clinical trials.

Latifi's book *The Modern Hospital* explains how, and why, patient-centered care is important in modern hospital settings and for improved patient outcomes [26]. Some of his ideas, and those of his co-authors, on patient-centered care can be extended to patients' homes and even to direct-to-consumer telehealth [1, 2, 26].

The aim of this chapter is to provide perspective on Patient Center Outcomes Research Institute (PCORI) extramural dissemination and intervention (D&I) funding for telemedicine and telehealth-related research. Hopefully, this data analysis provides new ideas for PCORI funding priorities, program review criteria, and ways to potentially be successful in competing for patient-centered clinical intervention effectiveness funding going forward.

Background of Dissemination and Intervention Science in the United States

In the USA today, there is an array of funders interested in patient-centered comparative clinical effectiveness research (CER). The list includes, but is not limited to, the National Institutes of Health (NIH), the PCORI, the US Department of Veterans Affairs (VA), and the Center for Disease Control and Prevention (CDC) [27–29]. The expansion of interest in (D&I) science and the creation of a funding base to support extramural activities in recent years have evolved on several fronts. In recent years, notable extramural-funding programs have been offered by both the NIH and PCORI [27, 30]. The US Congress sets both the NIH and PCORI budget allocations, monitors spending and progress, and for PCORI included a de facto sunset clause in its initial appropriation a decade ago to ensure adherence to the agreed upon vision and mission.

PCORI is a mission-specific medical science/service research enterprise that extends across the borders of drug and medical device innovation; D&I science;

patient-centered clinical effectiveness research; and interdisciplinary team-based clinical care delivery. Its website is data-rich and provides clinical researchers and healthcare strategists with up-to-date information on the patient-centered research landscape [27].

Origins of Dissemination and Intervention Science

Historically, NIH programs in D&I science grew out of President Richard M. Nixon's National Cancer Act (1973) which, for the first time, specified a role for the National Cancer Institute (NCI) that included a focus on cancer control [4]. This resulted in a transition of the cancer control program from a "diffusion of innovations" professional education model to a cancer prevention and control intervention research model. The new Division for Cancer Prevention and Control was charged with developing a framework for cancer control research that included the creation of a linear series of phases from hypothesis generation to development and implementation projects [4, 31, 32]. Beginning in 2005, NIH began soliciting applications to develop an implementation science knowledge base and to build capacity for studies to increase quality and quantity of implementation science knowledge [4].

In 2007, the NIH hosted its first annual conference on D&I research in health. An annual joint NIH and Veterans Administration (VA) D&I science meeting grew to over 1000 participants with over 700 abstract presentations by 2011. This meeting continues to draw a large number of participants each year and is currently co-sponsored by NIH, Academy Health, the Agency for Health Research Quality (AHRQ), PCORI, the Robert Wood Johnson Foundation, and the VA. In 2013, the NIH announced the expansion of its D&I research funding to include 15 other NIH institutes, in addition to the NCI, and the Office of Behavioral and Social Science Research. In 2014, the NCI began developing important international collaborations primarily focused on training D&I investigators. Within the NCI, although there was growth in implementation science funding from 2001 and 2016, it remains a very small proportion of the overall NCI funding [4].

The Patient-Centered Outcomes Research Institute

PCORI is a US-based non-governmental organization created by Congress as part of a modification to the Social Security Act, by clauses in the Patient Protection and Affordable Care Act. In comparison to the NIH, which is a very large federal agency with a broad mission to advance biomedical research that has close to $40 billion in annual research funding, PCORI is a relatively small organization with a narrowly focused mandate to advanced patient-centered outcomes research with approximately $300 million in annual research funding [33]. It is charged with leveraging principals of D&I science to move translational and clinical research findings into medical practices of practitioners everywhere, utilizing the results of CER. There has been a close working relationship between the PCORI organization and the NIH leadership since PCORI's inception [28, 30].

PCORI is supported by the Patient-Centered Outcomes Research (PCOR) Trust Fund, of which 80% is provided annually to PCORI to support its research funding and operations. The other 20% is provided to AHRQ and the Assistant Secretary for Planning and Evaluation (ASPE) to build data capacity for PCOR. The PCOR Trust Fund receives income each year from: (1) the general fund of the US Treasury; (2) transfers from the Centers for Medicare and Medicaid (CMS) trust funds; and (3) a fee assessed on private insurance and self-insured health plans [4].

An establishing concept for PCORI was that rigorous methodological standards help ensure that medical research produces information that is both valid and generalizable [4, 14, 34, 35]. This goes beyond the typical academic research medical center's vision, where clinical investigators typically strive to demonstrate validity for the uses of specific therapies and medical devices, but the diffusion of their discoveries into the general public is a secondary objective [7, 36–39]. Although academic medical centers housed federal-funded "clinical research units" for decades, in the past, community-implementation plans to encourage diffusion into the non-academic population were relatively uncommon.

PCORI was given important tools to accomplish its missions, including an independent, federally appointed Methodology Committee charged with developing methodological standards for patient-centered outcomes research. With oversight of the PCORI Board of Governors, this Methodology Committee, working with outside contractors, is charged with defining and prioritizing research questions [30, 36].

Analysis of the PCORI Telehealth-Related Research Portfolio Database (2010–2019)

PCORI Definitions of Telehealth and Telemedicine

PCORI has adopted a version of telemedicine and telehealth terminology defined by the American Telemedicine Association and the CMS. PCORI defines telehealth as the use of medical information exchanged between sites via electronic communication to improve a patient's health status. Telehealth includes a growing variety of applications and services using two-way video, smart phones, wireless tools, and other forms of telecommunications technology. The definition requires an exchange of information (bidirectional) across sites (e.g., not within clinics with the use of tablets). Telemedicine seeks to improve a patient's access to healthcare services by asynchronous data acquisition, transmission and subsequent consultation by a clinician, or alternatively by synchronous two-way, interactive communication, between two or more geographically separated locations where the patient and/or the patient's in-person clinicians are at one geographic location and the consulting clinicians are at one or more distant geographical locations. The interactive telecommunications equipment includes, at a minimum, audio and video equipment. Telemedicine patient encounters may also utilize peripheral devices such as vital signs measurement or monitoring devices, digital stethoscopes that support transmission of auscultation sounds to remote clinicians, and/or various imaging modalities with video outputs. This definition of telemedicine requires consultation with a licensed medical professional [40] (PCORI helpdesk, Ashlee Horn, personal correspondence, January 27, 2020).

PCORI uses an internally coded portfolio taxonomy for their own website project portfolio search tool filters. PCORI aims at providing researchers with the most comprehensive set of studies that might be relevant to any one of their questions about PCORI's work. In turn, the PCORI Science team uses this inclusive portfolio dataset as a starting place for PCORI's own work in portfolio analysis [40] (PCORI helpdesk, Ashlee Horn, personal correspondence, January 27, 2020).

Overview of PCORI Extramural Funding

PCORI provides extramural funding for 22 "Project Types" (Appendix A), ranging from "Engagement Award Conference" to "Research Project." All of the "telehealth-related funding" was in the "Research Project" category as of December 31, 2019. Eighty-eight out of a total of 655 funded research projects were classified as being "telehealth-related" by PCORI. The current analysis is restricted to examination of those 88 telehealth-related research projects.

PCORI Funding Opportunities

The PCORI website provides detailed information regarding each individual PCORI research project [39]. (Note: PCORI uses neither the terms "grant" nor "contracts" but prefers the term "project" to identify extramurally funded entities.) There have been 149 PCORI Funding Announcements (PFAs) since the inception of the PCORI extramural funding program in 2011. As of January 6, 2020, a total of 1606 projects, of which 655 are classified as "research projects," had been awarded by PCORI.

PCORI Telehealth-Related Research Project Themes

Generally, PCORI publishes PFAs in three cycles per year for the recurrent themes: "Addressing Disparities; Assessment of Prevention, Diagnosis and Treatment Options; Communication and Dissemination Research; Improving Healthcare Systems," and "Improving Methods for Conducting Patient-Centered Outcomes Research," constituting an "annual funding cycle." PCORI also publishes targeted and limited PFAs, many of which may be one-time funding opportunities. There are 51 distinct PFA titles listed on PCORI's funding webpages for PFAs published through the end of 2019. PCORI's 1606-project dataset (as of January 6, 2020) lists 45 distinct PFA titles associated with awarded projects. There are 35 distinct PFA titles associated with the subset of 655 awarded research projects [37–42].

What percentage of PCORI-funding research projects have been designated "telehealth-related projects"? Of 655 PCORI research projects funded prior to the year 2020, 88, or 13.4% of its research projects, were sub-classified by PCORI as "telehealth-related" projects [42]. Our database search showed that there were an additional 15 projects that included "telemedicine" as an "Intervention Strategy" in their program descriptions but were not included in PCORI's "Spotlight" list of 88 telehealth-related projects [40, 42, 43]. The reason for this omission is unclear. The PCORI website for telehealth-related research projects includes a listing of the project titles and hyperlinks for the 88 "official" PCORI "telehealth-related" research projects and PCORI's total funding awarded to these 88 telehealth-related research projects [42, 43].

PCORI Telehealth-Related Research Portfolio Analysis (2012–2019)

The PCORI website is rich in information about individual PCORI-funded research projects [42, 43]. We conducted a focused review of the 88 telehealth-related projects. We downloaded into an Excel database the publicly available PCORI research project dataset, and each of the individual telehealth-related project webpages from the PCORI website [42, 43]. These information sources included: (1) the PFA under which the project was awarded; and (2) attributes such as: the specific category, or categories that speak to the general goals for the specific program; organization; year awarded; actual or expected end date; budget; completion status; health conditions studied; patient population studied; intervention strategies; time frame; and, for the completed projects, articles published [42].

According to PCORI personnel, the information for the public PCORI website database was created by the PCORI organization using a process developed by PCORI staff with the help of an independent contractor. This involved a "systematic analysis and coding of PCORI's funded awards, based on a read of the research plan" [40] (PCORI Help desk, August 2019). The specific health conditions, patient populations, and intervention strategies studied as part of individual research projects are listed in the individual project profiles. For our analyses, we used data explicitly listed in the profiles carefully avoiding extrapolating based on assumptions of what we thought might be additional relevant categories for individual projects. Project funding amounts used in our analysis were included in the PCORI project profiles [42].

Telehealth-related D&I projects totaled $381 million dollars [42]. Included in the PCORI Telehealth Research Project Portfolio that lists 88 projects are 35 projects for which PCORI coded "Telemedicine" as one of their intervention strategies, and 53 projects that do not include "Telemedicine" as a PCORI-coded intervention strategy. The official telehealth-related component, 88 projects, represents 19% of total PCORI project research funding (2012–2019) and 13% of the total number of PCORI research projects. Since PCORI, and the awarded "telehealth-related" research projects, use the terms "telemedicine" and "telehealth" and a number of "telehealth-related" terms somewhat interchangeably, the complete set of telehealth-related projects is not retrievable by searching on any one of these terms thus requiring reading through entire project webpages in order to determine exactly how a project is "telehealth-related" in some instances.

Of the 88 telehealth-related research projects, 34.1% ($n = 30$) were listed as "completed," as of December 31, 2019 [43]. For the record, the 88 telehealth-related research projects, per individual project webpages and the data set downloaded from PCORI, had an exact total awarded funding of $379,591,036 and an average awarded budget of $4,313,535 (ranging from $716,243 to $15,201,613 for individual projects).

PCORI Research Project Themes

Telehealth-related research projects have been awarded under the following 13 thematic PFAs: (1) Assessment of Prevention, Diagnosis, and Treatment Options; (2) Communication and Dissemination Research; (3) Addressing Disparities; (4) Patient-Powered Research Networks (PPRN) Research Demonstrated Projects; (5) Symptom Management for Patients with Advanced Illness; (6) Improving Healthcare Systems; (7) Medication-Assisted Treatment (MAT) for Delivery for Pregnant Women with Substance Use Disorders Involving Prescription Opioids and/or Heroin; (8) Treatment of Multiple Sclerosis; (9) Management of Care Transitions for Emerging Adults with Sickle Cell Disease; (10) Partnerships to Conduct Research with PCORnet (PaCR); (11) Pragmatic Clinical Studies to Evaluate Patient-Centered Outcomes; (12) Community-Based Palliative Care Delivery for Adults with Advanced Illnesses and their Caregivers; and (13) Psycho-social Interventions with Office-Based Opioid Treatment for Opioid Use Disorder [41, 42]. These 13 "research themes" might have influenced the choices of some investigators regarding: (1) their interest in competing in the PCORI extramural funding process; and (2) the subject matter and research questions they chose to study.

It is interesting to note that our search of the 149 PFAs issued between 2011 and 2019 found the word "telemedicine" appears only in the "Improving Healthcare Systems" PFA, which was offered in 18 different funding cycles. The word "telehealth" appeared in only two targeted PFAs: "Treatment of Multiple Sclerosis" and "Management of Care Transitions for Emerging Adults with Sickle Cell Disease." A number of other telehealth-related terms appeared in various PFAs including, but not limited to, mHealth, mobile health, teleconference, telemonitoring, telephonic, teledelivery, telecare, telerehabilitation, and remote monitoring. Therefore, identifying telemedicine activities or telehealth funding opportunities can require searches on a broad set of telemedicine- and telehealth-related terms in addition to using umbrella terms such as "telehealth" and "connected health."

Figure 6.1 shows our tabulation of the percentage of the telehealth-related research project funding awarded to the 88 telehealth-related projects in each of the 13 PFA themes that telehealth-related research projects were awarded under. There is telehealth-related research project funding in 37% of the 35 distinct PFA themes under which the total of 655 research projects were awarded. The PFA theme with the most funding awarded to telehealth-related research projects is "Pragmatic

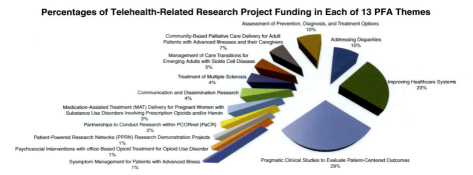

Fig. 6.1 PCORI telehealth-related research project themes with the percentages of total telehealth-related research project funding awarded under each of 13 PFAs that included a telehealth-related research project theme

Clinical Studies to Evaluation Patient-Centered Outcomes" (29%). "Symptom Management for Patients with Advanced Illnesses" had the least funding (1%). Low funding areas (0–5% of the total telehealth-related research) may represent areas of special opportunity for telehealth investigators moving forward.

The "Improving Healthcare Systems" (IHS) PFA "seeks to fund CER that addresses the same areas as those addressed by IOM" (Institute of Medicine; recently renamed the "National Academy of Medicine"). "IOM has addressed key aspects of systems improvement, including," the aims of, "making care: Accessible, Effective, Patient-centered, Timely, Efficient, Safe, Equitable, and Coordinated." Telemedicine is included in the IHS PFA as a "technology intervention" that research projects could potentially apply to achieve the IOM aims [41] (PCOR's Cycle 32,019 Funding Cycle; page 23).

Health Conditions, Patient Populations, and Intervention Strategies: Telehealth-Related Content Analysis (2010–2019)

Health Conditions

Five hundred twenty-eight of the 655 PCORI research projects, including the 88 telehealth-related projects, were coded by PCORI with one or more health conditions. The remaining 127 research projects were not coded with any health condition. Together, the 655 research projects contained a total of 139 unique health condition codes assigned by PCORI. There are 27 general health condition categories and 112 specific conditions coded as subcategories of the general health condition categories. Many research projects involved more than one health condition. The three highest frequency general health conditions in the telehealth-related project subset of PCORI research projects are: mental/behavioral health ($n = 32$), which included diseases such as substance addiction/abuse and depression; cardiovascular diseases ($n = 21$) including hypertension and stroke; and nutritional and metabolic disorders ($n = 17$) including diabetes and obesity (Fig. 6.2). In general, PCORI codes for both the general health condition categories and any specific disease subcategories for each research project.

6 Telehealth Dissemination and Implementation (D&I) Research: Analysis of… 85

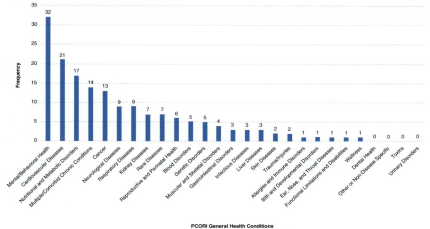

Fig. 6.2 Bar graph representing the number of times (frequency) each of the 23 "general health conditions" appears in the 88 PCORI-funded telehealth-related research projects [37]

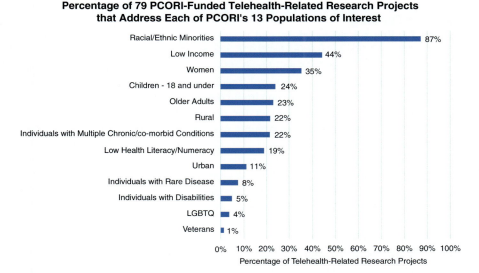

Fig. 6.3 Bar graph representing the percentages of 79 telehealth-related research projects that address each of the 13 PCORI-specified "Patient Populations of Interest." PCORI has not specified the target population(s) for the remaining 9 of the 88 telehealth-related research projects [37]

Patient Populations

Of the 13 categories of patient populations identified by PCORI as being disproportionately at risk for poorer healthcare outcomes, the groups most frequently targeted by telehealth-related research projects were Racial/Ethnic Minorities ($n = 69$), Low-Income Individuals ($n = 35$), and Women ($n = 28$) (Fig. 6.3).

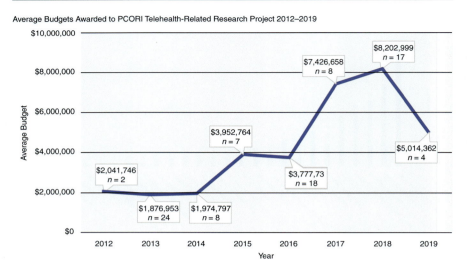

Fig. 6.4 Line chart representing the average budget awarded to telehealth-related research projects each year by PCORI from 2012 to 2019. The "*n*" represents the number of projects awarded each year [40]

Levels of Funding

PCORI funding for telehealth-related research projects averaged $1,911,786 for 2012, 2013, and 2014 combined, $3,826,744 for 2015 and 2016 combined, and $7,954,570 for 2017 and 2018 combined (Fig. 6.4). While these increases have not been steady, there is an overall upward trend. The average project award for 2017 and 2018 combined is more than quadruple the average award for 2012, 2013, and 2014 combined. The average budget for projects awarded in 2019 dropped to $5,013,909, perhaps reflecting uncertainty over reauthorization of the PCORI program funding until December 2019.

Of the 88 telehealth-related research projects (Fig. 6.5), 23 (26%) had budget awards between $0.0 and $2.0 million, 38 (43%) had budget awards between $2.0 million and $5.0 million, 18 (20%) had budget awards between $5.0 million and $10.0 million, and 9 (11%) had budget awards that exceeded $10.0 million dollars.

PCORI Research Study Designs

The PFAs identified, among other parameters, the general research theme (focus) and expected study design. For example, "Assessment of Prevention, Diagnosis, and Treatment Options" projects used randomized trials in clinical settings to compare the outcomes of at least two different healthcare options to address "gaps in the current evidence base" so patients could decide the most effective option for their individual circumstances [43]. In the years 2012 through 2019, telehealth-related research projects were awarded most commonly under the PFA themes for "Improving Healthcare Systems" ($n = 24$), "Addressing Disparities" ($n = 17$), and "Assessment of Prevention, Diagnosis, and Treatment Options" ($n = 17$). During the same time period, "Addressing Disparities" with average funding awarded per

Fig. 6.5 Stratification of the entire subset of 88 telehealth-related research projects according to total awarded budgets falling in each funding range (2012–2019)

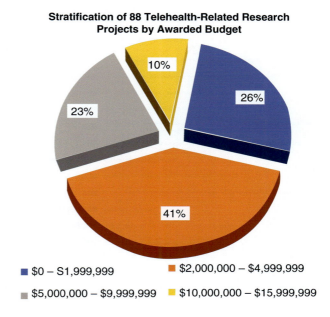

project of $2,331,198 and "Assessment of Prevention, Diagnosis, and Treatment Options" ($2,328,550) were two of the three PFA themes with the lowest average awarded budgets, while the PFA themes with the highest average awarded budgets were "Community-Based Palliative Care Deliver for Adult Patients and their Caregivers" ($n = 2$, average budget awarded of $12,372,111) and "Pragmatic Clinical Studies to Evaluate Patient-Centered Outcomes" ($n = 9$, average budget awarded $12,057,672) (Fig. 6.6).

Intervention Strategies

Included in the "PCORI Telehealth-Related Project Portfolio" are projects with as many as nine intervention strategies as coded by PCORI and its consultants. Thirty-five projects were coded specifically with "Telemedicine" as one of their intervention strategies. Figure 6.7 shows the percentage of telehealth-related projects utilizing each of the 15 "core" intervention strategies referenced by PCORI. The three most frequent intervention strategies associated with telehealth-related research projects were "Training and Education," "Technology," and "Other Health Services Interventions."

The 88 telehealth-related projects utilized one, or some combination, of the PCORI designated core "Intervention Strategies": Behavioral Interventions, Care Coordination, Complementary and Alternative Medicine, Device Interventions, Drug Interventions, Incentives for Behavior Change, Other Clinical Interventions, Other Health Service Interventions, Patient Navigation, Screening Interventions, Shared Decision-Making, Technology Interventions, Telemedicine, and Training and Education Interventions. On average, telehealth-related projects applied four to five intervention strategies (mean = 4.69; range 1–9).

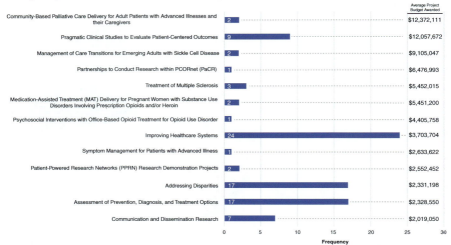

Fig. 6.6 Bar graph representing the frequency of PCORI-funded telehealth-related research projects in 13 PFA themes from 2012 to 2019. Numbers of projects in each group are listed, in white, at the left ends of each of the dark bars. Average dollar amounts for budgets awarded to each project within a PFA group are adjacent to each bar at the right. PFAs are listed in descending order (top to bottom) according to average project budget awards

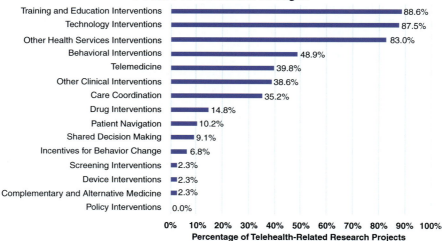

Fig. 6.7 Percentage of intervention strategies represented across the PCORI-funded telehealth-related research projects (individual projects can be listed in more than one intervention category)

Location and Organization

The majority of telehealth-related research projects were conducted at research universities, with others at non-university hospital systems and independent research institutes. With regards to location, organizations in 26 states received funding for telehealth-related projects (Fig. 6.8). California had the most telehealth-related projects at 14, followed by Massachusetts at 12 and Pennsylvania at 9. The current state and current organization specified by PCORI as of January 6, 2020, for each telehealth-related project were utilized for these tallies. Some telehealth-related projects included a descriptive footnote from PCORI that indicated that the project had originally been awarded to an organization in one state but then had been transferred to a new organization, often in a different state. From 2012 through 2019, the University of California (all campuses) was awarded six telehealth-related projects (three of which went to the University of California, San Francisco), and the Massachusetts General Hospital, in Boston, MA, was awarded five telehealth-related projects. The Feinstein Institute for Medical Research, Manhasset, NY, and University of New Mexico, Albuquerque, NM, were each awarded three telehealth-related projects. One project was awarded to the Sinai Health System (Toronto, Canada) with its study slated to recruit subjects in Toronto, Canada; Chapel Hill, North Carolina; and Chicago, Illinois.

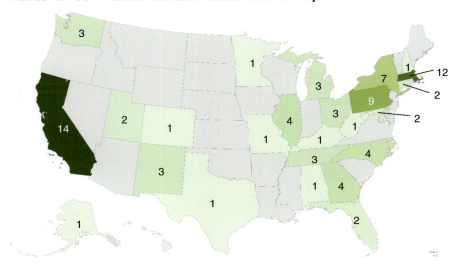

Fig. 6.8 State-by-state distribution of telehealth-related PCORI telehealth-related projects. Other PCORI projects, unrelated to telehealth, are not represented. Map produced with Microsoft Excel. "Microsoft product screen shot reprinted with permission from Microsoft Corporation"

Publications

In addition to PCORI's requirements for posting the final research report and final study protocol publicly on its website, PCORI encourages and permits publication of PCORI-funded research in any journal at any time [44]. PCORI requires that the awardees make their peer-reviewed publications publishing findings from PCORI research available in PubMed Central. PCORI will, upon request from the project awardee, pay the fees to make peer-reviewed articles published in journals freely available to the public [45]. Of the 30 completed PCORI telehealth-related research projects, 21 had their results published in peer-reviewed medical journals as of December 31, 2019. These journals are listed in Table 6.1. We queried the InCites

Table 6.1 Impact factors of journals in which 21 completed PCORI telehealth-related research projects have published their project results[a]

Journal	Impact factor (2018)	5-year impact factor (2018)
Journal of Spinal Cord Medicine	1.711	2.005
Telemedicine and E-Health (2)	1.996	2.339
Journal of Women's Health	2.009	2.694
Psychiatric Services	2.253	3.026
The Journal of Head Trauma Rehabilitation	2.667	3.645
Archives of Physical Medicine and Rehabilitation	2.697	3.618
PLoS One	2.776	3.337
Psycho-oncology	3.430	4.115
Medical Care	3.795	3.991
Nephrology, Dialysis, Transplantation	4.198	4.369
Circulation-Cardiovascular Quality and Outcomes	4.424	4.965
Arthritis Care & Research	4.530	4.439
Journal of General Internal Medicine	4.606	4.912
Osteoarthritis and Cartilage	4.879	5.701
Journal of Medical Internet Research	4.945	6.204
Pediatrics (2)	5.401	6.456
American Journal of Obstetrics and Gynecology	6.120	5.642
Clinical Journal of the American Society of Nephrology	6.243	6.175
American Journal of Kidney Diseases	6.653	7.065
Neurology	8.689	9.025
JAMA Pediatrics	12.004	12.268
JAMA	51.273	46.312
JAMA Network Open	Not ranked	Not ranked

[a]Only the journal articles listed immediately following the "Results of This Project" heading on individual PCORI project web pages were utilized to derive this journal list. Some projects have published results in more than one journal. *Journal* titles followed by "(2)" each published PCORI "Results of This Project" articles for two different PCORI telehealth-related projects [43]. "2019 Journal Citation Reports (Clarivate Analytics, 2020), last accessed Feb 24, 2020"

Journal Citation Reports database to obtain the 2018 impact factor and five-year impact factor (as of 2018) for each of the journals in Table 6.1 [46, 47].

Discussion

The original Congressional appropriation that created PCORI in 2010 provided 10 years of funding, expiring in 2019. In late 2019, the Congress re-appropriated federal funding for the PCORI foundation providing it with another 10 years of funding through 2028. The re-appropriate reflects the endorsements of PCORI by diverse constituencies including federal agencies, foundation, industry, and within the healthcare delivery community to attest to the successes of the strong founding leadership of PCORI [48–50].

PCORI was created to fund research projects focused on PCOR CER to provide high-quality, unbiased evidence enabling optimal decision-making between patients and caregivers, facilitate efficiency of healthcare systems at all levels of organization, and eliminate healthcare disparities for disadvantaged and minority groups [14, 47, 48]. A key Congressional mandate required patient-centeredness (the involvement of the patient in the management of their own healthcare) and collaboration with community stakeholders to ensure that research questions and study design would be relevant, feasible, and sustainable so that patients would have the ability to make the best evidence-based healthcare decision for themselves [6–8, 10–14]. PCORI-funded research projects involve comparing risks and benefits of at least two healthcare options, engage patients and other relevant stakeholders, follow methodology guidelines to ensure quality comparative effectiveness trials, and seek to improve healthcare outcomes—particularly in terms of conditions that place a heavy burden on society and populations disproportionately at risk for poor healthcare outcomes [48]. Additionally, much of the PCORI research has focused on improving CER methods and developing a network (PCORnet) to continue to advance patient-centered research capacity and infrastructure on a broader scale [45]. An additional expectation of PCORI-funded research was the publication of results in high-caliber academic journals [45, 46].

In line with PCORI's defined goals of using CER trials to establish a strong evidence base, the 88 telehealth-related research projects analyzed for this study utilized PCOR CER to study telehealth's impact on patient outcomes.

With regards to the health conditions studied, the most frequently referenced conditions included mental/behavioral health, nutritional and metabolic disorders, and cardiovascular diseases that disproportionately affect racial/ethnic minorities and low-income populations, and lack of insurance, lack of diversity among care providers, lack of culturally competent providers, and language barriers all pose as obstacles to these groups receiving adequate care [50, 51]. The leading causes of death in the USA in 2016, as outlined by the CDC, were heart disease, cancer, accidents, chronic lower respiratory diseases, stroke, Alzheimer's disease, diabetes, influenza and pneumonia, nephritis, nephrotic syndrome, nephrosis, and suicide [52]. In line with what we have already discussed about PCORI's focus on studying conditions that impact a large number of people and place a large burden on society, it seems logical that those were the most frequently studied categories of health conditions by PCORI awardees.

PCORI has effectively shown that there is value in having a term-limited quasi-governmental agency with a laser-sharp focus on promoting and supporting D&I research and education. Building a sunset clause in 2010 into the original Congressional funding undoubtedly encouraged the PCORI organization to stay on mission over the past decade. Community input into decision-making was strongly encouraged. Academia was forced to look outside of its own walls and seek council on what is important to the general public, the major consumers of healthcare. The recent re-appropriation of funding for another 10 years is good news and should be taken as an endorsement of the trajectory that PCORI is pursuing to identify and encourage implementation of new solutions to old problems in the delivery of healthcare [53].

While PCORI is filling a critical gap in the medical services innovation cycle by stimulating the creation of a sustainable, distributed D&I research enterprise that provides strong linkages between the PCORI-funded evidence-based clinical research teams and largely academic healthcare delivery systems, it remains to be seen how many of the improvements in patient outcomes identified by PCORI-funded research actually become incorporated into community healthcare practices. Only time will tell if PCORI actually "improved patient care and reduced the burden that some of our country's most pressing healthcare issues impose on individuals, their families, and the healthcare system," a commitment made to the US Congress by the PCORI Leadership [49, 50].

Finally, additional work is needed to establish the origins of the inclusion of telehealth-related projects in the PCORI telehealth-related research project portfolio. It is apparent that telehealth clinical research has benefitted significantly from PCORI funding—approximately $381 million dollars to date. The next step should be studying the long-term effects and outcomes of these projects. In particular, how does a PCORI-funded project change the current practice and does it advance improvements of clinical outcomes? Much remains to be done! (Fig. 6.9).

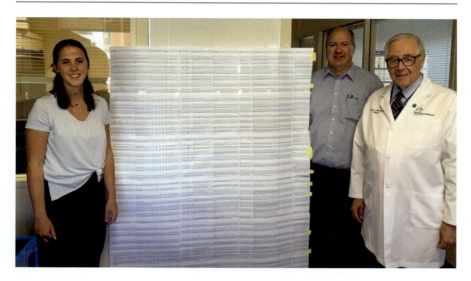

Fig. 6.9 Printouts of the mountain of Excel spreadsheets that formed the basis for the PCORI portfolio analysis described in this chapter. Left to right: Sir William Osler Summer Fellow Camryn Payne at the ATP headquarters, at The University of Arizona, Tucson, assembled this large database from publicly available information at the PCORI website and through the PCORI "Help Desk," in the summer of 2019. Michael J. Holcomb, the ATP's' Associate Director for Information Technology, worked closely with Dr. Weinstein to validate Camryn's data, and to study PCORI's entire research project portfolio. Ronald S. Weinstein, MD, Founding Director of the ATP and of the ATP's Sir William Osler Summer Program which he founded as a young Department of Pathology Chairman at Rush Medical College in Chicago, in the summer of 1978. He relocated the Osler Program to The University of Arizona, in Tucson, when he changed pathology chairs in order to continue his research on P-glycoprotein's role in multidrug resistance in cancer cells at the Arizona Cancer Center, in Tucson. This picture marked the 40th anniversary of Dr. Weinstein's Sir William Osler Summer Program for College and High School Students. Hundreds of college and high school students had benefitted from his Osler Summer Programs in Chicago and Tucson. Camryn Payne, a Tucson native, had finished her second year as a pre-medical college student at Washington University in St. Louis, Missouri

Appendix A: PCORI's 22 "Types of Projects"

1. Dissemination and Implementation Project
2. Engagement Award Conference
3. Engagement Award Conference, Conference: Dissemination
4. Engagement Award Project
5. Engagement Award Project, Dissemination Project
6. Implementation of Effective Shared Decision-Making Approaches Project
7. Implementation of Findings from PCORI's Major Research Investments
8. Implementation of PCORI-Funded PCOR Results (Limited Competition Project)
9. Other Evidence Products

10.	PCORnet Coordinating Center Phase II
11.	PCORnet Initiative on Health Plan/System Data Partnerships (A Stepwise Approach to Collaboration)
12.	PCORnet: Clinical Data Research Networks (CDRN) Phase I
13.	PCORnet: Clinical Data Research Networks (CDRN) Phase II
14.	PCORnet: Patient Powered Research Networks (PPRN) Phase I
15.	PCORnet: Patient Powered Research Networks (PPRN) Phase II
16.	Pipeline to Proposal, Tier A
17.	Pipeline to Proposal, Tier I
18.	Pipeline to Proposal, Tier II
19.	Pipeline to Proposal, Tier III
20.	PPRN Limited Competition Award
21.	Research Infrastructure Project
22.	Research Project

The 22 major categories of PCORI Project types encompass the total of 1606 funded PCORI projects (2012–2019). Of these 1606 funded projects, 655 were in the "Research Project" category. The 88 telehealth-related projects, discussed in this chapter, are a subset of the 655 projects in the "Research Project" category. There are an additional 15 projects searchable in the PCORI database as being "telemedicine-related" that are not listed among the 88 PCORI-identified "telehealth" and "telehealth-related" research projects featured on the PCORI "Telehealth" website [39, 40]

References

1. Daniel CY, Latifi R. Navigating and rebuilding. In: The modern hospital: patients centered, disease based, research oriented, technology driven. New York: Springer; 2019. p. 31.
2. Latifi R, Daniel CY. The modern hospital: patient-centered and science based. In: The modern hospital: patients centered, disease based, research oriented, technology driven. New York: Springer; 2019. p. 85–92.
3. Brownson RC, Golditz GA, Proctor EA, editors. Dissemination and implementation research in health. Translating science into practice. 2nd ed. New York: Oxford University Press; 2018.
4. Kerner J, Glasgow RE, Vinson CA. A history of the National Cancer Institute's support for implementation science across the cancer control continuum. Context counts. In: Chambers DA, Vinson CA, Norton WE, editors. Advancing the science of implementation across the cancer continuum. New York: Oxford University Press; 2019. p. 8–20.
5. Fernandez ME, Mullen PD, Leeman J, Walker TJ, Escoffery C. Evidence-based cancer practices, programs, and interventions. In: Chambers DA, Vinson CA, Norton WE, editors. Advancing the science of implementation across the cancer continuum. New York: Oxford University Press; 2019. p. 21–40.
6. Basch E, Aronson N, Berg A, et al. Methodological standards and patient-centeredness in comparative effectiveness research: the PCORI perspective. JAMA. 2012;307(15):1636–40.
7. Comparative effectiveness research: activities funded by the patient-centered outcomes research trust fund. https://www.gao.gov/assets/gao-18-311.pdf. Last accessed 23 Feb 2020.
8. Fischer MA, Asch SM. The future of the Patient-Centered Outcomes Research Institute (PCORI). J Gen Intern Med. 2019;34:2291–2. https://doi.org/10.1007/s11606-019-05324-9.
9. Tauber AI. Patient autonomy and the ethics of responsibility. Cambridge, MA: MIT Press; 2005.
10. Frank L, Basch E, Selby JV. The PCORI perspective on patient-centered outcomes research. JAMA. 2014;312(15):1513–4.
11. Selby JV. Interview: Patient-Centered Outcomes Research Institute seeks to find out what works best by involving 'end-users' from the beginning. J Comp Eff Res. 2014;3(2):125–9. https://doi.org/10.2217/cer.13.94.

12. Selby JV, Forsythe L, Sox HC. Stakeholder-driven comparative effectiveness research: an update from PCORI. JAMA. 2015;314(21):2235–6.25-9.
13. Sheridan S, Schrandt S, Forsythe L, Hilliard TS, Paez KA. The PCORI engagement rubric: promising practices for partnering in research. Ann Family Med. 2017;15(2):165–70.
14. Clinical Effectiveness and Decision Science. www.pcori.org/about-us/our-programs/clinical-effectiveness-and-decision-science. Last accessed 23 Feb 2020.
15. Kindig DA, Panzer AM, Nielsen-Bohlman L, editors. Health literacy: a prescription to end confusion. Washington, DC: National Academies Press; 2004. p. 1–345.
16. Schmitt MH, Gilbert JH, Brandt BF, Weinstein RS. The coming of age for interprofessional education and practice. Am J Med. 2013;126(4):284–8.
17. Weinstein RS, Lopez AM. Health literacy and connected health. Health Aff. 2014;33(6):1103B.
18. Weinstein RS. Reinventing the US Institute of Medicine: a second coming. Am J Med. 2015;128(11):e1–2.
19. Weinstein RS, Waer AL, Weinstein JB, Briehl MM, Holcomb MJ, Erps KA, Holtrust AL, Tomkins JM, Barker GP, Krupinski EA. Second Flexner Century: the democratization of medical knowledge: repurposing a general pathology course into multigrade-level "gateway" courses. Acad Pathol. 2017;4:2374289517718872.
20. Kohn LT, Corrigan J, Donaldson MS. To err is human: building a safer health system. Washington, DC: National academy press; 2000.
21. Berwick DM. A user's manual for the IOM's 'Quality Chasm' report. Health Aff. 2002;21(3):80–90.
22. Knebel E, Greiner AC, editors. Health professions education: a bridge to quality. Washington, DC: National Academies Press; 2003.
23. McDonald CJ, Weiner M, Hui SL. Deaths due to medical errors are exaggerated in Institute of Medicine report. JAMA. 2000;284(1):93–5.
24. Makary MA, Daniel M. Medical error—the third leading cause of death in the US. BMJ. 2016;353:i2139.
25. Rodwin BA, Bilan VP, Merchant NB, Steffens CG, Grimshaw AA, Bastian LA, Gunderson CG. Rate of preventable mortality in hospitalized patients: a systematic review and meta-analysis. J Gen Intern Med. 2020;21:1–8.
26. Latifi R. The modern hospital: patients centered, disease based, research oriented, technology driven. New York: Springer; 2019.
27. Primer: PCORI Background, Funding Streams, and Reauthorization. www.pipcpatients.org/blog/primer-pcori-background-funding-streams-and-reauthorization. Last accessed 2 Feb 2020.
28. Clancy C, Collins FS. Patient-Centered Outcomes Research Institute: the intersection of science and health care. Sci Transl Med. 2010;2(37):37cm18.
29. Washington AE, Lipstein SH. The Patient-Centered Outcomes Research Institute—promoting better information, decisions, and health. N Engl J Med. 2011;365:e31. https://doi.org/10.1056/NEJMp1109407.
30. Selby JV, Lipstein SH. PCORI at 3 years—progress, lessons, and plans. N Engl J Med. 2014;370(7):592–5.
31. Greenwald P, Cullen JW. The scientific approach to cancer control. CA Cancer J Clin. 1984;34(6):328–32.
32. Devita V, ed. Cancer control objectives for the nation: 1985–2000. NCI Monogr. 1986;(2):vii.
33. National Institutes of Health (NIH) Funding: FY 1994-FY 2020. Updated January 22, 2020. https://fas.org/sgp/crs/misc/R43341.pdf. Last accessed 2 Feb 2020.
34. Flay BR, Biglan A, Boruch RF, et al. Standards of evidence: criteria for efficacy, effectiveness and dissemination. Prev Sci. 2005;6:151–75. https://doi.org/10.1007/s11121-005-5553-y.
35. Kilbourne AM, Neumann MS, Pincus HA, Bauer MS, Stall R. Implementing evidence-based interventions in health care: application of the replicating effective programs framework. Implement Sci. 2007;2(1):42.
36. PCORI Board of Governors. https://www.pcori.org/about-us/governance/board-governors. Last accessed 2 Feb 2020.

37. What & Who We Fund. www.pcori.org/funding-opportunities/what-who-we-fund. Last accessed 2 Feb 2020.
38. About Our Research. www.pcori.org/research-results/about-our-research. Last accessed 23 Feb 2020.
39. Explore Our Portfolio of Funded Projects. https://www.pcori.org/research-results?f%5B0%5D=field_project_type%3A298. Last accessed 22 Jan 2020.
40. PCORI Help Center. https://help.pcori.org/hc/en-us/requests/new. Last accessed 2 Feb 2020.
41. PCORI Research Spotlight on Telehealth. https://www.pcori.org/sites/default/files/PCORI-Research-Spotlight-Telehealth.pdf. Last accessed 2 Feb 2020.
42. Telehealth-related PCORI-Funded Research Projects. https://www.pcori.org/topics/telehealth/telehealth-related-pcori-funded-research-projects. Last accessed 2 Feb 2020.
43. Closed PCORI Funding Announcements. https://www.pcori.org/funding-opportunities/awardee-resources/closed-pcori-funding-announcements. Last accessed 2 Feb 2020.
44. PCORI-Frequently Asked Questions. https://www.pcori.org/research-results/peer-review/peer-review-faq. Last accessed 24 Feb 2020.
45. PCORI Public Access to Journal Articles Presenting Findings from PCORI-Funded Research Policy. https://www.pcori.org/sites/default/files/PCORI-Policy-Public-Access-to-Journal-Articles-Presenting-Findings-from-PCORI-funded-Research.pdf. Last accessed 24 Feb 2020.
46. Journal Citation Reports. https://clarivate.com/webofsciencegroup/solutions/journal-citation-reports/. Last accessed 24 Feb 2020.
47. A Comparative Trial of Improving Care for Underserved Asian-Americans Infected with HBV. https://www.pcori.org/research-results/2014/comparative-trial-improving-care-under-served-asian-americans-infected-hbv. Last accessed 2 Feb 2020.
48. Healthcare Delivery and Disparities Research. www.pcori.org/about-us/our-programs/health-care-delivery-and-disparities-research. Last accessed 3 Feb 2020.
49. Keller AC, Flagg R, Keller J, Ravi S. Impossible politics? PCORI and the search for publicly funded comparative effectiveness research in the United States. J Health Polit Policy Law. 2019;44(2):221–65.
50. PCORI Statement on Congressional Reauthorization of Funding. https://www.pcori.org/news-release/pcori-statement-congressional-reauthorization-funding. Last accessed 3 Feb 2020.
51. Mental Health Disparities. https://www.ncbi.nlm.nih.gov/pmc/articles/PMC2759796/. Last accessed 3 Feb 2020.
52. FastStats – Leading Causes of Death. www.cdc.gov/nchs/fastats/leading-causes-of-death.htm. Last accessed 3 Feb 2020.
53. Weinstein RS, Holcomb MJ. Select healthcare transformation library. Healthcare Transform Artif Intell Autom Robot. 2020. https://doi.org/10.1089/hwR.2019.0009.

Open Access This chapter is licensed under the terms of the Creative Commons Attribution 4.0 International License (http://creativecommons.org/licenses/by/4.0/), which permits use, sharing, adaptation, distribution and reproduction in any medium or format, as long as you give appropriate credit to the original author(s) and the source, provide a link to the Creative Commons license and indicate if changes were made.

The images or other third party material in this chapter are included in the chapter's Creative Commons license, unless indicated otherwise in a credit line to the material. If material is not included in the chapter's Creative Commons license and your intended use is not permitted by statutory regulation or exceeds the permitted use, you will need to obtain permission directly from the copyright holder.

Standards and Guidelines in Teleheatlh: Creating a Compliance and Evidence-Based Telehealth Practice

Nina M. Antoniotti

How does a clinician new to Telehealth know how to practice via Telehealth? What are the standards by which a clinician is guided through a visit with a patient in traditional Telehealth, remote patient monitoring, or store-and-forward consultations? Where does one even go for such guidance?

These are the questions often posed to a clinician when he or she wants to start using Telehealth. These questions also get asked when a provider or health care organization who has been using Telehealth starts to bill for services. Oftentimes, the standard of care is not being met, due only to the lack of awareness that services delivered via telehealth are exactly the same as in-person care when it comes to standards of care. Telehealth is not a lower standard of care, nor does it demand a higher standard of care. Simply put, whatever is the standard of care for in-person services is the standard of care when those same services are delivered via Telehealth. For services that have been designed in the last decade as a new form of Telehealth, such as remote patient monitoring, brief video check-ins, or the use of patient portals for exchanging patient generated data, standards are developed as the industry and the service gains more experience.

Evidence-Based Practice

Masic et al. in 2008 indicated that "evidence-based medicine (EBM) is the conscientious, explicit, judicious and reasonable use of modern, best evidence in making decisions about the care of individual patients." Prior to evidence-based medicine, clinicians used their best guess based on literature, studies, and common practice of the day, to treat patients in a way that would hopefully produce the best outcomes.

N. M. Antoniotti (✉)
Interoperability and Patient Engagement, St. Jude Children's Research Hospital, Memphis, TN, USA
e-mail: nina@ninaantoniotti.com

© Springer Nature Switzerland AG 2021
R. Latifi et al. (eds.), *Telemedicine, Telehealth and Telepresence*,
https://doi.org/10.1007/978-3-030-56917-4_7

Memphis, Without the intent to do harm, many clinicians simply were not practicing based on scientific studies, and even some scientific studies were not rigorous enough on which to base clinical decisions about treatments or interventions for patients. Evidence-based medicine brought to the table a new approach for decision-making for clinicians, based on integrating their clinical experience, the wishes of the patient, and scientific research studies' outcomes, that promoted the best possible decisions. Often there is a gap between research and practice, with as much as 10 years span between the published results of scientific studies and the incorporation of those results into practice [1].

Evidence-based medicine is also predicated on the use of meta-analysis and a much more stringent method of analyzing results, giving rise to a higher level of evidence which lends to a higher level of care and clinical outcomes. As the researchers indicated in Masic et al. "[evidence-based medicine] requires a bottom up approach that integrates the best external evidence with individual clinical expertise and patients' choice, it cannot result in slavish, cookbook approaches to individual patient care."

The issue of quality in health care also impacts the concept of standards or guidelines. The early efforts in studying health care quality were born from the surgical disciplines. Essentially, surgeons wanted to understand why their patients died when death was not the expected outcome. Ernest Amory Codman, MD, a surgeon who worked at Massachusetts General Hospital, provided the first evidence of a patient database where specific factors and information about patients were collected. Dr. Codman kept a file card on every patient that included information such as demographics, diagnosis, treatment, and what happened to the patient [2]. Dr. Codman believed that unless he understood fully what was happening to and inside his patients as a result of treatments the patient received, he would not know how to improve his patient's outcomes. As a result, Codman and co-surgeon Edward Martin started the American College of Surgeons (ACS) in an effort to study outcomes and created committees to study the specific impact of standardizing care in certain patients. Dr. Codman is referred to as the founder of outcomes studies and evidence-based medicine and believed that it is the duty of hospitals to have follow-up systems to educate and inform other clinicians in order to improve quality and outcomes [3]. In addition, Florence Nightingale was credited with improving infection and loss of limb rates in the Crimean War by implementing sterilization of instruments and standardizing and educating nurses on nursing practice [4].

There is a fundamental difference between evidence-based practice and traditional medical practice and the issue is not that one is right and one is wrong. The difference is that evidence-based practice relies on a meta-analysis of all the best practices coupled with population-health specific data that has been collected and analyzed over years to produce the best predictable results for specific diagnoses, prognoses, and interventions and therapies provided to the patient population. Access to such information and the use of evidence in medical decision-making is the fundamental difference between evidence-based practice and traditional medicine. Clinicians who aim to be evidence-based in their practices have three tasks.

First, to use evidence summaries in clinical practice; second, to help develop and update selected systematic reviews or evidence-based guidelines in their area of expertise; and third, to enroll patients in studies of treatment, diagnosis, and prognosis on which medical practice is based [1].

Current Approaches to Standards and Guidelines

Standards and Guidelines in health care have long been the directives to clinicians and, subsequently, organizations to help clinicians treat and manage patients. In a report published by the Institute of Medicine in 1990, a taxonomy of standards was developed that remains principally the guidance for medical practice. This taxonomy has been adopted by other health care professions as well. The taxonomy includes:

1. Medical (or clinical) practice guidelines: systematically developed statements to assist practitioners in their decision-making in specific clinical settings.
2. Medical review criteria: statements used to assess the appropriateness of specific decisions, services, and outcomes in the delivery of health care.
3. Performance measures: specific measures of a quantitative nature that estimate or monitor compliance with medical quality standards, medical practice guidelines, and medical review criteria by health care professionals [5].

Standards by definition are something established by authority, custom, or general consent as a model or example [6]. Standards in clinical practice, regardless of the discipline, are typically set by consensus of an authoritative body on the evidence presented on a particular therapy, intervention, population-specific approach, drug therapies, surgical procedures, etc. A standard is considered the highest achievable level of care delivered, thus "the gold standard." Whereas a guideline is a general rule, principle, or advice that indicates or outlines policy or conduct [7]. Standards outline best practice and are the target for clinical decision-making. Guidelines outline the method by which best practice could be attained. Standards are meant to be followed closely, whereas guidelines are meant to be followed and individualized to the patient's situation.

Standards are set by such agencies and the Centers for Medicare and Medicaid, the Institute of Medicine, the National Institute of Medicine, the Centers for Disease Control, and the Agency for Health Care Research and Quality (government agencies). Private and public organizations such as the Institute for Clinical Systems Improvement (ICSI), the National Committee on Quality Assurance (NCQA), the National Quality Forum, the Joint Commission, the Commonwealth Fund, and the Leapfrog Group help to set standards of care as well. In addition, many for-profit consulting groups have taken on quality and assist organizations in achieving quality standards. These groups include such entities as Kaiser Permanente Medical Group (KPMG), Price-Gainey, and the Utilization Review Accreditation Committee (URAC).

It is important to also discuss the role of accreditation and certification within the concepts of standards and guidelines. Accreditation is the action or process of officially recognizing someone as having a particular status or being qualified to perform a particular activity, and with an acknowledgement of the person or entity's responsibility for or achievement of something [8]. A certification is the action or process of providing someone or something with an official document attesting to a status or level of achievement [9]. Accreditation is typically an annual or time-based achievement that must be renewed and requires a rigorous assessment and application process that results in an onsite evaluation process. Levels of accreditation may be given including sanctions or "findings" where the entity does not achieve specific standards. Certification is typically a one-time event that may or may not require renewal or retesting. Accreditation is given by a formal body such as the Joint Commission, and certification is typically awarded by an education institution or for-profit certifying body such as URAC.

There are two types of certifications, one a legal status awarded by a licensing or educational body for the purposes of practicing in a specialty such as pharmacy technician, psychiatric nurse practitioner, etc., and certification which shows that a person has attained a particular skill not necessarily required for a job but does make that person more attractive in skill set for a position. Such certifications include advanced life support or certifications in using a particular technology or software.

Position Statements

"A position statement is similar to a thesis or goal. It describes one side of an arguable viewpoint. When writing a position statement, the author(s) gather a list of reasons to support a particular viewpoint and make their stand clear to the audience" [10]. Position statements are often authored and issued by professional organizations who desire to make public their stand on certain issues, political, professional, operational, or legal. Health care professional associations often issue position statements (also called policy statements) on practices, therapies, or interventions, that have not risen to the standard of care but show promise, cause harm, or are in conflict or collaboration with other positions the professional organization has taken. Position statements help to set guidelines for practice when formal standards or guidelines have not been established.

The History of Standards and Guidelines in Telehealth

The first formal use of Telehealth in the United States was in Nebraska in 1954, between the Nebraska Psychiatric Institute and seven hospitals in Nebraska, Iowa, North and South Dakota. This network provided lectures with experts where the audience could ask questions. In addition, the network was used to connect the

Nebraska Psychiatric Institute with Norfolk State Hospital, to provide consultations and supervision of students, for the purposes of education and patient care. This linkage spans 112 miles and was one of the first networks to use "telepsychiatry." Over the next two decades, many other early projects were successful in demonstrating the use of a value of a distant care strategy including the same Nebraska project expanding to the Veterans Administration around Nebraska, Dartmouth Medical School and a rural hospital, and Massachusetts General Hospital and Logan Airport Medical Station in Boston [11].

These early programs were developed in a world where there were no practice standards or guidelines, no technology compatibility, and essentially, no agreement on how anything actually should have worked. The early programs were designed to test the effectiveness of using telemedicine to educate clinicians and care for patients. The question was "Does it actually work?" As the Federal government started to fund more programs in the early 1990s through grants from the Office for the Advancement of Telehealth (OAT), the focus began to shift from feasibility to sustainability. By 1997, telemedicine grant funding agencies were looking for lessons learned, best practices, and business planning for sustainability.

In 1997, the Balanced Budget Act formalized the concept that telemedicine was equal to in-person care for the purposes of payment for services delivered to Medicare beneficiaries [12]. Many states' Medicaid agencies and some private health plans were early adopters of telemedicine access and had payment policies already in place for their enrollees in health plan products, both Medicaid and commercial. As payment policies for telemedicine began to advance and calls for expanded reimbursement from telemedicine provider organizations began to be heard, the notion concept of telemedicine standards started to evolve. In addition, once CMS began to use the physician fee schedule as a modality to add new CPT codes to the list of approved Telehealth CPT codes, the need for guidelines and standards became even more important to prove Category II evidence. As the internet became more stable, affordable, and available, the rise of legitimate and not-so-legitimate telemedicine providers solidified the need for guidelines and standards. The professional organizations had also recognized the need for standards and guidelines and began to publish position papers in lieu of the needed evidence for a standard or guideline.

Along the way, in the 2000s, many scientific articles from research studies on telemedicine patient satisfaction, diagnostic accuracy, comparisons to in-person care, comparisons to no care, and other more specific telemedicine studies gave rise to the evidence needed to begin to write actual guidelines and standards. The early studies prior to the new century supported the use of telemedicine from a feasibility, practicality, and patient satisfaction standpoint, but did little to validate the standard of care experienced via telemedicine. The studies conducted in the early part of the new century gave rise to the evidence needed to support a standard of care that stated telemedicine encounters were at minimum equal to in-person care.

However, determining standards of care via telemedicine is not a simple task, as there are many modalities of telemedicine, different professional groups and clinicians who use telemedicine, different technologies, and different clinical outcomes desired. How then does one develop standards and guidelines for telemedicine? Krupinski states that "improving performance and accountability depends on having a shared goal that unites the interests and activities of all stakeholders" [13]. In developing a standard or guideline as an approach in health care, one must have a consensus of the experts that the standard or guideline as written supports agreement that the practice is safe, effective, can be used in most populations as intended, and legitimate, as well as should be held out as the attainable goal for anyone using that practice. The same is true for telemedicine.

Early work in position statements for telemedicine came from professional associations and other entities including the American College of Radiology (first in standards for teleradiology), the American Medical Association (one of the first on positions regarding telemedicine in general), and the European Code of Practice for Telehealth (one of the first international position papers on telemedicine and telehealth).

The early work in standards and guidelines was done by the American Telemedicine Association's (ATA) Standards and Guidelines Committee. The ATA's approach to development of standards and guidelines early on was to create Telemedicine Practice Standards based on the administrative, clinical, and technical approach to telemedicine by an organization (core standards) and telemedicine by specialty (Diabetic retinopathy, Dermatology, Psychiatry, and Mental Health). The first publication from ATA in the way of standards was the ATA Ocular Telehealth Special Interest Group's (SIG) guidelines for diabetic retinopathy. These guidelines set a standard for those who wished to use retinal imaging for screening patients at risk for early blindness from diabetes. The SIG effort in writing these standards identified a need to be reasonable and flexible in the standards and guidelines approach and to consider standards and guidelines as "required when feasible or practical" [14]. In addition, what became clear was the need to set a standard for wording in terms of how strongly should a person comply with the requirements of a standard or guideline when using telemedicine. *Shall, should, and may* were chosen as words to describe such responsibility of a program or clinician using telemedicine. *Shall* denotes the requirement is a requirement with no ability of the program or clinician to bend such rules. *Should* denotes a requirement that practitioners and organization strive to meet the standard, but some conditions might be present where full attainment of the standard is not achievable. *May* denotes a condition which makes a program or clinician's telemedicine initiative better and is good for the program but not required to meet the standard or guideline. For instance, a telemedicine program shall comply with all legal and regulatory requirements for patient safety, privacy, and confidentiality. There are no situations where a telemedicine program could skimp on these requirements. Therefore, the word *should* or *may* would never be used in the standard or guideline. Another example: A telemedicine program shall use H323 video connections through a 1.5 meg ISP connection. This standard could not be applied in all situations, and clinicians and programs could never meet this

7 Standards and Guidelines in Teleheatlh: Creating a Compliance and… 103

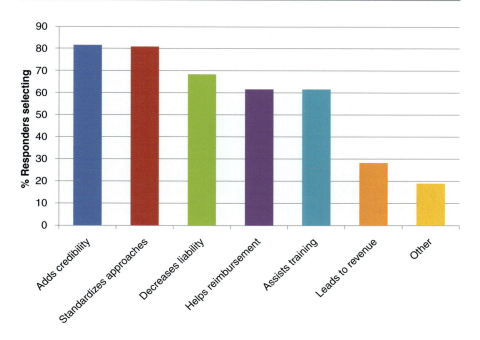

Fig. 7.1 Survey responses to why telemedicine should have guidelines. Responders could provide more than one response [15]

standard when the word *shall* is in place. *May* would be a more appropriate word to use for a standard that denotes technology requirements.

The question then becomes "why do we need standards and guidelines in telemedicine and telehealth?" Krupinski indicates through a survey conducted by the ATA's Standards and Guidelines Committee that people believed that standards and guidelines for telemedicine and telehealth added credibility, standardized approaches, decreased liability, assisted with training, and helped to increase reimbursement and revenue. Figure 7.1 shows the distribution of answers as to the reason standards and guidelines are valuable, and Fig. 7.2 shows the distribution of answers as to how standards and guidelines were used by the respondents. Antoniotti's research in 2002 in the publication "Rural Populations' Perceptions of the Institute of Medicine's Six Chasms of Quality" showed that rural populations are confident in the care they receive from their clinicians when those clinicians are practicing with quality and standards in mind.

The collaborative model used by ATA for consensus in building support from other professional associations such as the Association for Speech, Language, and Hearing and the American Academy of Dermatology led other associations to begin to develop their own set of standards and guidelines specific to the specialty practice. As more professional associations began their own collaborative efforts to write standards and guidelines for telemedicine practice, ATA's efforts became less important in the industry as others took up the charge.

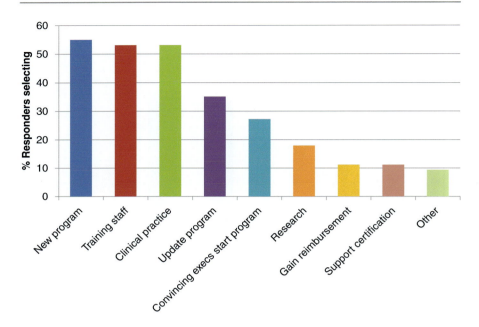

Fig. 7.2 Survey responses regarding top uses of guidelines. Responders could select more than one response [15]

Developing Standards and Guideline

As discussed earlier, standards and guidelines are based on a body of scientifically proven evidence that supports a particular method or approach to caring for patients (in the context of telemedicine). When such evidence was lacking, position papers were used to inform, educate, and guide clinicians and organizations in developing and implementing telemedicine. As the body of evidence grew, the feasibility of writing such standards and guidelines also grew.

Today, efforts to develop standards and guidelines follow a trajectory that includes purposeful steps to review the published scientific studies, quasi-studies, published articles, and opinion pieces, takes that published information, and applies a strict set of rules on how to determine strength and validity of the information. Most commonly used is the American Psychiatry Association's (APA) Practice Guideline development, which has a coding method for ranking a study on strength and validity [16].

The first step is to assemble a committee to write the standard or guideline, or in some cases a consensus document or position statement. The committee should ideally be a crossrepresentation of stakeholders in the specialty or telemedicine topic for which the standard is needed. In addition, inviting a wider participation from stakeholders outside of the organization, specialty group, or professional association produces greater consensus, a more valid product, a more generalizable document, and typically stands the test of time.

The committee then gathers and reviews the literature. Sometimes, a committee will appoint two or three members to gather, review, and score the literature. Scoring using APA's methods is not mandatory but does lend some validity to the selection of published studies and papers that support the end-product itself. The committee must decide on a method to identify legitimate published data that will be used to write the standards and guidelines. Even the true-and-tried "sniff test" is a process.

Once the literature is reviewed, and those results are identified as having results worthy of analysis for a standard or guideline, the committee's job is then to simply write the document. As the document is written, either in a workshop with all members present, or written part by part from different initial authors, or written by a writing subgroup, the initial document is written and cited with the literature chosen as the support for the actual standard or guideline being written. The committee reads and revises until a final draft is secured.

The decision as to whether or not the evidence used supports a standard (gold benchmark), a guideline (general rule), or a position paper (consensus of the experts on how to proceed). Once that determination is made, the document then would be named as such—a practice standard, a practice guideline, or a position statement on *xyz*.

Once the document is done, it is prudent for the authoring body to then shop the document to an even wider group of reviewers or to use a public comment period to get additional input on the standard or guideline. These efforts are useful to again run the agreed upon standard or guideline through a rigorous process of review and approval to gain validity and consensus throughout the industry. ATA's process for developing and getting to consensus on standards and guidelines is shown in Fig. 7.3.

Current Landscape for Telemedicine Standards and Guidelines

Today, standards and guidelines for telemedicine are as important as ever. With the increasing use of telemedicine, with telemedicine being a $4 billion-dollar investor industry, and the legal and regulatory environment tightening while reimbursement is loosening, standards are going to be the way organizations and clinicians justify the use of telemedicine, the modality being used, and technology and telecommunications deployment. With more and more start-ups filling the market with new and old ways of connecting with patients, and profits becoming more important to companies than quality patient care, the use of standards and guidelines to plan, develop, and implement a high-quality program is imperative. Congressional reaction to death, disruption of health care, illegal dispensing of prescriptions, etc., has been harsh, with restrictive legislative mandates that impede the progress of quality telemedicine programs. In addition, private for-profit companies' lobbying efforts impact the ability of the primary care and specialty provider in a multi-disciplinary practice to again, effectively move and expand a telemedicine program.

There are a variety of standards and guidelines that are consensus documents, that have been vetted properly, that are up-to-date, and should be in place to guide and maintain a telemedicine program.

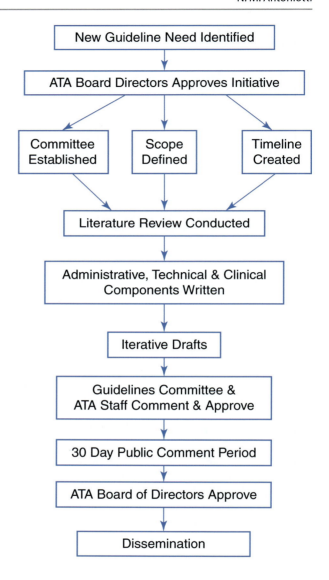

Fig. 7.3 Schematic of the ATA Guidelines development process [14]

Professional Associations

As of the date of this writing, the following professional associations have telemedicine standards or position statements. The reader would be wise to look up these and other references, ensure the copy is current, and use those references as a template to build the telemedicine program, and then use those resources as a guide for audits, accreditation, and certifications, especially for CMS and the Joint Commission.

American Medical Association
1. Ethical Practice in Telemedicine—also found at the end of the chapter [17].
2. "Your Questions Answered about Telemedicine"—a dynamic and up-to-date FAQ on telemedicine from AMA's point of view [18].
3. 50-state survey: Establishment of a patient–physician relationship via telemedicine. Establishes when a patient–physician relationship is established via telemedicine and is a position paper. This type of document is published by many different organizations, some of which are in error. One must always check the validity of the information in the document. These documents are good resources for getting started but are only a snapshot in time. The documents typically have links to original legislation and are a good place to start to find current information for each state. Be wary of statements that a particular state has a parity law. One must look up the parity law and read specific language to know if indeed, the law actually provides for parity.
4. Opinion 1.2.12, Physician Advisory or Referral Services by Telecommunication 2017. Defines and describes practice guidelines for telemedicine.

American Academy of Dermatology
1. Position Statement on Teledermatology (Approved by the Board of Directors: February 22, 2002; Amended by the Board of Directors: May 22, 2004; November 9, 2013; August 9, 2014; May 16, 2015; March 7, 2016). Defines and provides guidelines for TeleDermatology

American Academy of Family Practice
1. Telehealth and Telemedicine Policy and Position Statement—defines telemedicine and outlines good practice standards.

The Joint Commission
1. Environment of Care Standards
2. Element of Performance Standards
3. Medical Staff Services Standards
4. Leadership Standards
5. Others as updated annually

American Speech-Language-Hearing Association
1. TelePractice—overview and recommendations for Speech, Language, and Hearing professionals using Telehealth or telemedicine.

American Telemedicine Association
1. Standards Framework—Document that describes best in practice and evidence-based practice for telemedicine and telehealth 2017. Good working tool for starting and annual review of telemedicine programs.
2. Other specialty specific standards. ATA members have authored many practice guidelines since 2002 and have those guidelines available online. Many have not been updated since the original writing. However, these guidelines serve as a good resource for starting specialty telemedicine programs such as TelePsychiatry, Online TelePsychiatry, Tele-ICU, Tele-Urgent Care (DTC), etc.

Certification Pros and Cons

Today's telehealth and telemedicine environment has brought to the fore the certification question. For many years, telemedicine programs, telemedicine associations, and professional groups put little value in certification. However, once telemedicine became mainstream and was integrated into the way health care organizations did business, and the direct-to-consumer market took off, for-profit certification groups began to write their own standards and for a fee provide certification to telemedicine programs. In addition, certifications for telepresenters and site coordinators began to pop up from the Telehealth Resource Centers as a means to drive revenue. Online companies such as StarInstitute, a part of New College Institute, developed online certification courses that too 3–5 hours at a cost of $299 [18]. What basis, information, research, or best practice these certification programs are built upon is largely unknown.

Today, certification is a marketing and branding tool used in areas where there is heavy competition for patients or where status is valuable. There is little or no value in certification for telemedicine programs as such certification costs money, takes valuable resource time, and does little to improve patient care via telemedicine. Most programs simply start, run, and maintain a telemedicine program without certification, and most of the best programs in the country do not have certification.

Standard of Care

The question then becomes "what is the standard of care?" The standard of care for any telemedicine encounter is the same standard of care for in-person care by that specialty, profession, or function. A cardiologist has an ethical, moral, and practice responsibility to the patient to provide all components of a history and physical exam pertinent to the patient's condition. Those requirements do not change if the patient is seen via telemedicine. A psychiatrist has the same responsibility to the patient for safety and privacy when seen via telemedicine as the psychiatrist would have if the patient were in their office. No one practices telemedicine. Health care professionals practice dermatology and cardiology and neonatology and pediatrics. The same standards of care apply to these disciplines the same as in-person care.

A state will have standards of care for neonatal ICUs that must be followed when TeleNeonatology is used. The Joint Commission has standards on how to protect patient privacy that should be followed when a patient is seen via telemedicine. Professional associations have position statements on evidence-based care that must be followed when practicing via telemedicine. There is no certification program that can certify that a telemedicine provider is following a standard of care, as standards of care vary with each discipline, patient problem, patient location, and state of practice. Many telemedicine programs make this issue of standard of care more complicated than it needs to be. Simply put, the standard of care is the same as in-person care. If a program provides all the elements of care required from a legal and practice standpoint, then the standard of care is met. If a cardiologist is seeing patiets via telemedicine and does not have a digital electronic stethoscope to use, then the standard of care is not being met.

Writing Your Own Standards

What if the care or model of care desired is so innovative that no opinions, position statements, consensus documents, guidelines, or standards exist? The program still needs to compile the evidence that what is being proposed or done is safe, sound, generalizable to a larger population, and meets standards of care for in-person care. Gathering any scientific studies, pro or con, and authoring guidelines for what is being proposed based on the approaches outlined in this chapter puts the telemedicine initiative in a much better place than just "winging it!" Having explicit policies and procedures as to how the care delivery mechanism works (technology, connectivity, compliance with privacy and security regulations), what data is or is not stored, who can deliver the service, who can access the service, how is the care documented and shared with patient or others, helps to validate and document the organization's approach to quality care. The organization's documents serve as their "standards" for using telemedicine and engaging patients in health professions' practice. These documents should go through the approval process using the Medical Records Committees, Medical Staff Services, the Medical Executive Committee (or similar committees) for validation.

Once the policies and procedures are written and "guidelines" are documented, expanding the documents to a wider audience that may include professional associations, payers, or government review agencies such as the Quality and Payment side of Medicaid and the state's Office of Insurance Commissioner, and other telemedicine programs, helps to ensure due diligence in the review process. Consensus is the key to justifying the approach used in an innovative care delivery strategy via telemedicine that has no standards, guidelines, or evidence in the literature. Important also is to document and have retrievable information on any feasibility or pilot studies done to document efficacy and safety of the innovative telemedicine approach being taken.

Other Issues Not Necessarily Standards

When telemedicine providers or programs start, there are many legal and regulatory requirements not necessarily considered "standards or guidelines" but, nonetheless, are rules that need to be followed. Interstate health professions licensure, credentialing for practice and payment, scope of practice, supervision requirements, and e-prescribing and dispensing of medications are all requirements that must be evaluated for each telemedicine initiative. Payment and reimbursement are often tied to government regulations, scope of practice, and supervision requirements and also must be considered in the context of guidelines.

Summary

A prudent telemedicine initiative follows many of these recommendations for setting up a telemedicine program from a business need, a market need, and collects as many standards, guidelines, and position statements as are available pertinent to the program being developed. A thorough review of those standards, particularly those associated with professional practice, will assist the telemedicine program in having a high standard of care delivered via telemedicine. Setting up a telecardiology program without a digital electronic stethoscope at the patient site simply does not meet the standard of care. And unfortunately, there are some telemedicine programs who do exactly that. What happens in-person should happen over telemedicine when conducting a history and physical exam of the patient in order to meet the standard of care.

Addendum: American Medical Association Code of Medical Ethics Opinion 1.2.12 Ethical Practice in Telemedicine

Innovation in technology, including information technology, is redefining how people perceive time and distance. It is reshaping how individuals interact with and relate to others, including when, where, and how patients and physicians engage with one another.

Telehealth and telemedicine span a continuum of technologies that offer new ways to deliver care. Yet as in any mode of care, patients need to be able to trust that physicians will place patient welfare above other interests, provide competent care, provide the information patients need to make well-considered decisions about care, respect patient privacy and confidentiality, and take steps to ensure continuity of care. Although physicians' fundamental ethical responsibilities do not change, the continuum of possible patient–physician interactions in telehealth/telemedicine gives rise to differing levels of accountability for physicians.

All physicians who participate in telehealth/telemedicine have an ethical responsibility to uphold fundamental fiduciary obligations by disclosing any financial or other interests the physician has in the telehealth/telemedicine application or service and taking steps to manage or eliminate conflicts of interests. Whenever they provide health information, including health content for websites or mobile health applications, physicians must ensure that the information they provide or that is attributed to them is objective and accurate.

Similarly, all physicians who participate in telehealth/telemedicine must assure themselves that telemedicine services have appropriate protocols to prevent unauthorized access and to protect the security and integrity of patient information at the patient end of the electronic encounter, during transmission, and among all health care professionals and other personnel who participate in the telehealth/telemedicine service consistent with their individual roles.

Physicians who respond to individual health queries or provide personalized health advice electronically through a telehealth service in addition should:

(a) Inform users about the limitations of the relationship and services provided.
(b) Advise site users about how to arrange for needed care when follow-up care is indicated.
(c) Encourage users who have primary care physicians to inform their primary physicians about the online health consultation, even if in-person care is not immediately needed.

Physicians who provide clinical services through telehealth/telemedicine must uphold the standards of professionalism expected in in-person interactions, follow appropriate ethical guidelines of relevant specialty societies, and adhere to applicable law governing the practice of telemedicine. In the context of telehealth/telemedicine, they further should

(d) Be proficient in the use of the relevant technologies and comfortable interacting with patients and/or surrogates electronically.
(e) Recognize the limitations of the relevant technologies and take appropriate steps to overcome those limitations. Physicians must ensure that they have the information they need to make well-grounded clinical recommendations when they cannot personally conduct a physical examination, such as by having another health care professional at the patient's site conduct the exam or obtaining vital information through remote technologies.
(f) Be prudent in carrying out a diagnostic evaluation or prescribing medication by:
    - Establishing the patient's identity
    - Confirming that telehealth/telemedicine services are appropriate for that patient's individual situation and medical needs
    - Evaluating the indication, appropriateness, and safety of any prescription in keeping with best practice guidelines and any formulary limitations that apply to the electronic interaction
    - Documenting the clinical evaluation and prescription
(g) When the physician would otherwise be expected to obtain informed consent, tailor the informed consent process to provide information patients (or their surrogates) need about the distinctive features of telehealth/telemedicine, in addition to information about medical issues and treatment options. Patients and surrogates should have a basic understanding of how telemedicine technologies will be used in care, the limitations of those technologies, the credentials of health care professionals involved, and what will be expected of patients for using these technologies.
(h) As in any patient–physician interaction, take steps to promote continuity of care, giving consideration to how information can be preserved and accessible for future episodes of care in keeping with patients' preferences (or the decisions of their surrogates) and how follow-up care can be provided when needed. Physicians should assure themselves how information will be conveyed to the patient's primary care physician when the patient has a primary care physician and to other physicians currently caring for the patient.

Collectively, through their professional organizations and health care institutions, physicians should:

(i) Support ongoing refinement of telehealth/telemedicine technologies, and the development and implementation of clinical and technical standards to ensure the safety and quality of care.
(j) Advocate for policies and initiatives to promote access to telehealth/telemedicine services for all patients who could benefit from receiving care electronically.

(k) Routinely monitor the telehealth/telemedicine landscape to:
- Identify and address adverse consequences as technologies and activities evolve
- Identify and encourage dissemination of both positive and negative outcomes

References

1. Masic I, Miokovic M, Muhamedagic B. Evidence based medicine – new approaches and challenges. Acta Inform Med. 2008;16(4):219–25. Published online 2008 Dec. https://doi.org/10.5455/aim.2008.16.219-225.
2. Donabedian A. The end results of health care: Ernest Codman's contribution to quality assessment and beyond. Milbank Q. 1989;67(2):233–56; discussion 257–267.
3. Mallon B. Ernest Amory Codman: the end result of a life in medicine. Philadelphia: W. B. Saunders; 1999.
4. https://www.britannica.com/biography/Florence-Nightingale/Homecoming-and-legacy. Accessed online 1-10-2020.
5. Flexner A. Medical education in the United States and Canada. New York: Carnegie Foundation; 1910.
6. Merriam-Webster. Accessed online 1-10-2020 at https://www.merriam-webster.com/dictionary/standard.
7. Merriam-Webster. Accessed online 1-10-2020 at https://www.merriam-webster.com/dictionary/guideline.
8. https://www.bing.com/search?q=what+is+accreditation&form=EDGTCT&qs=DA&cvid=18 2b628a36a244e89c12e6fdcf16bc6b&refig=5a46853ff8764a46ec7e364583b8f0e8&cc=US& setlang=en-US&elv=AQj93OAhDTi*HzTv1paQdnjn17YCrDSDZ2papZZjXAjUv%21bPcS BZ98vYW5AQAGzv7vzRdW3ibSpDYBXc4dV8bvhWNaJHHq4fQ2VY5ZjgYyLa&plvar =0&PC=LCTS. Accessed online 1-10-2020.
9. https://www.google.com/search?sxsrf=ACYBGNSTeYBqizUuw14U3o1vVb_62bT7Hw% 3A1579060924583&source=hp&ei=vI4eXoiOIeq7tgW1t4rwCg&q=wjat+is+certification&oq= wjat+is+certification&gs_l=psy-ab.3..0i13l10.9113.14485..14849...2.0..0.91.1530.21......0....1.. gws-wiz.......35i39j0i67j0i131i67j0j0i131j35i305i39j0i10.zLcDgc-O0XU&ved=0ahUKEwiI3P Gr3ITnAhXqna0KHbWbAq4Q4dUDCAc&uact=5. Accessed online 1-10-2020.
10. American Academy of Ambulatory Care Nurses. https://www.aaacn.org/practice-resources/position-statements. Accessed online 1-10-2020.
11. Smith HA, Allison RA. Telemental health: delivering mental health care at a distance, a summary report. Washington, DC: US Department of Health and Human Services, Health Resources and Services Administration, Office for the Advancement of Telehealth; 1998. Also accessed online at http://nebhands.nebraska.edu/files/telemental%20health%20systems.pdf.
12. 105th United States Congress. H.R. 2015 Balanced Budget Act of 197 or Public Law No 105-33. Accessed online 1-10-2020 at https://www.congress.gov/bill/105th-congress/house-bill/2015/actions?KWICView=false.
13. Krupinski EA, Bernard J. Standards and guidelines in telemedicine and telehealth. Healthcare (Basel). 2014;2(1):74–93.
14. Krupinski EA, Bernard J. Standards and guidelines in telemedicine and telehealth. Healthcare (Basel). 2014;2(1):80.
15. Krupinski EA, Bernard J. Standards and guidelines in telemedicine and telehealth. Healthcare (Basel). 2014;2(1):85.

16. American Psychiatric Association Practice Guideline Development Process. Available online: http://psychiatryonline.org/content.aspx?bookid=28&sectionid=1674966 . Accessed online on 1-10-2020.
17. American Medical Association. https://www.ama-assn.org/delivering-care/ethics/ethical-practice-telemedicine.
18. STARHEALHT. CTC. Certified Telehealth Coordinator. Accessed online 1-10-2020 at http://www.startelehealth.org/ctc.

Federal and State Policies on Telehealth Reimbursement

8

Jordana Bernard and Mei Wa Kwong

Introduction

Over the past few years, the telehealth policy landscape has evolved as policy makers look for solutions to rising healthcare expenditures, limited healthcare resources, and the current opioid epidemic. More than ever before, legislators and regulators at both the federal and state levels have been turning to telehealth to play a greater role in both fee-for-service and transformation to value-based care. Although payer policies have been expanding, reimbursement continues to be a major barrier hindering telehealth adoption and realization of its fullest potential [1]. This chapter focuses on the current state of telehealth reimbursement policy in Medicare, Medicaid, and private plans.

> This chapter provides an overview of telehealth reimbursement policies prior to the COVID-19 pandemic. Many of the limitations on coverage and reimbursement of telehealth and other virtual care services were temporarily removed through waivers and interim rules at both the federal and state levels during the coronavirus public health emergency.

Medicare Reimbursement Policies

Medicare is the federal health insurance program that covers people who are 65 years of age or older, certain youths with disabilities, and people with end-stage-renal disease (ESRD). In 2017, Medicare's $705 billion budget covered 58 million

J. Bernard (✉)
InTouch Health, North Potomac, MD, USA

M. W. Kwong
Center for Connected Health Policy, Sacramento, CA, USA

© Springer Nature Switzerland AG 2021
R. Latifi et al. (eds.), *Telemedicine, Telehealth and Telepresence*,
https://doi.org/10.1007/978-3-030-56917-4_8

enrollees through Original Medicare (fee-for-service) which covers services and items in Medicare Part A (hospital) and B (medical) [2]. An enrollee can also receive Medicare benefits through a private, Medicare-approved private insurance company in a Medicare Advantage plan (Part C) that must cover the benefits in Medicare Part A and B, but may also offer additional benefits through supplemental plans. Medicare spending increased to $731 billion (60 million lives) in 2018 with per capita spending projected to grow at an average annual rate of 5.1% over the next 10 years (2018–2028), due to growing Medicare enrollment, increased use of services and intensity of care, and rising healthcare prices [3]. Through the use of telehealth technologies, reduced healthcare spending and cost savings can be achieved.

At the federal level, the reimbursement rules for telehealth under Medicare are defined in Section §1834(m) of the Social Security Act [4] (42 U.S.C. 1395m(m) (4)) which was created when Congress passed the Balanced Budget Act of 1997. In 2000 and 2008, Congress enacted legislation that expanded reimbursement of telehealth; however, the major constraints placed on payment of services included in the original statute remained intact. Between 2001 and 2018, under the 102nd to the 115th Congress, lawmakers introduced over 800 bills that included a provision(s) with telehealth [5] aiming to remove the existing restrictions to increase adoption (Fig. 8.1).

In 2018, Congress successfully passed telehealth legislation expanding telehealth reimbursement by enacting the Bipartisan Budget Act of 2018 (BBA) and the SUPPORT for Patients and Communities Act [6, 7]. These pieces of legislation created nationwide reimbursement for telehealth, for the first time ever, by removing the statutory "rural" geographic restriction for acute stroke, ESRD, and substance use disorders (SUDs). The BBA also expanded the use of telehealth in Medicare Advantage plans (MA) and for certain types of accountable care organizations (ACO). In an effort to further expand access to telehealth by removing the barriers to reimbursement in Medicare, Congress introduced the bipartisan, bicameral CONNECT for Health Act of 2019 in October 2019.

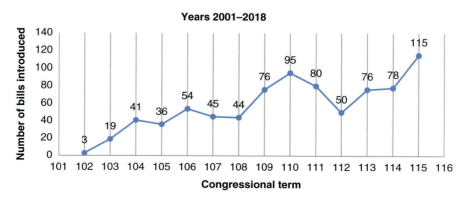

Fig. 8.1 Federal legislation with telehealth provisions introduced (102nd to 115th Congress, 2001–2018) [5]

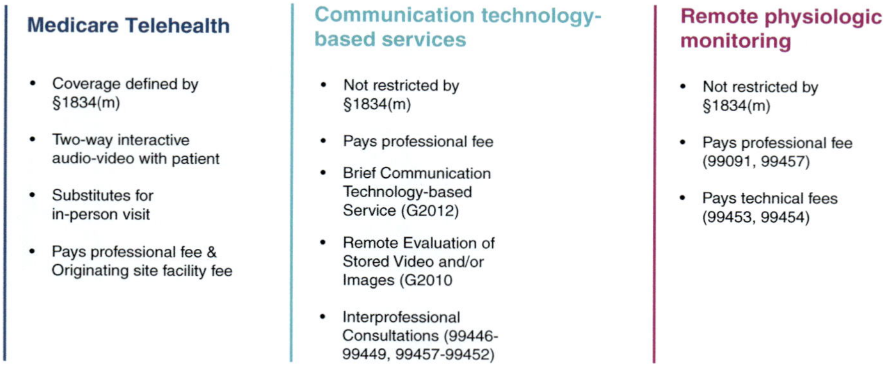

8 Federal and State Policies on Telehealth Reimbursement

Medicare Telehealth

- Coverage defined by §1834(m)
- Two-way interactive audio-video with patient
- Substitutes for in-person visit
- Pays professional fee & Originating site facility fee

Communication technology-based services

- Not restricted by §1834(m)
- Pays professional fee
- Brief Communication Technology-based Service (G2012)
- Remote Evaluation of Stored Video and/or Images (G2010
- Interprofessional Consultations (99446-99449, 99457-99452)

Remote physiologic monitoring

- Not restricted by §1834(m)
- Pays professional fee (99091, 99457)
- Pays technical fees (99453, 99454)

Fig. 8.2 CY 2019 Medicare payment categories

Current policies for reimbursement of virtual care services in Medicare fee-for-service fall into three payment categories: (1) Medicare telehealth, (2) communication technology-based services, and (3) remote physiologic monitoring. Reimbursement for Medicare telehealth services is defined by section §1834(m) in the Medicare telehealth law, whereas payments for communication technology-based services and remote physiologic monitoring are not considered to be "telehealth" by the Centers for Medicare and Medicaid (CMS), and therefore are not subject to the rural geographic, originating site, and other requirements in the statute (Fig. 8.2).

Medicare Telehealth Services

CMS reimburses Medicare telehealth services when the following requirements are met [8]:

- The originating site must be located in a defined rural geographic area,
- The Medicare beneficiary must be located in an authorized type of originating site when receiving services via telehealth,
- The healthcare practitioner providing services must be an eligible provider,
- The service provided is on the list of approved Medicare telehealth services, and
- The modality used to deliver services is two-way, interactive audio-video unless it is a demonstration project in Alaska or Hawaii in which case store-and-forward technology may be used (Fig. 8.3).

(See Table 8.1 for detailed summary of these conditions for payment of Medicare telehealth services.)

The BBA of 2018 and SUPPORT Act created exceptions to the rural geographic restriction for telestroke, ESRD, and SUD treatment services. The legislation also added mobile stroke units for treatment of acute stroke and the patient's home for ESRD and SUD treatment services as eligible originating sites. When these five

Fig. 8.3 Conditions for payment of Medicare telehealth services

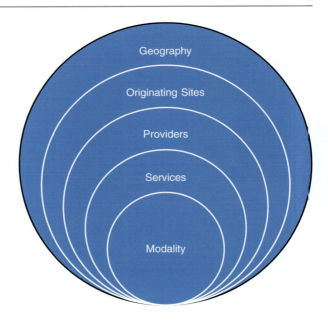

Table 8.1 2019 rules for Medicare telehealth reimbursement in fee-for-service [8]

Geographic limitation on the originating site where the patient can be located when the services take place	Rural HPSA or non-MSA Statistical area
Type of facility where the patient must be located when receiving services through telehealth	Offices of physicians or practitioners Hospitals Critical Access Hospitals Rural Health Clinics Federally Qualified Health Centers Hospital-based or CAH-based renal dialysis centers (including satellites) Skilled Nursing Facilities Community Mental Health Centers Renal Dialysis facilities (ESRD Services ONLY) Home (certain ESRD and SUD services ONLY) Mobile Stroke Units (acute stroke treatment ONLY)
Type of modality eligible to deliver the telehealth service	Live video unless it is a demonstration project in Alaska or Hawaii in which case store-and-forward was also eligible
Type of services that are reimbursed	Specific list of Medicare telehealth services noted by their CPT or HCPCS codes
Type of healthcare practitioner eligible to provide services and be reimbursed	Physicians Nurse practitioners Physician assistants Nurse midwives Clinical nurse specialists Certified registered nurse anesthetists Clinical psychologists & clinical social workers Registered dietitians or nutrition professionals

conditions for payment are met, under fee-for-service, Medicare reimburses the distant site practitioner a professional fee according to the Part B physician fee schedule and the originating site a facility fee (HCPCS code 3014). Currently, there are over 100 billing codes on the Medicare telehealth list with many describing general services that allow different specialists to be able to bill using the same code. For example, HCPCS code G0425 is a general consultation code that can be used by a stroke neurologist or a psychiatrist or cardiologist or other authorized Medicare provider for an initial visit with the patient in the emergency department, hospital inpatient setting, or skilled nursing facility. There are other codes on the list that describe more specific services such as psychotherapy and diabetes management; however, the ability to use the codes is constrained by the restrictions that are defined in the Medicare telehealth statute.

For 2020, CMS added a set of three bundled payment codes (G2086–G2088) to the Medicare telehealth list for office-based opioid use disorder treatment, as part of a monthly bundled episode of care. The bundle allows the therapy and counseling components to be delivered through telehealth without the rural restriction, and it allows services into the patient's home—both of these exceptions are the result of passage of the SUPPORT Act.

Communication Technology-Based Services

Currently, CMS reimburses for three types of communication technology-based services:

- Brief communication technology-based service—(HCPCS code G2012) Virtual check-in by a physician or other qualified healthcare professional who can report Evaluation/Management (E/M) services, provided to an established patient, not originating from a related E/M service provided within the previous 7 days nor leading to an E/M service or procedure within the next 24 hours or soonest available appointment; 5–10 minutes of medical discussion.
- Remote Evaluation of Pre-recorded Patient Information—(HCPCS code G2010) Remote evaluation of recorded video and/or images submitted by the patient (e.g., store and forward), including interpretation with verbal follow-up with the patient within 24 business hours, not originating from a related E/M service provided within the previous 7 days nor leading to an E/M service or procedure within the next 24 hours or soonest available appointment.
- Interprofessional Internet Consultation—(Current Procedural Terminology (CPT) codes 99446–99449, 99451–99452) Interprofessional telephone/Internet assessment and management service provided by a consultative physician including a verbal and written report to the patient's treating/requesting physician or other qualified healthcare professional. Commonly referred to as "eConsult" [9].

For 2020, CMS allows a single advance beneficiary patient consent for multiple communication technology-based services. In addition, CMS added reimbursement for online digital evaluation services for physicians, qualified healthcare professionals, and non-physician practitioners (eVisits) using CPT codes 99421–99423 and HCPCS G2061–G2063, respectively.

Remote Physiologic Monitoring

In 2018, CMS unbundled reimbursement (CPT code 99091) for the professional component of remote physiologic monitoring (RPM) for the first time. In 2019, CMS expanded payment for RPM professional services including reimbursement for the technical components of RPM, as well as allowing ancillary staff to provide "incident to" services under supervision of the billing provider.

- CPT code 99091 defined as the collection, interpretation of physiologic data, 30 minutes or more per 30-day period by physician or other qualified healthcare professional (QHP)
- CPT code 99453 defined as "Remote monitoring of physiologic parameter(s) (e.g., weight, blood pressure, pulse oximetry, respiratory flow rate), initial; set-up and patient education on use of equipment"
- CPT code 99454 defined as "Remote monitoring of physiologic parameter(s) (e.g., weight, blood pressure, pulse oximetry, respiratory flow rate), initial; device(s) supply with daily recording(s) or programmed alert(s) transmission, each 30 days"
- CPT code 99457 defined as "Remote physiologic monitoring treatment management services, 20 minutes or more of clinical staff/physician/other qualified healthcare professional time in a calendar month requiring interactive communication with the patient/caregiver during the month"

Beginning in 2020, CMS (1) considers RPM to be under the care management program, (2) redefines CPT code 99457 to describe the initial 20 minutes of time spent providing RPM services, (3) adds new payment code 99458 for each additional 20-minute blocks of time, and (4) allows RPM services billed "incident to" under general supervision for codes 99457 and 99458 (Fig. 8.4).

Medicare Telehealth	Brief communication technology-based services	Remote physiologic monitoring

Adds 3 bundled payment codes G2086-G2088 for treatment of opioid use disorders
 	
• Allows therapy and counselling component by telehealth
 	
• Implements SUPPORT Act, waiver of rural geographic restriction adds home as originating site
	• Adds online digital evaluation services (eVisits)
	• Patient-initiated, established patients
	• Cumulative time spent during 7-day period
	  • 99421-99423 for physicians and QHPs
	  • G2061-G2063 for non-physicians pracitioners
	• Modifiers requirement to obtain patient consent to once/yr (G2010, G2012, 99446 - 99449, 99451-99452)
		• Redefines pro fee code 99457 to describe initial 20 min
		• Adds new payment code 99458 for each addl 20 min
		• Allows RPM services billed "incident to" under general supervision for codes 99457 & 99458

Fig. 8.4 CY2020 policy changes by payment category

Medicare Capitated and Value-Based Payment

Fundamentally, telehealth can play a big role in value-based care because it allows all entities to work together to drive better, more efficient, cost-effective care. With approximately 34% of Medicare enrollment in Medicare Advantage (MA) plans (22 million beneficiaries in 2019), these plans offer the largest opportunity to leverage telehealth in a value-based payment model. Furthermore, beginning January 1, 2020, new rules defining the use of telehealth in these plans significantly improved due to passage of the MA provision in the BBA of 2018.

Historically, MA plans have been required to cover the same telehealth delivered services found in Medicare fee-for-service and with the same 1834(m) restrictions discussed above. Should the plans offer telehealth coverage that goes beyond what is in fee-for-service, the plan or the enrollee would need to cover the cost through a supplemental premium or through rebates. With passage of the BBA, MA plans have the flexibility to build additional telehealth benefits beyond what is in fee-for-service into their basic plan bids rather than requiring them to do this as supplemental benefits. Furthermore, plans have the ability to determine which services will be covered by telehealth, as long as the services are covered under Medicare [10].

Another way to leverage telehealth in the Medicare program is in Medicare ACOs (Medicare Shared Savings Program) [11]. However, the ability to use telehealth has been limited except for a few types of ACOs, such as the Next Generation ACOs. The BBA also changed this beginning January 1, 2020, when other types of performance-based ACOs were given increased flexibility to use telehealth to treat their patient populations in urban areas and at home. Under the CMS Innovation Center (CMMI), there are a number of alternative payment models that allow the use of telehealth [12]. Two bundled payment programs offer a telehealth waiver that allows providers to deliver services in urban areas and into the patient's home: (1) Comprehensive Joint Replacement (CJR) bundled payment program and (2) Bundled Payments for Care Improvement Advanced Program (BPCI Advanced) with inpatient and outpatient episodes. The Medicare Advantage Value-Based Insurance Design (VBID) model is testing increased access to telehealth services to meet requirements for provider network adequacy. Two other models launched in 2020 to pilot the use of telehealth: (1) Emergency Triage, Treatment and Transport model (ET3) for EMS personnel to use telehealth in the field as a way to prevent trips to the ED and (2) the Kidney Care Choices (KCC) model to manage the care of beneficiaries with ESRD. Lastly, CMMI is targeting primary care practices and other providers with five new risk-sharing payment models options under two paths: (1) Primary Care First and (2) Direct Contracting (capitated and partially capitated payments). These models build on lessons learned from initiatives involving Medicare ACOs, Medicare Advantage, and private sector risk-sharing arrangements. As the government drives the industry toward capitated and VBC models, it offers the industry more flexible use of telehealth.

Reimbursement policy at the state level has developed at a faster pace than federal policy. However, with 51 different jurisdictions (including the District of Columbia), it has also led to the development of telehealth policies that vary from state to state. No two states are alike in telehealth Medicaid policies, laws, and regulations setting up a confusing landscape for providers who operate in multiple states. The remainder of this chapter will discuss the evolution of state telehealth reimbursement policies.

State Reimbursement

State telehealth reimbursement policies fall into two categories: Medicaid reimbursement and private payer reimbursement. Medicaid is a federal and state health coverage program for individuals with limited income and resources. While it has both federal and state funding, Medicaid is administered by the state. State Medicaid programs also have great leeway in how they structure their telehealth policies. This flexibility allows each state the ability to adjust to the needs of its respective population.

Medicaid Fee-for-Service

As of September 2019, all state Medicaid fee-for-service programs reimburse for some services delivered via telehealth. In January 2019, Massachusetts became the last state Medicaid program to officially adopt a policy of telehealth reimbursement (only for mental and behavioral health services delivered via live video) [13]. State Medicaid telehealth policies have evolved considerably over the past decade. Live video is the most common modality being reimbursed in Medicaid programs. Reimbursement policies for the other modalities of store-and-forward and RPM have not been adopted as readily as live video and are limited to use in certain conditions. In the period from 2012 to 2019, there was a steady increase in live video reimbursement policies being enacted in Medicaid programs, but less movement for store-and-forward and RPM (Fig. 8.5).

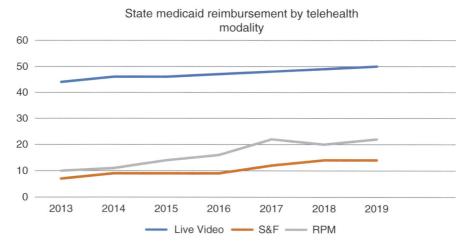

Fig. 8.5 State Medicaid reimbursement by modality 2013–2019

Such a result is not surprising as live video is the most likely substitute for an in-person interaction. Part of the difficulty in adopting reimbursement policies for store-and-forward and RPM is that there may not be a comparable, currently reimbursed service in the Medicaid program. For example, a Medicaid program may not be reimbursing for the continuous monitoring of a patient's chronic condition, as that service may not be done in-person. The services these two modalities deliver may be new services to the program that may make it more difficult to adopt a reimbursement policy.

In the last decade, Medicaid telehealth programs began to remove the limitations on the use of telehealth that were similar to the ones seen in Medicare. As noted earlier, federal telehealth policies in Medicare contain restrictions on geography and location where telehealth services can take place, the type of practitioner providing the service, the specific services themselves, and what modality can be used. Early on, some state Medicaid programs had replicated these restrictions such as the originating site must be located in a rural area. Over the past decade, Medicaid programs have been removing some of these caveats, particularly the rural requirements. Other limitations, such as types of providers eligible to be reimbursed, the services, and the type of location, have changed over the years becoming broader, but have not been removed with as much finality as the geographic limitations.

Partly why states have been able to alter their telehealth Medicaid reimbursement policies may be due to the greater administrative flexibility these programs have to enact changes. Unlike Medicare where much of the restrictive policies are in federal statute, most states do not require legislation to be passed to enact a change in their Medicaid policies. There have been state legislatures that have passed laws requiring Medicaid programs take certain actions regarding telehealth, but for the most part, if a Medicaid program decides to change its policies on telehealth, there is very little found in state statutes that prevent the program from acting.

However, there has been some confusion in how much the federal requirements and regulations may inhibit or affect the use of telehealth in a Medicaid program. For example, in 2016 CMS issued a statement to clarify that state Medicaid programs did not have to submit a state plan amendment (SPA) to begin reimbursing for telehealth if certain conditions have been met. To that point, some states believed that any change it made to incorporate telehealth into its Medicaid programs would require approval from CMS and were delaying any changes to create a SPA.

Other states with a long history of telehealth reimbursement within Medicaid have charged forward without hesitation. For example, California Medicaid, Medi-Cal, has been reimbursing for telehealth-delivered services for nearly two decades. In the summer of 2019, Medi-Cal updated its telehealth policies to allow providers to decide what services would be delivered via live video or store-and-forward. This policy put decision-making power into the provider's hands, allowing the clinician to determine when telehealth would be appropriate to use. To date, Medi-Cal has implemented the most advanced telehealth policy of any other public payer in the United States. (Vermont Medicaid does give the provider this decision-making power, but only for live video encounters.) However, even with this progressive policy, California Medicaid has yet to adopt a policy to reimburse for RPM.

Private Payer Laws

States legislatures have also promulgated policies that address coverage and reimbursement through private payer laws. These are laws that direct how health plans operating in the state must deal with telehealth. As with Medicaid programs, the telehealth private payer laws vary widely from state to state. While not all, many of the existing private payer laws do not impact Medicaid Managed Care programs or carve out exceptions for other plans such as state employee plans. Generally, telehealth private payer laws target policies related to private health insurance.

As of October 2019, 42 states and the District of Columbia have a telehealth private payer law. The requirements of the laws range from simply clarifying that health plans "may" reimburse for telehealth delivered services to "mandating" coverage and payment parity of services to the same extent as in-person care. At this time, the only states without a telehealth private payer law are Alabama, Idaho, North Carolina, Pennsylvania, South Carolina, West Virginia, Wisconsin, and Wyoming (Fig. 8.6).

Due to the wide variation of what each state's law requires, providers who operate in multiple states face the same issues as they would when looking toward Medicaid for reimbursement—a wide variation on what is reimbursed. Complicating matters further is that variations may occur from plan to plan operating within a single state. Depending on what is required of health plans in the state statute, there may be no commonalities between health plans on their reimbursement policies. Therefore, a provider operating in one state may still encounter the problem of multiple reimbursement policies that impact the services to be delivered via telehealth.

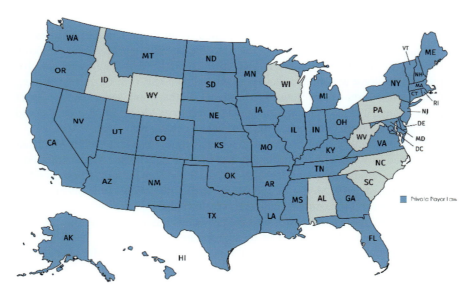

Fig. 8.6 States with a private payer telehealth law (as of October 2019)

Generally, states do not include a specific consequence mechanism should a health plan refuse to comply with the law. While a health plan would be in violation of a law that says the plan must cover services delivered via telehealth in the same manner as it would had the service been delivered in-person, no state attaches a specific penalty, such as a fine, should a plan fail to do so. However, there has been one case of a state regulatory body fining a plan for improperly denying telehealth claims. The North Dakota Insurance Department levied a fine of $125,000 on Blue Cross Blue Shield of North Dakota for several violations including not reimbursing for telehealth delivered services. It was noted that not keeping up with current laws contributed to the violations [14]. Thus far, this has been the only case of a health plan being penalized for not abiding by a telehealth private payer law.

Medicaid Managed Care

Medicaid managed care is another avenue in which telehealth reimbursement may be available. Unlike the previous discussion of fee-for-service Medicaid policies, what Medicaid Managed Care plans are required to cover for telehealth delivered services may not be as readily apparent. Generally, state Medicaid managed care plans will follow the telehealth reimbursement policies in fee-for-service. A managed care plan's willingness and ability to go beyond the fee-for-service policies will depend upon the rules in the state and the plan's own inclination. Most states do not prohibit a managed care plan from having a more expansive telehealth reimbursement policy than what is seen in fee-for-service.

Telehealth private payer laws may also have an impact on the Medicaid managed care plans. For example, in recently passed legislation in California that updated the state's telehealth private payer law, an exception for Medicaid managed care plans was carved out [15].

As with private payers, most states are silent on Medicaid managed care plans sharing their telehealth policies with the public, and as a result, a good number of plans do not make that information readily accessible. This has led to difficulty in understanding just how expansive Medicaid managed care telehealth reimbursement policies are for the various states, especially if there are multiple plans operating.

Other Non-reimbursement State Policy Issues

Reimbursement policies are only a portion of the telehealth-related policies that states may promulgate that impact the use of telehealth. Other areas where states have been active in the last few years in establishing state policies have included establishing a patient–provider relationship via telehealth, prescribing when using telehealth, licensing, and various requirements made by state regulatory boards on licensees. While this chapter has focused on reimbursement policy, the reader must keep in mind that there are other policy topics that will also determine how and to what extent telehealth can be used and that it will vary from state to state.

Conclusion

As evidenced by the legislative and regulatory progress made over the past few years at both the federal and state levels, the industry has reached an inflection point where policy makers' attitudes and innovative technologies are coming together in significant ways to improve the reimbursement paradigm to accelerate adoption. Reimbursement changes for virtual care services will continue to evolve incrementally in both fee-for-service and value-based care delivery models.

References

1. U.S. Government Accounting Office, GAO [Internet]. Health care: telehealth and remote patient monitoring use in Medicare and selected federal programs. 2017-365. [cited 17 November 2019]. Available from: http://www.gao.gov/assets/690/684115.pdf.
2. Center for Medicare and Medicaid Services, CMS [Internet]. Medicare program general information; [cited 17 November 2019]. Available from: https://www.cms.gov/Medicare/Medicare-General-Information/MedicareGenInfo/index.
3. Kaiser Family Foundation, KFF [Internet]. The facts on Medicare spending and financing; 20 August 2019; [cited 22 October 2019]. Available from: https://www.kff.org/medicare/issue-brief/the-facts-on-medicare-spending-and-financing/.
4. U.S. House of Representatives, Office of the Law Revision Counsel, U.S. Code [Internet]. 42 USC 1395m: Special payment rules for particular items and services; [cited 22 October 2019]. Available from: https://uscode.house.gov/view.xhtml?req=(title:42%20section:1395m%20edition:prelim).
5. Congress.gov [Internet]. [cited 22 October 2019]. Available from: www.congress.gov.
6. Bipartisan Budget Act of 2018 [Internet]. Bipartisan Budget Act of 2018, Title III, Subtitle C, Section 50323. 2018 [cited 26 April 2018]. Available from: http://bit.ly/2JS35P1.
7. SUPPORT for Patients and Communities Act of 2018 [Internet]. Pub. L. No. 115-271, §§ 2001, 7162, 7172, 8072 (2018). See also H.R. Con. Res., 115th Cong. (2018); [cited 22 October 2019]. Available from: https://www.congress.gov/115/plaws/publ271/PLAW-115publ271.pdf.
8. MLN Booklet Telehealth Services [Internet]. CMS.gov. 2019 [cited 17 November 2019]. Available from: https://www.cms.gov/Outreach-and-Education/Medicare-Learning-Network-MLN/MLNProducts/downloads/TelehealthSrvcsfctsht.pdf?utm_campaign=2a178f351b-EMAIL_CAMPAIGN_2019_04_19_08_59&utm_term=0_ae00b0e89a-2a178f351b-353229765&utm_content=90024810&utm_medium=social&utm_source=facebook&hss_channel=fbp-372451882894317.
9. Federal Register [Internet]. Medicare Program; revision to payment policies under the physician fee schedule, 83 Fed. Reg, 35,704 (July 27, 2018); [cited 17 November 2019]. Available from: https://www.federalregister.gov/documents/2018/07/27/2018-14985/medicare-program-revisions-to-payment-policies-under-the-physician-fee-schedule-and-other-revisions.
10. Federal Register [Internet]. Medicare and Medicaid Programs; policy and technical changes to the Medicare advantage, Medicare prescription drug benefit, program of all-inclusive care for the elderly (PACE), Medicaid fee-for-service, and Medicaid managed care programs for years 2020 and 2021, 83 Fed. Reg. 54982, 55010, 55051-57 (proposed Nov. 1, 2018); [cited 17 November 2019]. Available from: https://www.federalregister.gov/documents/2018/11/01/2018-23599/medicare-and-medicaid-programs-policy-and-technical-changes-to-the-medicare-advantage-medicare.
11. Center for Medicare and Medicaid Services, CMS [Internet]. Medicare Shared Savings Program [cited 17 November 2019]. Available from: https://www.cms.gov/Medicare/Medicare-Fee-for-Service-Payment/sharedsavingsprogram/index.

12. Center for Medicare and Medicaid Services, CMS [Internet]. Innovation Models [cited 17 November 2019]. Available from: https://innovation.cms.gov/initiatives/#views=models.
13. Massachusetts Executive Office of Health and Human Services, Office of Medicaid [Internet]. MassHealth All Provider Bulletin 281, January 2019. [cited 15 November 2019]. Available from: https://www.mass.gov/files/documents/2019/01/23/all-provider-bulletin-281.pdf.
14. North Dakota Insurance Department. Insurance Commissioner fines Blue Cross Blue Shield of North Dakota $125,000 as a result of market conduct examination, July 9, 2019; [cited 13 November 2019]. Available from: https://www.nd.gov/ndins/news/insurance-commissioner-fines-blue-cross-blue-shield-north-dakota-125000-result-market-conduct.
15. California Legislation AB 744 (Aguiar-Curry). [Internet] October 2019. [cited 17 November 2019]. Available from: https://leginfo.legislature.ca.gov/faces/billTextClient.xhtml?bill_id=201920200AB744.

Legal and Regulatory Implications of Telemedicine

Geena George and Brandon E. Heitmann

Introduction

Telemedicine can generally be defined as the use of medical information exchanged electronically from one site to another to improve patients' health status [1, 2]. This care can be anything from the sharing of pictures or video to remote patient monitoring [3]. Telehealth is a broader term, including additional modalities. Typically, there are four basic types of telehealth: real-time video (synchronous), store-and-forward transmission (asynchronous), remote patient monitoring, and mobile health [4, 5]. As internet use and technology are increasingly intertwined in daily life, the use of telemedicine and telehealth is increasing. According to the American Hospital Association (AHA), more than 50% of hospital systems utilized some form of telehealth in 2013 [6]. One reason for this increase is that patients are using it to address issues such as a lack of appointment times, requiring care outside of regular business hours, and the inability to see providers that are located far away [7].

The recent 2019 Coronavirus (COVID-19) outbreak has demonstrated yet another reason to use telemedicine and telehealth—protection from exposure. The World Health Organization (WHO) declared COVID-19 a pandemic on March 11, 2020 [8]. Due to the infectious nature of the virus, responding to the outbreak required patient isolation, monitoring of contacts, and quarantining. The efforts to control the virus consequently interrupted routine care for non-COVID-19 patients. As a result, the use of telemedicine and telehealth became a viable alternative to provide care to these patients while reducing the risk of transmission.

G. George
Department of Surgery, Clinical Research Unit, Westchester Medical Center, Valhalla, NY, USA

B. E. Heitmann (✉)
Fitzpatrick & Hunt, Pagano, Aubert, LLP, New York, NY, USA

© Springer Nature Switzerland AG 2021
R. Latifi et al. (eds.), *Telemedicine, Telehealth and Telepresence*, https://doi.org/10.1007/978-3-030-56917-4_9

Though telemedicine and telehealth can improve a patient's access to health care, it can also present legal and health information challenges. Its use can present licensure, privacy, security, and confidentiality obstacles [9, 10]. Although addressing these factors is often time-consuming and cumbersome, legislation and policy has been identified as one of the five main determinants for successful telemedicine implementation [11]. As telemedicine and telehealth become more conventional, understanding the legal and regulatory aspects of telehealth is crucial for both providers and patients.

Licensing

The practice of medicine—like many other professions—requires the issuance of a license by the state in which the professional is practicing and where the patient resides [5, 12–15]. In the US, each state has the power to establish and enforce licensing standards and regulate the practice of medicine within its own borders [15]. For example, California's Licensing Law, found in §2052 of the Business and Profession Code, prohibits any person from diagnosing, treating, operating on, or prescribing for patients without a valid medical license [16]. Many other States have statutes that proscribe variations on this same general rule. These licensing regulations are often seen as barriers to the use of telemedicine [17]. Physicians risk sanctions if they practice telemedicine across state lines without appropriate licenses [18]. Examples of the "interstate" practice of telemedicine, among other things, can include reviewing an out-of-state patient's imaging, answering questions on a medical website, video conferencing with patients in different states, or consulting with other physicians in order to diagnose an out-of-state patient. One example of the unlicensed practice of telemedicine across state lines is *Hageseth v. Superior Court of California* [16].

Hageseth v. Superior Court of California

In 2007, a California court addressed interstate licensing issues in *Hageseth v. Superior Court of California*. There, Dr. Hageseth, a Colorado-licensed psychiatrist, was charged with the felony offense of practicing medicine in California without a license. Dr. Hageseth challenged the California court's jurisdiction over him by arguing that all the alleged unlawful conduct took place outside of California. John McKay, a California resident, attempted to buy fluoxetine online. McKay filled out a purchase request and questionnaire that identified him as a California resident and submitted it to the operators of a website in Texas. The operators forwarded the purchase request and questionnaire to Dr. Hageseth in Colorado for approval. After review, Dr. Hageseth issued a prescription for the medication and returned it to the site operators. The operators subsequently forwarded the prescription to a pharmacy in Mississippi where the prescription was filled and mailed to McKay at his California address. Shortly thereafter, "intoxicated with alcohol and with a detectible amount of fluoxetine in his blood, McKay committed suicide by means of carbon monoxide poisoning." At no point did Dr. Hageseth communicate with anyone in California regarding this prescription.

Ultimately, the court denied Hageseth's jurisdictional challenge, stating that "without having at the time a valid California medical license, [Hageseth] prescribed fluoxetine for a person he knew to be a California resident, knowing that act would cause the prescribed medication to be sent to that person at the California address he provided." Dr. Hageseth pled guilty and served 9 months in prison [17]. The *Hageseth* case presents a cautionary tale for physicians who attempt to practice medicine via the internet or other electronic means. It also illustrates how strict some courts can be when interpreting their State's licensing laws.

Interstate Medical Compact

Since the *Hageseth* decision, States have shown a willingness to relax some of their licensing laws to allow the practice of telemedicine. According to the Federation of State Medical Boards (FSMB), 14 state boards allow for doctors to operate across state lines. Nine states issue "special licenses or certificates related to telehealth." These states allow practitioners from different states to provide telemedicine services even in a state where they are not physically located [17]. These nine states include Alabama, Louisiana, Maine, Minnesota, New Mexico, Ohio, Oregon, Tennessee (osteopathic board only), and Texas. Perhaps the most comprehensive of these allowances is the Interstate Medical Licensure Compact (IMLC). The IMLC is a legal agreement among states that addresses interstate physician licensure. Under this agreement, physicians that meet the IMLC eligibility requirements can practice medicine among the states within the compact [19]. Think of it as the "European Union" of telemedicine. As of December 2019, 29 states along with the District of Columbia and the territory of Guam participate in the IMLC.

However, participation in the IMLC is not without its own risks. For each state that a physician acquires an unrestricted license for, the physician is bound to abide by that individual state's laws and medical boards [20]. These responsibilities can include maintaining continuing medical education (CME), annual licensure renewal requirements, as well as state laws/regulations regarding the practice of medicine in that state. Should a physician fail to meet these responsibilities, he or she can be held responsible in not only the state in which the violation occurred, but also the other states for which the physician is licensed through the ILMC [20]. Therefore, a physician should review all the laws and regulations related to the practice of medicine (and telemedicine) in a particular state, prior to obtaining a license and practicing medicine. As telemedicine and the internet become more and more intertwined in the practice of medicine, it is imperative that States continue to adopt regulations that permit or provide guidance on the practice of telemedicine. Since there is no federal legislation addressing telemedicine, it is necessary for individual providers to be informed about their state's telemedicine licensure rules.

Informed Consent

Once doctors meet the appropriate licensing requirements in a particular state, the next legal hurdle is obtaining informed consent from the patient. Failure to obtain informed consent is considered a crime [4]. Appropriate informed consent should identify the patient, the physician, the physician's credentials, the types of transmission that are allowed by the use of telemedicine, details of security measures, and documentation of release of protected health information to any third party [21]. In other words, informed consent for telemedicine requires consent for the treatment itself, as well as the transmission of digital data [4, 22]. Liabilities for informed consent in telemedicine must consider the ways in which it varies from face-to-face consent. A telemedicine consent form will always include the standard aspects of non-telemedicine consent; however, it must also consider potential complications due to the nature of the communication. For example, a telesurgical procedure would include standard risks; however, the consent form must also consider risks such as loss of communications or the damages resulting from converting a telesurgical procedure into a traditional one [23]. Telemedical risks that go beyond the control of the health care providers such as system crashes, power outages, or other software glitches should also be considered [24]. In addition to disclosing all potential risks on the informed consent document, another legal consideration arises when telemedicine is utilized by a referring physician. The question becomes which physician should be the one to obtain consent. Depending upon which state a physician practices, there may be laws regarding who can be the one to obtain consent. As such, in some states, it may be necessary to have both the referring physician as well as the remote physician to separately document consent.

In two different cases, we see the impacts of a physician's failure to properly document consent. In *Knight v. Department of Army,* the plaintiff, Joseph Knight, a resident of Alabama, was treated for a heart condition in Georgia [25]. Knight required a bypass surgery which he chose to receive in Texas, where he received a blood transfusion that contained the human immunodeficiency virus (HIV) [25]. The patient later sued his physicians for failure to be informed about the risk of HIV infection from a blood transfusion [25]. In this case, the court first had to determine choice of law, to establish which state's informed consent laws applied. The patient was treated in Texas and Georgia, but ultimately passed away in Alabama. The court reasoned that Texas law should apply for liability because the plaintiff's infection and surgery occurred in Texas despite his subsequent medical care and death occurring in Alabama. Next, the Court had to determine the merits of the case. In this case, the court found that under Texas law, the plaintiff did not bring a proper informed consent claim because a reasonable person would still have undergone the bypass surgery even after being informed of the remote possibility of an HIV infection. As such, the Court concluded that the doctor complied with his duties and obtained proper consent under Texas law.

In the second case—*Blakesely v. Wolford*—Terri Blakesely, a Pennsylvania resident, had her wisdom teeth removed but during the operation her lingual nerve was damaged [26]. The nerve damage caused numbness and shocks to her mouth and tongue. Eventually, Blakesely sought relief by consulting with two Pennsylvania surgeons who eventually referred her to Dr. Larry Wolford, a Texas oral surgeon. Dr. Wolford evaluated Blakesely while he was in Pennsylvania on business. The Texas surgeon suggested that a nerve graft surgery may help to alleviate her discomfort but noted that removal of a portion of her auricular nerve for the graft may cause slight numbness. Blakesely agreed and the surgery was conducted in Texas. However, during the surgery, Dr. Wolford opted to use a graft from another nerve as opposed to the patient's greater auricular nerve. The surgery was unsuccessful and left Blakesely with an additional feeling of strangulation any time her neck was touched [26].

Blakesely sued Dr. Wolford in Pennsylvania for malpractice and failure to obtain her informed consent for the surgery. Once again, the court had to determine choice of law. Should the stringent Pennsylvania standard for informed consent or the more relaxed Texas standard apply? Pennsylvania law requires physicians to disclose all feasible possibilities and alternatives of a surgical procedure. Whereas, Texas law only requires the doctor to disclose information that the doctor believes is necessary. The Court found that Texas law should apply because the surgery and injury occurred there and because Blakesely signed a consent form while in Texas.

As these cases make clear, courts will give great deference to the place of injury or the place of consent when determining what State's law should apply for informed consent. For telemedicine, the place of injury or consent is less clear, but the courts will likely evaluate where both parties were situated at the time of the alleged injury and determine which state had the most significant relationship to the claims. These cases also highlight that differences in states' informed consent law can greatly impact a physician's liability. Thus it is vital for any physician attempting to see patients from various states via telemedicine to be knowledgeable of their patient's states' consent laws.

"Selfie" Telemedicine

As technology advances, remote access to care is becoming increasingly popular. Rather than having to wait for an appointment, a patient can simply send an e-mail or an instant message and communicate with a doctor instantly. Although this technology offers obvious advantages, this form of patient–provider communication opens the door for new concerns about privacy and confidentiality. One method of e-communication between patients and providers is the use of the "selfie." A selfie is typically a photograph or video that one takes of his or herself. As we experience the increasing intersection between technology and medicine, the medical selfie is becoming relatively common place. As medical selfies diffuse throughout the field of telemedicine, there are various patient privacy and confidentiality issues to consider. All correspondences between a patient and a provider are important for documentation purposes. When these correspondences are electronic, the necessity of maintaining records is less clear.

To examine the potential legal issues, one must consider the form this medical selfie takes. Who initiated the selfie—the patient or the provider? The initiation of care is important to consider because the patient–provider relationship is how legal responsibility is determined. The patient–provider relationship will be described in more detail below. In patient-initiated communication, the patient is giving consent by sharing information or images with a health care provider. The provider is then ethically responsible for keeping that information confidential [26]. In this type of interaction, there may be two subgroups. In the first, the patient is seeking care from a doctor whom they have a prior relationship. In the second, the patient is seeking care from a previously unknown doctor [27].

Once this relationship is established, confidentiality of patient information is the next legal hurdle. Maintaining patient privacy requires security in both the transmission of the data and the storage of data. One author described transmissions as either formal or informal. Formal transmission includes those utilizing Health Insurance Portability and Accountability Act (HIPAA) compliant platforms. Informal transmissions include those that are not secure [28]. Insecure transmissions may unknowingly lead to breaches in security. Maintaining security is paramount as threats to medical information are becoming more frequent. One study reported that cyber-attacks that targeted medical information was increasing 22% a year, with millions of records being compromised [29].

Medical Records

The initiation of the doctor–patient relationships begins the start of the medical record. The medical record should contain the informed consent documentation, all communications between the patient and the provider, any evaluations, prescriptions, laboratory results, other test results, instructions, and/or educational materials [21]. These records must follow the established laws and regulations for the jurisdiction where care is being administered. These documentation requirements vary from state to state. A good resource to look at documentation standards by state is the National Consortium of Telehealth Resource Centers (NCTRC), funded by the US Department of Health and Human Services. The NCTRC provides information and assistance regarding specific state policies [30]. Physicians are responsible for knowing their state's applicable privacy, confidentiality, security, and medical retention laws. The US Department of Health and Human Services provides guidelines on these requirements [31].

The American Health Information Management Association (AHIMA) is a national organization that provides widely cited health information practices. AHIMA offers its own guidelines of what information should be included in a telemedical record. The recommendations suggest including the following information in the patient's medical record: patient name, identification number, date of service, referring physician, consulting physician, provider organization, type of evaluation performed, informed consent, evaluation results, diagnosis/impression, and recommendations for future treatment [13]. These records may be in any form: hard copy, video, audiotape, etc., unless specified by states laws and regulations. Unless there are policies specifically addressing disclosures of telemedical documents, disclosures should only be allowed with the written authorization of the patient or legally authorized representative. Other acceptable reasons to disclose this information include court orders, subpoena, or statue.

Physician–Patient Relationship

Prior to the widespread adoption of telemedicine, it was relatively easy to determine when a physician–patient relationship existed and when it did not. The introduction of telemedicine raises interesting questions about if and when a physician–patient relationship starts. Typically, "[f]or a physician to be liable for medical negligence, the defendant-physician and plaintiff-patient must have a physician-patient relationship" [32]. In a typical case, a doctor could be held liable for any negligence that occurred within the "episode of care" [32]. Further, "any additional consultations with specialists" could also fall within the physician–plaintiff relationship. In other words, this relationship forms a contract that serves as the basis for bringing suits against providers [33].

Telemedicine, however, distorts this relationship. It is much more difficult to track the "episode of care." For example, a case may involve multiple physicians and consultants simultaneously reviewing a patient's records, or involve stored images and data that the primary or secondary providers review at a later, undefined time. Essentially, a physician could be providing care to patient that the physician has never had any interaction with. In regards to telemedicine, the following considerations are important to determine whether a physician–patient relationship exists: did the physician and patient see each other during the telemedicine visit, did an actual exam take place, did the physician provide a diagnosis, treatment, or other care on which the patient relied, did the physician have access to the patient's medical records, and did the physician accept a fee for the telemedicine consultation? [34]

Unsurprisingly, the case law surrounding when a telemedicine physician–patient relationship forms is still developing. Though courts seem to find that a relationship existed whenever a physician gives medical advice and the patient relies on that advice. For instance, in *Bienz v. Central Suffolk Hospital,* the court found that a physician–patient relationship existed when a doctor gave medical advice to a patient over the phone and the patient relied on that advice. Conversely in *Clanton v. Von Haam*, a patient with back pain called a doctor and listed her complaints. The doctor listened but refused to see her that night. The court found that this did not constitute a physician–patient relationship because she did not rely on the phone conversation.

Extrapolating this line of case law to telemedicine, it seems that courts will focus on two factors when determining if a physician–patient relationship exists. First, the physician must actually render medical advice. Second, the patient must rely on that advice. Given that courts have found a physician–plaintiff relationship via telephone conversations, whether advice was rendered via phone, email, text, blog post, or video chat will likely be immaterial so long as the other elements are met. Therefore, physicians who engage in these types of consultations or evaluations should be aware that they can be subjected to liability for any opinion they render over the internet, phone, etc.

Risks to Privacy

Telemedicine requires the same privacy requirements as a face-to-face visit would under the HIPAA of 1996. The HIPAA sets standards for handling health care information. The HIPAA Privacy Rule sets standards for health plans, health care clearinghouses, and health care providers who conduct electronic health care transactions. However, since most health care providers also rely on a variety of other persons or business, the Privacy Rule also covers these "business associates" [35]. The HIPAA Security Rule sets standards for the protection of electronic protected health information (PHI). These protections include confidentiality, integrity, and availability of PHI [36]. The standards set forth in these two rules represent only some of the protections that are needed when utilizing telemedicine. The American Academy of Allergy Asthma & Immunology summarizes some of the guidelines from the HIPAA Rules as follows:

1. Only authorized user should have access to electronic PHI (ePHI).
2. A system of secure communication should be implemented to protect the integrity of ePHI.
3. A system of monitoring communications containing ePHI should be implemented to prevent accidental or malicious breaches [37].

However, there are additional considerations when the care rendered is via telemedicine. Protection of privacy cannot only apply to the telemedicine itself but also the technology and systems used to accomplish this care. Data storage is an example of technology used to provide telemedicine. Medical professionals that have ePHI that is stored by a third party must have a Business Associate Agreement (BAA). A BAA consists of individuals or entities that a health care professional can contract with to assist in the practice of telemedicine. Typically, the assistance of the BAA requires access to PHI [37]. A valid BAA should include the permitted and required uses of PHI and agreements from the Business Associate to take the appropriate measures to safeguard the PHI to which they will be given access. Other factors to be included in the BAA include the following: agreement that business associates will not use or disclose PHI beyond what is permitted or required by contract/law, should a covered entity know of a security breach, reasonable steps will be taken to solve the breach and if such measures are unsuccessful, then the contract or agreement with the business associate will be terminated, and finally if a contract is unable to be terminated, the covered entity will report the problem to the Department of Health and Human Services Office for Civil Rights [37]. After completing the appropriate BAA, it is necessary to ensure that the Business Associate only uses the PHI in a secure and established manner [36]. A health care provided may only disclose this PHI to a business associate if it is necessary for a covered entity to carry out a health care function.

Physician Liability

In the US, physician liability is generally governed by states [15]. Physicians have a duty to provide care within an accepted standard to all their patients. Failure to do so can subject physicians to lawsuits. The two main theories of liability by patients against their physicians are medical malpractice and medical negligence. Though similar, the difference revolves around intent. For medical malpractice cases, the patient must show that the physician deviated from accepted professional standards. For instance, failing to follow accepted surgical procedures or failing to order tests to aid in a diagnosis can form the basis of a malpractice suit. Negligence cases arise when a doctor fails to act as a reasonably prudent person would under similar circumstances. Negligence claims are often premised on carelessness, mistakes, or a lack of attention.

Malpractice

Upon the establishment of a patient–doctor relationship, the doctor now has a responsibility for duty of care and treatment that is considered standard of care [4, 38]. Duty of care establishes the responsibility of the patient/caregiver and other involved health care providers. Duty of treatment requires health care providers to define their roles and responsibilities regarding treatment [4]. In addition to establishing these roles and responsibilities, a practice should have a clear risk assessment in addition to written policies or procedures. After duty of care is established, the next consideration in a malpractice case is whether a physician breached this duty. Typically, a breach of duty means that the physician failed to meet the expected treatment standards [33]. In the US, there are two ways to determine the "standards" for a physician. These standards include the "community standard" and the "national standard." The community standard holds physicians accountable to what other similarly trained local physicians would do in a similar situation. The national standard holds physicians accountable to nationally recognized standards of medicine [33]. For example, the District of Columbia follows the national standard [39], whereas New York [40] and Idaho follow community standards [41].

Frazier v. University of Mississippi Medical Center

An example of potential liability through telemedicine is *Frazier v. University of Mississippi Medical Center*. In this case, a young Mississippi girl with congenital hydrocephalus was treated in New Orleans, Louisiana, after complications from a procedure she underwent in Mississippi [42]. Following surgery, the neurosurgeon arranged for her discharge to a Mississippi home health care provider. The girl continued to suffer symptoms and was subsequently treated in both New Orleans and Jackson, Mississippi. Ultimately, the girl was sent home with "permanent brain injuries requiring tube feeding and home nursing care 16 hours per day" [42]. After returning home to Mississippi, her Louisiana neurosurgeon continued to follow up with her.

The patient's family subsequently filed a complaint (in Mississippi) on her behalf in December 2016 alleging medical malpractice and negligence, among other things, against her Mississippi home health care providers and her Louisiana neurosurgeon. The Louisiana neurosurgeon moved to dismiss the claims against her for lack of personal jurisdiction. Personal jurisdiction is the court's ability to hear claims against a defendant based on their connections with the state in which the court sits. In order for a state's court to subject a non-resident to jurisdiction, the claims must "relate to or arise out of a nonresident's contacts" with the state. Accordingly, the neurosurgeon argued that, all of her contacts with her patient were while the patient was still in Louisiana. The court agreed and dismissed the claims with respect to the Louisiana neurosurgeon. The court reasoned that the claims mostly arise out of allegedly deficient discharge instructions to the home health care providers in Mississippi. Importantly, these discharge instructions were signed and ordered entirely in Louisiana. Further, the court also found that even though the neurosurgeon supervised treatment in Mississippi via telemedicine, it was unclear how this harmed the girl in any way.

The *Frazier* case stands as an important example of how physicians may limit their malpractice liability if they perform telemedicine to out-of-state patients. If they are able to confine their treatment plans and diagnoses to their home state, they limit their exposure to lawsuits brought in states across the country. Physicians that are not able to limit their care to their home state should be diligent in knowing another state's legal requirements regarding patient care.

Conclusion

In summary, the integration and use of telemedicine and telehealth will continue to expand. Though the law and regulatory guidance surrounding the practice of telemedicine is still developing, it will undoubtedly grow as well. It should be expected that governments will continue to implement new regulations, and courts will continue to define the scopes and duties of physicians practicing telemedicine and telehealth. Thus, practitioners should continue to stay abreast of all changes as it will allow themselves to best position their practice for the future while also mitigating their exposure to potential liability or sanctions.

Disclaimer This information has been prepared for informational purposes only and does not constitute legal advice. Reading of this information does not create an attorney–client relationship.

References

1. *U.S. v. Valdivieso Rodriguez,* 532 F.Supp.2d 316, 326 (D. P.R. 2007).
2. Parimbelli E, Bottalico B, Losiouk E, et al. Trusting telemedicine: a discussion on risks, safety, legal implications and liability of involved stakeholders. Int J Med Inform. 2018;112:90–8.
3. ATA. State telemedicine gap analysis. Coverage and reimbursement. 2017. Available at http://www.americantelemed.org/policy-page/state-telemedicinegaps-reports. Last accessed 15 May 2018.

4. Ateriya N, Saraf A, Meshram VP, Setia P. Telemedicine and virtual consultation: The Indian perspective. Natl Med J India. 2018;31(4):215–8.
5. Marcoux RM, Vogenberg FR. Telehealth: applications from a legal and regulatory perspective. P T. 2016;41(9):567–70.
6. Trendwatch: The promise of telehealth for hospitals, health systems, and their communities. Washington, DC: American Hospital Association; 2015. Available at: www.aha.org/research/reports/tw/15jan-tw-telehealth.pdf. Last accessed 12 Mar 2020.
7. National Public Radio/Robert Wood Johnson Foundation/Harvard T.H. Chan School of Public Health. Patients' perspectives on health care in the United States. A look at seven states and the nation. 2016. Available at https://www.rwjf.org/content/dam/farm/reports/surveys_and_polls/2016/rwjf427031. Last accessed 15 May 2018.
8. Ohannessian R, Duong TA, Odone A. Global telemedicine implementation and integration within health systems to fight the COVID-19 pandemic: a call to action. JMIR Public Health Surveill. 2020;6(2):e18810.
9. Brous E. Legal considerations in telehealth and telemedicine. Am J Nurs. 2016;116(9):64–7.
10. Friedberg R, Daniel K. Telehealth, remote monitoring & medical records: What data must providers include in a patient medical record. TechHealth Perspectives Web site. https://www.techhealthperspectives.com/2013/07/30/telehealth-remote-monitoring-medical-records-what-data-must-providers-include-in-a-patient-medical-record/. Published July 30, 2013. Updated 2013. Last accessed 31 Mar 2020.
11. Broens TH, Huis in't Veld RM, Vollenbroek-Hutten MM, Hermens HJ, van Halteren AT, Nieuwenhuis LJ. Determinants of successful telemedicine implementations: a literature study. J Telemed Telecare. 2007;13(6):303–9.
12. Silverman RD. Regulating medical practice in the cyber age: issues and challenges for state medical boards. Am J Law Med. 2000;26(2–3):255–76.
13. AHIMA Practice Brief. Telemedicine services and the health record (2013 update). (Updated May 2013).
14. Documentation requirements. American Academy of Allergy Asthma & Immunology Web site. https://www.aaaai.org/practice-resources/running-your-practice/practice-management-resources/Telemedicine/documentation. Last accessed 2 Apr 2020.
15. Sokolovich N. Legal and regulatory considerations in expanding telemedicine services across international borders. In: Doarn CR, Latifi R, Hostiuc F, Arafat R, Zoicas C, editors. A multinational telemedicine systems for disaster response: opportunities and challenges. 1st ed. Amsterdam: IOS Press; 2017. p. 59–75.
16. *Hageseth v. Sup. Ct. of Cal*, 150 Cal.App.4th 1399 (2007).
17. Becker CD, Dandy K, Gaujean M, Fusaro M, Scurlock C. Legal perspectives on telemedicine part 1: legal and regulatory issues. Perm J. 2019;23:18–293. https://doi.org/10.7812/TPP/18-293.
18. Guttman-McCabe C. Telemedicine's imperiled future? Funding, reimbursement, licensing and privacy hurdles face a developing technology. J Contemp Health Law Policy. 1997;14(1):169–70.
19. The IMLC. Interstate Medical Licensure Compact Web site. https://imlcc.org/faqs/. Last accessed 31 Mar 2020.
20. Stewart M. The risks of multi-state licensure for telemedicine providers. The University of Arizona Web site. https://telemedicine.arizona.edu/blog/risks-multi-state-licensure-telemedicine-providers. Published July, 18, 2019. Updated 2019. Last accessed 4 Apr 2020.
21. Kmucha ST. Physician liability issues and telemedicine: part 2 of 3. Ear Nose Throat J. 2015;94(12):466–9.
22. Chaet D, Clearfield R, Sabin JE, Skimming K, Council on Ethical and Judicial Affairs American Medical Association. Ethical practice in Telehealth and Telemedicine. J Gen Intern Med. 2017;32(10):1136–40.
23. Siegal G. Telemedicine: licensing and other legal issues. Otolaryngol Clin N Am. 2011;44(6):1375–84, xi
24. Kane B, Sands DZ. Guidelines for the clinical use of electronic mail with patients. The AMIA Internet Working Group, Task Force on Guidelines for the Use of Clinic-Patient Electronic Mail. J Am Med Inform Assoc. 1998;5(1):104–11.

25. *Knight v. Department of Army,* 757 F. Supp. 790 (W.D. Tex. 1991).
26. *Blakesely v. Wolford,* 789 F.2d 236 (3d Cir, 1986).
27. Mars M, Morris C, Scott RE. Selfie telemedicine – what are the legal and regulatory issues? Stud Health Technol Inform. 2018;254:53–62.
28. Fofel AL, Sarin KY. A survey of direct-to-consumer teledermatology services available to US patients: explosive growth, opportunities and controversy. J Telemed Telecare. 2017;23(1):19–25.
29. Kruse CS, Frederick B, Jacobson T, Monticone DK. Cybersecurity in healthcare: a systematic review of modern threats and trends. Technol Health Care. 2017;25(1):1–10.
30. About our consortium. National Consortium of Telehealth Resource Centers Web site. https://www.telehealthresourcecenter.org/about-us/. Last accessed 2 Apr 2020.
31. Health information privacy. U.S Department of Health and Human Services Web site. https://www.hhs.gov/hipaa/for-professionals/privacy/guidance/introduction/index.html. Updated 2015. Last accessed 2 Apr 2020.
32. O'Conner MC. The physician-patient relationship and the professional standard of care: reevaluating medical negligence principles to achieve the goals of tort reform. Tort Trial Insur Pract Law J. 2010;46:109.
33. Granade PF. Malpractice issues in the practice of telemedicine. Telemed J. 1995;1(2):87–9.
34. Hoffman LC. Telehealth, children, and pediatrics: should the doctor make house calls again, digitally? Nova Law Rev. 2019;43(3):321–51.
35. Business Associates. U.S Department of Health and Human Services Web site. https://www.hhs.gov/hipaa/for-professionals/privacy/guidance/business-associates/index.html. Updated 2019. Last accessed 3 Apr 2020.
36. HIPAA for professionals. U.S Department of Health and Human Services Web site. https://www.hhs.gov/hipaa/for-professionals/index.html. Updated 2017. Last accessed 2 Apr 2020.
37. Security and HIPAA. American Academy of Allergy Asthma & Immunology Web site. https://www.aaaai.org/practice-resources/running-your-practice/practice-management-resources/Telemedicine/HIPAA. Last accessed 2 Apr 2020.
38. Wade VA, Eliott JA, Hiller JE. A qualitative study of ethical, medico-legal and clinical governance matters in Australian telehealth services. J Telemed Telecare. 2012;18(2):109–14.
39. *Kordas v. Sugarbaker,* 990 A.2d 496, 500 (D.C. 2010).
40. *Korszun v. Winthrop University Hospital,* 172 A.D.3d 1343, 1344 (2d Dep't 2019).
41. *Phillips v. Eastern Idaho Health Services,* 2020 WL 1164508, at *5 (Sup. Ct. Id. Mar. 11, 2020).
42. *Frazier v. University of Mississippi Medical Center,* 2018 WL 5289907 (S.D. Miss. Oct. 24, 2018).

Business Aspects of Telemedicine

10

Nina M. Antoniotti

History of Telemedicine Business Planning

For many years, organizations have struggled to understand business planning for telemedicine programs. In the early 1990s, starting in 1991, the federal government funded telemedicine programs through grants administered from the Office of Rural Health Policy, the Health Care Financing Administration (HCFA), now the Centers for Medicare and Medicaid (CMS), the Agency for Healthcare Research and Quality (AHRQ), and the National Institute of Health (NIH). These early funding programs gave multi-million-dollar grants to rural health care organizations to set up telemedicine programs in rural areas with little or no access to specialty health care services such as cardiology, pulmonary medicine, neurology, and others. Early telemedicine programs were successful in implementation and proving the feasibility and practicality of using distance-care technologies, but paid little or no attention to the business aspects of a telemedicine program or how to sustain the program after grant funding. Many early telemedicine programs also paid clinicians a stipend of $60.00, which was a part of the grant-funded budget, to incentivize clinicians to provide consults via telemedicine in a world of little or no health plan reimbursement. In the early years of telemedicine, few health plans, including government and private payers, reimbursed for care delivered via telemedicine. Therefore, it was imperative that telemedicine programs in the early 1990s paid clinicians from grant funds. The resulting problem was that when grant funds ran out, clinicians stopped using telemedicine. Rural communities who began to depend on the services provided via telemedicine found themselves suddenly without the specialty health care. Over time, federally funded telemedicine programs began to fall by the wayside after the 3-year grant funding cycle, unless additional grant funding was secured.

N. M. Antoniotti (✉)
Interoperability and Patient Engagement, St. Jude Children's Research Hospital, Memphis, TN, USA
e-mail: nina@ninaantoniotti.com

© Springer Nature Switzerland AG 2021
R. Latifi et al. (eds.), *Telemedicine, Telehealth and Telepresence*,
https://doi.org/10.1007/978-3-030-56917-4_10

In 1997, the Office for the Advancement of TeleHealth (OAT), Health and Human Services (HHS), Washington, D.C., offered a grant funding cycle with the intent to look at programs that could test the feasibility and practicality of implementing TeleHealth in an integrated health care delivery system, such as Marshfield Clinic, Intermountain Health, and others. This grant funding cycle, called the 1997 TeleHealth Network Grant Program (TNGP), included a 3-year grant that required an initial application and Year 02 and Year 03 business plans to be developed and implemented, thus paving the way for business planning in TeleHealth for the first time.

The early business plans focused mainly on sustainability plans to ensure that services started as a result of grant funding were carried on after the grant cycle completed. Sustainability plans included activities that implemented billing and coding for telemedicine services, converting grant-funded positions to enterprise-funded full-time equivalent (FTE) positions, and initiating contracts for network, services, and other functions of the infrastructure that supported the delivery of care via telemedicine.

Another early program that helped to bring in additional revenue was the Universal Services Administration Company, a private enterprise dedicated to administering the Rural Health Care (RHC) fund, the Federal Communications Commission (FCC) Pilot Program, and the newer FCC Health Care Connect Fund. These FCC programs attempted to add a fiscal impact to telemedicine programs by rebating back to the health care organization monies paid to telecommunications carriers for broadband access. Although these federal rebate programs infused badly needed dollars back into telemedicine programs, the monies were not a long-term solution to financial stability or business planning.

The early business plans from OAT's TNGP grantees assisted telemedicine programs in moving toward a business approach but did not result in many organizations reaching sustainability. A few programs took business planning seriously and actually started telemedicine initiatives with a business plan in place, primarily focused on covering costs associated with an operating budget. Little was done to project revenue based on growth potential or increasing opportunities through increased market share.

It was not until the mid-2000s that organizations began searching for the perfect business plan for telemedicine. Early business models focused on traditional revenue/expense budgeting financial modeling, which rarely posed a positive revenue case for moving forward with a telemedicine initiative. What has been learned over the years is that traditional budgeting methods of telemedicine do not work to justify a telemedicine program and organizations must look to other methods of justifying and sustaining a telemedicine initiative.

In addition, modern-day telemedicine programs have a variety of business planning approaches specific to the individual model of telemedicine being used. Models of telemedicine include traditional, online, store-and-forward, concierge, self-help, artificial intelligence (AI), and remote monitoring. Other health care services that use telemedicine include health coaching, care management and coordination, and transitions of care. Today's modern business planning approaches use modern big data analytics, market analysis, value-based purchasing, and traditional fee-for-service reimbursement to calculate the financial impact of a telemedicine initiative.

Current Telemedicine Business Planning

What telemedicine organizations have finally understood is that business planning for a telemedicine initiative is *exactly the same* as planning for any other health care service. The same fundamental business planning steps apply in determining a go-no-go decision for telemedicine, which also includes the critical steps of writing down what is known and putting it all together!

The Small Business Association recommends that a business plan must include the following elements:

- Executive summary—a snapshot of the business
- Company description—describes what the business does
- Market analysis—research on the industry, market, and competitors
- Organization and management—the business and management structure
- Service or product—the products or services being offered
- Marketing and sales—how the business will be marketed and the sales strategy
- Funding request—how much money will be needed for next 3–5 years
- Financial projections—supply information like balance sheets
- Appendix—an optional section that includes résumés and permits [1]

To apply these principles to telemedicine, one just needs to think of the program at hand and then think through, research, plan, and design, based on the elements listed above. In addition, the telemedicine program would also apply these elements with a health care organization in mind. What telemedicine organizations often fail to do is plan for 3–5 years, or underestimate the market, or incorrectly gauge capacity of providers to use the service or have time to see patients. Let us begin to apply these principles to some of our telemedicine models described above.

Traditional Live Two-Way Interactive Audio and Video

The most common use of telemedicine prior to the development of direct-to-consumer (DTC) messaging and email consults was traditional telemedicine. Traditional telemedicine is when the patient and provider are present at the same time but are in different locations, and are using two-way audio and video at bandwidths sufficient to mimic in-person care. In traditional telemedicine visits, the practitioner is able to conduct a history and physical exam appropriate to make a diagnosis for a new patient and evaluate and gauge progress of established patients. Typically, traditional telemedicine is used by practitioners for services that are reimbursed in a fee-for-service environment, but may also be used in contractual services, which are explained further in the chapter. Using our business plan model, we apply the principles to traditional telemedicine in this manner. Table 10.1 outlines a template to develop a business plan using the principles noted above.

Table 10.1 Traditional telemedicine business plan

Element	Research data/examples/summary
Summary of the program	Examples: To extend the organization's service area in a specific specialty; to reduce the cost of outreach; to provide services without brick-and-mortar expenses or conducting outreach; to assist with retaining certification in such programs as Bariatric Surgery
Program description	Examples: To convert or provide services via TeleHealth (traditional live interactive) through broadband connections to other health care organizations, referring partners, affiliates, outreach sites, using full exam capabilities, for the purposes of maintaining or improving access, lowering cost, and improving retained earnings.
Market analysis	Examples: Is there a market for the telemedicine specialty service? Is expensive outreach being converted to economical telemedicine? Is there a need that exceeds capacity and can telemedicine help alleviate that need by practicing more efficiently? Do you have Is there competition for the same service in the marketplace? Is someone already providing the service in the same area? Can the telemedicine organization do it better? How?
Organization and management	Examples: Traditional telemedicine works the same as in-person care is the most efficient and economical in that manner. Use the same scheduling system, with the same appointment master with a telemedicine appointment type, book the same amount of time as in-person care, use the same documentation tools/system/EHR, bill and code the same as in-person care (unless regulatory requirements are for different CPT/HCPCs codes or modifiers)
Service or product	Examples: Live interactive two-way audio and video telemedicine consultations, encounters, visits, and care to referred or primary patients of specialty practices.
Marketing and sales	Examples: May not be applicable in situations where cost avoidance is the biggest driver of the service. To build practices, using the organization's marketing strategy is the same for telemedicine as in-person with different messaging. Wider catchment area, need to network with primary care practices, and making it easier for patients to get care are the primary marketing pitches for traditional telemedicine.
Funding	Examples: Funding for traditional telemedicine includes funding for telemedicine clinical video for providers and full exam telemedicine carts for patient sites. Once the initial investment in telemedicine technology is made, ongoing funding includes funding for operations (Telehealth coordinator, support technical staff) and maintenance and support for technology.
Financial projections	Examples: The cost of traditional telemedicine is calculated through activity-based costing that calculates the cost of the resources consumed by the telemedicine consult. Most financial cost projections for traditional telemedicine are in the form of cost savings and cost avoidance. Examples are shown later in the chapter.

Table 10.2 Cost of 30-min telemedicine versus in-person visits

Resources	In-person	Telemedicine
Physician – average salary per hour = $250 = $4.16 per minute	$125	$125
Support staff – average salary + benefits = $65,000 = $.52 per minute	$15.66	$0
Scheduling/reception – average salary $35,000 = $.28 per minute	$8.41	$8.41
EHR costs	$.25	$0.25
Technology software license	$0.00	$1.00[a]
TelePresenter costs	$0.00	$0.00[b]
Indirect costs[c]	$5.00	$2.00
Total	$154.32	$141.66

[a]Cost for concurrent use video license per use
[b]Telepresenter costs are added only when the provider organization owns the patient site
[c]Indirect costs are always lower when telemedicine is used as the exam rooms, consumables, HVAC, etc. are not consumed as the patient is not present

Activity-Based Costing

Activity-based costing is a method to calculate the actual cost of an activity based on the number and type of resources consumed [2]. The use of activity-based costing allows for and includes the financial calculations of all costs associated with the activity. Most health care organizations use revenue over expense for financial projects. However, a revenue over expense calculation does not consider actual resources consumed by a single activity, but rather calculates all expenses incurred applied to all revenues earned.

In telemedicine, calculating how much a single telemedicine visit costs considers all activities and resources consumed. For instance, in a 15-min telemedicine consult (activity), one would calculate the costs associated with the resources used (practitioner, nurses, telepresenters, EHR, reception, scheduling, technology, etc.), broken down into one (1)-min increments. Table 10.2 shows an example of calculations based on activity-based costing of a telemedicine consult versus an in-person visit.

One can see that providing services to patients over telemedicine is less costly to the organization than seeing the patient in-person. Many clinicians also comment that seeing a patient over telemedicine is more efficient than in-person care, taking less time, with higher patient satisfaction. Even when one pays for the telepresenter (health care person assisting the patient at the patient end) in situations where the same corporate entity owns both locations, the costs are still comparative to in-person care (adding back in the support staff costs at $23.45 [45 min of time] only raises the costs $7.79, which is significantly lower than the costs associated with outreach). In addition, providers who use traditional telemedicine interspersed into their daily in-person schedule see more patients per clinic day than in physical outreach, which decreases the number of hours in an outreach clinic day due to travel. If one considers all these factors, the financial impact of traditional telemedicine is calculated in Table 10.3.

Table 10.3 Total financial impact of telemedicine visits versus in-person care

Resources	In-person	Telemedicine	Outreach
Physician – average salary per hour = $250 = $4.16 per minute	$125	$125	$125
Support staff – average salary + benefits = $65,000 = $.52 per minute	$15.66	$0.00	$15.66
TelePresenter (same as support staff) 45 min	$0.00	$23.75	$0.00
Scheduling/reception – average salary $35,000 = $.28 per minute	$8.41	$8.41	$8.41
EHR costs	$.25	$0.25	$0.25
Technology software license	$0.00	$1.00*	$0.00
TelePresenter costs	$0.00	$0.00**	$0.00
Indirect costs***	$5.00	$2.00	$50.00
Travel costs	$0.00	$0.00	$100.00
Lost productive time****	$0.00	$0.00	$800.00
Total	$154.32	$165.41	$1099.32

* Per unit cost for visit
** Only paid when the organization owns the patient site
*** HVAC, sq ft lease, etc
**** Loss of time in office (revenue) when provider has to travel to outreach site

One can see that conducting outreach is infinitely more expensive than staying at the home base clinic and seeing patients via telemedicine. In addition, the revenue model is equally compelling. When one looks at the different payer sources and the contractual revenue produced per visit, clearly outreach costs the organization more in expenses that are not covered by revenue. The model is "reducing losses" versus trying to gain additional revenue. In addition, when the remote site (patient site) is not owned and operated by the consulting organization, the cost of the telepresenter is eliminated, making the case even better for economic savings when telemedicine is used. For clinicians who are interventionalists, such as interventional cardiologists or surgeons, who do outreach to sites where interventions or surgery are not possible, the potential losses for conducting physical outreach become extreme.

Typically, organizations do not use activity-based costing to conduct the financial analysis of outreach versus staying at the home office and using telemedicine instead. In addition, activity-based costing is rarely used to analyze the financial component of any health care initiative in general. Understanding how much something costs is paramount to a good financial analysis of a telemedicine initiative.

Using activity-based costing to identify the true costs of telemedicine initiatives supported by a sound business plan using the business plan elements listed above for any telemedicine initiative results in a successful go-no-go decision and plan for moving forward. Applying these elements to any of the models of telemedicine leads to success.

Scaling a traditional telemedicine program thus is dependent on provider access and is calculated to grow with the same formulas as used to simply grow an office practice. The higher the demand and time commitment needed to cover the patient sites, the more providers are needed. Typically, a provider is added when practices are 98% full and time to next available appointment goes beyond a set number of days, typically three.

Remote Patient Monitoring

Remote patient monitoring (RPM) is the use of technologies to monitor patients wherever the patient may reside or live temporarily or permanently. The technologies collect physiological data or answers to questionnaires, and transmit that data to the health care team electronically. Some RPM provides a communication chat feature, reminder systems for medication, appointments, and activities, and provides patients with educational materials and videos. Such RPM features and functionality are focused on early symptom management and reducing complications in a high, at, or near-risk patient populations. Risk populations are those persons who are at risk for developing a complication that may go untreated for some time and then result in a lengthier more costly treatment course or hospitalization. Grouping such patient populations and providing a care team that coordinates and communicates health care needs to and with the patient is commonly called care coordination and is typically a part a primary care-based patient-centered medical home (PCMH) approach.

The value of the fundamental tenets of primary care is well established. This value includes higher health care quality, better whole-person and population health, lower cost, and reduced inequalities compared to health care systems not based on primary care. The PCMH moves beyond primary care as it is practiced now, to include new approaches to organizing practice to enhance its responsiveness to local patient needs [3]. RPM fits well into a PCMH approach to managing risk populations.

Planning for a remote patient monitoring program is not different than traditional live interactive telemedicine, when considering the business plan elements and activity-based costing. One must first start with the costs associated with the program. Most costs fall into two categories of resources consumed—nursing staff and equipment. There are several reimbursement models for RPM which are imbedded in the fee-for-service world or in the new approaches CMS has taken in 2019 to the use of RPM as a non-telemedicine initiative to improve quality and reduce complications in its high-risk Medicare population [4]. The financial impact of using RPM in all models can be seen in Table 10.4.

One can see that with one registered nurse monitoring 125 high-risk patients in one month, the revenue potential versus the actual cost of 41 hours of nursing time to review data shows a profit. In addition, there are 38 hours of care left over in the month for other nursing activities that may or may not draw additional revenue.

Now add in the cost of technology and one can see that with the lease cost of $99 per month for technology, a 30-day episode of care generates an additional cost of $12,375 for RPM equipment. As technology innovation continues, the cost of such RPM devices is going down rapidly as more consumer devices are being used appropriately and with good validity, to monitor patients in the home. With our example of the basic care coordination fee-for-service 99486–99489 CPT codes revenue minus the cost of equipment, the cost of the RPM care coordination program is $8,971.89 to the health care system.

Table 10.4 Financial impact of the use of RPM with activity-based costing

Activity-Based Costing Calculation of Cost/Revenue Without New 99091		
RN salary	$65,000 salary and benefits	($31.25/h, $.52/min)
Time spent with patient per month	20 min	$10.42
# of patients	125	125 × 20 min = 2,500 min = 41 h of care = × 1.5 = 61.5 h of care/month
Payment	125 patients × $42.60	$5,325
Total cost of RN	(61.5 h at $31.25/h)	$1,921.87
Net revenue	$5,325–$1,921.87	$3,403.13
Hours of care left over	38 h (1 week)	
Total cost of equipment	$99 monthly lease fee	$12,375

Table 10.5 Additional RPM revenue potential: 125 high-risk patients

Activity-Based Costingm Calculation of Cost/Revenue CCM with new 99091		
RN salary	$65,000 salary and benefits	($31.25/h, $.52/min)
Time spent with patient	20 min per month	$10.42
# of patients	125	125 × 20 min = 2500 min = 41 h of care = × 1.5 = 61.5 h of care/month
CCM payment	125 patients × $42.60	$5,325
Remote monitoring pmt.	125 patients × $59	$7,375 ($12,700 total)
Total cost of RN	(61.5 h at $31.25/h)	$1,921
Net revenue	$5,325–$1,921.87	$10,778
Hours of care left over	38 h (1 week)	Value = $1,187
Cost of equipment	$99 per month	$12,375
Net revenue		−$1,957

But, not all is lost. With additional revenue sources for RPM for 2018 and 2019 and forward, care coordination programs now have additional revenue potentials. Starting with adding in the revenue for 99091, Table 10.5 shows the additional cost benefit of using RPM in a care coordination or PCMH strategy.

For the value that RPM brings to the health and well-being of the patient and for clinical and population health outcomes metrics for the health care organization, a cost of $1,957 per month is pennies considering the overall benefit. However, the entire financial impact is not yet finished.

10 Business Aspects of Telemedicine

Many health organizations have risk contracts with payers and CMS or state Medicaid agencies to improve quality while reducing costs associated with a specific high-risk population. Shared savings programs in health care result in a split of the savings health plans experience when providers, who typically shoulder the majority of the risk, also are paid back a part of the health plan savings. In a 30% shared savings agreement, the bonus or incentive payment back to the health care organization can be quite impressive, and certainly make up for the $1,957 in cost.

CMS talks about shared savings in relation to its Accountable Care Models (ACO).

The Shared Savings Program offers providers and suppliers (e.g., physicians, hospitals, and others involved in patient care) an opportunity to create an Accountable Care Organization (ACO). An ACO agrees to be held accountable for the quality, cost, and experience of care of an assigned Medicare fee-for-service (FFS) beneficiary population. The Shared Savings Program has different tracks that allow ACOs to select an arrangement that makes the most sense for their organization.

The Shared Savings Program is an important innovation for moving CMS' payment system away from volume and toward value and outcomes. It is an alternative payment model that:

- Promotes accountability for a patient population.
- Coordinates items and services for Medicare FFS beneficiaries.
- Encourages investment in high quality and efficient services [5].

Table 10.6 shows the cost benefits of a RPM strategy with care coordination in a shared savings program with payers. The calculations assume one kit per patient and add-in cost of one RN for 125 high-risk patients at $125,000 salary and benefits (regional).

One can see that in a shared savings or bonus/incentive program contract with health plans or government payers, the use of RPM can be used successfully to garner millions of dollars in additional retained earnings above and beyond the cost of the program itself.

Scaling a RPM program is based on calculating the number of patients the health care team can care for in terms of risk stratification. One RN can care for 125 high-risk patients in a care coordination and RPM program. As the need increases, the

Table 10.6 Shared savings calculations in RPM for 125 patients

Number of patients	Average cost of hospitalization	# of hospitalizations per year	Cost burden to health plan	Shared savings program at 30%	Average cost of remote monitoring
1	$17,000	3	$51,000	$16,830	$1,900
125	$17,000	3	$6,375,000	$2,103,750	$190,000
125 + RN	$17,000	3	$6,375,000	$2,103,750	$290,000
1	$17, 000	7	$119,000	$39,270	$1,900
125	$17,000	7	$14,875,000	$4,908,750	$190,000
125 + RN	$17,000	7	$14,875,000	$4,908,750	$290,000

number of nurses increases as well. One Medical Director is needed for the program, and one advanced registered nurse practitioner is needed per daytime shift for a care coordination and RPM program (2.4 FTEs annually).

Direct-to-Consumer

Direct-to-consumer telemedicine is the most rapidly growing model of telehealth and is driven and dominated by the for-profit sector [6]. Direct-to-consumer (DTC) telemedicine allows patients from their home, office, school, and even their cars, to access a provider online and on-demand. Typically, DTC is a cash-based health care system where the patient uses a credit card or other e-payment option to pay for care, usually around $49 to $95 depending on the type and level of care desired. Primary care, urgent care, and behavioral health are the most common specialty services using online DTC with dermatology, a growing service as well. While DTC is a subset of telemedicine, in 2019, DTC represents the largest segment of telemedicine.

DTC is a model where any person in any state can access a provider licensed in that state, without having a previously established patient–provider relationship. Patients go online, search the internet for a health care visit "now," and select among a plethora of online care providers. Some providers are companies whose sole purpose is to provide online care and have no brick and mortar offices or locations. These types of DTC companies are typically investor driven with the need to increase value for shareholders. Other forms of DTC include direct-to-enrollee (employee) (DTE) and direct-to-patient (DTP). DTE strategies are often employed by health plans and third-party administrators (on behalf of self-ensured employers), who are looking to decrease costs by diverting enrollees from primary care, urgent care centers, and the emergency department, when sudden illnesses occur, such as colds, flu, rashes, pinkeye, etc. If a health plan can spend a nominal per member per month rate or a fixed fee per click (per online visit), then the health plan typically can save $100 to thousands of dollars by avoiding the primary care provider visit or a visit to an emergency department.

DTP is often used as a strategy for meeting metrics for programs such as Accountable Care Organizations, Merit-based Incentive Payment System (MIPS), or the Medicare Access and CHIP Reauthorization Act of 2015 (MACRA) or any other quality/cost merit payment system. When health care systems are paid or incentivized by keeping an assigned patient population healthy or on a health continuum, out of the hospital and emergency department, and better connected to primary care, the health system benefits from a DTP strategy. By using online care, patient portals, and other messaging systems for patients to contact their providers first before accessing care through high-cost access points, the health care system keeps costs down while increasing quality and avoids patient leakage. Most often, emergency department and urgent care visits are avoided, and patients are treated at home through self-care strategies and sometimes, with the addition of a called-in prescription. By avoiding hundreds of thousands of dollars of costs to the payer(s) by diverting these emergency department and urgent care visits to telephonic or online care, the health plan experiences a higher incentive payment at the annual reconciliation.

A DTC telemedicine program is one of the costliest telemedicine initiatives to start. The issue is that 24×7×365 day coverage or some portion thereof needs to be staffed by a minimum of registered nurses and advanced practice registered nurses in order to provide the customer service expected and the level of professional expertise to deal with the patient's problems and to prescribe if needed. Calculating the number of calls per hour on a bell-shaped curve is another challenge and is dependent on market needs. At a minimum, one registered nurse and one back-up registered nurse and one nurse practitioner and one back-up nurse practitioner are needed to start the service. To cover all shifts, 8.4 full-time equivalents (FTEs) are needed per professional group. In addition, physician providers should be available for on-call support to nurse practitioners, thus increasing the overall costs. For a DTC start-up, these professional providers must be in place in order to start a program and to ensure coverage and quick response to patient requests for a visit.

In addition, a DTC initiative needs software that can on-board patients, collect fees, conduct insurance verification and collect co-pays, and provide all the necessary components for patients to enter health information and for clinicians to schedule, document, and respond. Management and quality reporting are often requirements for such online software products. Fees for software can range from $100 per provider per month for unlimited calls to thousands of dollars per year for organizations, with additional fees per click.

Some health care organizations who desire a DTC program partner with existing for-profit DTC companies. In this relationship, a health care organization will sign a contract with a DTC company to cover all or a portion of the 24 hour day or the seven day week. Again, the financial impact is a cost to the budget with no guaranteed revenue stream until calculations can be made after the first year.

In a DTP or DTE program, the value can be calculated as the avoidance of high-cost access points and diverting patients back to primary care or to the health plan's own DTE program. In these models, staffing has the same requirements, but in the DTP programs, many of the professional staff needed for the program are already on-call for primary care and internal medicine practices, staffing urgent care centers, or are interested in staffing extra shifts for the DTP program. The most cost-effective way to implement DTP in an existing health care organization is to staff from existing resources while building the financial outcomes over the first year. Nurse triage call centers with nurse practitioner back-up can handle most of what is needed in a DTP program. Any organization with care coordination in place or the PCMH model can benefit from implementing simple software to allow the patient to connect with the health care team and request a visit. Transitional care programs experience the same benefit from using a DTP strategy in the first 60 days post discharge to avoid re-admissions and give the patient an alternative to emergency visits if complications arise.

Using the same business planning principles from traditional telemedicine, one can put together a strategy and plan for implementing a DTC/DTP/DPE program. Table 10.7 outlines the business elements to consider and some comments on each.

Table 10.7 Business planning elements for DTC

Element	Research data/examples/summary
Summary of the program	Examples: To extend the organization's market share by providing DTC options; to increase competitive advantage in the market by offering a DTC program; to compete with other health systems and online care providers in the market and prevent patient leakage; to increase the quality outcomes of MIPS and MACRA incentive payment programs.
Program description	Examples: To provide online urgent and primary care services to patients in the regional market place (or patients of the health care system or patients enrolled in chronic care management, etc.) and avoid unnecessary urgent care and emergency department visits.
Market analysis	Examples: Is there a market for the online DTC service? Is there competition in the marketplace? Is someone already providing the service in the same area? Can you do it better? How?
Organization and management	Examples: Online DTP telemedicine requires a 24×7×365 staffing plan similar to nurse triage centers. A Director is required to manage the program and to oversee staffing, quality, clinical standards and guidelines, and all components of a health care service. Registered nurses would answer the first call and escalate when needed to an APN or physician. Documentation is typically inside the DTC software program as an abbreviated visit note or in the organization's EHR. Revenue cycle management is dependent on the billing philosophy, but typically involves a credit card or other electronic payment system.
Service or product	Examples: Artificial intelligence, telephonic, or live interactive two-way audio and video telemedicine visits.
Marketing and sales	Examples: To build practices, using the organization's marketing strategy is the same for telemedicine as in-person with different messaging. Wider catchment area, better access, lower cost, and convenience primary marketing pitches for DTC.
Funding	Examples: Funding for DTC is required for staffing, software, malpractice insurance, some indirect building costs, and other health care service related costing. The biggest funding need is for staffing which initially will be much higher than revenue for the first year. Investment funding is most often used to start a DTC program. DTP and DTE programs are started with enterprise funding and existing staffing until revenue streams, including incentive and bonus payments, are received.
Financial projections	Examples: Financial metrics for DTP, DTC, and DTE are typical revenue/expense and the use of break-even analysis. Essentially, the financial impact is the number of widgets provided at what cost as compared to the actual revenue. Organizations implementing a DTC program should calculate the break-even (BE) point, the time to get to BE and at one point positive cash flow is expected. Secondly, the DTC program must calculate at what point in revenue is it anticipated to pay-back investors. For a DTP or DTE program, the BE point is that point at which revenue is covering costs, and is typically the goal, as the bonus and incentive payments are the key revenue.

Although activity-based costing is important in all health care initiative, the break-even point is of greater value in the DTC program. Calculating costs and price can be done via activity-based costing using the same calculations as above. Table 10.8 represents the resources and costs associated with one online care visit (typically taking 7–12 min, calculated at 10 min).

10 Business Aspects of Telemedicine

Table 10.8 Calculating the cost of a 10-min DTC visit

Resources	DTC online visit cost physician	DTC online visit cost for APN	DTC online visit cost per click MD	DTC online visit cost per click APN
Physician – average salary per hour = $250 = $4.16 per minute (APN salary per hour = $85 = $1.42 per minute or $14.20 per visit)	$40.16	$14.20	$0	$0
Physician per click rate = $25.00 and APN per click rate = $15.00			$25.00	$15.00
Online care software costs	$7.00	$7.00	$7.00	$7.00
RN staffing costs – $65,000 salary and benefits ($31.25/h, $.52/min)	$5.20	$5.20	$5.20	$5.20
Indirect – management, overhead, etc.	$7.00	$7.00	$7.00	$7.00
Total	$59.36	$33.40	$44.20	$34.20

In a pure model of financial analysis, one would set the price of the online consult higher than the costs of doing the consult, to gain a profit. In other situations, where just covering the cost of the consult is the goal, one would set the price near the cost point. However, in DTC programs, typically, the cost of the professional provider is calculated based on the need to pay the provider either to be on call and a per click rate, or a higher per click rate and no call. When the telemedicine program can pay the provider a per click rate with no on-call stipend, the costs are less.

In most DTC programs, a provider can conduct about five to seven visits per hour. With a projected price of $49 per consult (based on industry average), the DTC program could generate $294 of revenue per hour. Costs are outlined in Table 10.9, showing the difference in revenue and break-even for a DTC program based on professional staffing and payment models.

As can be seen, increasing the price per visit in a for-profit DTC program decreases the number of required visits to get to break-even. In addition, changing any one of the variables produces a different result in the number of visits required for break-even. Each individual program must do this analysis in order to determine the financial impact and drivers of the decisions being made. DTP and DTE programs may have different needs based on economics of the program but certainly should know how much the program costs to run and what potential incentive and bonus payments, as well as avoidance of penalties, can be actualized through implementation of the program. A shared savings program that pays a bonus or incentive payment of $2.5 million dollars per year more than covers the cost of the DTP program.

Scaling a DTC program is based on the number of calls per hour, documentation requirements, ease of use of the software, the number of states to be covered, and the time from patient contact to connecting with a provider. Patients use online care options for the convenience and timeliness of care, "I want it today, and I want it now."

Online care patients do not want to wait hours or at times, even 20 min to reach a provider. DTC programs must be staffed and scaled to meet the consumer demands.

Table 10.9 Break-even and revenue analysis for DTC

Cost of online consult salaried provider	
Physician Salary $59.36 × # of visits/h (5) = $296.80 Revenue $49 × # of visits (5) = $294.00 Net Loss $2.80	*APN* Salary $14.20 × # of visits/h (5) = $71.00 Revenue $49 × # of visits (5) = $294.00 Net Gain $223.00
Cost of online consult per click rate	
Physician Salary $25.00 × # of visits/h (5) = $125.00 Revenue $49 × # of visits (5) = $294.00 Net gain $169.00	*APN* Salary $15.00 × # of visits/h (5) = $75.00 Revenue $49 × # of visits (5) = $294.00 Net gain $219.00
Break-even points on type of provider and price	
DTC online visit physician staffed	Salary = $240,000 + indirect costs of the program ($832,000) = $1,072,000 Break even = $1,072,000/$49 per visit = 21,877 visits
DTC online visit APN staffed	Salary = $185,000 + indirect costs of the program ($832,000) = $1,017,000 Break even = $1,017,000/$49 per visit = 20,755 visits
DTC online visit per click MD	Salary = 5 visits per hour × 2080 h of work (1 FTE) = $260,000 + indirect costs of the program ($832,000) = $1,092,000 Break even = $1,092,000/$49 per visit = 22,285 visits
DTC online visit per click APN	Salary = 5 visits per hour × 2080 h of work (1 FTE) = $156,000 + indirect costs of the program ($832,000) = $988,000 Break even = $988,000/$49 per visit = 20,163 visits

Metrics to use are the minimum staffing requirements noted above for each state of licensure (providers need to be licensed in each state where the patient resides, either through a licensure compact agreement or primary sourced licensure applications), the length of time from initial visit request to contact with a provider, and the market expectations. DTP and DTE programs may have slightly different goals for scaling a program as the populations are often more limited than a DTC program, and can be oftentimes, more predictable. Holidays, weekends, nights, and other special events often generate more requests for visits for all three direct-to-care options. Staffing and scaling for these episodic events must be considered in addition to volume scaling when expansion is desired or experienced.

And What If None of That Matters!

There are times when telemedicine just makes good business sense. There are times when setting the price lower than the costs makes good business sense. There are times when logic flies out of the window. Good practical business decision making in health care at times defies the best of business and financial planning.

For instance, a psychiatrist used telemedicine in his practice in Northern Wisconsin despite the ability to get paid for the service, because it was the right thing to do for patients. The health care organization billed when it could, collected what it could from the patient, but otherwise, provided the service regardless of the patient's ability to pay.

A health care system in Central Illinois decided to launch a DTC program for urgent and primary care and use its own clinicians to staff the program. When the planning committee was asked at what price point would they like to be at, the Vice President of Operations said "$27." When the consultant said that $27.00 was a bit low for the market, the Vice President indicated that the health care system across the street had DTC for $27 a visit and there was no ability to go higher. Twenty-seven dollars was it, even though the health system would lose money on every visit.

An emergency department initiated DTC for patients who showed up during high peak times and had non-urgent conditions identified in triage. These patients were diverted to a DTC company who had a kiosk at the entrance of the Emergency Department. Although the health care system lost revenue from diverting these patients to DTC, the value gained in reducing the backlog and risk associated with patients waiting far outweighed the lost revenue.

Home health agencies have been using RPM for decades without a penny of reimbursement, as RPM helps to improve efficiencies, reduce the number of unnecessary trips to patient homes, and identify early changes in a patient's condition, without traveling to the home. In any situation, where patients' conditions may be unpredictable, where populations are at risk, or where readmission potential is high, RPM is of value despite the ability to get paid for the actual service itself.

Sometimes, it just makes good sense to use a distance-care strategy to help alleviate the burden of access on patients, backlogged practices, and costs of outreach. When health care becomes too difficult to access or provide in a physical environment, one needs to look at strategies in telemedicine initiatives to determine value and cost. It's not always about the money.

References

1. United States Small Business Administration. Business guide: write your business plan. 2019. Retrieved from https://www.sba.gov/business-guide/plan-your-business/write-your-business-plan on 8-14-2019.
2. Kaplan R, Cooper R. Cost & effect: using integrated cost systems to drive profitability and performance. Boston: Harvard Business Review Press; 1997.
3. Stange KC, Nutting PA, Miller WL, et al. Defining and measuring the patient-Centered medical home. J Gen Intern Med. 2010;25:601–12. https://doi.org/10.1007/s11606-010-1291-3.
4. Centers for Medicare and Medicaid Services. Summary of policies in the calendar year (CY) 2018 Medicare physician fee schedule (MPFS) final rule, Telehealth originating site facility fee payment amount and Telehealth services list, and CT modifier reduction list. MLN 10393 Dec 22, 2017. Bethesda, MD.
5. https://www.cms.gov/Medicare/Medicare-Fee-for-Service-Payment/sharedsavingsprogram/about. Accessed 12-3-2019.
6. Elliott T, Shih J. Direct to consumer telemedicine. Curr Allergy Asthma Rep. 2019;19(1):1. https://doi.org/10.1007/s11882-019-0837-7.

Advancing Telehealth to Improve Access to Health in Rural America

11

Charles R. Doarn

Background

We live in an amazing time, where the whole world is at our finger tips. With a few keywords typed into a search engine, we can visit anywhere in the world. We can get information about the best place to eat, to stay, the sites to see while we are there, the current news feeds, and, of most importance, access to health information. We may be searching for a doctor, the best cure for whatever ails us, or we may in fact be able to virtually link to our physician from our home to the big city. Telemedicine and telehealth, which are not entirely the same, do encompass the intent of providing healthcare when there is a distance between the provider and patient. There are a wide variety of definitions for telemedicine and its various synonyms [1]. Some of these definitions come from professional societies like the American Telemedicine Association,[1] the American Medical Association,[2] and the American Academy of Family Medicine.[3] The federal government has several definitions based on the legislative intent of the department or agency that utilize it for unique populations and/or then general public, which makes a single definition somewhat allusive [2].

---

[1] American Telemedicine Association – https://www.americantelemed.org/resource/why-telemedicine/

[2] American Medical Association – https://www.ama-assn.org/practice-management/digital/how-definitions-digital-health-differ

[3] American Academy of Family Physicians – https://www.aafp.org/about/policies/all/telemedicine.html

---

C. R. Doarn (✉)
Department of Environmental and Public Health Sciences, College of Medicine, University of Cincinnati, Cincinnati, OH, USA
e-mail: charles.doarn@uc.edu

© Springer Nature Switzerland AG 2021
R. Latifi et al. (eds.), *Telemedicine, Telehealth and Telepresence*,
https://doi.org/10.1007/978-3-030-56917-4_11

Regardless of how telemedicine and telehealth are defined, it has spread across the landscape of American healthcare unevenly. Like traditional healthcare, there is a maldistribution of resources and the equity and access are extremely dissimilar [3]. Khairat et al. indicated that rural residents have significantly lower health status than urban counterparts, but this can be ameliorated via virtual urgent care [3]. What then is virtual urgent care and can it be applied to the management of chronic disease? Virtual care is when a patient receives care from a physician or healthcare provider when they are separated by some distance. Davis et al. reported in 2019 that virtual care was shown to be highly effective in treatment of sinusitis and in fact antibiotic utilization drops when telemedicine is used [4]. Bashshur et al. indicated that telemedicine intervention in chronic conditions such as congestive heart failure, stroke, and chronic obstructive pulmonary disease has proven to be useful [5].

Over the past several decades, telemedicine and telehealth have become more widespread due in part to higher speed broadband and cellular phone service. It has been applied to nearly every clinical discipline. This phenomenon has been realized in rural areas on a global scale [6]. Telemedicine in rural areas has been shown to be valuable tools in rural hospitals [7], and according to a Speyer et al.'s systematic review and meta-analysis in 2018, telehealth services can be just as effective as face-to-face encounters concomitant with access, and time and cost savings to the patient and the overall health system [8].

Here we are in the twenty-first century, and significant differences still remain between rural and urban areas. The vastness of the American West (Fig. 11.1) illustrates the stark differences to those of the big city. Douthit et al. discuss some of the important barriers to healthcare in rural America such as supply chains, lack of trained physicians, and insufficient transportation [9]. Health disparities continue to exist throughout the USA [9], and while the integration of technology in these areas can be quite effective, there still remain challenges of individuals accepting care this way. While Call et al. reported in 2015 that technology, regulations, and physician buy in are often cited as barriers [10]. While academic institutions around the USA

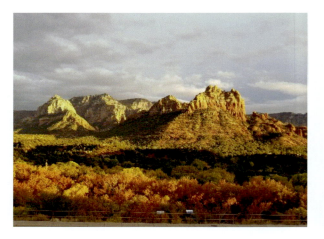

Fig. 11.1 Rural areas near Sedona, Arizona. (Courtesy C Doarn collection)

are beginning to grasp the possibilities that telemedicine and telehealth bring to healthcare, it is often challenging to accept paradigm shifts that they are too disruptive [11, 12].

While this section could go on and on, it is best to lay out the remainder of this chapter along specific and relevant points including policy, payment, trust, transportation, access, applications of technology, and future healthcare delivery systems for rural America.

Rural Health Policy

The majority of the US population lives within urban settings or close enough to gain access to a wide variety of services, including health services. It is estimated that approximately 19% of the US population live in rural areas. A rural area is defined by the US Census Bureau[4] as those areas that are sparsely populated. We think of farmland and large swathes of forested and unforested land, which equates to more than 95% of the entire US landmass. Figure 11.2 illustrates the 2010 US

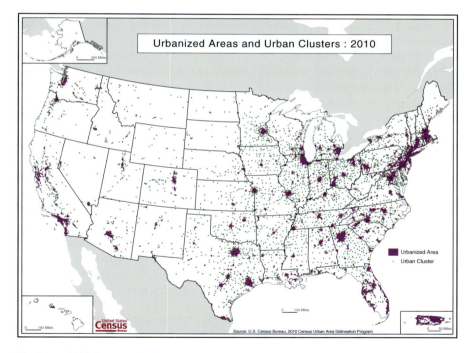

Fig. 11.2 2010 Census urbanized areas and urban clusters. (Courtesy: U.S. Census Bureau)

---

[4] United States Census Bureau – https://www.census.gov/library/stories/2017/08/rural-america.html

Census for Urbanized Areas and Urban Clusters. Those areas that are not green or purple are designated rural, and while there are more than 3000 counties across the US, a little over 1800 are mostly or completely rural. It is the population in these counties that has limited access to care, including emergency services and specialty care. This is key in America's frontier state of Alaska and for American indigenous populations [13]. The health of this population is managed by the Indian Health Service. Advanced telemedicine technology has been demonstrated effectively in rural Arizona as a direct result of US Government interaction [14].

Access to simple services like childbirth care is at a clear disadvantage in rural areas [15] as is primary care [16]. Bashshur et al. commented on the empirical foundations of telemedicine interventions in primary care that showed telemedicine could be as effective as face-to-face interactions [17].

So, if there is a need and it has been shown to work and can alleviate costs, what are the last barriers to overcome wide distribution? [9, 13] Cary et al. discuss their work on the benefits and challenges of delivery rehabilitation via telemedicine to Veterans who live in rural areas [18]. Furthermore, Adcock et al. developed a model for acute stroke care in West Virginia, which has a scarcity of services and resources to address stroke patients [19]. Is it bandwidth, is it fear, is it quality, is it access to technology what is it really that is limiting the widespread adoption in rural America? Lin et al. address some of these—cost reimbursement and technical issues—in their 2018 *Health Affairs* article [20].

While each state is responsible for its citizenry, the US Government sets Federal policy that drives state and territorial policies and regulations. This task is accomplished by vetting economic, political, social, legal, ethical, and administrative factors; and involves a whole host of individuals and organizations. One area is health information technology (HIT), which involves electronic health records, decision support systems, telehealth, etc.

The Office of the National Coordinator (ONC), which is part of the US Department of Health and Human Services (HHS), supports broadband penetration and connectivity to rural areas. The Federal Office of Rural Health Policy (ORHP) provides training and curriculum resources for communities to adapt technologies to meet the needs of rural communities. Programs exist to showcase and to encourage communities to adopt HIT, and according to Buntin et al., "HIT has the potential to improve the health of individuals and the performance of providers, yielding improved quality, cost savings, and greater engagement by patients in their own health care" [21]. HIT helps all healthcare professionals remain current on health information and support efficiency in healthcare delivery, patient engagement, and management of patients and their health.

The ORHP was established in 1987 as Section 711 of the Social Security Act and has four main tasks:

1. Keep HHS apprised of issues related to rural health and rural hospitals;
2. Coordinate with HHS activities related to rural health;
3. Establish and maintain rural health information resource (like a clearinghouse); and

4. Administer grants, cooperative agreements, and contracts to support technical assistance and rural health activities.

There are several other Federal organizations that work with ORHP, including the Agency for Healthcare Research and Quality, the Centers for Disease Control and Prevention, the Centers for Medicare and Medicaid Services, the Health Resources and Services Administration, the Indian Health Services, the Medicaid and CHIP Payment and Access Commission, the Medicare Payment Advisory Commission, the US Department of Agriculture, the US Department of Housing and Urban Development, the US Department of Transportation, and the Veterans Health Administration Office of Rural Health.

Each of the Federal agencies, departments, and offices advocates for rural health issues. In addition, there is a whole host of organizations that have an interest in rural health at the national and state levels.

In summary, there are organizations at the federal, state, and local levels that formulate policy in regards to rural populations and healthcare services available for that populace. While rural areas represent significant challenge, including remoteness, lack of resources, and other social determinants of health, telemedicine and telehealth show great promise in helping ameliorate the challenges rural American experiences [22–24].

Payment

Healthcare expenses are not universally the same across the American healthcare landscape. When resources are scarce, the price often is much higher (e.g. pineapples are cheap in Hawaii but quite expensive in Maine). Of course, the cost of care is based on the kind of care sought. If you live in rural America and require emergent care, ambulance or air car (helicopter) will be very expensive. Figure 11.3 is illustrative of a road in Wyoming about 200 miles from Yellowstone National Park. The people that live near this road will require several hours drive in any direction to get definitive care at a level 2 or 3 trauma center and even longer to a level 1 trauma center.

Fig. 11.3 Rural road in Wyoming

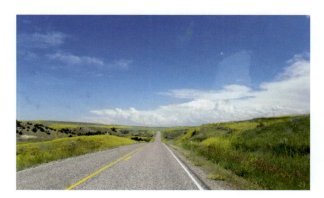

Healthcare cost can be episodic or continuous. Managing acute or chronic diseases is based on a wide variety of factors including access to care, access to information, access to appropriate technology, and access to pharmaceuticals. In March 2020, during the COVID-19 pandemic, simple medical instruments such as ventilators were in short supply. But this pandemic cemented the rationale that telemedicine could be highly effective in managing many patients from their homes. In fact, the Centers for Medicare and Medicaid Services (CMS) issued a broad wavier to support telehealth reimbursement. This was laid out in the recent legislation *P.L. 116-123 "Coronavirus Preparedness and Response Supplemental Appropriations Act, 2020."*[5]

In rural areas, individuals with sufficient bandwidth can be remotely monitored [12, 25]. Stensland et al. reported that rural healthcare provider's payment policies from CMS are influenced by the shortage of skilled physicians or services as compared to urban areas [26]. Furthermore, Conway et al. posited that care coordination in the frontier (rural) communities helps improve patient outcomes and reduce costs [27].

Trust

Face-to-face interactions between patients and their providers encompass an underlying element of trust that the healthcare providers are trained and know exactly what they are doing. Telemedicine and telehealth are both synchronous and asynchronous, and while the synchronous may be face to face, it is across a video-based platform. So, the patient and provider must be comfortable with this kind of interaction. Velsen et al. used the Patient Trust Assessment Tool (PATAT) to quantitate patient's trust in telemedicine services [28]. While Velsen et al. applied this in an anticoagulation web service, they stated the PATAT could be used as a benchmark to any service [28].

There are also ethics involved as well. Voeman et al. discussed the idea that patients should receive good reasons to trust telecare services [29]. While telemedicine and telehealth can be seen as cost cutting or cost savings, the quality of care must remain the same or better. In research by Mort et al., a framework and the ethical implications for elder individuals were reviewed [30].

The key part of telemedicine and telehealth in rural or urban areas is that the interaction between the patient and provider is of the same standard and quality as a face-to-face interaction and convenience to the patient. Zholudev et al. conducted a study of 400 hematuria evaluations with 300 via teleurology and 100 face to face. They compared three criteria: transportation, clinic operations, and patient time. The result indicated a cost savings of $124/encounter [31].

---

[5] Coronavirus Preparedness and Response Supplemental Appropriations Act, 2020. Wikipedia, March 17, 2020.

Transportation

As shown in Fig. 11.2 above, there are significant distances for many Americans to gain access to definitive care. Transportation is challenging for many in states like Alaska, where it might take a chartered plane to get to a hospital. In New Mexico, Del Rio et al. performed a Health Impact Assessment in Dona Ana County along the border with Mexico [32]. They found that providing a bus service would add benefit to the population, including access to care, food, education, and economic opportunity.

In Bashshur et al., the authors cover a wide range of subjects that can be ameliorated with solving transportation challenges in rural areas [33]. There are known inequities in care with uneven quality and fragmentation of services. While some of this is related to distribution of services and the demographics of the population, much of it can be solved with access. This was shown to be effective with the Papago Indians in southern Arizona in early 1970s [14]. Access via broadband can in many cases reduce the unnecessary and expensive transportation of patients. Telestroke and telemental health are excellent examples of this paradigm [5, 17, 19, 23, 31, 34, 35].

Applications

Telemedicine and telehealth have been and continue to be applied in every clinical discipline and in every corner of the world. While rural areas may not see the level of complexity as a large academic medical center, there has been a number of unique applications.

Telemedicine and telehealth have been applied in pediatrics in rural areas in traumatic brain injury [36], pediatric obesity [37], and pediatric surgery [38]. In South Carolina, Sundstrom et al. used telehealth to increase contraceptive access [39], and in Oklahoma, Sorocco et al. looked a home-based primary care by integrating home telehealth [40]. Oest et al. reviewed emergency department services to understand the perceived utility of telemedicine. They found at high demand psychiatric care, cardiology, and neurological services in the rural hospital in the Midwest [41]. An Australian study by Scriven et al. demonstrated a need for remote pain management through a multisite review [42].

Teledermatology [43], teledentistry [44], diabetes [45], and telemental health in Alaska among Veterans [46] are but a few successful examples of the utility of telemedicine and telehealth in rural America.

Future Applications

While telemedicine and telehealth are firmly entrenched in America's healthcare landscape, challenges and barriers remain. Chandrashekar et al. discuss the elimination of barriers of portable licensure [47]. The issue with cross state licensure continues to evolve, and the state compacts have provided some help, but nevertheless it remains an issue. The recent COVID-19 pandemic has the potential to greatly alter medical care and specifically access to it. The response we have seen worldwide would not be possible without advanced technology in computing power, information technology, sensors, artificial intelligence, and robotics. Robots have been applied in medicine and in rural settings [48], and some researchers in Arizona have studied the use of smartphones in surgery [49].

Each of these tools that have been presented and the wide variety of applications are only a small sample of what has been occurring in rural America and in other parts of the world. The fundamentals of medicine have not changed; it is just the new tools that have been applied [50]. As healthcare continues to evolve with these tools, it will become more integrated such that rural healthcare will be in lockstep with urban care [51].

Conclusion

The frontier of America can be defined in many ways, and regardless of how it is defined, it is always rural. Traditionally, urban areas have much more of everything than rural areas. There have been document fragmentation issues with healthcare, in quality, quantity, access, and equity. However, telemedicine and telehealth concomitant with other advancing technologies show great promise in ameliorating these issues. These tools, applied correctly, can be beneficial to all Americans, regardless of geography or zip code. After all, every American was provided access to electrical power as early as 1935 with the Rural Electrification Act. Nearly 90 years later, no American should be without access to appropriate medical care.

References

1. Sood S, Mbarika V, Jugoo S, Dookhy R, Doarn CR, Prakash N, Merrell RC. What is telemedicine? A collection of 104 peer-reviewed perspectives and theoretical underpinnings. Telemed J E Health. 2007;13(5):573–90.
2. Doarn CR, Pruitt S, Jacobs J, Harris Y, Bott DM, Riley W, Lamer C, Oliver AL. Federal efforts to define and advance telehealth--a work in progress. Telemed J E Health. 2014;20(5):409–18.
3. Khairat S, Haithcoat T, Liu S, Zaman T, Edson B, Gianforcaro R, Shyu CR. Advancing health equity and access using telemedicine: a geospatial assessment. J Am Med Inform Assoc. 2019;26(8–9):796–805.
4. Davis CB, Marzec LN, Blea Z, Godfrey D, Bickley D, Michael SS, Reno E, Bookman K, Lemery JJ. Antibiotic prescribing patterns for sinusitis within a direct-to-consumer virtual urgent care. Telemed J E Health. 2019;25(6):519–22.
5. Bashshur RL, Shannon GW, Smith BR, Alverson DC, Antoniotti N, Barsan WG, Bashshur N, Brown EM, Coye MJ, Doarn CR, Ferguson S, Grigsby J, Krupinski EA, Kvedar JC, Linkous J, Merrell RC, Nesbitt T, Poropatich R, Rheuban KS, Sanders JH, Watson AR, Weinstein RS, Yellowlees P. The empirical foundations of telemedicine interventions for chronic disease management. Telemed J E Health. 2014;20(9):769–800.
6. Durupt M, Bouchy O, Christophe S, Kivits J, Boivin JM. Telemedicine in rural areas: general practitioners' representations and experiences. Sante Publique. 2016;28(4):487–97. Article in French

7. Coffey B. Telemedicine in small-town America. A game changer for rural hospitals. Health Manag Technol. 2014;35(11):24.
8. Speyer R, Denman D, Wilkes-Gillan S, Chen YW, Bogaardt H, Kim JH, Heckathorn DE, Cordier R. Effects of telehealth by allied health professionals and nurses in rural and remote areas: a systematic review and meta-analysis. J Rehabil Med. 2018;50(3):225–35.
9. Douthit N, Kiv S, Dwolatzky T, Biswas S. Exposing some important barriers to health care access in the rural USA. Public Health. 2015;129(6):611–20.
10. Call VR, Erickson LD, Dailey NK, Hicken BL, Rupper R, Yorgason JB, Bair B. Attitudes toward telemedicine in urban, rural, and highly rural communities. Telemed J E Health. 2015;21(8):644–51.
11. Doarn CR, Dorogi A, Tikhtman R, Pallerla H, Vonder Meulen MB. Opinions on the role of telehealth in a large Midwest academic health center: a case study. Telemed J E Health. 2019;25(12):1250–61.
12. Hollander JE, Davis TM, Doarn C, Goldwater JC, Klasko S, Lowery C, Papanagnou D, Rasmussen P, Sites FD, Stone D, Carr BG. Recommendations from the first national academic consortium of telehealth. Popul Health Manag. 2018;21(4):271–7.
13. Cromer KJ, Wofford L, Wyant DK. Barriers to healthcare access facing American Indian and Alaska natives in rural America. J Community Health Nurs. 2019;36(4):165–87.
14. Simpson AT, Doarn CR, Garber SJ. Interagency cooperation in the twilight of the great society: telemedicine, NASA and the Papago nation. J Policy Hist. 2020;31(1):25–51.
15. Shah NT. Eroding access and quality of childbirth care in rural US counties. JAMA. 2018;319(12):1203–4.
16. Selby-Nelson EM, Bradley JM, Schiefer RA, Hoover-Thompson A. Primary care integration in rural areas: a community-focused approach. Fam Syst Health. 2018;36(4):528–34.
17. Bashshur RL, Howell JD, Krupinski EA, Harms KM, Bashshur N, Doarn CR. The empirical foundations of telemedicine interventions in primary care. Telemed J E Health. 2016;22(5):342–75.
18. Cary MP Jr, Spencer M, Carroll A, Hand DH, Amis K, Karan E, Cannon RF, Morgan MS, Hoenig HM. Benefits and challenges of delivering tele-rehabilitation services to rural veterans. Home Healthc Now. 2016;34(8):440–6.
19. Adcock AK, Choi J, Alvi M, Murray A, Seachrist E, Smith M, Findley S. Expanding acute stroke care in rural America: a model for statewide success. Telemed J E Health. 2020;26:865–71.
20. Lin CC, Dievler A, Robbins C, Sripipatana A, Quinn M, Nair S. Telehealth in health centers: key adoption factors, barriers, and opportunities. Health Aff (Millwood). 2018;37(12):1967–74.
21. Buntin MB, Burke MF, Hoaglin MC, Blumenthal D. The benefits of health information technology: a review of the recent literature shows predominantly positive results. Health Aff (Millwood). 2011;30(3):464–71.
22. Zhau J, Weber T, Hanson J, Nelson M, Birger C, Puumala S. A county-level health index to capture geographic variation in health conditions in North Dakota, South Dakota, and Minnesota. S D Med. 2019;72(5):206–13.
23. Harrington RA, Califf RM, Balamurugan A, Brown N, Benjamin RM, Braund WE, Hipp J, Konig M, Sanchez E, Joynt Maddox KE. Call to action: rural health: a presidential advisory from the American Heart Association and American Stroke Association. Circulation. 2020;141(10):e615–44.
24. Probst JC, Barker JC, Enders A, Gardiner P. Current state of child health in rural America: how context shapes children's health. J Rural Health. 2018;34(Suppl 1):s3–s12.
25. Haselkorn A, Coye MJ, Doarn CR. The future of remote health services: summary of an expert panel discussion. Telemed J E Health. 2007;13(3):341–7.
26. Stensland J, Akamigbo A, Glass D, Zabinski D. Rural and urban Medicare beneficiaries use remarkably similar amounts of health care services. Health Aff (Millwood). 2013;32(11):2040–6.
27. Conway P, Favet H, Hall L, Uhrich J, Palche J, Olimb S, Tesch N, York-Jesme M, Bianco J. Rural health networks and care coordination: health care innovation in frontier communities to improve patient outcomes and reduce health care costs. J Health Care Poor Underserved. 2016;27(4A):91–115.

28. Velsen LV, Tabak M, Hermens H. Measuring patient trust in telemedicine services: development of a survey instrument and its validation for an anticoagulation web-service. Int J Med Inform. 2017;97:52–8.
29. Voeman SA, Nickel PJ. Sound trust and the ethics of telecare. J Med Philos. 2017;42(1):33–49.
30. Mort M, Roberts C, Pols J, Domenech M, Moser I, EFORTT investigators. Ethical implications of home telecare for older people: a framework derived from a multi-sited participative study. Health Expect. 2015;18(3):438–49.
31. Zholudev V, Safir IJ, Painter MN, Petros JA, Filson CP, Issa MM. Comparative cost analysis: teleurology vs conventional face-to-face clinics. Urology. 2018;113:40–4.
32. Del Rio M, Hargrove WL, Tomaka J, Korc M. Transportation matters: a health impact assessment in rural New Mexico. Int J Environ Res Public Health. 2017;14(6):629.
33. Bashshur RL, Shannon GW, Krupinski EA, Grigsby J, Kvedar JC, Weinstein RS, Sanders JH, Rheuban KS, Nesbitt TS, Alverson DC, Merrell RC, Linkous JD, Ferguson AS, Waters RJ, Stachura ME, Ellis DG, Antoniotti NM, Johnston B, Doarn CR, Yellowlees P, Normandin S, Tracy J. National telemedicine initiatives: essential to healthcare reform. Telemed J E Health. 2009;15(6):600–10.
34. Fairchild RM, Ferng-Kuo SF, Laws S, Rahmouni H, Hardesty D. Telehealth decreases rural emergency department wait times for behavioral health patients in a group of critical access hospitals. Telemed J E Health. 2019;25(12):1154–64.
35. Marcin JP, Shaikh U, Steinhorn RH. Addressing health disparities in rural communities using telehealth. Pediatr Res. 2016;79(1–2):169–76.
36. Yue JK, Upadhyayula PS, Avalos LN, Cage TA. Pediatric traumatic brain injury in the United States: rural-urban disparities and considerations. Brain Sci. 2020;10(3):135.
37. Hosseini H, Yilmaz A. Using telehealth to address pediatric obesity in rural Pennsylvania. Hosp Top. 2019;97(3):107–18.
38. Kohler JE, Falcone RA Jr, Fallat ME. Rural health, telemedicine and access for pediatric surgery. Curr Opin Pediatr. 2019;31(3):391–8.
39. Sundstrom B, DeMaria AL, Ferrara M, Meier S, Billings D. "The closer, the better:" the role of telehealth in increasing contraceptive access among women in rural South Carolina. Matern Child Health J. 2019;23(9):1196–205.
40. Sorocco KH, Bratkovich KL, Wingo R, Qureshi SM, Mason PJ. Integrating care coordination home telehealth and home-based primary care in rural Oklahoma: a pilot study. Psychol Serv. 2013;10(3):350–2.
41. Oest SER, Swanson MB, Ahmed A, Mohr NM. Perceptions and perceived utility of rural emergency department telemedicine services: a needs assessment. Telemed J E Health. 2020;26:855–64.
42. Scriven H, Doherty DP, Ward EC. Evaluation of a multisite telehealth group model for persistent pain management for rural/remote participants. Rural Remote Health. 2019;19(1):4710.
43. Coustasse A, Sarkar R, Abodunde B, Metzger BJ, Slater CM. Use of teledermatology to improve dermatological access in rural areas. Telemed J E Health. 2019;25(11):1022–32.
44. Martin AB, Nelson JD, Bhavsar GP, McElligott J, Garr D, Leite RS. Feasibility assessment for using telehealth technology to improve access to dental care for rural and underserved populations. J Evid Based Dent Pract. 2016;16(4):228–35.
45. Siminerio L, Ruppert K, Huber K, Toledo FG. Telemedicine for Reach, Education, Access, and Treatment (TREAT): linking telemedicine with diabetes self-management education to improve care in rural communities. Diabetes Educ. 2014;40(6):797–805.
46. Goss CW, Richardson WJB, Dailey N, Bair B, Nagamoto H, Manson SM, Shore JH. Rural American Indian and Alaska Native veterans' telemental health: a model of culturally centered care. Psychol Serv. 2017;14(3):270–8.
47. Chandrashekar P, Jain SH. Eliminating barriers to virtual care: implementing portable medical licensure. Am J Manag Care. 2020;26(1):20–2.
48. Murray C, Ortiz E, Kubin C. Application of a robot for critical care rounding in small rural hospitals. Crit Care Nurs Clin North Am. 2014;26(4):477–85.

49. Zangbar B, Pandit V, Rhee P, Aziz H, Hashmi A, Friese RS, Weinstein R, Joseph B. Smartphone surgery: how technology can transform practice. Telemed J E Health. 2014;20(6):590–2.
50. Weinstein RS, Krupinski EA, Doarn CR. Clinical examination component of telemedicine, telehealth, mHealth, and connected health medical practices. Med Clin North Am. 2018;102(3):533–44.
51. Bashshur RL, Krupinski EA, Doarn CR, Merrell RC, Woolliscroft JO, Frenk J. Telemedicine across time: integrated health system of the future-a prelude. Telemed J E Health. 2020;26(2):128–30.

Part II

Strategies for Building Sustainable Telemedicine and Telehealth Programs

Innovative Governance Model for a Sustainable State-Wide University-Based Telemedicine Program

12

Ronald S. Weinstein, Nandini Sodhi, Gail P. Barker, Michael J. Holcomb, Kristine A. Erps, Angelette Holtrust, Rifat Latifi, and Elizabeth A. Krupinski

Introduction

Forms of governance and arrangements for oversight can be critically important determinants of the successes and sustainability of telemedicine programs regardless of their sizes, which range from large multi-national programs down to small programs involving a small cluster of telemedicine service providers and/or service users [1–4]. Fine-tuning of a telemedicine services' organization chart regarding the political realities of the environments in which stakeholders will deliver or utilize telehealth services can have long-term rewards. This may be especially true in the United States where experience shows that university-based telemedicine programs' priorities can be misaligned with the priorities of their parent university's healthcare entity. Experience has shown that unless suitable bi-directional communication with higher authorities, such as a state legislature or a state department of health services, is established at the time of the founding of a telemedicine program, and baked into the telemedicine program's organization chart and oversight mechanisms, the telemedicine program is more likely to fail than succeed.

In 1996, Arizona embarked on an experiment in governance (little more than a "tweak" in existing university's state government policy) for its recently funded university-based state-wide telemedicine program. The Arizona State Legislature took the initiative of creating the state-wide Arizona Telemedicine program with the

---

The original version of this chapter was revised. The correction to this chapter is available at https://doi.org/10.1007/978-3-030-56917-4_30.

R. S. Weinstein (✉) · N. Sodhi · G. P. Barker · M. J. Holcomb · K. A. Erps · A. Holtrust
Arizona Telemedicine Program, The University of Arizona's College of Medicine, Tucson, AZ, USA
e-mail: rweinstein@telemedicine.arizona.edu

R. Latifi
Department of Surgery, New York Medical College, School of Medicine and Westchester Medical Center Health, Valhalla, NY, USA

E. A. Krupinski
Department of Radiology, Emory University, Atlanta, GA, USA

© The Author(s) 2021, corrected publication 2021
R. Latifi et al. (eds.), *Telemedicine, Telehealth and Telepresence*,
https://doi.org/10.1007/978-3-030-56917-4_12

specific aims of: (1) encouraging, and supporting, the build-out of a dedicated healthcare telecommunications network to support the delivery of specialty medical services to Arizona's underserved rural communities; and (2) to promote the expansion of Arizona's rural healthcare workforce. The first step was the creation of a rural telecommunications infrastructure for healthcare [5–7].

In 1996, broadband telecommunications were virtually non-existent in rural Arizona. Several Arizona Governors, including Fife Symington III and Rose Mofford, had been unsuccessful in attracting large telecommunication companies to do business in rural Arizona. In the early 1990s, the state's only medical school was in Tucson, Arizona, 115 miles southeast of the state capitol in Phoenix. The legislature tasked the University of Arizona's College of Medicine's Dean with finding a solution to the telecommunications challenges.

In 1996, initial enabling legislation created funding for what the state legislature labeled the "Arizona Rural Telemedicine Network (ARTN)," a name that stuck and is still attached to the annual funding of the program. The Medical College's then Dean James Dalen created the Arizona Telemedicine Program (ATP), a new administrative unit at the University of Arizona, to house the ARTN. ATP has a large portfolio of healthcare services, innovative educational programs, research activities, and federal grants [7].

The Arizona Telemedicine Council's (ATC) creation was agreed upon by the Chairs of the Appropriations Committees of Arizona House of Representatives and Arizona Senate. The ATC was designed to provide the ATP with a direct reporting relationship to the Arizona State's Legislature, on the Arizona State Capitol Campus. The general principles for the ATC had been conceived by the director-designate of the ATP, Ronald S. Weinstein, MD, as a requirement for his recruitment as ATP Founding Director (Fig. 12.1). It was understood that the ATP was to be a part time job, in addition to his responsibilities as Head of the Department of Pathology in the University of Arizona's College of Medicine-Tucson and Pathologist-in-Chief at University Medical Center in Tucson. However, it eventually became his full-time job 11 years later, in 2007, when he stepped down as a pathology department head after 32 years in that position at two different medical schools, first in Chicago and then in Tucson, AZ.

Mr. John Lee, an Assistant Director at the AZ State Legislature's Joint Legislative Budget Committee (JLBC), who had state university budgets in his portfolio, discussed Dr. Weinstein's requirement for a direct channel though which to communicate with the Arizona State Legislature with him by telephone. Dr. Weinstein outlined what he wanted to accomplish and expressed his concerns over the capability of research universities to accommodate some programs' whose primary constituencies resided outside of the walls of the university, such as rural communities and the Arizona state prisons where telemedicine was expected to address access to care issues, which were a healthcare concern in the state at that time. Dr.

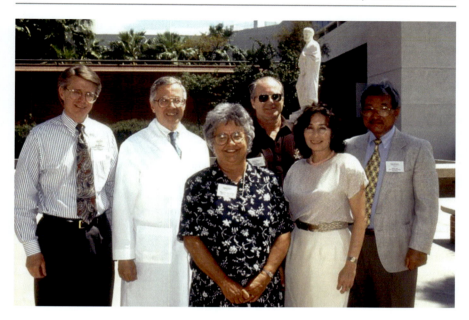

Fig. 12.1 Founders of the Arizona Telemedicine Program, June 1996 at the Arizona Health Sciences Center, Tucson, Arizona. Left to right: Richard A. McNeely, Director, Biomedical Communications and Co-Director of the Arizona Telemedicine Program, Ronald S. Weinstein, MD, Co-founder and Director, Arizona Telemedicine Program, Arizona Representative Lou Ann Preble, Arizona Representative Robert "Bob" Burns, Co-founder Arizona Telemedicine Program and Chair, and Co-founder of the Arizona Telemedicine Council, Rachel Anderson, Director, Arizona Health Sciences Medical Library, and John Lee, Assistant Director, Joint Legislative Budget Committee, Arizona State Legislature. A statue of Hippocrates is seen in the background. (Reproduced with permission from [8])

Weinstein trained as a cancer scientist and pathologist at Harvard and the Massachusetts General Hospital in Boston and regarded these institutions as being insular in the 1960s when he had trained there. Having worked with university budgets, Mr. Lee understood his concerns.

Their invention was the Arizona Telemedicine Council (ATC). To address these concerns, Mr. Lee and Dr. Weinstein came up with the idea of creating the ATC as a *blue ribbon* "non-statutory overarching authority." Dr. Weinstein insisted that ATC meetings be on the Arizona State Capitol Campus. He had worked at the US Capitol in Washington, DC, as a college student and appreciated the value of the "halo effect" of state and the federal capitol campuses. Since academic, governmental, and commercial buildings are designed with large atriums at the fronts of buildings, often for the singular purpose of gaining "public trust," Dr. Weinstein reasoned that holding ATC quarterly meetings on the Arizona Capital Campus, especially in the

JLBC Board Room, would add to the perceived legitimacy of the ATC and its implied authority. In addition, Mr. Lee and Dr. Weinstein also agreed that the ATC would meet quarterly (January, April, July, and October) for 2-hour lunch meetings. ATC meetings would have all the trappings of a "public meeting." The JLBC has its own small red brick building across the street from the Arizona State Capitol, 1.6 miles from downtown Phoenix. Mr. Lee would propose to Representative Bob Burns that the current chairs of the Arizona State Legislature's House and Senate Appropriations Committees, or their successors, chair these two-hour meetings. Dr. Weinstein would create the agenda, with input from stakeholders. Agendas would be pre-published before the meetings, as is required for "public meetings" at the State Legislature, and minutes of the previous ATC meeting would be presented to the Director of the ATC at the time of the next meeting.

At the time of the creation of the ATC, Representative Bob Burns, the co-sponsor for the enabling legislation for the ATP, and his counterpart in the Arizona State Senate both agreed to co-chair these meetings. To his great credit, Representative Burns (ret.) has continued to do so for the next 23 years, even after he termed out of the House, was elected to the AZ State Senate, and was immediately selected as Chair of Senate Appropriations, and State Senate President, in his fourth term as a Senator, and then elected onto the Arizona Corporation Commission, for which he is currently Chairman. Bob Burns remains the face of telemedicine in Arizona today from the perspective of the Arizona state government. Governance of the ATP was divided up in a highly creative manner. The ATP would report to the ATC for programmatic oversight and to the Arizona College of Medicine for fiduciary oversight.

Under the joint leadership of Dr. Weinstein and (currently) Arizona Corporation Commission Chairman Bob Burns, the ATP has expanded into one of the largest, most comprehensive university-based telemedicine and telehealth programs in the United States (Fig. 12.2).

The ATC meetings serve as a showcase for current independent telemedicine programs in operation throughout Arizona as well as emerging telemedicine technologists and innovative healthcare service delivery models. It provides a forum for discussing legal, regulatory, and reimbursement issues, and prospective legislation (Fig. 12.3). In addition, the ATC provides a platform for presentations by telemedicine medical devices and telehealth, robotics, Artificial Intelligence, and automation advances in the healthcare industry. Arizona-based telemedicine companies are encouraged to make presentations on their visions for the industry. The ATP's federally funded programs, as well as state and federal funding opportunities are openly discussed. The ATP has been a magnet for federal grant and contracting funding.

The following analysis of the interrelated ATP and ATC covers a 15-year period (2003–2018).

12 Innovative Governance Model for a Sustainable State-Wide University-Based...

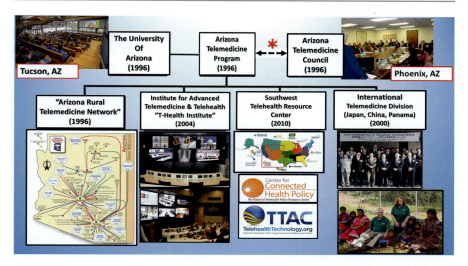

Fig. 12.2 Activities Chart for the Arizona Telemedicine Program (upper tier, center). The Arizona Telemedicine Program (ATP), founded in 1996, reports to The University of Arizona, in Tucson, AZ (upper tier, left) for fiduciary purposes and the Arizona Telemedicine Council (ATC) (upper tier, right) for programmatic review. The ATC, also founded in 1996, is a non-statutory over-arching authority (red asterisk/dotted bi-directional arrow) which meets quarterly on the AZ State Capitol Campus, in Phoenix. The "Arizona Rural Telemedicine Network" (lower tier left) is operated by ATP. By 2006, it linked 160 sites in 70 communities. The ATP's T-Health Institute, in downtown Phoenix, AZ, houses its T-Health Amphitheater (lower tier, 2nd from the left (Upper photo–Video-wall layout for an Interprofessional Education and Collaborative Practice [IPECP] exercises; Lower photo–"Community Briefing on Telemedicine" for Phoenix-area executives)), a multi-purpose video-conferencing facility used by dozens of organizations each year. In addition, In addition, the T-Health Institute developed innovative medical science curriculum for K-12 and college students [9–12]. The HRSA-funded Southwest Telehealth Resource Center (lower tier, 3rd from the left) is also operated by the ATP. Its territory (map; red box) includes Arizona, Colorado, New Mexico, Nevada, and Utah. National components of the Telehealth Resource Center consortium are the Center for Connected Health Policy (CCHP) and the Telehealth Technology Assessment Center (TTAC). The International Telemedicine Division of the ATP was organized in 2000 [13, 14]. The ATP provided technical assistance for the Republic of Panama's Telemedicine and Telehealth Program, from 2000 to 2009. Dr. Weinstein in Kyoto, Japan, (lower tier, right, upper photo; Dr. Weinstein is in the front row, 2nd from the right, next to Dr. Jame McGee, Chair of pathology at Oxford University, UK, who 1st to the right) at a meeting of leaders in telepathology from Japan, Poland, Germany, United States, and Great Britain, in 2000. Dr. Weinstein and an ATP associate director are pictured with families at a telemedicine clinic on a native Panamanian reservation in rural Panama (lower tier, right, lower photo) [15]

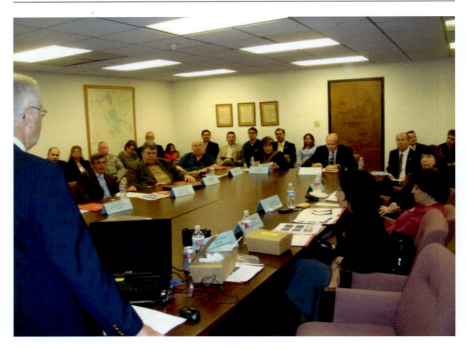

Fig. 12.3 Quarterly meeting of the Arizona Telemedicine Council in the Board Room of the Joint Legislative Budget Committee of the Arizona State Legislature on the Arizona State Capitol Campus, in Phoenix, Arizona. State Senators Robert "Bob" Burns (Chairing the meeting) and Amanda Aguirre are at the far end of the table. Ronald S. Weinstein, MD, Director of the Arizona Telemedicine Program, is speaking at the head of the table (left, standing)

ATC Membership

The members of the ATC serve for open-ended terms. Many come from the governmental, agency, public, and/or educational sectors (Fig. 12.4). Membership of the Arizona Telemedicine Council is regarded as a significant honor in Arizona. Corporate Commissioner Burns and Dr. Weinstein select, and invite, members. Mr. Burns and Dr. Weinstein keep two factors in mind: (1) maintaining a balance of individuals with "corporate memory" of the development of the Arizona telemedicine programs and of the telemedicine industry; and (2) the value of having members with a broad range of relevant job descriptions and skill sets. Candidates are often invited to attend ATC meetings before they are recruited as members. One litmus is the capability of an individual to leave one's "corporate identity outside the door" of the JLBC conference room.

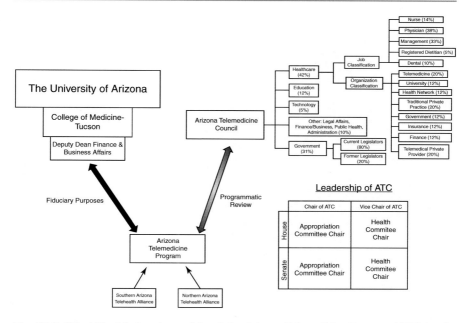

Fig. 12.4 "Dual Track" shared oversight of the Arizona Telemedicine Program (ATP) by the University of Arizona's College of Medicine and Arizona Telemedicine Council (ATC). Birds eye view of this hybrid set-up is shown in this figure. Upper right shows the distribution of ATC current 39 members. Lower right shows the leadership of the ATC. Mr. Burns, as co-founder of the ATP and ATC, substitutes for the House Appropriation Committee Chair when available, which is most of the time for the past 23 years

Analysis of the Arizona Telemedicine Council

Industries represented on the ATC. Figure 12.5 shows the distributions of industry classifications of the current 39 members of the ATC. The single largest percentage of ATC members had jobs in the healthcare industry.

The largest percentages of healthcare industry workers came from telemedicine service organizations (20%), private telemedicine practices (20%), healthcare networks (12%), and universities practices (12%) (Fig. 12.6).

Over half of the healthcare slice consisted of practicing physicians, nurses, dentists, and dietitians, while hospital management also well represented (Fig. 12.7).

Government Attendees

The second largest category of ATC members (12%) had jobs in government (Fig. 12.8). The government job sub-classifications (Fig. 12.8) included current and former legislators (71%) and government agency employees (29%).

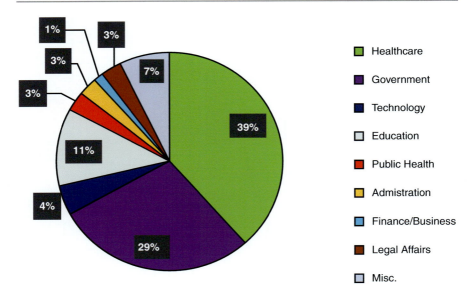

Fig. 12.5 Industry classifications of all ATC members for a 15-year period (2003–2018). It shows the distributions of job classifications of the current 39 members of the ATC and illustrates the fact that ATC members are drawn from a broad spectrum of industries

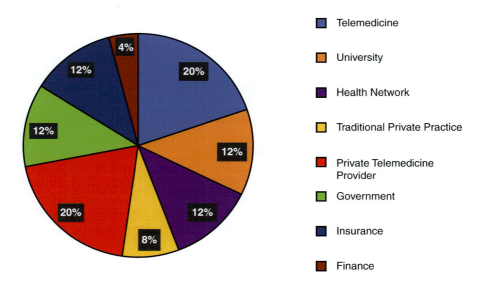

Fig. 12.6 Business sectors for ATC members working in the healthcare industry (2003–2018)

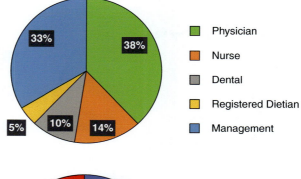

Fig. 12.7 Breakout, by position, of health workers employed in the health sector

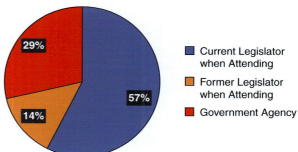

Fig. 12.8 Status of government ATC attendees (2003–2018)

The presence of current, and former, legislators present at the ATC meetings provides an opportunity for open communication between the professionals in the field, such as physicians, nurses, insurers, and the state legislature.

ATC Presenters

ATC quarterly meeting agendas consist of ATP updates by the ATP Director and ATC moderator, Dr. Weinstein; presentations on a series of legislative, regulatory, and reimbursement issues; overviews of newer telehealth applications; and telehealth industry updates. Over half of the speakers are invited one-time speakers (Fig. 12.9).

Figure 12.10 shows the number of meetings members on the council have attended with some attending for more than a decade (Fig. 12.11). Over the 15-year period, over half of ATC members have attended a minimum of six meetings, Dr. Weinstein being at all 58 meetings and Corporate Commissioner being at 52 of the 58 meetings.

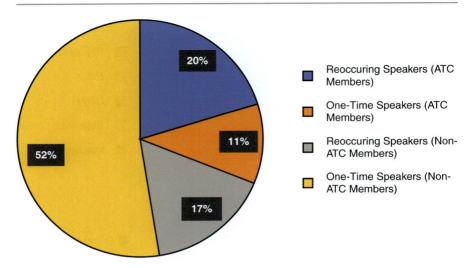

Fig. 12.9 Frequencies of ATC meeting speakers (2003–2018)

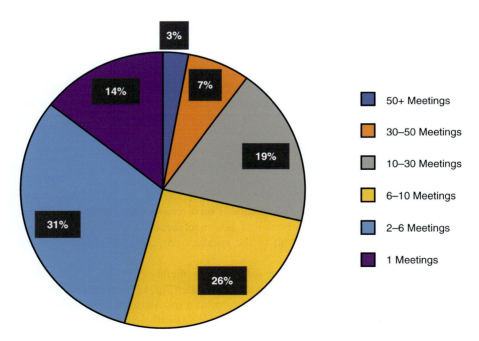

Fig. 12.10 Numbers of meetings attended by ATC members (2003–2018)

Fig. 12.11 Ranges of years of ATC membership (2003–2018)

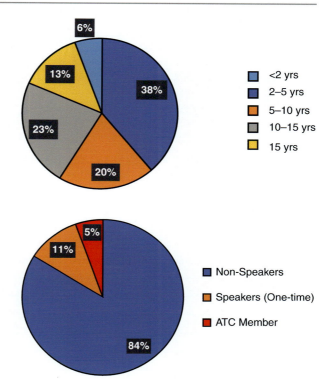

Fig. 12.12 Profiles of single ATC meeting attendees (2003–2018). The ATC meetings serve as a showcase for the telemedicine industry. Often attendees from industry come to a single ATC meeting. Not infrequently, other employees of an individual company come on other occasions

Having the same leadership present in the council was also critical. This continuity of the same leadership in the council has allowed for the maintenance of goals and provided a foundation for the relationships within the council to develop.

The ATC meetings have an important role in showcasing telemedicine, telehealth, and digital medicine to a very broad spectrum of interested groups ranging from community leaders and healthcare advocacy groups, to principals in healthcare related start-up companies. The ATP is a national leader in federally funded digital medicine research and in telehealth-enabled distance education. Many different interested individuals and groups are invited to attend ATC meetings as spectators to learn about diverse facets of the telehealth and digital medical industries (Fig. 12.12).

Retrospective Longitudinal Analysis of ATC Attendance

Meeting attendance per meeting by attendees (blue line in Fig. 12.13) and members (orange line in Fig. 12.13) reflects the interest and commitment made by their communities to guide telemedicine in Arizona to help alleviate the healthcare disparities

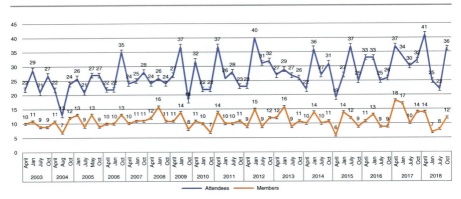

Fig. 12.13 Numbers of member (orange line) and total attendees (blue line) at ATC meetings over time (2003–2018)

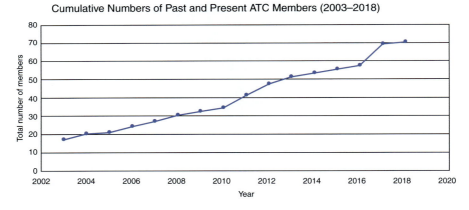

Fig. 12.14 Cumulative numbers of individuals who have served as ATC members (2003–2018)

and make a difference in their communities. On average, meetings have 28 attendees in the room (room seats 43 people) and 11 are ATC members. Some meetings, however, have reached 41 attendees of which 15 are ATC members. There is no apparent correlation between meeting quarters (January, April, July, or October) and the level of attendance.

Overall, the consistency of the same leadership and members has strongly contributed to the impact made by this council since it has provided a foundation for friendships and understanding within the ATC along with stability and structure. Without stability and long-lasting relationships, the ATP wouldn't have been able to integrate into the capital as easily since consistency turned out to be the key. Cumulatively, ATC has had 70 members (Fig. 12.14).

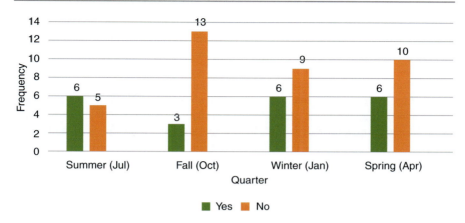

Fig. 12.15 Bar graph showing the frequency with which legislation was discussed at ATC meetings, by quarter (2003–2018). *Note: the following ATC meetings were cancelled: January 2014, July 2004, and July 2006–2010. This accounts for the lower net numbers of ATC summer meetings

Frequency of ATC Consideration of Legislation

Lastly, since legislation is addressed in the ATC repeatedly through presentations and discussions, the ATC remains closely linked with the Arizona Legislature. This link helps preserve the council since it provides current and past legislators a motivation to continue to attend the meetings. More importantly, it allows for the council to communicate to the healthcare legislators what is needed for the industry and what currently is working or not. The legislators benefit from knowledge that the ATC members bring while the ATC members benefit from being able to directly communicate with current Arizona legislators.

It was concluded via this longitudinal 15-year study, overall, legislation is discussed in over half the summer, winter, and spring meetings. In the fall meeting though, legislation is not as frequently discussed as the legislative session is adjourned for the year. Per year there are approximately four quarterly meetings, though some were not held (Fig. 12.15).

ATC Leadership: The Burns–Weinstein Partnership

We acknowledge that the Burns–Weinstein partnership is unusual in terms of the ranges of shared interests of Mr. Burns and Dr. Weinstein coming into their leadership roles for the ATP. They are also the same age and perceive that they are at the similar stages in their careers.

Mr. Burns and Dr. Weinstein were schooled in government, although at different stages of their lives and from somewhat different perspective. They understood the important roles that legislative staffs have in linking constituents to governmental resources.

Mr. Burns entered politics to deal with regulatory issues negatively affecting the chain of pre-K education centers he operated with his wife. Dr. Weinstein had a lifelong interest in government. He had been a student leader and actively participated in mock legislatures in high school. In college, although a pre-medical student, he competed successfully for a Ford Foundation-funded summer internship in the US House of Representatives which was awarded to the Union College (Schenectady, New York) student with the highest grade in the "Introduction to Government" course. Dr. Weinstein spent the summer of 1959 in Washington, DC, participating in the management of constituent relations in the office of an up-and-coming Congressman from Upstate New York. As a bonus, he attended the hearings of Senator McClellan's "United States Senate Select Committee on Improper Activities in Labor and Management" featuring Senator John F. Kennedy, a member of the committee and its select subcommittee (on "racketeering") and candidate for the US Presidency in 1960, and his 34-year-old younger brother Bobby Kennedy, Chief Council of the Select Committee and future Attorney General and then New York Senator. Weinstein shared a birthday with Bobby Kennedy (November 20) who was just 13 years his senior. Jimmy Hoffa, the President of the Teamsters' Union, testified at length, and the mob of his Teamster supporters were in the audience over a period of several days. These were "showcase" hearings which were electrifying theater from Dr. Weinstein's perspective. For three consecutive days, Dr. Weinstein, a 21-year-old soon-to-be college senior, sat behind Jackie Kennedy, Senator Kennedy's wife, seated in the front row of the audience, who had spent her 30th birthday the weekend before the hearings at the Kennedy family horse farm in Virginia. He chatted with members of the Kennedy family entourage who surrounded him in the audience. Later in life, he served on the Board of Directors of a Kennedy family foundation.

Mr. Burns and Dr. Weinstein both had long standing interests in computers nurtured during their respective US military services, Mr. Burns as an Aviation Electronics Technician, in the US Navy, and Dr. Weinstein as a Major in the US Air Force Medical Corp during the Vietnam War. In 1962, after completing his stint in the US Navy, Mr. Burns became a computer programming analyst at the General Electric Company, in Phoenix, Arizona. Ironically, Dr. Weinstein's father had worked as a mechanical engineer at the General Electric Company's headquarters in Schenectady, New York, during World War II. Family rumor had it that his father, H. Edward Weinstein, may have worked on designing the trigger mechanism for the atom bomb exploded in Hiroshima. As a lead programmer, Mr. Burns successfully wrote computer code for a broad range of clients including software systems for plants in the electrical generation, fuel distribution, paper, petrochemical, and steel industries. Dr. Weinstein received his training in computer science auditing courses at the Air Force Institute of Technology at the Aerospace Medical Researcher Laboratories at Wright-Patterson Airforce Base in Fairborn, Ohio, while he was in service as a Major in the US Air Force with a day-time job as Vice Chair of Pathology in the Division of Toxicology at the Aerospace Medical Research Laboratories. He gained experience with BASIC, FORTRAN, and COBOL programming languages, computer system design, and the use of a relatively portable Hewlett-Packard 9700 computer with punched paper reels for data input, and a Burroughs B-3500 computer, with IBM punch cards used for their data input. While he was stationed at the Aerospace Medical Research Laboratory in his role as a toxicologist, he found that a fuel oxidizer, mono-methyl hydrazine, exposure was causing hemolytic anemias in young airmen working in Titan missile silos [16]. After completing his military service, he became Chair of Pathology at Rush Medical College and Rush-Presbyterian St. Lukes' Medical Center in Chicago, Illinois, at age 36. His focus was on cancer research. In Chicago, his research group published often cited papers: (1) linking P-glycoprotein expression to invasion and metastasis in human colon cancers; and (2) demonstrating that perturbation of the lipid bi-layer in cancer cell membranes can reverse P-glycoprotein-induced multi-drug resistance, a potential pharmacological breakthrough [17, 18].

With the encouragement of the Rush leadership, which was promoting university technology transfer in the early 1980s, Dr. Weinstein, partnering with his businesswoman sister, Beth Newburger, co-founded one of the first PC-based high school education software companies. They caught the crest of the early personal computer wave of activity in computer-based education in the early 1980s. Dr. Weinstein personally designed the software for one of the first successfully marketed Scholastic Aptitude Test (SAT) preparation course study products, incorporating one of the first computer study games and including a ground-breaking product manual. Their OWLCAT company was acquired by Digital Research Inc., a pioneering California software company, in 1984.

Next, responding to a crisis in National Cancer Institute clinical trials, involving high levels of interobserver variability in surgical pathology diagnosis being rendered by expert uropathologists supporting urinary bladder cancer clinical trials, Dr. Weinstein had invented, patented, and successfully commercialized computer-driven robotic telepathology in the mid-1980s, and is known today as the "father of telepathology." His Corabi International Telemetrics, Inc. (i.e., "Corabi" is Dr. Weinstein's wife's family name), and a companion family-owned company, Apollo Telemedicine, became suppliers of telepathology equipment to the United States Department of Veterans of Affairs, in 1996. This was adopted as the telepathology platform for the longest sustainable telepathology service in the United States [19–21]. Therefore, Mr. Burns and Dr. Weinstein each had years of prior experience in developing computer applications and, in addition, decades of experience as small business owners, by the time they met in 1996.

Their shared interests in public service were also significant components of both of their careers. Mr. Burns is one of the most successful politicians in Arizona history (approximately 28 years of service as an elected official). Dr. Weinstein has been president of six professional organizations and is President-Emeritus of the American Telemedicine Association as a "pioneer" in the field of telemedicine. Mr. Burns, and his wife, ran a successful pre-school education business for

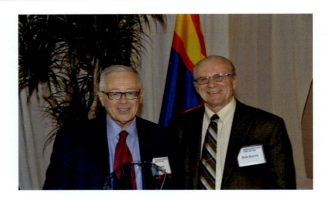

Fig. 12.16 Ronald S. Weinstein, MD (left) and Robert "Bob" Burns (right: as an AZ State Senator) acknowledging receipt of the highly regarded The University of Arizona's "2012 Technology Innovator Award" for their work in creating and developing the state-wide Arizona Telemedicine Program. Three hundred invited guests, faculty members, and graduate students attended the University of Arizona's "Innovation Award Luncheon" which honored the Arizona Telemedicine Program's co-founders, at The University of Arizona Student Union, in Tucson, Arizona, with a glass artists plaque (being held by Dr. Weinstein) and a monetary award of $10,000. This was used to support the ATPs' Sir William Osler Summer Fellowship Program for College and High School Students and the development, testing, and implementation of regular school year K-12 medical science courses [9, 11–13, 22, 23]

27 years. Dr. Weinstein was awarded his first National Institutes of Health grant as a first-year resident at the Massachusetts General Hospital and was an academic department head for 32 years. He has had continuous federal research support for 54 years, nearing a record in that category. He also had a long-time interest in university technology transfer and spun out five start-up companies while a full-time employee of universities (Fig. 12.16).

Challenges

Inventing a robust but nuanced form of governance for a telemedicine and telehealth program can be challenging for creators of telemedicine programs, both large and small [1–5]. Alignment of the expectations and needs of future stakeholders within the framework imposed by governance arrangements for a lead organization can be a daunting task.

Is the ATC Zoom Compatible?

COVID-19 will put the institutionalization of the ATC as an Arizona quasi-agency, dedicated to maintaining a communication channel between the university-housed ATP, in Tucson, and the AZ State Legislature, in Phoenix, to the test. The ATC held its April 2020 quarterly meeting as a "virtual" meeting, over Zoom, for the first time. This ATC meeting on Zoom had 70 attendees which set an attendance record for the ATC but, noticeably, with a reduced number of ATC members in attendance. On the one hand, ATC was no longer constrained by the 43-seat capacity in the Board Room in the JLBC building on the state capitol campus. Also, the ATC was readily available for rural participants hundreds of miles away, if they had access to the broadband internet. On the other hand, using Zoom, the ATC sacrificed almost all of the personal networking that typically took place at in-person ATC quarterly meetings in the past and, arguably, even kept the ATC focused on its "primary mission" of supporting rural telemedicine for over two decades. Lively discussions and the questioning of presenters were notably absent. The 10-minute ATC lunch breaks, during which time even "frantic networking" took place in-person, were sorely missed by the "virtual" attendees. Not only were the shared commitments to the telemedicine mission highly valued by the ATC members and non-member attendees alike over many years, the thought of losing long-term professional and personal friendships, the by-products of these ATC meetings, is sad to contemplate.

It remains to be seen if ATC "virtual" meetings will become the new normal for the ATC. In fact, we will see if this shift in strategy, going "virtual," negatively impacts the long-term viability of the ATC itself. One way or the other, our initial impression is that Zoom has its limitations with regards to professional networking. The unique environment created within the ATC over the years is, already, sorely missed! Hopefully that's limited to the "old-timers."

References

1. Hashiguchi TC. Bringing health care to the patient: an overview of the use of telemedicine in OECD countries. Paris: OECD Publishing; 2020.
2. Jenkinson D. Governance issues for telemedicine in acute stroke. NHS Improvement Stroke. 2010.
3. Arkwright B, Jones J, Osborne T, Glorioso G, Russo Jr J. Telehealth governance: an essential tool to empower today's healthcare leaders. Telehealth Med Today. 2017;2.
4. Giorgio F. European eHealth governance initiative: a new way forward. In: eHealth: legal, ethical and governance challenges. Berlin, Heidelberg: Springer; 2013. p. 371–85.
5. Arizona Telemedicine Council. https://telemedicine.arizona.edu/about-us/atc. Last accessed 8 Feb 2020.
6. Weinstein RS, Barker G, Beinar S, Holcomb M, Krupinski EA, Lopez AM, Hughes A, McNeely RA. Policy and the origins of the Arizona statewide telemedicine program. In: Whitten P, Cook D, editors. Understanding health communications technologies. San Francisco: Jossey-Bass; 2004. p. 299–309.
7. Krupinski EA, Weinstein RS. Telemedicine in an academic center—the Arizona Telemedicine Program. Telemed e-Health. 2013;19(5):349–56.
8. Weinstein RS, Lopez AM, Krupinski EA, Beinar SJ, Holcomb M, McNeely RA, Latifi R, Barker G. Integrating telemedicine and telehealth: putting it all together. Current Principles and Practices of Telemedicine and e-Health. IOS Press. 2008;131:23–8. Available at: http://ebooks.iospress.nl/publication/11413.
9. Weinstein JB, Weinstein RS. Brush up your Shakespeare! Democratization of medical knowledge for the 21st century. Am J Med. 2015;128(7):672–4.
10. Briehl MM, Nelson MA, Krupinski EA, Erps KA, Holcomb MJ, Weinstein JB, Weinstein RS. Flexner 2.0—longitudinal study of student participation in a campus-wide general pathology course for graduate students at The University of Arizona. Acad Pathol. 2016;3:1–13.

11. Weinstein RS, Krupinski EA, Weinstein JB, Graham AR, Barker GP, Erps KA, Holtrust AL, Holcomb MJ. Flexner 3.0—democratization of medical knowledge for the 21st century: teaching medical science using K-12 general pathology as a gateway course. Acad Pathol. 2016;3:1–15.
12. Weinstein RS, Waer AL, Weinstein JB, Briehl MM, Holcomb MJ, Erps KA, Holtrust AL, Tomkins JM, Barker GP, Krupinski EA. Second Flexner Century: the democratization of medical knowledge: repurposing a general pathology course into multi-grade level "gateway" courses. Acad Pathol. 2017, 4:1–12.
13. Weinstein RS. Foreword. In: Latifi R, editor. Establishing telemedicine in developing countries: from inception to implementation. Amsterdam: IOS Press; 2004. p. v–vi.
14. Weinstein RS, Lopez AM, Krupinski EA, Beinar SJ, Holcomb M, Barker G. Integrating telemedicine and telehealth: putting it all together. In: Latifi R, editor. Current principles and practices of telemedicine and e-health. Washington, DC: IOS Press; 2008. p. 23–38.
15. Vega S, Marciscano I, Holcomb M, Erps KA, Major J, Lopez AM, Barker GP, Weinstein RS. Testing a top-down strategy for establishing a sustainable telemedicine program in a developing country. The Arizona Telemedicine Program-U.S. Army-Panama initiative. Telemed J eHealth. 2013;19:746–53.
16. Weinstein RS, George J. Interrelationship of methemoglobin, reduced glutathione and Heinz bodies in monomethylhydrazine-induced anemia. In: Third conference on environmental toxicology. Fairborn, Ohio; 1972. p. 281–301.
17. Weinstein RS, Jakate SM, Dominguez JM, Lebovitz MD, Koukoulis GK, Kuszak JR, Kluskens LF, Grogan TM, Saclarides TJ, Roninson IB, Coon JS. Relationship of the expression of the multidrug resistance gene product (P-glycoprotein) in human colon carcinoma to local tumor aggressiveness and lymph node metastasis. Cancer Res. 1991;51:2720–6.
18. Coon JS, Knudson W, Clodfelter K, Lu B, Weinstein RS. Solutol HS 15, nontoxic polyethylene esters of 12-hydroxystearic acid, reverses multi-drug resistance. Cancer Res. 1991;51:897–902.
19. Dunn BE, Choi H, Almagro UA, Recla DL, Krupinski EA, Weinstein RS. Routine surgical pathology in the Department of Veterans Affairs: experience-related improvements in pathologist performance in 2200 cases. Telemed J. 1999;5:323–37.
20. Bashshur RL, Krupinski EA, Weinstein RS, Dunn MR, Bashshur N. The empirical foundations of telepathology: evidence of feasibility and intermediate effects. Telemed J e-Health. 2017;23:155–91.
21. Weinstein RS, Holcomb MJ, Krupinski EA. Invention, and early history of telepathology (1985–2000). J Pathol Inform. 2019;10:1.
22. Weinstein RS, Holcomb MJ. Case study: congenital toxoplasmosis diagnosis and a pair of Myers-Briggs Type Indicator® (MBTI®) test results for an academic pathologist. JSM Clin Pathol. 2019;4:6.
23. Weinstein RS. On being a pathologist: a pathway to pathology practice; the added value of supplemental vocational training and mentoring in college and medical school. Hum Pathol. 2018;82:10–9.

Open Access This chapter is licensed under the terms of the Creative Commons Attribution 4.0 International License (http://creativecommons.org/licenses/by/4.0/), which permits use, sharing, adaptation, distribution and reproduction in any medium or format, as long as you give appropriate credit to the original author(s) and the source, provide a link to the Creative Commons license and indicate if changes were made.

The images or other third party material in this chapter are included in the chapter's Creative Commons license, unless indicated otherwise in a credit line to the material. If material is not included in the chapter's Creative Commons license and your intended use is not permitted by statutory regulation or exceeds the permitted use, you will need to obtain permission directly from the copyright holder.

Telehealth Patient Portal: Opportunities and Reality

13

Ronald C. Merrell

Introduction

A patient portal is defined as a secure website that offers patients a convenient access to personal health information with an Internet connection secured by username and password or some other security step. This information can include a long list of pertinent and personal information. The portal is a gateway to the aggregate medical information of the patient with the conviction that medical information is the property of the patient who has right to access and interact with the medical personnel generating the information. At the basic level, the portal is an access for patient to their electronic health record. The most basic interactions are to update contact information, review charges, make payments, confirm insurance benefits and coverage, and download and complete necessary forms [1].

The effort to have patients maintain their own records electronically has not been very successful. Simply storing your own records apparently did not meet patient expectations, and it is not entirely clear why! The portal is more, richer, a dialogue and guide through the complexity of health care [2]. The electronic data will include recent medical encounters, discharge summaries, medications prescribed, allergies, and immunizations. The data set also includes laboratory results, radiology reports, and pathology findings. Patients can interact with medical personnel and arrange elective appointments or request prescription refills. The patient can also report interim changes in their status, symptoms, and interventions that might be unknown to the portal site. They can securely correspond with their doctors and nurses and may message to ask for clarification of reports. They can also report apparent errors in their data and visits as they read their reports. They are provided with medical information about their condition, information about upcoming procedures and

R. C. Merrell (✉)
Virginia Commonwealth University, Mentone, AL, USA
e-mail: ronald.merrell@vcuhealth.org

© Springer Nature Switzerland AG 2021
R. Latifi et al. (eds.), *Telemedicine, Telehealth and Telepresence*,
https://doi.org/10.1007/978-3-030-56917-4_13

tests, and behavior modification programs of worth in improving their condition, compliance, and well-being.

The power of the patient portal to improve health care and personal involvement is enormous. The portal offers *information, engagement,* and *empowerment* for patient-centered care. It may seem that the introduction of the patient portal is only eclipsed by sliced bread as a positive good in our era. But are there any challenges? Portals are offered by essentially every health system in the United States and in Europe where there are even considerations for national portals. The decision-makers really like this portal thing, but reservations remain with caregivers and patients [3, 4]. Many of the concerns have been addressed in the 15 or so years of portal development and applications. This chapter explores some of the special issues, challenges met, those that remain, and the opportunities yet to be realized.

There was a long-held belief that medical records were the private property of doctors and hospitals. That belief is no longer valid. Records are the property and responsibility of health-care entities, but patients have every right to access and sharing. Decades ago, when records were paper, the MD Anderson Cancer Center took a bold approach to records management by giving patients full access. When patients checked in for appointments, they went to medical records, and their complete charts were pulled and given to the patient. Newly diagnosed patients had a thin record, and this they carried by hand to their appointments. The heroes of the center were those who were long-term survivors whose records were of such duration and consequent volume that they had to be carried about in little red wagons! These patients were held in high esteem by those just beginning their trek into cancer survival and gave visible proof that the trek might be toward a happy outcome.

Despite the advantages of portals, there is always the matter of patient use. Build it and it may be thoroughly ignored. I recall the situation at a major VA hospital when electronic records were scheduled to launch. Months had been spent on teaching, cajoling, and refining the excellent record ready for use. However, the medical staff was reluctant and combative. I recall as a member of the staff that it was generally agreed that the senior physicians would just transfer the responsibility to house staff. Certainly, there was frustration in the administrative offices. There turned out to be no problem at all at launch date. The staff was informed ever so gently that in order to demonstrate their role in patient care and thereby qualify for their income the record would be completed as indicated by the staff member personally. When even the most curmudgeonly of the senior staff saw the innovation as necessary for employment, they quickly joined in, and no problems ensued. It is difficult to imagine giving patients no choice, but the use of the portal can certainly be presented in an inescapably advantageous way!

In a similar vein, the record should never be seen as a way to extract additional labor and time from a busy staff. Revolt or disuse might follow. Talk, survey, convince, and make it real that the portal is going to save time and permit more meaningful allocation of time with patients. Then not only is the patient engaged, informed, and empowered, but that mantra extends to all users of the technology. Just as patients should be invited to interact with quality surveys, so should all the users in order for the portal to evolve gently toward an ever more useful tool. Thus, the health-care and administrative users feel a sense of ownership.

The access to records has important features distinct from personal notes of caregivers that might be reviewed by insurance carriers or courts. The records must recognize that the words should be understandable to the patient and never disparage. The record is an open statement of the best in professional assessment and should reflect the clinician's respect for patient and devotion to accuracy. The best records recognize the reader and the needs of the reader whether that reader is a patient, colleague, administrator, or regulator. Common advice to medical personnel just starting to create records is they should pretend the entry is to be read out in court to a hostile jury! Similar advice would be to pretend you are reading the material out loud to your patient and family members.

The purpose of the portal should be understood by all from the outset. The purpose is to facilitate interactions with patients and meet the high objective to engage, inform, and empower patients. The outcome is clear. The portal should reflect and seek an improvement in care. Certainly, an effective portal should be expected to be a tool for patient recruitment and retention. Indeed, the portal should also be a tool to enhance effective business practices for billing and collection. It should be obvious in the portal what the patient is being charged for what service. The portal should be a device to effectively manage the time of clinicians through facile appointments and follow-up. Indeed the material on the portal document should be in compliance with all pertinent regulations for care and billing. None of these objectives is particularly paramount and all may be considered in balance. A portal designed to maximize collections at the expense of patient information will fail. The portal must serve all involved effectively and easily.

How should the portal be designed and made useful? First the portal should be of value to health-care personnel, management people, and the patient. It should be easy to use, timely, and highly interactive. The interfaces should be intuitive and cover many levels of patient sophistication. The benefits of the portal to patients should be obvious and reinforced regularly. The information on the portal must be timely. Notes from clinicians should be posted promptly preferably on the day of service, and transcription should be of the highest quality. Dictating notes later or any reliance on handwritten information should be abandoned. Thus, a patient can review what transpired and be reinforced in the recommendations. Should the note lead to questions on the part of the patient, interactive components should encourage patients to correspond with the clinician and clarify issues recognized by the patient based upon the visit and encourage to request clarification of anything confusing or not recalled from the visit. The portal is not a way to protect clinician time from patient intrusion but to make the interactions more efficient and effective. This is a bold new way to create and edit clinical information. The interaction should allow patients to promptly make arrangements for follow-up appointments or plans for inpatient care. Preoperative instructions and instructions for upcoming tests should be clear and concise. The portal should encourage patients to evaluate their recent care and make suggestions. This interaction could be a powerful element of quality control and assessment of patient outcomes from patient perspective.

Furthermore, patients should be encouraged to send messages if they feel they have a change in their status such as a change in symptoms, interim operations, or other critical events such as cardiac or hospitalizations that would otherwise be unknown to the managing clinicians at the portal site. Certainly, patients should report adverse reaction to medications or apparent lack of effectiveness of what was been prescribed and the addition of other medications by other clinicians to their regimen. Messaging to the site is obviously beneficial as well as messages emanating from the portal site. Reminders about appointments, timely notes to prepare for care, timely requests for current perceived status, and simply queries as to well-being can be accommodated. This can be marvelously personal! Messaging can also alert patients to new reports and science about their condition, changes in recommendations, recalls, and educational materials. The portal can and should be a rich and highly personal conversation with and for our patients. That is one of the strengths that has invited creativity from all parties and made the portals acceptable.

A successful portal should be extensively tested and validated before introduction. This is the time to expand the inquiry as to purpose, acceptability, and implementation. Certainly, the portal should be assessed regularly for quality and needed revision. However, patients do not like improved and therefore now unfamiliar websites. There should be few changes over time if the portal is well designed. Changes might be out of sight but not a regular interruption of cues. The adage should be recalled. The enemy of good is better! It should be clear in portal design that there is every effort to maintain privacy. In order to achieve this, the portal should require a username and password. However, invitation to hacking can be minimized. The greatest asset to hackers is name, birthday, and social security number. Can these not be eliminated in terms of access? Recent legislation has made the Medicare number different from social security number [5]. The portal at the time of design can address the important matters of compliance for insurance and regulators and needed interface for meaningful use. The portal should be designed to accept imported medical information from other caregivers and send data to other caregivers at different sites with the agreement of the patient. Patients should be notified that their information relevant to an upcoming appointment was received and that correspondence with other caregivers has happened. The portal ideally represents a very busy place for exchange between patients, various caregivers, and data sources to limit the waste of time at the actual physical interview and examination. Insurance numbers need not be posted up front but stored at an appropriate part of the file. The same may be said of birthdays [6]. I recently reported the highly inappropriate questions asked by a prominent portal such as confirming remote real-estate transactions for self and family [7]. What has that to do with username and password to the portal? There is a temptation to recruit enormous amounts of information that might be of much greater interest to the scoundrels of the Internet than pertinent to patient care. Calls to patients from office personnel may not be effective or best represent the desire of caregivers to be thorough and helpful. Recently I had an arrhythmia. I was sent for an ultrasound study and waited a few days for a report. When I got the call back, the nurse told me my study was normal. What about the arrhythmia that I still had? I asked for a copy of the report and picked it up at the office. I indeed had frequent premature atrial contractions and occasional ventricular contractions. The ejection fraction was normal in fact, and the heart wall was moving in an acceptable manner. I never had contact with the cardiologist who interpreted the study. Never met her. Never had a call from primary care physician suggesting things I might do to alleviate the situation. Being a physician, I knew pretty much what to do. What if I had been a mechanic? Patients should receive reports on major tests from people qualified to interpret the data and advise. It is unreasonable to assume that patients can look at complex metabolic data and understand the implications, reassuring or otherwise. Radiology reports can be obtuse to other physicians simply by their nature. Explaining the implications of a brain lesion, cardiac catheterization, computed tomogram of the pancreas, etc. should be done by a competent physician. This is necessary not only when the report says something that will change a life such as tumor margin or type but also the robust and lengthy reports on lab values where the news may not be so bad but indeed subject to outrageous interpretation by a frightened patient. Now the data are posted on the electronic health record in real time. What keeps the patient from seeing it before the physician has called? Aha! The flagged items on lab reports, path reports, etc. should come to the attention of the ordering physician promptly and allow at least early notification and interpretation with a personal phone call. Now would it not be great to have a videoconference in these circumstances?

The patient is the consumer of the information in the portal. What happens if the patient needs help from a caregiver or family member? I know a man 75 years of age in our area who has a powerful family history for dementia. Of late he has been showing signs of dementia with forgetfulness and difficulty with conversation and ordering his priorities. He continues to drive, shop, and manage his financial affairs. Recently matters took a turn. He had some symptom and called to make an appointment with a specialist in a city some several hours drive from his home in rural America. He told his family he had an appointment, and no one thought much of it since he had multiple medical conditions and many doctors. He returned from the day trip and his wife asked him for a report. He could not remember the symptom that prompted the call for an appointment. He could not remember the specialty of the consultant or name. He could not remember what he asked the doctor or what the specialist told him. His wife reconstructed the situation by finding his appointment card and calling the office. Thereafter the family including RN daughter is committed to accompany him to all medical encounters. How would this have worked as the patient became more confused and is communicating through a portal? With patient permission and periodic review, family members and caregivers really need to have access through the portal with the same assurance of privacy as the patient.

There are numerous providers of software for patient portals. Most are highly reputable purveyors of electronic medical records. Electronic record programs do not automatically translate into workable patient portals. There should be planning starting with the purpose and usability of the interface. The user is not a highly trained medical caregiver or medical record expert. The user is of varied levels of skill and little can be assumed as to ability to interface. For success extensive testing and modification is required. Legal, business, and medical professional people as well as panels of potential users should work with programmers and designers. Certain portions of the portal data should be accessible for downloading, and interaction with primary care and other caregivers should be carefully programmed into the software. The early efforts at patient portals faced many challenges, but it may be said that now the portals are largely excellent although there are many shortcomings in the expectations outlined above [8–11].

Current reports about portals most often deal with specialty applications and populations [12, 13]. Pediatrics, geriatric, chronic disease management, pregnancy, cancer, and rehabilitation are all areas of active application. Preoperative instruction and postoperative surveillance put patients and surgeons in a continuum of care not in place previously. There is no apparent solution for the illiterate, poorly informed, naive, and generally underserved. Efforts for portals that expand beyond health systems to national programs are underway and will prove difficult. Extension to small offices and remote sites and response to alerts or red flags will continue to require great attention.

There are opportunities beyond special application that invite vigorous attention. Patient portals could be embellished by the best in telemedicine videoconference clinics. Data from home monitoring could readily be fed into the database for review as well as instant analysis and trending analysis. The portals could also be the object of artificial intelligence to anticipate needs of the individual patient. Also, games and other behavioral tools could be appended to the information aspects of the portals. These are applications of proven worth as free-standing health initiatives.

There are numerous research opportunities to aggregate portal data with protection of privacy to explore best practices, disease trends, population statistics, and signs of illegal behavior on the part of health-care groups. Practice compliance research should be of great interest.

Patient portals are not new. They have not reached their potential and steadily deflect their detractors with increasingly favorable performance. The structure of the portals should not be simply accepted in any way that might compromise patient care. They are so important that they simply must be held to a high expectation and continually improved to be a seamless link between patients and caregivers with the objective of improved care and efficiency.

References

1. https://www.healthit.gov>faq> what is a patient portal. Last accessed 25 Aug 19.
2. https://medcitynews.com/2019/04/microsoft-healthvault-is-officially-shutting-down-in-november/.
3. https://patientengagementhit.com>news>patient-portal-access.
4. Annenworth E, Hoebrst A, Lannig S, Mueller G, Siebert U, Schnell-Inderst P. Effects of adult portal on patient empowerment and health-related outcomes. Stud Health Technol Inform. 2019;264:1106–10.
5. www.congress.gov/bill/114thcongress/house-bill2. HR2 medicare access and CHIP reauthorization act of 2015.

6. Merrell RC, Doarn CR. Medical insecurity. Telemed J E Health. 2015;21:599–600.
7. Merrell RC, Doarn CR. Identity theft, a reprise. Telemed J E Health. 2017;23(8):619–20.
8. Wildenbos GA, Peute L, Jaspers M. Facilitators and Barriuers of electronic health record patient portal adoption by older adults. Stud Health Technol Informat. 2017;235:308–12.
9. Tieu L, Sarkar U, Schillinger D, Ralston JD, Ratanawongsa N, Pasick R, Lyles CR. Barriers and facilitators to online portal use among patients and caregivers in a safety net health care system: a qualitative study. J Med Internet Res. 2015;17(12):e275.
10. Irizarry T, DeVito Dabbs A, Curran CR. J Med Internet Res. 2015;17(6):e148.
11. Kruse CS, Bolton K, Freriks G. The effect of patient portals on quality outcomes and its implications to meaningful use: a systematic review. J Med Internet Res. 2015;17(2):e44.
12. Miller DP Jr, Latulipe C, Medius KA, Quandt SA, Arcurry TA. Primary care providers' views of patient portals: interview study of perceived benefits and consequences. J Med Internet Res. 2016;18:e8.
13. https://www.medicaleconomics.com/business/future-patient-portals.

Technology Enabled Remote Healthcare in Public Private Partnership Mode: A Story from India

14

K. Ganapathy and Sangita Reddy

Introduction to Technology-Enabled Remote Healthcare (TeRHC)

A solution is not a solution unless it is universally available to anyone, anytime, anywhere at an affordable cost without compromising quality. This is easier said than done. It is universally known and accepted that providing healthcare in suburban and rural areas, particularly in developing countries, is more than a challenge. Paradoxically the "third world" does not have to follow the advanced countries, not even piggyback or even leap frog. After all, how much can a frog leap! Today emerging economies like India are pole-vaulting. There are no technology-enabled legacy systems to disinherit. Advances in information and communication technology are mind-boggling. The Jugaad approach is making *TeRHC* a reality. This flexible approach to problem-solving, using limited resources in an innovative way or a simple work-around, signifies creativity – a form of frugal engineering at its peak.

Telehealth in India: The Beginnings

The challenges in evangelising the very concept of telehealth, creating the necessary awareness and persuading the various stakeholders in a then non-existing ecosystem, to agree to even pilot projects, were so daunting that it was extremely difficult at that time, to collect reliable data, analyse the data and publish the observations. Publications then were limited [1–6]. In what subsequently became a highly downloaded article [7], the principal author demonstrated that as of Sep 2014,

K. Ganapathy (✉)
Apollo Telemedicine Networking Foundation, Chennai, Tamil Nadu, India
e-mail: drganapathy@apollohospitals.com

S. Reddy
Apollo Hospitals Group, Hyderabad, Telangana, India

© Springer Nature Switzerland AG 2021
R. Latifi et al. (eds.), *Telemedicine, Telehealth and Telepresence*,
https://doi.org/10.1007/978-3-030-56917-4_14

935 million Indians lived in areas where there was not a single neurologist or neurosurgeon. This confirmed the general observation that specialists' distribution in India is totally lopsided. Two decades ago the authors among others realised that telemedicine would be the only way to bridge the enormous urban-rural health divide. Passion and persistence have at last started yielding dividends. Telehealth is slowly being accepted in the community. India's 11th Five-Year Plan (2007–2012) allocated about US$50 million to telemedicine. In the subsequent 12th Five-Year Plan, telemedicine has been recognised as a distinct entity. The major telemedicine service providers/supporters in India include Apollo Hospitals, Arvind Eye Care System, Sankara Nethralaya, Sanjay Gandhi Postgraduate Institute of Medical Sciences, Sri Ramachandra Medical College and Narayana Hrudayalaya among many others. Indian Space Research Organisation had initially played a major role in providing satellite connectivity [8]. The primary author [9] had earlier pointed out that awareness, perception and attitude of healthcare providers, even in relatively isolated states like Himachal Pradesh, towards mobile health (mHealth), suggested that healthcare providers were ready to use information and communication technology to provide virtual healthcare. In spite of major operational challenges, non-availability of quality healthcare in mountainous isolated, inaccessible, sparsely populated regions has been addressed successfully, deploying telehealth [10].

Public Private Partnerships in Healthcare: An Introduction

To have access to the highest attainable standard of healthcare is a fundamental right of every human being. In this context, universal access to healthcare assumes prime importance. The World Health Organization advocates that health systems adopt universal coverage. This is to ensure that everyone can avail health services and are protected from associated financial risks. However, universal healthcare delivery poses a significant challenge for policymakers. The public sector is generally perceived to have reduced innovative skills. The private sector on the other hand is perceived to look for compensation, for additional efforts and taking higher risk. Technological features are becoming so sophisticated that public authorities may not possess the know-how to conceive, build and operate them in a future-ready mode. Synergies with private players are therefore recommended. Fortunately, investors are now looking at investments that in addition to financial returns also yield social benefits. Government has a choice of being a provider, contributing to building infrastructure and directly managing operations or pay for healthcare services provided by private players. Given the changing landscape, incorporating technology solutions into PPP projects is a complex undertaking, particularly for long-term contracts, which integrate care across multiple levels.

A PPP is a government service or private business venture, which is funded and operated through a partnership of government and one or more private sector companies. Governments are encouraged to adopt several key factors while initiating PPP, to ensure sustainability. These include (1) building of trust; (2) having clearly defined objectives and roles; (3) time commitment; (4) transparency and candid information, particularly in relation to risk and benefit; (5) contract flexibility; (6) technical assistance or financial incentive behind procedural arrangements; and (7) the awareness and acceptability of structural changes related to responsibility and decisions (power and authority) [11].

Partnership is a synergistic relationship between two or more individuals or organisations that share mutual liabilities with some expected benefits. Availability of resources in terms of manpower and finance, legal and regulatory framework, transparency, accountability, commitment and mutual understanding is most needed. Neither public nor private sectors alone have been perspicacious enough to attain the goals and objectives of the healthcare industry. Constant surge in healthcare costs has made it difficult for any single organisation to provide quality and affordable services independently. This has enhanced scope for public and private sectors to collaborate [12]. PPPs in healthcare are an important element of the World Bank Group's response to country health challenges. These are reflected in various reports. From 2004 to 2015, the Bank Group had approved 78 projects that provided support for health-related PPP operations [13].

The next big "PPP health" would include the microelectronics sector, pharma, biotech and medtech. The PPP Innovative Medicines Initiative (IMI) was funded by the European Commission and through in-kind contributions from pharmaceutical companies has a budget of more than €3 billion. This confirms that solutions to health challenges do not lie with one specific group. The future is patient-centred and integrated, with a significant role for digital technologies [14]. PPP as a solution for integrating genetic services into healthcare of countries with low and middle incomes has also been proposed [15].

According to the projections of the ICT Health Observatory of the Milan Polytechnic, savings of at least 6.8 billion euros for a year could be achieved through extensive use of digital healthcare in critical areas of the National Health Service. Savings made possible by deploying technology may be partially used to finance PPP smart investments. The transition to smart technologies is inevitable and will have a significant impact on healthcare processes and their governance. New actors, networks and innovation are already challenging consolidated health governance practices [16]. International organisations like the World Health Organization, European Union and the Organisation for Economic Co-operation and Development promote PPPs in order to ensure the construction of a national e-health infrastructure [17].

Establishment and management of robust telemedicine and digital health PPP programmes presupposes a focus on overall digital health framework, financing and affordability, data standards, information security, project planning and implementation, evaluation and establishing a transparent procurement process [18]. By leveraging private sector expertise, financing, capacity, systems and management discipline, public health systems have been able to revive many aborted projects. PPPs must be designed within the local context and aligned with a country's national or local healthcare policies and delivery strategy. Clearly defined and measurable output-based performance standards will need to be defined that specify the end goal. Private partners want flexibility to incorporate new ways of achieving desired patient and financial outcomes as conditions evolve [19]. Both public and private providers deliver health services, each with their particular virtues and liabilities.

Nigel Crisp has pointed out in his book *Turning the World Upside Down* [20] that advanced countries could benefit from technologies/solutions developed *in and for* low-resource settings. Incorporating technology into PPP projects requires expertise across clinical, legal, technology and contract management. Decision-makers must think long-term and consider how technology can be used to take healthcare delivery to new levels, e.g. deploying telemedicine systems to extend access to healthcare to remote populations, with little access to transportation, and allowing clinicians to monitor and treat patients in lower-cost distributed clinic settings. Political will is arguably the most critical enabling condition for PPP projects. Changes in political philosophies when a new political party takes over after an election can have significant impact – up to and including halting of projects. The private sector will not invest resources and time into bidding on PPP projects if public sector commitment is not assured. Governments worldwide have undertaken some or even all of the responsibility for financing and delivering health services, either at subsidised rates or free of cost, at the point of utilisation. Given systemic deficiencies in government health programmes as well as the spiralling costs of an expensive, inequitable and often unregulated private sector, the concept of PPPs has emerged as a policy option in which the healthcare needs of people could be met more effectively if both sectors worked together [21]. Genesis of most PPPs is the inability of the public sector in reaching out to a particular target group by virtue of its geographical position or difficulty in working with high-risk groups [22].

A United Nations Economic Commission for Europe (UNECE) standard on best practice in relation to the management of PPP programmes in telemedicine and digital health has been advocated. This would include (a) providing guidance on efficient and effective project delivery of telemedicine and digital health PPP projects and (b) assessing different models of PPP in telemedicine and digital health – using feedback from markets where PPP programmes have been established.

PPP in Healthcare: A Global Perspective

Literature review reveals that many countries have started adopting PPP in healthcare. In Ireland primary care centres, network has been increasingly implemented by relying on the private sector. This has resulted in a more commercialised network subject to financial risks associated with PPP [23]. Experiences of institutional PPPs within the Italian National Health Service (*Sistema Sanitario Nazionale*) have been reported [24]. Public-private sector partnership has helped make available telemedicine in Jamaica [25]. Kenya Healthcare Federation through its PPP is now focusing on scaling up delivery of healthcare [26]. In a study executed in Korea, Lee concluded that non-profit, non-governmental organisations, the central government, the private sector and public healthcare services were the groups interested in PPP healthcare [27]. In New Zealand PPP has been introduced for specific diagnostic procedures. Sakowska et al. have reported that wait times for both specialist outpatient assessment and colonoscopy were significantly reduced in the province of Geelong [28]. Several reports on PPP and healthcare have originated from Pakistan [29–31]. Reports on PPP and healthcare have been published from the Philippines [32, 33]. In recent decades, Portugal witnessed the private sector increasingly extending their engagement in health services with the public sector. This relationship originated from the legal framework enabling agreements and PPP [34]. In an interesting observation, Purcărea et al. opine that "marketing" is an essential and important component of PPP in healthcare. They point out that Romanian medical system is in the process of a cultural change, which takes time, patience and perseverance, despite the unpredictability and resistance that it faces inevitably. A painful period of transition with total quality management is essential before PPP in healthcare is accepted [35]. Telemedicine has been enabled in rural Yakutia Sakha, Republic of Russia, through a PPP [36]. Kula et al. in a study of PPP in healthcare in South Africa opined that private for-profit sector is engaged in projects closely aligned to current health system reform priorities. Factors that increase the likelihood of interactions being successful included (a) increasing the government's capacity to manage PPP; (b) choosing PP interactions that are strategically important to national goals; (c) building a knowledge base on what works, where and why; (d) moving from pilots to large-scale initiatives; and (e) harnessing the contracting expertise in private providers and encouraging innovation and learning [37]. Since the inception of the Spanish National Health System, hospital care has also been purchased from private not-for-profit or for-profit providers, usually complementing public provision. Administrative concessions awarded to the private provider in 1999 were not renewed in April 2018. The authors reiterate that it is another example that PPP in healthcare is to a large extent governed by changing political considerations [38]. Kamugumya et al. discussed various barriers hindering implementation of PPP for reproductive and child health services at the district level in Tanzania [39]. A study from Turkey evaluated opinions and evaluations of stakeholders in the implementation of PPP models in integrated health campuses (city hospitals). Majority interviewed believed that PPP was relevant in Turkey with an appropriate finance model. Most positive views were expressed by public and private sector stakeholders, while some negative views were voiced by NGO representatives [40]. Interestingly Turkey's largest PPP in healthcare is an integrated health campus costing US$1.3 billion [41]. In 2005, the Turkish Ministry of Health allowed the private sector to build and operate new hospitals under build-lease-transfer model. A PPP department was established, to share risks and to utilise experience of the private sector. With launch of the PPP Integrated Health Campuses Programme in 2007, the Turkish Ministry of Health has its own PPP management system to design, build, finance and operate large-scale, regional hospitals and trauma centres around the country with a 10 billion USD investment [42]. In a study from Uganda, Joloba et al. demonstrated the potential of PPP collaborations to assist patient care by strengthening laboratory systems. Increased access to drug-susceptibility testing was achieved by integrating specimen transport networks to maximise resources [43]. In a publication in 2016, Sadeghi et al. after reviewing publications on PPP in healthcare from the United Kingdom, Spain, Canada, Turkey,

Australia, Lesotho and one project in Iran conclude that duration of the projects ranged from 12 to 40 years in different countries, depending on the model [44]. Some experts opine that the crisis in the National Health Service, United Kingdom, has been created by a mixture of government underfunding and privatisation and marketisation of services, which have left services fragmented and profits diverted out of healthcare to promote PPPs [45]. Generally, implementing PPP projects in healthcare had valuable outcomes for governmental hospitals. Healthcare spending in the Gulf Cooperation Council (GCC) is about $69.4 billion in 2018, according to Deloitte. Understandably, a significant beneficiary of PPP in the GCC and around the world should be, and is, healthcare. As healthcare costs increase, there is added pressure on governments to look for private capital and expertise. According to an estimate in PwC's 2018 "PPPs in Healthcare" report, there are roughly 600 healthcare infrastructure projects or assets in the world, of which the vast majority are PPPs [46]. According to a report from the Ministry of Foreign Affairs of the Netherlands, the Dutch government spent 48.3 million euros on 54 PPPs with African countries like Mozambique, Rwanda and Burundi as well as other countries like Indonesia and Mongolia [47]. Even a backward country like Afghanistan has an e-health network supported physically and financially through a PPP. With just 2 doctors for every 10,000 people, it is difficult for the country's 32 million people to obtain timely access to quality healthcare. The French Medical Institute for Mothers and Children and the Aga Khan University Hospital in Karachi provide the clinical expertise; the Aga Khan Health Service in Afghanistan manages the hospitals in the provinces of Bamyan and Badakhshan for Afghanistan's Ministry of Public Health, and the private sector, through Roshan Telecom, supplies the telecommunication services. Aga Khan Development Network health resource centre provides the technical expertise underpinning the initiative [48]. Many governments in Africa are seeking to establish PPPs for financing and operation of new healthcare facilities and services [49]. The planning and operation of a high-profile case in Maseru, Lesotho, has been evaluated to discuss problems specific to low-income and middle-income countries [50]. PPP has demonstrated significant contributions in developing a more competent laboratory workforce, reinforced laboratory systems and improved treatment efficiencies by significantly reducing turnaround time to provide accurate laboratory results to patients afflicted by deadly diseases, such as multidrug-resistant TB and HIV. Such PPPs have not just improved efficiencies in the countries where they exist; it has also provided a successful model for other low-income countries to consider [51, 52]. Sajani in a paper on PPP in Bangladesh points out that the country has achieved near universal coverage in immunisation thru PPP [53]. A PPP project deploying telemedicine in the design-build-finance-operate (DBFO) mode where the private sector designs, finances and operates the facility during the term of the lease and charges user fees for the lease period has been described in Belarus, Russia [54]. Successful pilot studies have led to a country-wide mobile telemedicine project in a PPP mode between the Botswana government, a private telecommunications partner and a local IT company [55]. PPP projects in healthcare from Brazil, Canada and China have been reported [56–58]. Beijing New Century International Hospital for Children was the first specialised children's hospital operating on international standards. This PPP model was dedicated to providing comprehensive and quality healthcare service to newborns, infants, schoolchildren and teenagers. It has yielded many benefits enabling efficient use of resources to better serve patients with more targeted care [59]. PPPs have been most successful in Canada, where they work well with the country's single-payer health system. In the United States, the PPP market is still in its early stages, but it shows promise. The new $2 billion Centre Hospitalier de l'Université de Montréal (CHUM) is the largest healthcare project in North America. Canada has a strong record in healthcare PPPs. Between 2003 and 2011, more than 50 public-private hospital projects alone, valued at more than 18 billion Canadian dollars, have taken place. In Ethiopia PPPs for specific healthcare services (e.g. malaria control) through partners and the national malaria prevention control programme have been suggested [60].

PPP in Healthcare: The Indian Scenario

India has a long history of PPPs in health with most of the national health programmes partnering with non-profit and for-profit organisations. In India, the new Companies Act of 2013 mandates corporates to spend 2% of their profits on CSR activities. The government is now partnering with the private sector, leading to improvement in healthcare delivery through a combination of good infrastructure, current technology and the best available medical expertise [61]. Global management-consulting firm McKinsey & Company has recommended PPP for improving healthcare delivery in India by 2022. A possible road map to achieving healthcare objectives under the Five-Year Plan was presented. Adopting the payer role could slow down growth of public beds. However, this could be resolved by adopting PPP models [62].

PPP in the Indian healthcare sector is growing exponentially. Impressive technological innovations and advancements, complemented by favourable government policies, have considerably helped improve quality of life. Several parts of India still remain at a disadvantage, lacking affordable access to healthcare services. High operational costs and insufficient investments have affected quality of healthcare services and accessibility. The confluence of resources of the private sector and the organisational capacities of the public sector are making PPP a potential game changer. If utilised well, the government, through this model, could successfully standardise healthcare, while maintaining a high quality of services [63].

The National Health Policy (NHP) 2017 of India envisages building a strong partnership between the government and private organisations to strengthen overall functioning and efficiency of the health system. An investment of Rs 150,000 crore (US $20 billion) is required, of which 80 per cent is likely to come from the private sector, primarily under the PPP model. The Indo UK Institute of Health (IUIH) the largest PPP project in India in healthcare believes that PPP is the way forward to improve healthcare in India. PPPs in health segment can work when the risk is shared. It cannot be a one-sided game with benefits taken by one partner and risks borne by the other. In many cases, the private sector is the dominant provider. A real PPP is one on a level-playing field. Terms have to be fair, and the risks have to be equally divided, only then will it be a level-played game [64]. Scope of PPP initiatives in India includes disease surveillance, purchase and distribution of drugs, national disease control program, management of primary health centres, medical education and training, engaging private sector consultants, pay clinics, R&D investments, telemedicine, health cooperatives and accreditation. Opportunities for private player participation in PPP models in Indian healthcare system include facility development, management and operations management (MOM), capacity building, training, financing mechanism, IT infrastructure development and inventory management [65]. Pleas for promoting PPP model for healthcare services have been made at a ministerial level. A mechanism of single-window clearance involving different ministries has also been proposed [66]. PPPs in India deploying technology to enable remote healthcare (telehealth) is a recent phenomenon [67]. Recent publications are optimistic that telemedicine is set to grow in India over the next 5 years [68] and e-health in India will result in reaching the unreached [69].

India has become a vibrant testing ground for health market innovations. The Indian government is looking at PPPs, as one of the key vehicles to meet India's vast health challenges and capitalise on existing private sector capacity. PPPs can combine government-level patient volumes with private efficiency, providing lower-cost and higher-quality care. The road to establishing a successful PPP is filled with challenges – from identifying the right stakeholders and models and managing partnerships and expectations to contracting, payment systems and legal protections [70]. PPP in digital health is addressing many key challenges. National eHealth Authority (NeHA) and Integrated Health Information Program (IHIP) are some of the new initiatives in the field of digital health. These have led to the notification of EHR standards in 2013 (revised in 2016). In a concept note on PPP issued by the Ministry of Health and Family Welfare, government of India, in 2005, it was stressed that attention should be paid to accessibility and coverage in rural areas, better management of existing infrastructure and ensuring adequate number and quality of healthcare professionals. It was pointed out that private sector provision of healthcare was as high as 70%. The health service market had evolved into two distinct streams: private sector for those who could afford to pay and public sector for those with limited means. The health sector has represented a significant investment market for PPPs since the inception of private finance initiative (PFI) in 1992. The same note referred to three key health PPP procurement programmes in the United Kingdom (UK). All of them were driven by a range of different public sector requirements, policy initiatives and outcomes – PFI hospitals, National Health Service (NHS) Local Improvement Finance Trust (LIFT) and independent sector treatment centres (ISTCs) [71].

India is well positioned to give exemplary digital health solutions through PPPs. The world's largest healthcare programme, Ayushman Bharat, is one such example [72]. PPP initiatives taken by the Indian government include (a) Yeshasvini health scheme in Karnataka, (b) Arogya Raksha scheme in Andhra Pradesh and (c) telemedicine initiative by Narayana Hrudayalaya in Karnataka.

The government of Karnataka, the Narayana Hrudayalaya hospital in Bangalore and the Indian Space Research Organisation initiated a telemedicine project called "Karnataka Integrated Telemedicine and Tele-health Project" (KITTH), which is an online healthcare initiative in Karnataka [73]. Teleradiology Solutions a Bengaluru-based company was accredited by the Singapore Ministry of Health to provide teleradiology services to hospitals and diagnostic centres in Singapore. This joint venture had dramatically reduced the report turnaround time in Singapore from 2 to 3 days to less than an hour. Tripura a state in a remote part of northeastern India have their X-rays contemporaneously interpreted in real time from 23 sites by 50 specialist radiologists from a central reporting centre located in southern India. Similar PPPs have made remote radiology available 24/7 to healthcare providers across tier 2 cities and remote markets in India. Other PPP initiatives started by the Indian government include (a) emergency ambulance services scheme in Tamil Nadu (b); Urban Slum Health Care Project, Andhra Pradesh; and (c) Rashtriya Swasthya Bima Yojana – the last has been implemented in 25 states of India [74].

Inadequacies in outreach and unaffordability coupled with escalating healthcare costs have aggravated the problem of receiving healthcare. PPP model has the potential to ease the impasse. Deficiencies in infrastructure, human resources (HR) and financial inability are being addressed by the spread of Rashtriya Swasthya Bima Yojana and National Rural Telemedicine Network (NRTN) jointly. Fair price shops are also an effective tool in reducing cost of treatment. The NRTN covered three levels: networking primary health centres (PHCs) to district hospitals (level I), district hospitals to state/super-specialty hospitals (level II), interconnected state/super-specialty hospitals (level III) and also mobile units connected to nearest PHCs and district hospitals (level M), all connected through high bandwidth fibre-optic/satellite connection. Medical opinions, consultation, diagnosis and surveillance are possible at a very cost-effective and efficient manner through telemedicine network spread across the country [75].

The present system of providing rudimentary services in the government sector, leaving high-tech care largely to the private sector, has been questioned, especially when public funds are used to subsidise private providers. PPP can be an effective means of providing rational, affordable and comprehensive care to the entire population, provided that the private partners are chosen with care. Current evidence suggests that the best private partners are the not-for-profit entities like self-help groups. Some authors opine that medical care privatisation can result in adverse health impacts [76]. Others contend that private participation is sought not for lack of funds but for lack of managerial and technical ability [77]. After identifying gaps in public health delivery in rural areas, the Confederation of Indian Industry (CII) reported that PPP can help improve the healthcare delivery system [78]. In a study of 13 states where PPP was used in managing PHC, Pal et al. conclude that PPP has now become an increasingly popular option in healthcare delivery system in India [79]. Corporates are actively participating in health programmes utilising mandatory corporate social responsibility funds. This increases opportunity for improving healthcare delivery through PPP [80].

The government of India has laid down guidelines for facilitating entry of the private sector in the healthcare space at the district level, through PPP models. Public think tank NITI Aayog, along with technical assistance from the World Bank, has charted out guidelines for PPP that states can choose to opt for, as health is a state subject. The decision to create model concessionaire agreements (MCA) for PPP in health sector was taken in March 2016. The centre of the MCAs is the district hospitals, and the focus is on preventing, diagnosing and treating non-communicable diseases (NCDs) like heart and lung diseases and cancer in tier 2 and 3 cities [81].

Variations in level of access and quality of healthcare service delivery have led to massively disparate outcomes among states and even districts in India. Accessibility and coverage in rural areas are difficult, given the diversity in geographical terrain. Inaccessible areas are also the most backward areas. Providing medical services to these regions is indeed a challenge. In this context, networking the existing facilities through telemedicine facilities will immensely help in reaching out to even a remote primary health centre. Availability of demographic and clinical information at the point of care can significantly influence the choice of clinical intervention and consequently the clinical outcome. Regional and national data repositories can be made accessible through web-based smartcard applications or an IT backbone. Private players with expertise and managerial experience in deploying huge ICT networks to link the healthcare units across the country can significantly contribute to increasing the access and improving quality of healthcare across India [82]. Defining parameters to evaluate PPP projects in healthcare will enable conditions for the success of a partnership, enhancing the probability of better implementation, intended outcome and improved resource utilisation [83].

Specific State Government Initiatives in Healthcare PPP

In the state of Jharkhand – an area characterised by a low average income, high tribal population, high incidence of poverty and little social development – PPPs in healthcare are starting to make a difference [84]. The state's medical infrastructure faced severe constraints, with demand for specialists outpacing supply by 95 per cent. New advanced diagnostic centres are now located in small tier 2 and tier 3 towns, providing much needed health services to a mostly rural and tribal poor population. Twenty-four district hospitals and the three state-owned medical colleges were part of this PPP. In 2014, the government of Jharkhand set out to change this. With International Finance Corporation of the World Bank Group, the state structured its first health PPP and set up a network of modern diagnostic centres to provide comprehensive radiology and pathology. With better technology, efficiency, skilled health staff and speedy service, 3.5 million residents per year benefited from better primary and preventive healthcare, including basic and advanced diagnostics in oncology, cardiology, urology and other pathology services at affordable prices.

A "hub and spoke" PPP model – in which services are distributed and routed into and out of a central location – was used. Two leading pathology service providers, SRL Limited and Medall Healthcare, signed 10-year concession contracts to build, operate and transfer the facilities back to the state government. A joint venture between Manipal and Philips signed a concession contract with the state government to set up radiology services across all the state districts [85].

Chiranjeevi Yojana (CY) is a PPP between the state and private obstetricians in the state of *Gujarat*, which commenced in 2007. The state pays for institutional births of most vulnerable households (below poverty line and tribal) in private hospitals. An innovative remuneration package has been designed to disincentivise unnecessary caesareans. The target beneficiary group is widened through this initiative [86]. The government of Karnataka issued a formal policy on PPP in 2000 for NGOs to manage PHCs. This enabled Dr Sudarshan of the Karuna Trust to start doing yeoman service [87]. Karnataka also demonstrated the impact of a PPP on the continuum of HIV care among adults enrolled at a private hospital/ART link centre. PPP models of ART delivery improved HIV treatment initiation and loss to follow-up without compromising the effectiveness of treatment [88].

Similar initiatives of people like retired Colonel CS Pant (Uttaranchal mobile health clinic), Dr KJR Murthy (Mahavir Trust Hospital in Hyderabad), Mr MA Wohab (boat-based mobile health services in the Sundarbans of West Bengal) and Dr Haren Joshi (Shamlaji Hospital in Gujarat) have inspired partnership initiatives. Geographical and topographical limitations in accessing health services by the people in Uttaranchal and in the Sundarbans prompted innovative health delivery mechanisms by local private agencies [89]. OTTET telemedicine network with the support of the government of *Odisha* has successfully been implementing telemedicine project throughout the state to bridge the gap of demand-supply mismatch, doctor-wise and facility-wise, to provide healthcare at the doorsteps to a population living in far-flung areas of 51,000 villages of Odisha. OTTET rolled out a platform in technical collaboration with School of Telemedicine and Biomedical Informatics (The National Resource Center), SGPGI, Lucknow [90].

Bihar a low-income and third most populous state in India involved the private sector in partnerships through the National Rural Health Mission as early as 2005. During 2006–2007, PPP in radiology (X-ray and ultrasound) was implemented across 38 districts, from primary health centres to the district hospitals. In addition, many other ancillary services were also provided. The authors however point out serious issues in quality of services and non-adherence to the contractual agreement [91]. West Bengal government initiated an innovative PPP telemedicine pilot venture in Mousani, a small island in the Sundarbans with 30,000 inhabitants. It is being implemented through a partnership with the Namkhana Panchayat Samiti (of which Mousani is a part), the South 24 Parganas district magistrate and a private firm Global Healthcare on a sustainable low-cost model [92]. It has brought healthcare within the reach of every consumer by optimum use of technologies enabling connected health and providing continuum of care.

Technology-Enabled Remote Healthcare: Challenges on the Field

TeRHC: Conceptualisation

As there was no precedent whatsoever and nothing to fall back on, frugal innovation was the key word. Programme implementation started with planning optimum human resources and proper training. Improving stakeholder participation, increasing problem assessment capacities and developing local leadership to promote the programme in the community were critical. Tools used for community outreach included deploying banners and hoarding for promotion of awareness cum screening camps and door to door universal health screening. The aim was to achieve a radical cultural transformation. Technology and clinical management resources alone would not have sufficed. Following a need assessment study, a turnkey solution, end-to-end, on a programme management approach with measurable milestones and monthly reports was initiated. A devoted passionate team of telemedicine specialists, clinicians and programme managers using HR from the local community identified and circumvented hosts of issues. This resulted in delivery of affordable quality healthcare to anyone, anytime, anywhere. Standard operating procedures (SoP), service-level agreements, accountability, responsibility, defining measurable goals, regular auditing, deploying objective impact assessment tools, performance indicators, grievance redressal mechanisms and escalation and evaluation matrices were used. Creating a motivated team to administer and implement well thought out SoPs, with good "man management", helped fulfil primary objectives of delivering remote healthcare.

As this was a first of its kind initiative, strategic decision-making was deployed. To compound the concerns, the beneficiaries, who had been living in a world of their own for decades, were at the "bottom of the pyramid". The consultants were urban super-specialists working in a state-of-the-art, future-ready, JCI-accredited hospital. A major cultural transformation had to be effected. Challenges included (a) convincing the community that a healthcare provider could appear on a screen, make a diagnosis and advise treatment; (b) convincing the beneficiaries that virtual consultants would be able to empathise with them; (c) convincing the very few complacent doctors at the remote centre that this new service would not undermine their status and importance and that instead of being a threat, the new service would only be helping them; and (d) convincing the government that a radical exponential cultural transformation among all the stakeholders could be executed, (e) that the programme would be cost-effective and need based using appropriate technology and (f) that the programme would be totally transparent, accountable, responsible and open to external third-party audit.

Delivering hitherto undelivered services was a major challenge for Apollo TeleHealth Services (ATHS). This highly technical project required considerable inputs from telemedicine specialists with an in-depth domain expertise. No information was available on how an isolated community, totally unfamiliar with virtual healthcare, would accept this new delivery system. Concept of "staying healthy" was alien to the existing culture. Proactive measures had to be introduced to modify health-seeking behaviour. Technology acceptance was a major concern. Apollo Hospitals was staking its reputation spending considerable human resources, effort and time without the usual return on investment. Benefitting the community and making the impossible possible were the primary objective. Several indirect costs were absorbed by ATHS.

Strategy and Planning to Introduce TeRHC

These included:

(a) Creation of virtual OPs at predetermined times and days, depending on local convenience. Specialist telecamps would ensure maximum utilisation of the specialist's limited time. Generally, a specialist gets "turned on" by seeing more patients.
(b) Tele-OP clinics for comprehensive primary and preventive healthcare services.
(c) Tele-super-speciality consultation services, tele-emergency services, tele-laboratory services, community outreach and tele-social health education programmes and teleradiology reporting were additional services.
(d) Customised electronic medical records systems would enable detailed analytics and impact analysis.
(e) For emergency patients, the primary objective was to avoid expensive, logistically complex transfers to higher centres especially if they could be managed at the tele-emergency centre itself. The proposed Apollo tele-emergency system would be linked in real time to support the front-line medical system. Initial stabilisation before transferring the patients to the nearest higher centre was a secondary objective.
(f) A list of deliverables was offered to the government. Non-functioning of telemedicine equipment for more than 5 working days, even in the remote isolated mountainous areas, would be considered as failure in delivery of services.
(g) In practice, it would be extremely difficult, if not impossible, to get Hindi-speaking consultants available at short notice for highly subsidised compensation from quaternary centres. Enthusiasm and willingness of younger doctors would be more. They would also see in this an opportunity for increasing their own knowledge, experience and popularity. It was decided to build redundancy into the system, so that at no time would there be a shortage of consultants.
(h) A list of all drugs available and *not* available in the remote centres would be provided to the teleconsultants.
(i) Backup plans were made for mobilising equipments in time, facing treacherous roads and landslides and temperatures of −25C during winter. Figure 14.1 shows the way to reach the telehealth centre at Kaza; Fig. 14.2 shows telehealth centre at Kaza, Keylong, Pangi and Bharmour.

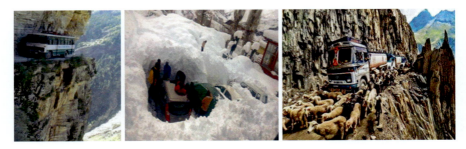

Fig. 14.1 Way to reach telehealth centre at Kaza

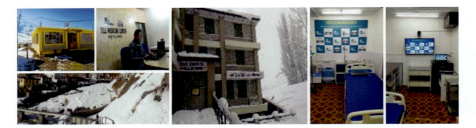

Fig. 14.2 Telehealth centres at Himachal Pradesh – Kaza, Keylong, Pangi, Bharmour

(j) Total transparency ensured accountability to the government, who could also monitor the programme. Remote consultations would ensure functional learning, with a scope for improvement at all levels.

Supportive Steps to Ensure Utilisation of Services in a PPP Mode

This was addressed by having a full-time employee in each centre dedicated exclusively for community outreach. Mass communication methods, with customised, cost-effective, need-based information, were deployed. A rigorous, detailed standard operating procedure ensured that all factors were taken into account. Non-familiarity with hardware and software and reluctance to use the new tools were addressed by training and retraining, ensuring constant skilling and upskilling. Relearning and unlearning were emphasised. Government employees are transferrable. Newly trained resources may get transferred or may go on leave, and this may affect the stringent deliverables of ATHS. Even at the conceptualisation stage, the government was requested to permit human resources for this project, to be employees of ATHS. Managers would not be able to ensure accountability and responsibility from existing government employees, who could even view the telehealth service as an additional work. As a private organisation, ATHS could provide performance-based incentives. The resources would be closely monitored remotely and a carrot and stick policy actually implemented.

Training

Training and re-training was a major component of the project for ATHS staff and government employees associated with the project.

Subjects covered included (a) clinical areas, (b) IT, (c) community linkage, (d) attitudinal change and (e) patient delight aspects. Change management and workflow process re-engineering were new to the staff in the centres where telehealth was to be introduced. As telehealth services were hitherto non-existent in the conventional government health system, it was proposed to blend this and create a workflow process, which would be integrated with the existing government healthcare system. The SoP included a section on training, with details on course content, method of delivery and method of evaluation. HR provisioning included inducting an existing medical resource team into a training programme for capacity building. After an intensive 3-month training at Chennai, a telehealth coordinator/facilitator and two telehealth community linkage coordinators, all initially recruited from the local community, were posted in the mountainous areas of Kaza and Keylong. Training components include fundamentals of information and communication technology, clinical induction, simulation and soft skills. Field teams were inducted into the system after 3 months of training in basics of telehealth. Training covered basics of telemedicine and telemedicine equipment, familiarity with tele-emergencies, trouble shooting for managing Internet connectivity, petty cash accounting, management information system (MIS) and reporting and community linkage programmes. The staff were taught the nuances of presenting a clinical problem, in an emergency situation, thru videoconferencing. Figure 14.3 shows general training in progress at Chennai; Fig. 14.4 shows medical training of staff before deployment in remote areas.

Setting up Tele-Emergency Services

A comprehensive ideal list of 113 items was provided for setting up tele-emergency services. It was emphasised that as time was of the essence and a good emergency response centre should be well-equipped as a stand-alone unit, it would be prudent to have duplication of some equipments. A well-integrated teleconsultation unit with remote diagnostic devices (digital 12 lead ECG, spirometer, stethoscope, point of care diagnostics) and seamless Internet connectivity of 512 Kbps enabled tele-emergency service (TES) implementation. X-ray films developed at the remote casualty centre (digital X-ray machines were not available) were scanned and sent. The TES system blended seamlessly with the very limited emergency services theoretically available. The emergency set-up followed Joint Commission International-prescribed protocols. The telemedicine solution had to take into account enormous cultural differences, language issues, patient and doctor requirements, inclement weather and isolated geographical location. No reliable statistical data was available to even guestimate the types of specialties that need to be provided, or even a very rough incidence and prevalence of secondary/tertiary diseases in the community.

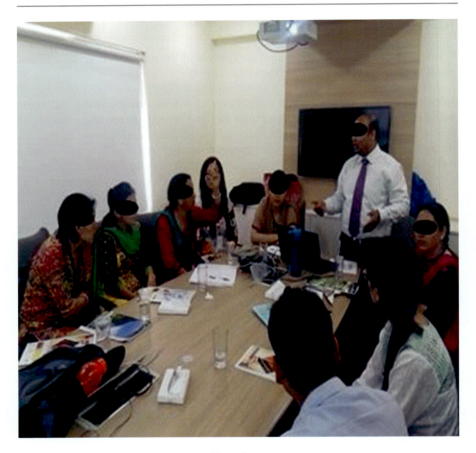

Fig. 14.3 General training in progress at Chennai

Though attendance at the existing government OP was high, 150–300 people daily, it was felt that for the majority, a hospital visit was more an outing and an occasion for social intercourse rather than for attending to medical problems per se. As this was a new initiative which neither the doctor nor the patient is familiar with, it was felt that there would not be more than 20–30 requests for emergency teleconsultations per month from each centre at least during the first few months. Providing immediate services for such a very small number only compounded the problem.

Contact with Community

Resource persons would make as many physical visits as possible to the community members and distribute simple, public-friendly, profusely illustrated information booklets, which would highlight and simplify the entire telemedicine process and explain at length its advantages. They would provide information, which would

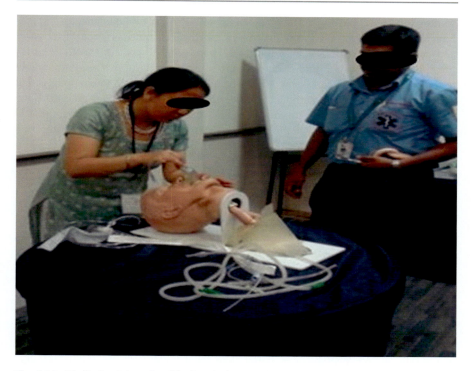

Fig. 14.4 Medical training of staff before deployment in remote areas

assist the community in reducing travel to distant locations saving money and enabling the community to access seamless healthcare services, through the existing government health system. Major change management issues were initially faced with the local staff, who perceived telehealth as a threat. Limited infrastructure, multiple dialects, poor health-seeking behaviour and total unawareness of telehealth compounded the challenges. Technology provided virtual specialists on a screen – but making available drugs prescribed and tests requested was extremely difficult. Making sophisticated urban teleconsultants constantly use generics for limited medicine available and avoiding multiple and sophisticated investigations were also difficult.

Cost-Effectiveness

The government had been willing to spend INR 25 million annually (355,000 US$ as compensation to make available 10 specialists for the district.) These salaries were almost triple of what is normally paid. In spite of these inducements, it was not possible to persuade doctors to physically reside in the district. Additional expenses were incurred on helicopter evacuations for ill patients. The total cost of the telehealth project during the first 15 months, with its major societal impact, for two centres was INR 23 Million. A sample survey of 105 users of the telehealth services indicated that in addition to saving considerable effort, time, physical discomfort and emotional stress INR 8.7 Million would have been spent in travel alone for obtaining perhaps suboptimum healthcare for this small group. The non-tangible benefits are literally priceless and cannot be quantified including the happiness that a caring government has facilitated quality accessible healthcare, at no cost to the end user. Benefits to the environment include reducing carbon print, as about 100 ambulance trips of 150 km and probably 5 helicopter evacuations have already been avoided in the initial 9 months.

Challenges in Communication

Dedicated customised highly subsidised *very small aperture terminal* (VSAT) satellites were provided by BSNL (largest network provider of the government of India (www.bsnl.co.in). The authors implemented a novel reliable 24/7 premium package with a committed bandwidth of 512 Kbps uplink and 512 Kbps downlink. Normally, expensive C-band satellite or intermediate Ku-band satellite connectivity would have been other options. Ku-band is less reliable in terms of committed bandwidth. 24 × 7 seamless, totally dependable, reliable broadband high-speed Internet connectivity was ensured. Minimum bandwidth compatible hardware and software were deployed. From a clinical patient management perspective, "just enough" bandwidth always available was better than ideal bandwidth not totally reliable. Redundancy was built into the system with an additional independent backup network. Due to security reasons, as these centres were very close to the Indo China border, private network operators are not allowed to provide services here. Measuring performance is essential in understanding, if the network is working as intended and its effect.

Assessing Performance

All telemedicine systems should provide information about set-up and running costs, as understanding cost-effectiveness is crucial for ensuring sustainability. Measuring the performance of a system is only one aspect of its overall evaluation. A telemedicine network does not exist in isolation. It is a component or subsystem within an organisation. Measurement includes selecting the characteristics to be measured, choosing a suitable method to measure that characteristic, collecting the data, analysing the collected data, making decisions on the basis of the results and implementing those decisions. "Performance" criteria would differ for each stakeholder – perspective being different for the patient, telehealth coordinator, teleconsultant and financial officer. Societal perspective could be totally different. *The context is critical in measuring the impact of a telehealth network.* To the inhabitants of an isolated sparsely populated district like Lahaul and Spiti, ATHS has made a tremendous difference, for the simple reason that there was no other option. From an audit perspective, the absolute numbers (of money spent and patients who have utilised this service) may not, in the first few years, fully justify the cost incurred. One could customise a wide range of indicators and metrics that might be relevant to the measurement of performance. Indicators "indicate" impact, but they do not attempt to quantify that impact, whereas metrics are "numerical indicators" that allow the impact to be quantified. A combination of indicators and metrics is therefore needed. Indicators could include (a) utilisation (how busy is the network?), (b) quality (how good are the responses?), (c) usability (how easy is the system to use? trouble shooting technical problems?) and (d) patient outcomes.

Societal Influences

Local champions play an important part in overcoming barriers, through opportunistic exploitation of technological and financial options. Telehealth usage fluctuates between medical and administrative operations, in response to internal needs and contextual dynamics. Sustainability of telehealth is affected by existing structures and processes of the healthcare delivery system, policy frameworks, communication and technology costs and physician and patient acceptance. A telehealth service is sustainable when it has been absorbed into the routine healthcare delivery system. Collaboration within the institution, developing alliances within the community, developing external partnership, identifying critical services, engaging external specialists, developing shared vision, exploiting funding opportunities, exploring technological options and improving administrative processes are all equally important. This approach makes the whole greater than the sum of its parts. Implementation of telemedicine requires rethinking and redesigning of the functions, structure and culture within the organisation to achieve major improvements in cost, quality, service and speed. The main objectives should include developing new business processes that support and improve the delivery of services and continually evaluating the enterprises' structure and operations to achieve more responsive systems.

Barriers to Adoption of Telemedicine

These include technology integration, interoperability, standardisation, security, time constraints and financing. As the history of telemedicine depicts, governments can provide technology, but unless health professionals are proactive, the equipment will not be used. Health professionals' perceptions, together with organisational and cultural structures affecting health, legal issues, technical difficulties, time, convenience and cost, are critical. Hurdles relate to reimbursement, policies governing telecommunication and information technologies, development and licensure. Issues pertaining to healthcare organisations influence telehealth adoption. Telehealth adoption is a complex behaviour determined by a large set of psychosocial factors [93]. Studying telemedicine quality from a patient perspective, as consumer and indirect user, is needed from a healthcare business perspective. Patient opinions shape the marketplace and may be missed by an organisation or provider if not specifically studied. One reason for low utilisation rates could be dissatisfaction with the telemedicine encounter experience.

Illustrations of Mega TeRHC Projects in PPP Mode in India, Executed by ATHS

Figure 14.5 shows distribution of TeRHC projects in PPP mode in India.

Telehealth in the Himalayas

The Himachal Pradesh government telehealth services programme operationalised by ATHS was a first of a kind PPP telehealth care programme in South Asia [94]. This programme provides much-needed primary, secondary, specialty, super-specialty and emergency consultations virtually, from Chennai and Hyderabad up to 2950 km away. The remote telemedicine centres are physically located in four isolated locations situated at heights of 12,500–7000 feet in the Himalayan mountain range.

At Kaza and Keylong, temperatures go down to −25C. During winter, the roads are blocked for 4–5 months due to major snowstorms and landslides. Established initially as a proof of concept technology-enabled service delivery model, it is now a time-tested program. The programme allows patients to get remote videoconference-based consultations supported by online, real-time and remote peripheral

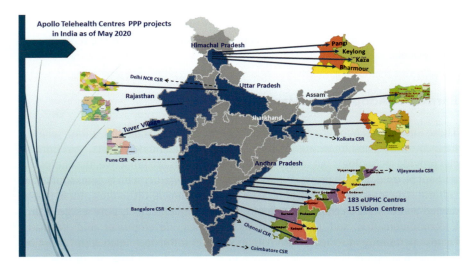

Fig. 14.5 Shows distribution of the various PPP projects deploying Telehealth spread over India

14 Technology Enabled Remote Healthcare in Public Private Partnership Mode... 217

diagnostics. This programme links emergency and specialty experts from Apollo Hospitals with state-of-the-art telehealth centres set up by ATHS in the regional government hospitals using dedicated satellite bandwidth connectivity. In a first of its kind publication, it was shown that delivering tele-emergency services in inhospitable terrains in a public-private partnership mode is doable and is welcomed by the community [95]. Preventive healthcare services like tele-cervical cancer screening, under the supervision of obstetrician and gynaecologist from Apollo Hospitals, are also being provided at Kaza and Keylong. Figure 14.6 gives details of the various milestones achieved in this project. The objective of this telemedicine programme is to create a conducive environment in remote and difficult to access areas and to provide the required healthcare support system. This programme has reduced, difficult travel for patients to distant locations seeking healthcare, saving effort, time and money.

Telehealth in Andhra Pradesh Mukhyamantri Arogya Kendram (e-UPHC) (182 Centres)

To address the need for providing essential primary and specialist healthcare services for the urban poor, living in slum areas, selected urban primary health centres (UPHCs) were upgraded to electronic UPHCs by incorporating telehealth services. These centres provide basic services and, harnessing technology, deliver a spectrum of remote specialist services including cardiology, orthopaedics, endocrinology and general medicine through telemedicine. Spread across nine districts in the state of Andhra Pradesh, 182 e-UPHCs were commissioned [96]. Each centre is remotely connected to Apollo Hospitals, Hyderabad. By leveraging benefits of communication

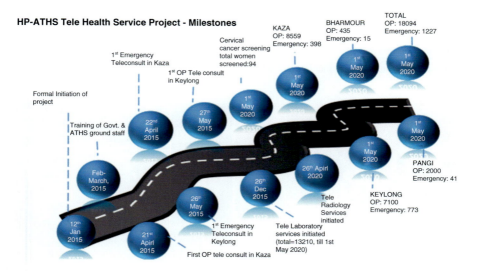

Fig. 14.6 Milestones in HP ATHS TeRHC as of 01 May 2020

technology, this first of a kind PPP initiative has extended the outreach of a quaternary care hospital, bringing specialised care to the doorsteps of the underprivileged. The initiative is a part of the National Health Mission (NHM), a government of India programme. NHM envisages meeting healthcare needs of the urban population with focus on urban poor, thus reducing out-of-pocket expenses for treatment. In recognition of the benchmarks set up, 18 more centres have been added to this project by the government. Table 14.1 gives details of various services rendered from October 2016. Figure 14.7 shows patients waiting and a teleconsultation in progress.

Tele-Ophthalmology (MeEK): 115 Centres

Another major PPP project executed by ATHS for the government of Andhra Pradesh is the Mukhyamantri e-Eye Kendram or MeEK project. One hundred fifteen existing community health centres/vision centres run by the Department of Health and Family Welfare, government of Andhra Pradesh, in 13 districts were identified. State-of-the-art tele-ophthalmology services were introduced by

Table 14.1 MAK services snapshot – as of Apr 2020

MAK services snapshot – Apr 2020			
Parameter	Mar'20	Apr'20	Cumulative
Total consultations	2,58,020	1,03,481	1,03,42,380
General op consultations	2,31,563	99,420	93,51,018
Specialist teleconsultations	26,457	4061	9,91,397
Unique patients treated	41,571	18,859	24,66,124
Repeat consultations	2,16,449	84,622	78,76,256
Lab referrals	46,967	11,245	17,83,091
Lab tests	1,88,312	35,795	72,17,4538
ANC visits	11,936	6208	4,23,600
Immunization visits	16,608	8147	9,33,713

Source: Government of Andhra Pradesh http://www.euphc-ap-gov.in/

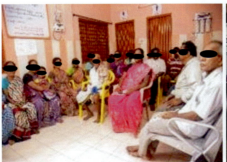 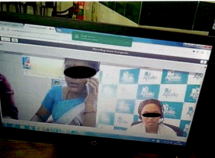

Fig. 14.7 e-UPHC in Andhra Pradesh: outpatient waiting and teleconsultation

ATHS. The low ophthalmologist-patient ratio of 1:10,000 is further compounded by the urban-rural health divide. Acute shortage of optometrists in rural India results in millions developing visual impairment, unnecessarily, due to lack of access to eye care services in their community. Early diagnosis and initiation of corrective measures could prevent the irreversible condition at which individuals often present themselves now. By making available free, quality eye care services in the community itself, the government is fulfilling a major requirement. The specific problems addressed include high-quality evaluation of refractive errors for tens of thousands of individuals, providing them with quality-monitored spectacles and remote fundus screening to enable early referral to higher centres for definitive treatment. Implementing this in 115 rural centres in 13 districts and maintaining a "customer delight" milieu were indeed a humongous task. Being a first of a kind initiative in a PPP mode made the problem even more challenging. Ensuring continuous quality control, constant compliance and adherence to strict deliverables closely monitored by the government in a consortium environment, to about 2000 individuals a day, 8 hours daily, 6 days a week, would aptly describe the scenario.

Each tele-ophthalmology unit has a paramedical ophthalmic officer (PMOO). One equipment assistant (EA) per centre ensured maintenance of the automated digital equipment including non-mydriatic fundus camera, auto-refractometer, lensometer and other equipments. Administrative support from district managers supervised by a programme manager ensured achievement of all objectives. Apollo TeleHealth manages the project electronically through electronic medical record keeping, digital transmission of images captured from the equipment for eye screening and digital reports sent remotely. Practical measures to comply with the strict TAT (turnaround time) are deployed. The impact, 1,460,786 have had their eyes screened during the last 24 months. 1,132,154 spectacles have been distributed. 1,372,446 refraction checks have been done and 351,643 fundus images examined remotely. Figure 14.8 shows eye evaluation in a remote centre and Table 14.2 gives details of services rendered. Figure 14.9 illustrates the real-time dashboard in the public domain.

Other Telehealth PPP Projects

Jharkhand Digital Dispensaries Programme [97]
The government of Jharkhand understanding the need for more doctors and improved medical facilities decided to launch telemedicine through digital dispensaries (Fig.14.10). Consultants in general medicine, dermatology, gynaecology and paediatrics would initially be available virtually. Basic laboratory investigations would be provided. One hundred digital dispensaries in 22 districts were identified. ATHS was chosen as the service provider to implement, operate and manage the digital dispensaries for 5 years. The service commenced on 20 Feb 2019. As in other PPP projects with ATHS, a dashboard (http://jhdd.ind.in/) gets updated in real time. This total transparency ensures confidence among all stakeholders that public money is well spent. It also ensures credibility of the healthcare provider and their

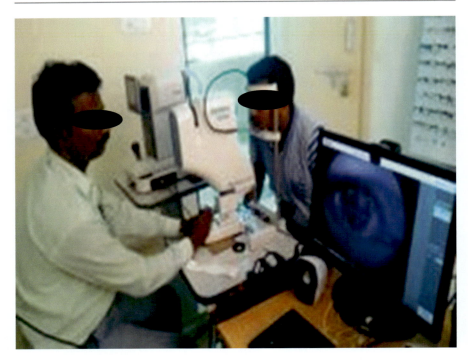

Fig. 14.8 Eye evaluation in remote centre

Table 14.2 Tele-ophthalmology data as of 23 May 2020

S. no	Data	Cumulative
1	No. of patients registered	1,460,786
2	Fundus examination done	351,643
3	Reports finalised	318,312
4	Patients referred to higher centre	90,428
5	Spectacles ordered	1,132,154
6	Spectacles delivered to patients	1,098,518

Source: Government of Andhra Pradesh http://enethraap.phc.ind.in/

operational competence. Numbers speak for themselves. They reflect the satisfaction of the beneficiaries. In the first 15 months alone, 328,648 teleconsultations were done. Figure 14.10 displays a typical dispensary; Fig. 14.11 shows screenshot from real-time government dashboard – details of remote healthcare in 100 digital dispensaries in Jharkhand.

Uttar Pradesh Telemedicine Programme

In order to provide timely and quality specialty healthcare services, the Department of Medical Health and Family Welfare, Government of Uttar Pradesh (UP),

14 Technology Enabled Remote Healthcare in Public Private Partnership Mode... 221

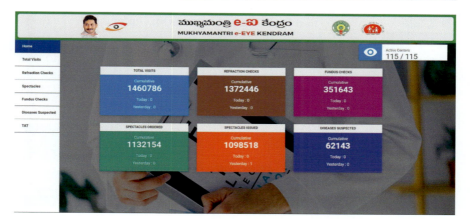

Fig. 14.9 Example real-time dashboard MeEK project as of 23 May 2019. (Source: Government of Andhra Pradesh http://enethraap.phc.ind.in/)

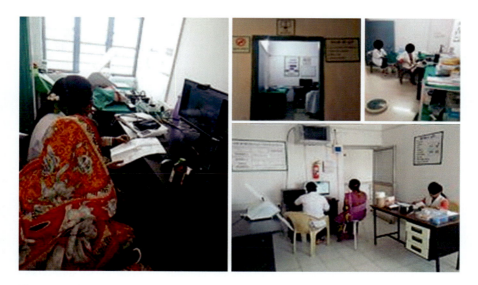

Fig. 14.10 Typical digital dispensary at Jharkhand

overcame existing challenges by deploying Telemedicine. ATHS was selected as the "Service Provider", to render Specialty Teleconsultations at specified Community Health Centres (CHCs) in the State. The primary objective of the UP telemedicine programme was to provide specialist healthcare services, especially in rural areas. The programme is currently being implemented by ATHS across 114 Community Health Centres (CHCs). Secondary (specialty) healthcare services are made available virtually through CHCs. This results in reduction of out of Pocket (OOP) expenditure, unnecessary travel and cost. From 20 May 2019 when the services

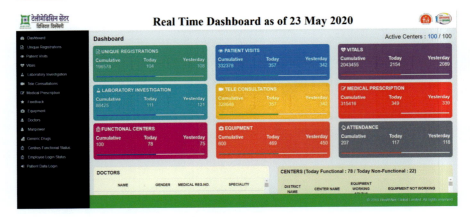

Fig. 14.11 Government dashboard – details of remote healthcare in 100 digital dispensaries in Jharkhand. (Source: Government of Jharkhand http://jhdd.ind.in/)

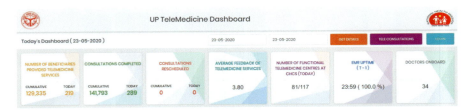

Fig. 14.12 Snapshot of UP Telemedicine Dashboard updated in real time as of 23 May 2020. (Source: Government of Uttar Pradesh http://uptm.ind.in)

commenced till 23 May 2020, 141793 specialty teleconsultations were provided. Only 5% were referred to a higher centre. Reducing the number of patients at higher centres, one of the objectives of the telemedicine programme, appears to have been achieved. Figures 14.12 and 14.13 shows Snapshots of UP Telemedicine Dashboard

Uttar Pradesh teleradiology PPP program With increased acceptance and application of technology in healthcare and acute shortage of radiologists throughout India particularly in suburban and rural India, teleradiology thru a PPP mode would bring immense benefits. The UP teleradiology programme provides access to expert and specialist radiology reporting services, especially for the rural areas. Systematic implementation of operational activities, beginning from site development and installation of IT equipment to training of human resource and trial testing for assessing functional status of centres, has led to commissioning of 127 teleradiology centres in rural UP – a mammoth undertaking by any standards. Figure 14.14 shows training of teleradiology facilitators.

Stringent Tturnaround Ttime (TAT) is an important parameter to evaluate success of the programme. To maintain consistency in service delivery, TAT for interpreting, diagnosing and reporting for non-emergency cases was fixed at 6 hours. For

14 Technology Enabled Remote Healthcare in Public Private Partnership Mode... 223

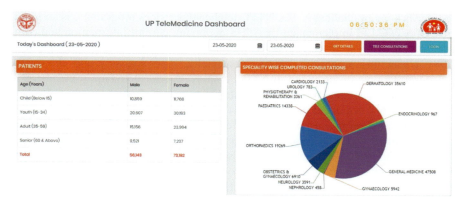

Fig. 14.13 Snapshot of UP Telemedicine Dashboard updated in real time as of 23 May 2020. (Source: Government of Uttar Pradesh http://uptm.ind.in)

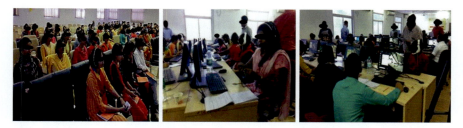

Fig. 14.14 127 Teleradiology centres – training of teleradiology facilitators

emergency cases TAT was 2 hours. This was achieved in 97.3% Continuous training to radiographers stationed at all teleradiology centres and continuous quality checks reduced the number of studies that could not be reported, because of deficiencies in the uploaded X-ray images, to 2.7%. Attempts are being made to reduce this further. However, considering the age of the X- ray machines and the suboptimal infrastructure in the isolated geographical areas, this is not surprising. A real- time Ddashboard link http://uptr.ind.in ensures transparency and opportunity for instituting immediate corrective measures. About 33,000 X-ray images have been scanned and transmitted digitally for remote reporting (average 360 images per day). Service uptime has been 99.1%.

National Thermal Power Corporation (NTPC)

NTPC is one of the biggest public sector units in India. The NTPC Bongaigaon Thermal Power Plant (BgTPP) located in Salakati village of Kokrajhar district in the state of Assam provides a significant part of India's thermal energy. Providing quality, affordable, accessible, 24/7 healthcare including specialties for only 2500 families inside an isolated remotely located, disturbed area close to the Indo China border is a major challenge. The NTPC telehealth services programme is an initiative of NTPC Ltd implemented by ATHS deploying current information and communication technology (ICT) coupled with trained human resources and diagnostics [98]. Under this programme, primary, specialty, super-specialty and emergency teleconsultations are provided to NTPC employees and their family members. A pharmacy with essential medicines operated by a trained pharmacist, physiotherapy services with a dedicated physiotherapist and a digital X-Ray unit with a trained radiographer complement the services offered. X-ray images are remotely evaluated from Chennai 2500 km away. To promote preventive health-seeking behaviour, health profiling of NTPC employees and social health education sessions are organised. Risk categories are identified based on specific health parameters and residents grouped into one of four risk categories. High- and medium-risk patients are monitored continuously. The objective is to provide a personalised *continuum of care* health model. Figure 14.15 shows telehealth services rendered at NTPC as of 07 May 2020; Fig. 14.16 shows the telehealth centre at NTPC.

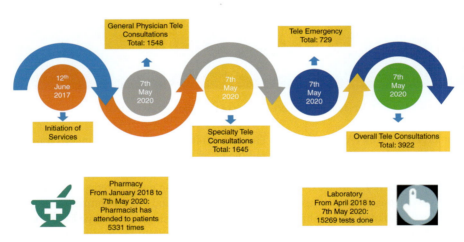

Fig. 14.15 Telehealth services rendered at NTPC as of 07 May 2020

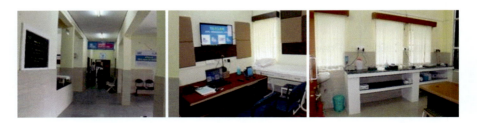

Fig. 14.16 Telehealth centre NTPC

14 Technology Enabled Remote Healthcare in Public Private Partnership Mode…

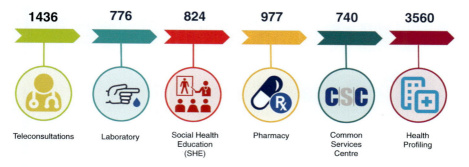

Fig. 14.17 Pictogram detailing services at Tuver as of 30 April 2020

TUVER: Beneficiaries of TeRHC at Tuver

With a vision to provide sustainable, comprehensive and quality healthcare services, the University of Pittsburgh (UoP) Business of Humanity (BoH) in association with Apollo Telemedicine Networking Foundation (ATNF), Safeworld Rural Services (SRS) and Narottam Lalbhai Rural Development Fund (NLRDF) has initiated Tuver Health and Wellness Centre (THWC) project [99]. The THWC project envisages to promote health and wellness among the rural communities in and around Tuver village, Gujarat. The THWC project is unique, as it is a combination of healthcare and digital services. It not only looks at improving access but also aims at achieving self-sustainability, especially with inclusion of solar power. The final goal of the project is to empower "bottom of the pyramid" individuals, to improve quality of life and contribute towards overall development. Remote healthcare is provided to a far-flung isolated area using Internet services. The pictogram below (Fig. 14.17) summarises what has been achieved in the last 15 months. Figure 14.18 shows promotion of health literacy in progress.

Technology-Enabled Mega Screening thru CSR Funding: NCD Screening Programme

To facilitate a paradigm shift from "illness to wellness", ATHS focused on promoting preventive healthcare deploying technology-enabled selective NCD screening for specific populations. Screening camps were conducted for hypertension, diabetes, obesity and anaemia. ATHS is the implementation partner of a "get active" programme. This programme is for prevention and control of NCDs, using screening and health education tools. This programme is being implemented across seven cities in India – Bangalore, Chennai, Delhi NCR, Pune, Kolkata, Vijayawada and

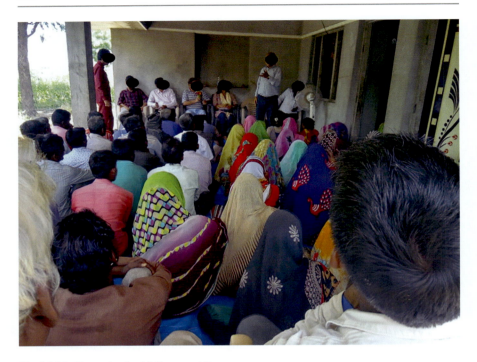

Fig. 14.18 Promoting health literacy at Tuver

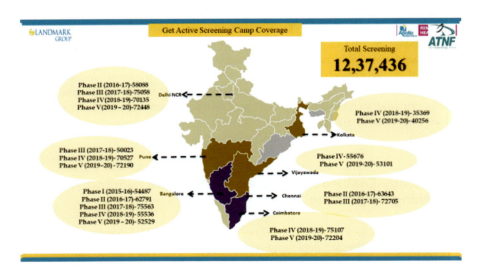

Fig. 14.19 Details of technology-enabled screening camps pan-India as of 31 Jan 2020

Coimbatore. Stakeholders or social groups targeted under this initiative include individuals from lower-income groups in urban slums and industrial workers. Features unique to this service include data collection through integration of information technology (IT) and clinical decision support software module. Figure 14.19

14 Technology Enabled Remote Healthcare in Public Private Partnership Mode… 227

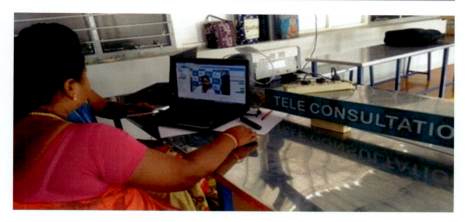

Fig. 14.20 Teleconsultation from camp

gives details of the number of beneficiaries pan-India, Provision of real-time onsite teleconsultations in the camps, to participants who are identified "at risk" and participants already affected with NCDs is a first. Health education sessions are regularly conducted, using customised audio-visual content (in local vernacular language) on NCDs, to women participants in urban slums along with assessment of knowledge retention.

The programme is a "corporate social responsibility" initiative of a multinational company "Landmark" [100].

34,302 Teleconsultations were done in camp mode (Fig. 14.20) as of 19 October 2019. Teleconsultations are provided in the screening camp for participants identified with elevated HbA1C and lipid profile values. Teleconsultations are being provided to allay fears and improve adherence to treatment. All processes are performed through an online-automated system, which enables capturing of data at source and provides decision support. Participants provided with teleconsultations are being followed up for adherence to treatment and initiation of preventive measures. This study of 34,302 update beneficiaries from six centres pan-India has proved that providing teleconsultations in a camp mode is doable [101]. Connecting in real time, to a doctor remotely, in an NCD screening camp, offering immediate counselling, advice and even an e-prescription, is a value-added service and a differentiator.

Lessons Learnt and Conclusions

Nothing can stop an idea whose time has come. It has taken two decades, but we believe that we are reaching that critical mass essential for a successful take off. Persistence, passion and a continuing belief in oneself is what keeps one going, in spite of what at one time appeared to be unsurmountable odds. What started as a hobby today has become a large division of a mega conglomerate corporate hospital group. This would not have been possible but for the enormous vision of the leadership, who like Nostradamus, were able to look into the future. The confidence reposed in the operational team acted as a stimulus for the latter. Today the team consisting of almost 3000 individuals (including all project staff) facilitates about 5000 teleconsults a day. Ten million lives have been touched by the remote healthcare division of the Apollo Hospital Group. We are pleased that we have been an evangelist par excellence motivating many, many other organisations to embrace telehealth and make remote healthcare a reality in India. We are confident that soon telehealth will be integrated into the core of the healthcare delivery system in India.

Acknowledgements It is impossible to enumerate the scores of individuals who in the last two decades are making our dream and vision come true. Dr Prathap C. Reddy, founder and chairman of the Apollo Hospital Group, as early as 1998 had realised that telehealth was here to stay. Along with Dr Preetha Reddy, vice chairperson, all the members of the board of directors have given carte blanche to the operational team. This has gone a long way. Vikram Thaploo CEO is managing an outstanding team of dedicated professionals for whom the words "not possible" do not exist. S Premanand vice president programme management, Dr Ayesha Nazneen chief medical officer, Lakshminarayan Chebolu head of IT, V Krishnamurthy deputy general manager, Tamilmaran manager and dozens of section managers and their assistants are all part of the team who made this possible. We also wish to place on record the secretarial assistance rendered by Lakshmi executive secretary.

References

1. Ganapathy K. Telemedicine and neurosciences in developing countries. Surg Neurol. 2002;58:388–94.
2. Ganapathy K. Telemedicine and neurosciences – a review. J Clin Neurosci. 2005;12:851–62.
3. Ganapathy K, Ravindra A. Healthcare for rural India: is telemedicine the solution? J eHealth Technol Appl. 2007;5:203–7.
4. Ganapathy K. Telehealth for one sixth of humankind. Making it happen. In: Malina Jordanova editor. The Apollo story in global telemedicine and eHealth updates: knowledge resources. ISSN 1998-5509. Publishers ISfTeH Belgium; 2015;8: 128–133.
5. Mohan V, Deepa M, Pradeepa R, Prathiba V, Datta M, Ravikumar S, Rakesh H, Sucharita Y, Webster P, Allender S, Kapur A. Prevention of diabetes in rural india with a telemedicine intervention. J Diabetes Sci Technol. 2012;6:1355–64.
6. Bali S, Gupta A, Khan A, Pakhare A. Evaluation of telemedicine centres in Madhya Pradesh, Central India. J Telemed Telecare. 2016;22:183–8.
7. Ganapathy K. Distribution of neurologists and neurosurgeons in India and its relevance to the adoption of telemedicine. Neurol India. 2015;63:142–54.
8. Praveen KB, Ali SS. Telemedicine in primary health care: the road ahead. Int J Prev Med. 2013;4:377–8.
9. Ganapathy K, Kanwar V, Bhatnagar T, Uthayakumaran N. m-Health: a critical analysis of awareness, perception, and attitude of healthcare among providers in Himachal Pradesh, North India. Telemed J E Health. 2016;22:675–88.
10. Ganapathy K, Chawdhry V, Premanand S, Sarma A, Chandralekha J, Kumar KY, et al. Telemedicine in the himalayas: operational challenges-a preliminary report. Telemed J E Health. 2016;22:821–35.
11. Wong LY, Yeoh E-k, Chau YK, Yam HK, Cheung WL, Fung H. How shall we examine and learn about public-private partnerships (PPPs) in the health sector? Realist evaluation of PPPs in Hong Kong. Soc Sci Med. 2015;147:261–9.
12. Public-private partnerships in health promotion. https://www.jliedu.com/blog/public-private-partnerships-in-health-promotion/. Last accessed 15 Aug 2019.

13. Public-private partnerships in health – World Bank group – Engagement in health PPPs – IEG synthesis. https://ieg.worldbankgroup.org/evaluations/public-private-partnerships-health. Last accessed 15 Aug 2019.
14. The EU's future public-private partnership for health marks a new era for medtech innovation. http://www.medtechviews.eu/article/eu%E2%80%99s-future-public-private-partnership-health-marks-new-era-medtech-innovation. Last accessed 15 Aug 2019.
15. Meier F, Schöffski O, Schmidtke J. Public–private partnership as a solution for integrating genetic services into health care of countries with low and middle incomes. J Community Genet. 2013;4:309–20.
16. Moro Visconti R, Martiniello L, Morea D, Gebennini E. Can public-private partnerships foster investment sustainability in smart hospitals? Sustainability. 2019;11:1704. https://doi.org/10.3390/su11061704.
17. Lang A. Government capacities and stakeholders: what facilitates ehealth legislation? Glob Health. 2014;10:4. https://doi.org/10.1186/1744-8603-10-4.
18. Standard on PPPs in telemedicine and digital health. http://www.temdec.med.kyushu-u.ac.jp/img/katsudo/domestic/2016PH/Opening/Standard%20for%20PPP%20in%20Telemed.pdf. Last accessed 15 Aug 2019.
19. PPPs in healthcare models, lessons and trends for the future healthcare public-private partnerships series, no. 4 by PWC & Institute for Global Health Sciences. https://www.pwc.com/gx/en/industries/healthcare/publications/trends-for-the-future.html. Last accessed 15 Aug 2019.
20. Crisp N. Turning the world upside down: the search for global health in the 21st century. 1st ed. London: CRC Press; 2010. https://doi.org/10.1201/b13481.
21. Venkat Raman A, James Warner Björkman. Public-private partnerships in healthcare. The Palgrave International Handbook of Healthcare Policy and Governance; 2015;376–392. https://doi.org/10.1057/9781137384935_23. Last accessed 15 Aug 2019
22. Chakravarty N, Sadhu G, Bhattacharjee S, Nallala S. Mapping private-public-partnership in health organizations: India experience. Int J Med Public Health. 2015;5:128–32.
23. Mercille J. The public-private mix in primary care development: the case of Ireland. Int J Health Serv. 2019;49:412–30.
24. Cappellaro G, Longo F. Institutional public private partnerships for core health services: evidence from Italy. BMC Health Serv Res. 2011;11:82. https://doi.org/10.1186/1472-6963-11-82.
25. Public private sector partnership brings telemedicine in Jamaica to reality. http://go-jamaica.com/pressrelease/item.php?id=644. Last accessed 17 Aug 2019.
26. Public-private partnership in Kenya. http://khf.co.ke/public-private-partnership-in-kenya/. Last accessed 17 Aug 2019.
27. Lee HS. A. Study on the Public-Private Partnership to Global Health Issues in Korea. Public Health Res Perspect. 2013;4:308–15.
28. Sakowska MM, Cole JAM, Watters DA, Guest GD. Impact of public-private partnership on a regional colonoscopy service. ANZ J Surg. 2019;89:552–6.
29. Imtiaz A, Farooq G, Haq ZU, Ahmed A, Anwar S. Public private partnership and utilization of maternal and child health Services in District Abbottabad, Pakistan. J Ayub Med Coll Abbottabad. 2017;29:275–9.
30. Khan NN, Puthussery S. Stakeholder perspectives on public-private partnership in health service delivery in Sindh province of Pakistan: a qualitative study. Public Health. 2019;170:1–9.
31. US forms telemedicine public-private partnership in Pakistan. https://fp.brecorder.com/2008/10/20081021823544/. Last accessed 17 Aug 2019.
32. The Philippine health sector is set to grow through a number of public-private partnerships. https://oxfordbusinessgroup.com/analysis/philippine-health-sector-set-grow-through-number-public-private-partnerships. Last accessed 17 Aug 2019.
33. Proposed National eHealth System and Services Act approved by house panel in the Philippines https://www.healthcareitnews.com/news/proposed-national-ehealth-system-and-services-act-approved-house-panel-philippines. Last accessed 17 Aug 2019.
34. Fernandes AC, Nunes AM. Hospitals and the public-private combination in the Portuguese health system. Acta Medica Port. 2016;29:217–23.

35. Purcărea VL, Coculescu BI, Coculescu EC. The concept of marketing in the public-private partnership in the medical system in Romania. J Med Life. 2014;7:20–2.
36. PPP in rural areas: Another hospital with telemedicine built in Yakutia Sakha Republic of Russia https://investyakutia.com/en/posts/65. Last accessed 17 Aug 2019.
37. Kula N, Fryatt RJ. Public-private interactions on health in South Africa: opportunities for scaling up. Health Policy Plan. 2014;29:560–9.
38. Comendeiro-Maaløe M, Ridao-López M, Gorgemans S, Bernal-Delgado E. Public-private partnerships in the Spanish National Health System: the reversion of the Alzira model. Health Policy. 2019;123:408–11.
39. Kamugumya D, Olivier J. Health system's barriers hindering implementation of public-private partnership at the district level: a case study of partnership for improved reproductive and child health services provision in Tanzania. BMC Health Serv Res. 2016;16:596. https://doi.org/10.1186/s12913-016-1831-6.
40. Top M, Sungur C. Opinions and evaluations of stakeholders in the implementation of the public-private partnership (PPP) model in integrated health campuses (city hospitals) in Turkey. Int J Health Plann Mgmt. 2019;34:e241–63. https://doi.org/10.1002/hpm.2644.
41. Bilkent campus public-private partnership: the right prescription for turkey's healthcare. http://middleeast.geblogs.com/en/stories/bilkent-campus-public-private-partnership-the-right-prescription-for-turkeys-healthcare/. Last accessed 17 Aug 2019.
42. An analysis of public-private-partnership (PPP) hospital campuses construction programme of Turkey. https://ww2.frost.com/frost-perspectives/analysis-public-private-partnership-ppp-hospital-campuses-construction-programme-turkey/. Last accessed 17 Aug 2019.
43. Joloba M, Mwangi C, Alexander H, Nadunga D, Bwanga F, Modi N, et al. Strengthening the tuberculosis specimen referral network in Uganda: the role of public-private partnerships. J Infect Dis. 2016;213:41–6.
44. Sadeghi A, Barati O, Bastani P, Jafari DD, Etemadian M. Experiences of selected countries in the use of public-private partnership in hospital services provision. J Pak Med Assoc. 2016;66:1401–6.
45. UK pushing dodgy public-private partnerships. https://newint.org/blog/2018/01/18/UK-exporting-PPPs. Last accessed 15 Aug 2019.
46. Why public-private partnerships can provide flexibility to GCC's healthcare sector. https://www.entrepreneur.com/article/314152. Last accessed 17 Aug 2019.
47. Khushbu Thadani B. Public private Partnership in the Health Sector: Boon or Bane. Procedia Soc Behav Sci. 2014;157:307–16.
48. How e-health is changing lives in Afghanistan. https://www.akdn.org/project/how-e-health-changing-lives-afghanistan. Last accessed 15 Aug 2019.
49. Cohen G. Role of public-private partnerships in meeting healthcare challenges in Africa: a perspective from the private sector. J Infect Dis. 2016;213:S33. https://doi.org/10.1093/infdis/jiv578.
50. Hellowell M. Are public-private partnerships the future of healthcare delivery in sub-Saharan Africa? Lessons from Lesotho. BMJ Glob Health. 2019;4(2):e001217. https://doi.org/10.1136/bmjgh-2018-001217.
51. Hader SL. Role of public-private partnerships in meeting healthcare challenges in Africa: a perspective from the public sector. J Infect Dis. 2016;213(Suppl_2):S34. https://doi.org/10.1093/infdis/jiv575.
52. Diarra A. Making a public-private partnership work--an insider's view. Interview by John Maurice. Bull World Health Organ. 2001;79:795–6.
53. Sajani TT, Alo K. Aktaruzzaman. Public Private Partnership (PPP) in Health Sector of Bangladesh. AKMMC J. 2014;5:42–5.
54. Public private partnership in ICT infrastructure: the case study on telemedicine in Belarus. https://www.unece.org/fileadmin/DAM/SPECA/documents/kdb/2011/International_Conference/Presentations/Andrianova.pdf. Last accessed 15 Aug 2019.

55. Ndlovu K, Littman-Quinn R, Park E, Dikai Z, Carrie Kovarik L. Scaling up a Mobile telemedicine solution in Botswana: keys to sustainability. Front Public Health. 2014;2:275. https://doi.org/10.3389/fpubh.2014.00275.
56. A PPP encore in Brazil: two healthcare partnerships boost Bahia's ability to care for citizens. https://blogs.worldbank.org/ppps/ppp-encore-brazil-two-healthcare-partnerships-boost-bahia-s-ability-care-citizens. Last accessed 15 Aug 2019.
57. How public-private partnerships can boost innovation in health care. https://knowledge.wharton.upenn.edu/article/public-private-partnership-enabled-innovation-healthcare/. Last accessed 15 Aug 2019.
58. Zhang JY, Long RY, Yan H, Yang Q, Yang B. Policy and Practice Model of Public-Private Partnership in Public Hospitals during the New Medical Reform Period. J BUON. 2016;21:478–81.
59. Role of private enterprises in making government healthcare services better. https://telradsol.com/role-of-private-enterprises-in-better-healthcare-services/. Last accessed 15 Aug 2019.
60. Argaw MD, Woldegiorgis AG, Abate DT, Abebe ME. Improved malaria case management in formal private sector through public private partnership in Ethiopia: retrospective descriptive study. Malar J. 2016;15:352. https://doi.org/10.1186/s12936-016-1402-7.
61. Partner the private sector: PPP is win-win, government cannot deliver universal healthcare on its own. https://timesofindia.indiatimes.com/blogs/Plainspeak/partner-the-private-sector-ppp-is-win-win-government-cannot-deliver-universal-healthcare-on-its-own/. Last accessed 15 Aug 2019.
62. PPP is the way forward to improve healthcare in India: McKinsey. https://www.downtoearth.org.in/news/ppp-is-the-way-forward-to-improve-healthcare-in-india-mckinsey-39883. Last accessed 15 Aug 2019
63. The need for public private partnership in healthcare in India. https://www.zhl.org.in/blog/the-need-for-public-private-partnership-in-healthcare-in-india/. Last accessed 15 Aug 2019
64. Fast-tracking PPPs. https://www.expresshealthcare.in/features/fast-tracking-public-private-partnerships/390503/. Last accessed 17 Aug 2019.
65. PPP model: a right impetus on healthcare delivery. https://ehealth.eletsonline.com/2018/12/ppp-model-a-right-impetus-on-healthcare-delivery/. Last accessed 17 Aug 2019.
66. Press Information Bureau, Ministry of Personnel, Public grievances & pensions, Government of India. http://pib.nic.in/newsite/PrintRelease.aspx?relid=155540. Last accessed 17 Aug 2019.
67. Telangana – TeleOphthalmology (Mukhyamantri e-Eye Kendram). http://enethraap.phc.ind.in/. Last accessed 17 Aug 2019.
68. Solberg KE. Telemedicine set to grow in India over the next 5 years. World Report. 2008;371:17–8.
69. eHealth for India: reaching the unreached. https://assets.aspeninstitute.org/content/uploads/files/content/docs/pubs/2010%20India%20Text%20FINAL.pdf. Last accessed 17 Aug 2019.
70. Spotlight on ACCESS health-facilitating public private partnerships for health. https://healthmarketinnovations.org/blog/spotlight-access-health-facilitating-public-private-partnerships-health. Last accessed 15 Aug 2019.
71. Concept note on public-private partnerships. https://www.adb.org/sites/default/files/publication/27495/health-education-delivery-india-ppp.pdf. Last accessed 16 Aug 2019.
72. PPP in digital health can provide affordable access and quality in Indian healthcare and catalyse Ayushman Bharat: commerce secretary. http://ficci.in/pressrelease-page.asp?nid=3367. Last accessed 16 Aug 2019.
73. Public-private partnerships in India by KPMG. https://www.ibef.org/download/PublicPrivatePartnership.pdf. Last accessed 15 Aug 2019.
74. Dawra A, Jagtap MS. Public-private partnership (PPP) role in health care in India. AdvEcon Bus Manage. 2015;2:1434–7.

75. Dutta S, Lahiri K. Is provision of healthcare sufficient to ensure better access? An exploration of the scope for public-private partnership in India. Int J Health Policy Manag. 2015;4:467–74.
76. Thomas G, Krishnan S. Effective public-private partnership in healthcare: apollo as a cautionary tale. Indian J Med Ethics. 2010;7:2–4.
77. Das A. Public-private partnerships for providing healthcare services. Indian J Med Ethics. 2007;4(4):174–5.
78. Public-private partnerships can plug gaps in delivering rural healthcare: CII. https://www.livemint.com/Science/kYKDNIE9JjEWvFi4CeScXK/Publicprivate-partnerships-can-plug-gaps-in-delivering-rura.html. Last accessed 15 Aug 2019.
79. Pal R, Pal S. Primary health care and public-private partnership: an Indian perspective. Ann Trop Med Public Health. 2009;2:46–52.
80. Ranganadhan S. Public-private partnership in health sector – opportunities for better health care delivery. IOSR J Nurs Health Sci. 2018;7(25):33.
81. Niti Aayog frames PPP guidelines for district hospitals. https://www.thehindubusinessline.com/economy/policy/niti-aayog-frames-ppp-guidelines-for-district-hospitals/article25249012.ece. Last accessed 15 Aug 2019.
82. The emerging role of PPP in Indian healthcare sector – Prepared by CII In collaboration with KPMG. https://www.ibef.org/download/PolicyPaper.pdf. Last accessed 15 Aug 2019.
83. Public-private partnership in healthcare in India: analysis of success factor using quantitative content analysis. http://vslir.iima.ac.in:8080/jspui/bitstream/11718/14115/1/CMHS_IC-15-030.pdf. Last accessed 15 Aug 2019.
84. How India is using public-private partnerships to expand healthcare. https://www.weforum.org/agenda/2016/01/creating-a-sustainable-health-diagnostics-network-for-low-income-populations-in-india-through-private-sector-participation/. Last accessed 15 Aug 2019.
85. India's new health care PPP mends medical infrastructure. https://www.ifc.org/wps/wcm/connect/news_ext_content/ifc_external_corporate_site/news+and+events/news/impact-stories/health-care-ppp-jharkhand-india. Last accessed 15 Aug 2019.
86. Iyer V, Sidney K, Mehta R, Mavalankar D, De Costa A. Characteristics of private partners in Chiranjeevi Yojana, a public-private-partnership to promote institutional births in Gujarat, India Lessons for universal health coverage. PLoS One. 2017;12(10):e0185739. https://doi.org/10.1371/journal.pone.0185739.
87. Sudarshan H, Innovations in primary health care through public-private partnerships hon. Secretary, Karuna Trust, India. http://www.karunatrust.com/wp-content/uploads/2011/03/KT_FINAL_ANNUAL_Report_17-18.pdf. Last accessed 16 Aug 2019.
88. Waldrop G, Sarvode S, Rao S, Swamy VHT, Solomon SS, Mehta SH, et al. The impact of a private-public partnership delivery system on the HIV continuum of care in a south Indian city. AIDS Care. 2018;30:278–83.
89. Public/private partnership in health care services in India by Dr. A Venkat Rama and Prof. James Warner Björkman. http://medind.nic.in/haa/t08/i1/haat08i1p62.pdf. Last accessed 15 Aug 2019.
90. We believe in public private partnership with people. https://ehealth.eletsonline.com/2013/05/we-believe-in-public-private-partnership-with-people/. Last accessed 15 Aug 2019.
91. Public private partnerships in healthcare outsourcing of radiology services in Bihar a case study. https://www.oxfamindia.org/sites/default/files/2018-10/Bihar_Radiology_PPP%20Study%20Report.pdf. Last accessed 15 Aug 2019.
92. Access to primary healthcare for people in rural areas of West Bengal got a fillip with a new initiative known as G1 Digital Dispensary. https://economictimes.indiatimes.com/news/politics-and-nation/west-bengal-governments-latest-effort-to-spread-healthcare-in-rural-areas/articleshow/51269602.cms?from=mdr. Last accessed 17 Aug 2019.
93. Gagnon M-P. Telehealth adoption in hospitals: an organisational perspective. J Health Organ Manag. 2005;19:32–56.
94. Himachal pradesh tele health services. https://www.thestatesman.com/cities/tele-health-services-come rescue-tribals-1502621402.html. Last accessed 17 Aug 2019.

95. Ganapathy K, Alagappan D, Rajakumar H, Dhanapal B, Rama Subbu G, Nukala L, et al. Tele-emergency services in the himalayas. Telemed J E Health. 2019;25:380–90.
96. Telangana – eUrban Primary Health Centre (eUPHC). http://www.euphc-ap-gov.in/. Last accessed 17 Aug 2019.
97. Jharkhand. https://timesofindia.indiatimes.com/city/ranchi/e-health-services-launched-for-rural-areas/articleshow/68085735.cms. Last accessed 17 Aug 2019.
98. https://www.apollohospitals.com/apollo_pdf/apollo-excellence-report-2018-e-version.pdf. Last accessed 14 Oct 2019.
99. http://www.dcpower.pitt.edu/opening-business-humanity-project-s-tuvar-village-initiative-gujarat-india. Last accessed on 14th Oct 2019.
100. CSR Activities supported by Landmark. http://www.landmarkcares.in/partners.html. Last accessed 05 Oct 2019.
101. Ganapathy K, Nukala L, Premanand S, Tamilmaran P, Aggarwal P, Saksena S, et al. Telemedicine in camp mode while screening for noncommunicable diseases: a preliminary report from India. Telemed J E Health. 2019;26(1):42–50. https://doi.org/10.1089/tmj.2018.0300.

International and Global Telemedicine: Making It Work

15

Dale C. Alverson

Spectrum of Telehealth Platforms and Applications, a Continuum of Health Services

The global community is facing the "digital transformation of healthcare" with the integration of telehealth and telemedicine, incorporation of electronic health records, and interoperable health information exchange. This remarkable transformation is having an impact on countries around the world and for patients of all ages [1–3]. There are several international and national organizations with an interest in promoting telehealth, sharing knowledge, and assisting in ongoing development of telehealth programs in the global community and with individual countries (Fig. 15.1).

These associations include the International Society for Telemedicine and eHealth [4]; American Telemedicine Association (ATA) and its international chapters [5]; the Swinfen Charitable Trust (SCT) [6]; Doctors Without Borders or Medecins Sans Frontieres (MSF) [7]; regional telehealth associations, such as the "Asociacion Iberoamericana de Telesalud y Telemedicina" (AITT) [8]; and telehealth associations or societies in specific countries, such as in Australia, European countries, Russia, China, Japan, the Middle East, Africa, and many others. The time zone differences between countries create challenges and opportunities for telehealth collaboration. Providing 24-hour coverage is possible, for example, when providers in time zones that are 12 hours apart, so that night coverage in one time zone can be covered by providers 12 hours apart when it is daytime in their location. Teleradiology programs such as NightHawk [9] took advantage of those time zone differences using radiologists in the different time zones in Australia, the United States, and Europe. Emory University in Atlanta is placing their own faculty and

D. C. Alverson (✉)
Health Sciences Center, University of New Mexico, Albuquerque, NM, USA
e-mail: dalverson@salud.unm.edu

© Springer Nature Switzerland AG 2021
R. Latifi et al. (eds.), *Telemedicine, Telehealth and Telepresence*,
https://doi.org/10.1007/978-3-030-56917-4_15

Fig. 15.1 Global health. (Reproduced from https://earthobservatory.nasa.gov/images/565/earth-the-blue-marble, NASA)

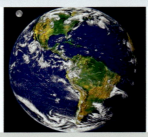

nurses in Perth, Western Australia, to cover the night call monitoring in the Atlanta area hospitals for which they are responsible and relieving some of the night call burden of the Georgia-based critical care staff [10].

Telehealth can be used to address global health issues as outlined by the World Health Organization (WHO) [11–13] and the 17 Sustainable Development Goals (SDGs) published in 2015 [14]. These SDGs replaced the Millennium Development Goals (MDG) published in 2008 [15]. The SDGs that are particularly relevant for telehealth application include Goal 3, "Ensure healthy lives and promote well-being for all at all ages"; Goal 4, "Ensure inclusive and equitable quality education and promote lifelong learning opportunities for all"; and Goal 17, "Strengthen the means of implementation and revitalize the global partnership for sustainable development." For telehealth to have an impact, other issues need to be addressed, including access to clean water, adequate nutrition, waste management, access to power, electricity, and the Internet (Fig. 15.2).

Telehealth can also be used in dealing with life-threatening or debilitating infectious communicable disease outbreaks, epidemic or pandemics, as well as endemic infections and diseases, such as HIV/AIDS, malaria, dengue, tuberculosis, hepatitis, leishmaniasis, Chagas, and other tropical diseases. The spread of those disease can be mitigated through rapid sharing of knowledge and appropriate interventions. The threats of Ebola, Zika, SARS, and other outbreaks can utilize telehealth networks in addressing those life-threatening outbreaks and the serious associated morbidities and mortality.

Telehealth and telemedicine can be used for disaster response and useful when there is a need for international response and availability of expertise to address the medical issues encountered, or triage, particularly when the existing healthcare infrastructure is damaged or the medical issues become overwhelming for local providers or there is a need to transfer patients to other facilities or other countries that have the capacity to manage those medical problems or injuries [16, 17]. These

15 International and Global Telemedicine: Making It Work

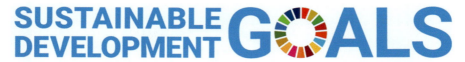

17 Goals that can create significant transformation globally that address improving the quality of life and health of people around the world

Fig. 15.2 The United Nations (UN)/World Health Organization (WHO) Sustainable Development Goals (SDGs): (https://www.un.org/sustainabledevelopment/)

approaches have been applied effectively after earthquakes, hurricanes, flood, and other natural or man-made disasters. To more effectively and efficiently use telehealth in a disaster, telehealth should be included in disaster preparedness planning so that systems and the needed infrastructure needed can be deployed and quickly put in place for adequate response.

There is a wide spectrum of ways to utilize telehealth that represents a continuum of care. Each approach should be complimentary in the coordination and continuity of care in the international community. Furthermore, appropriate and effective international collaboration can build better relationships and strengthen mutual understanding. Those applications include (1) education, case reviews, and simulations, (2) telementoring and tele-supervision, (3) teleconsultation and e-consults including specialty services along with direct patient evaluation and management, (4) Web-based second opinions, (5) mobile health (mHealth) and Internet of Medical Things (IoMT), (6) asynchronous store and forward, (7) remote patient monitoring, and (8) future development of artificial intelligence along with decision support. All of these approaches apply to international telehealth as well outlined below.

Education, Case Reviews, and Simulation

(a) The ECHO model

   The Extension for Community Health Outcomes (ECHO) is an example of a model using telehealth technologies for education and case reviews directed toward primary care providers related to common complex health problems that improve knowledge and confidence in managing patients with a spectrum of medical disorders [18–23]. This model is being adopted by countries around the world and offers an important component of the spectrum of telehealth and can be part of the continuum of providing and extending access to healthcare knowledge and services using communication and information technologies (Fig. 15.3).

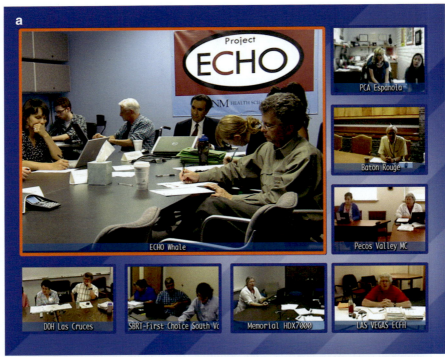
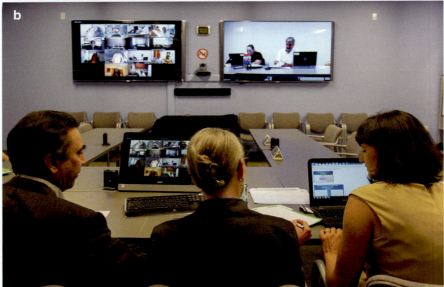

Fig. 15.3 (**a**) A typical ECHO session with a panel of experts interacting with multiple primary care providers (*Used with permission from Project ECHO/ECHO Institute*). (**b**) TeleECHO session. (*Used with permission from Project ECHO/ECHO Institute*)

When this model exceeds the knowledge, time, and skills of the primary care provider, specialty electronic consults and direct patient evaluation and management can also play an important role in providing care locally and fill gaps in specialty care not otherwise available.

(b) Simulations

Simulations have been used with high-fidelity mannequins and virtual reality environments to allow a safe environment to learn, reinforce training, and provide a safe environment to make mistakes and learn from those mistakes and thus be better prepared for actual events in which they may not commonly encounter. A program called "child ready" helps local providers in their community use simulation for education and training in dealing with life-threatening emergencies in children such as serious medical problems or trauma [24]. Experts can observe, advise, and provide feedback during the virtual simulation exercises. This can be part of a telemedicine program for consultation and triage and when and how to access real-time consultation with pediatric emergency experts (Fig. 15.4).

Virtual reality environments can also be used with participants joining in the virtual world from different locations and other countries over distance to provide opportunities for team interaction and again create a safe environment to make mistakes and learn with expert observation, advise, and feedback [refs and images]. There is evidence that these experiences can also improve knowledge and performance during actual events [25–31] (Fig. 15.5).

1. Telementoring and tele-supervision
   (a) There are several models of providing virtual mentoring and supervision using telehealth technologies. Experts can transmit their procedures for education and training for students or providers with less experience interested in applying these procedures to their patients. Furthermore, real-time supervision can be provided virtually by having experts available to view and advise others when doing the procedure, as if they were present in-person during the procedure and virtually looking over the shoulder of those

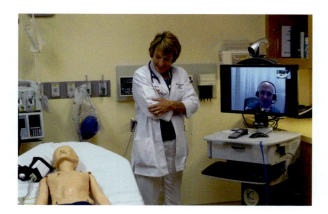

Fig. 15.4 Child ready: providing simulation training and direct consultation in the emergency room of distant hospitals

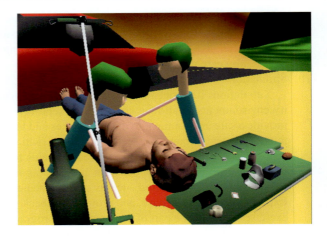

Fig. 15.5 Virtual reality: collaborative team training across international boundaries with participants entering the virtual reality environment from locations around the world

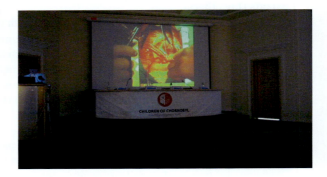

Fig. 15.6 Tele-supervision/telementoring in the operating room during open-heart surgery on an infant (Kiev, Ukraine)

performing the procedure. The Children's Heart Hospital in Ukraine has used this approach in the operating room during open-heart operations where a more experienced expert surgeon can observe and supervise a more junior surgeon during the surgical procedure (Fig. 15.6).
  (b) Similar procedures using telehealth have been applied in critical care for demonstrating a procedure or supervising other providers during the procedures that are emergent but where there may not have been significant experience.
2. Teleconsultation/e-consults and direct patient evaluation and management
  (a) Specialty services
     Real-time video has also been used to evaluate, diagnose, and assist in management of patients with experts from other countries or facilitate specialty interaction within a country from a medical center to providers and their patients in distant rural or remote locations. Videoconferencing systems provide the means to interact with patients directly in real time for evaluation, diagnosis, and management. These systems also can provide methods for follow-up and ongoing care particularly when those services are not

available locally. In addition, emergent and urgent needs for evaluation and treatment can be facilitated through videoconferencing interactions and also support more appropriate triage decisions [32–39] (Figs. 15.7 and 15.8).
3. Web-based second opinions

Asynchronous systems have also been applied for evaluation and management recommendations, as well as second opinions from experts in support of

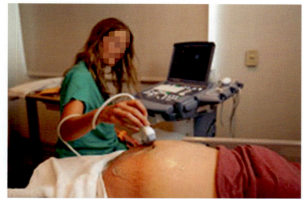
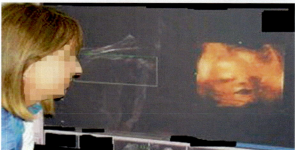

Fig. 15.7 Real-time teleconsultation for maternal-fetal medicine transmitting fetal ultrasound in real time

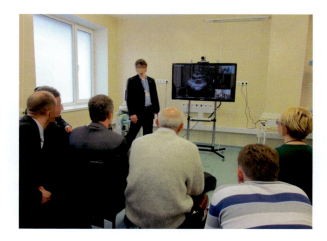

Fig. 15.8 Demonstrating real-time videoconferencing in Ukraine

primary care providers facing unusual or complex medical problems with which they may not have adequate knowledge or experience or simply desire reinforcement regarding their diagnosis or management approach. As noted earlier, Web-based programs, such as the Swinfen Charitable Trust (SCT) [6] and Doctors Without Borders (MSF) [7], use this type of platform for locations round the world, particularly in low- and middle-income countries and where connectivity may be limited. Primary care providers can transmit patient information and even images to assist the expert consultants to assess the patient and make diagnostic and management recommendations in context with the capabilities available locally (Figs. 15.9 and 15.10).

4. mHealth, use of cell phones, and Internet of Medical Things:

The mobile cellular phone and associated communication networks are being applied in countries around the world [40–56]. A multitude of cellphone applications have been developed to build upon these cellular phone networks. In some countries this may be the most effective communication network for telehealth or certainly complimentary to other broadband options.

5. Store and forward

Capturing images, storing them, and forwarding to an appropriate expert for evaluation also can play an important role and may be the best option when real-time interaction may not be necessary and improve efficiency in timely evaluation. This can be particularly useful in bandwidth limited environments. Applications for store and forward have included (1) radiology for evaluation of

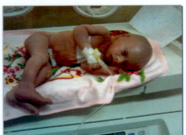
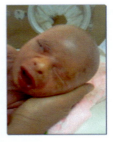

Fig. 15.9 Swinfen Charitable Trust expert consultation Web site

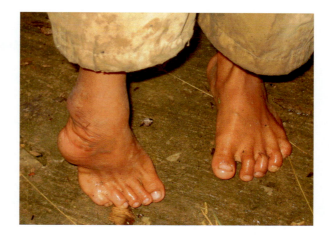

Fig. 15.10 Specialty consultations are possible via telemedicine such as evaluation of this child with a club foot

radiologic images, such as X-rays, CT scans, MRI, mammography, or ultrasound, (2) pathology and evaluation of macro- and microscopic specimen images, (3) dermatology for evaluation of skin abnormalities such as rashes or possible skin cancers such as melanoma, and (4) retinal images in the evaluation of potential diabetic retinopathy or retinopathy of prematurity. These approaches have provided more timely and effective evaluation leading to earlier diagnosis and subsequent appropriate intervention without which delays in consultation and evaluation may be significantly long [57, 58].

6. Remote patient monitoring

    Remote patient monitoring (RPM) is playing a more important role in monitoring and surveillance of individual patient medical data to provide improved detection of abnormalities and better continuity of care. An increasing array of wearable devices provides the means to capture that data and transmit to other providers for evaluation and response when necessary. Creating systems for pattern recognition and appropriate thresholds for detection of abnormalities also can assist in more effective screening and involve healthcare professionals only when needed for evaluation and intervention and thus lessen the burden of data overload [59, 60].

Steps in Planning and Implementing an International Telehealth Program

There are several steps in planning and implementing a telehealth program in specific countries and effective integration into their health system:

1. Identifying a collaborative partner or partners within the country
2. Performing a needs assessment and identifying gaps that can be addressed through telehealth

3. Assessment of existing conditions
4. Determining workforce needs
5. Integration into workflow
6. Technical plans
7. Documentation and integration into health information systems
8. Addressing legal and regulatory issues
9. Development of a business and sustainability plan
10. Determine the metrics and measures that demonstrate the impact of telehealth and return on investment (ROI)
11. Development of a continued quality improvement (CQI) plan

These steps are critical in the successful implementation and maintenance of a telehealth program within a country and between countries. This outline can be used as a checklist when developing a collaborative international telehealth program with other countries and is similar to previously published guideline for humanitarian international telehealth program development [61].

1. *Finding a collaborative partner(s) from the country with which you plan to work*

   Each country is unique, and a collaborative partner or partners from the country with which one is working should be identified since they would know the culture, health and wellness perspectives, the existing healthcare system, and political infrastructure necessary to effectively integrate telehealth into the country's healthcare delivery system. This partner can facilitate interaction with appropriate authorities and existing government agencies and leadership, such as the ministry of health, the ministry of foreign affairs, interested academic centers and universities, and other stakeholders ensuring appropriate integration in current and longer-term strategic plans for ongoing development of the country's healthcare system (Fig. 15.11).

2. *Needs assessment and identifying gaps that can be addressed through telehealth*

   A systematic assessment and determination of the priority healthcare needs and identification of gaps in care within the country are critical in the appropriate application of the tools of telehealth that can be effectively addressed. Often the ministry of health has data on specific causes of mortality and morbidity in the population and assists in prioritizing the targets for using telehealth. In many countries, their aging population and associated noncommunicable chronic diseases, such as diabetes, chronic heart failure, chronic obstructive pulmonary disease, asthma, cancer, psychiatric disorders, and dementia, become existing challenges that can be addressed via telehealth and enhance access to care. Other issues include enhancing maternal and children's services [3] that improve the outcomes of pregnancy, including improved approaches to managing delivery and maternal emergencies through sharing knowledge and appropriate treatment that can be realistically applied within a specific country and newborn resuscitation, with education and training programs such as Helping Babies Breathe/Helping Babies Survive [62]. In countries such as Nigeria, seven hundred newborn babies die per day. Basic resuscitation techniques can be taught and applied that can significantly improve survival.

15 International and Global Telemedicine: Making It Work

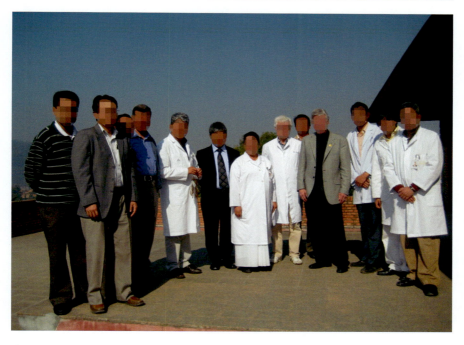

Fig. 15.11 Kathmandu University School of Medicine international collaborative team

3. *Existing conditions assessment*
   (a) Health system capabilities
       It is important to determine the existing healthcare and information technology and communication workforce that is available to support the telehealth program and technologies. Without an adequate workforce, the telehealth program cannot be implemented and used effectively. If there are identified gaps, a plan for training the needed workforce should be developed and could be approached through collaborative relationships with other countries with the training and care skills required as noted in the workforce planning, #4.
       Also, there should be an understanding of the use of traditional healers and healing practices in each country and how they can be incorporated and made complimentary to conventional medical practice. Traditional medicine has usually been accessed for hundreds of years and utilized by many in the population. An example of successful integration of traditional and conventional medicine is demonstrated in clinics such as "La Clinica Alternativa" in Otovalo, Ecuador, and proves to be widely accepted by the community for accessing healthcare (Figs. 15.12 and 15.13).
       This should be recognized when applying telehealth in a specific country. Furthermore, it is important to realize that "one size doesn't fit all" and there is a need for flexibility in defining and addressing healthcare needs [63].

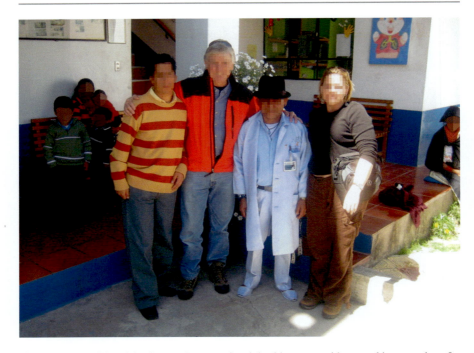

Fig. 15.12 Traditional healers and conventional healthcare providers working together: La Clinica Alternativa in Otovalo, Ecuador

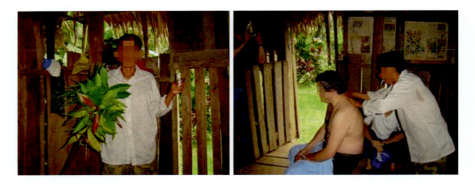

Fig. 15.13 Traditional healers in the jungles of Ecuador and Peru

(b) Communication network options

A major challenge in implementing telehealth programs is having adequate communication networks or broadband that can support the technology and connect the providers and users of the telehealth application being considered. Investigation regarding the existing communication infrastructure and networks is also critical to determine the capacity to support the program

or needs for enhancement. Access to the Internet may be difficult or only intermittent. Options can be addressed in the technical planning.
  (c) Access to power for the devices being considered
    Another challenge is understanding access to power and electricity that exists to support the technologies being considered. Many countries may have only intermittent access to electricity, and in more remote rural communities, it is even more difficult and they rely upon generating electricity if connection to a power grid may not exist.
  (d) Other possible in-country telehealth programs and opportunities for collaboration
    It is common to find that there are other telehealth-related efforts within a country, and a careful survey is needed to determine what other programs are in place or being developed. This creates opportunities for collaboration, better coordination, complementary initiatives, and avoidance of unnecessary duplication of efforts
4. *Determine workforce needs: internal and external to that country*
    As noted in the existing conditions assessment, if gaps in the workforce are identified that would be required to support the telehealth program, a plan for filling those workforce needs should be developed through further training and educational efforts that could be supported through the telehealth program and possible filling of those gaps with medical expertise from other countries, particularly for gaps in specialty care. Using a collaborative approach, the need to transfer patients to other countries for evaluation and care or follow-up care after a procedure in another country could be avoided which offers better support for patients and their local healthcare providers and avoids expensive travel expenses, alleviating a burden on the country's healthcare system and costs.
    Additionally, telehealth platforms provide a system for e-consults and second opinions to determine the best options for evaluation and management of patients in the country, and that can be realistically applied considering the resources available. Ongoing training of the users becomes important in maintaining and sustaining the telehealth system and the technology being utilized.
5. *Integration into workflow*
    For telehealth to be effectively implemented and used, these systems need be integrated in the common and routine processes and procedures of the local and distant healthcare providers. This can include scheduling and registering patients for telehealth encounters that follow methods for in-person encounters. In addition, access to patient healthcare information and documentation of the encounter should be considered, including integration with any existing or planned electronic health record as noted in #7. The healthcare staff and providers need to be familiar with the telehealth system and determine how best to fit into their workflow.
6. *Technical plan*
  (a) Determine the most appropriate and affordable technology needed to support the telehealth applications. Consider a technology industry partner familiar with the spectrum of technologies that can be best applied to sup-

port a defined need and be integrated into the environment using these tools, including adequate trained individuals at both the consulting and patient/provider sites and adequate connectivity and electricity to support those tools. Whatever technology is implemented, appropriate and ongoing training in the use of the equipment or software is critical to ensure sustainability and address the anticipated turnover in personnel using the telehealth systems. Training and education in the use of the technologies being deployed as an ongoing effort that supports utilization address turnover and onboarding of new users.

(b) Determine communication networks needed to support the telehealth technologies and programs: cellular networks, satellite, microwave, and fiber and hybrid connections related to middle and last mile links from networks to the local or rural sites using the telehealth technologies being applied or considered. This communication infrastructure is critical in supporting the overall telehealth system and its usability.

(c) Determine scalability and potential expansion of sites and specific health applications. Many telehealth programs appropriately start with pilot applications to determine the feasibility of using the technologies to address a specific health issue. Thus, changes can be made as needed and provide the data to demonstrate the effectiveness of the telehealth application. When successful, these pilots can serve as a model for expansion of the program to other sites or for addressing other health needs.

7. *Documentation and integration with possible health information platforms*

An electronic health record (EHR) and a system for health information exchange (HIE) to provide interoperability across different EHRs may need to be considered if they exist. Often, in many countries, documentation is still done in writing, and methods of accomplishing this, when telehealth is used, should be determined. However, more countries are planning or implementing EHRs or HIEs, and this can be addressed and planned for integration into the telehealth program being developed.

8. *Address medical-legal and regulatory policies, procedures, and requirements: licensure, credentialing, and malpractice insurance*

Each country may have unique regulatory and legal requirements for providing telehealth services, particularly when services are bring provided by out-of-country healthcare providers. It is mandatory that those requirements be appropriately addressed. This may include appropriate licensing, credentialing, and privileging of healthcare professionals providing care via telehealth. It is also prudent for telemedicine that healthcare providers have adequate malpractice insurance and risk management systems that cover them in the event of an untoward patient outcome.

9. *Develop a business plan that considers sustainability*

The resources required for maintaining and expanding the telehealth system and its health applications should be developed. Often humanitarian efforts are initially used to support a telehealth application or pilot project. Some vendors may initially offer technology for a project. However, a business plan to sustain or enhance the program should be developed. Options may include ongoing support through the country's social security health system or other subsidies. Other options may include ongoing support from humanitarian organizations. Billing and reimbursement for the services may be possible, as well as specific contracts between government or academic institutions for receiving or providing telehealth services. Although grants can be a useful catalyst to initiate a telehealth program, without a business plan for sustainability, programs cannot be maintained after the grant is completed.

10. *Determine the metrics and measures that demonstrate the impact of the telehealth program*

    It is important to determine the metrics and measures that demonstrate the impact of the telehealth program and return on investment (ROI). Those measures can include improvement in the patient's and provider's experience, improvement in healthcare outcomes for patients and populations being served, and cost savings or avoidance through the use of telehealth.

    The National Quality Forum (NQF) outlined the guidelines for evaluation and the domains that should be addressed [64].

    The World Health Organization (WHO) has also outlined Sustainable Development Goals (SDGs) [14]. Many of these can be addressed and telehealth applied to assist in meeting those goals. Appropriate data, collection, and analysis can be extremely useful in demonstrating the effects of a telehealth program and ROI that also supports the importance of sustaining or expanding the telehealth program. Collaborative research and evaluation can also involve exchange of faculty, healthcare providers, and students (Figs. 15.14 and 15.15).

11. *Develop a continued quality improvement (CQI) plan*

    The ongoing evaluation to ensure possible enhancements in the telehealth program and technologies used requires an ongoing effort. Identifying problems and need for improvement is important to ensure the quality of the program. Additionally, new and improved technologies and software can be anticipated and should be applied as appropriate. Future advances in health information systems and use of artificial intelligence are likely to play an important role in enhancing healthcare diagnosis and management and should be incorporated in future telehealth programs.

    These steps as outlined are critical in planning, implementing a sustainable international telehealth program, and making it work. Although many healthcare issues are common across the international community, each individual country's healthcare needs, cultural perspectives, and systems for delivery are often unique. Those components should be addressed when developing a telehealth program for each country [65–71]. When integrated successfully, telehealth can enhance the quality of life and health of people around the world.

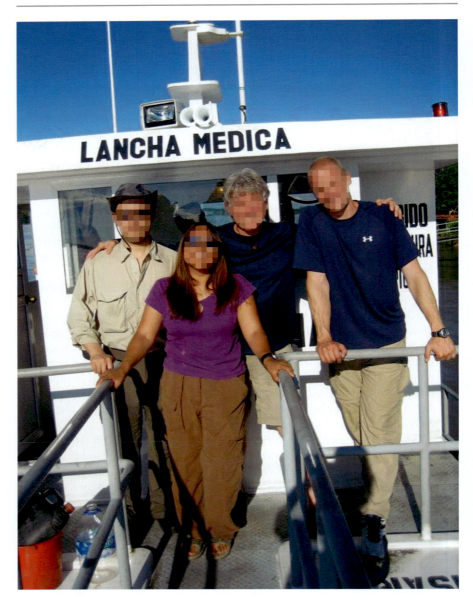

Fig. 15.14 Exchange of students

15 International and Global Telemedicine: Making It Work

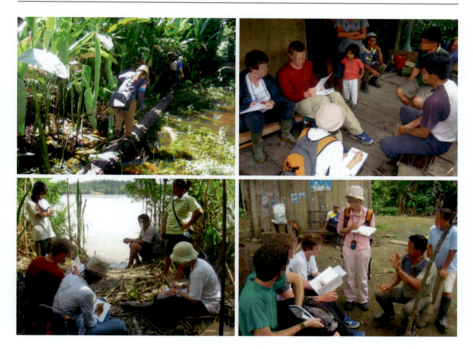

Fig. 15.15 Students conducting research in the jungles of Ecuador

References

1. Wootton R, Patil NG, Scott RE, Ho K, editors. Telehealth in the developing world. London: Royal Society of Medicine Press and Ottawa: International Development Research Center; 2009.
2. Mills A. Health Care Systems in low- and Middle-Income Countries. N Engl J Med. 2014;370(6):552–7.
3. Alverson DC, Mars M, Rheuban K, Sable C, Smith A, Swinfen P, Swinfen R. International pediatric telemedicine and eHealth: transforming systems of care for children in the global community. Pediatr Ann. 2009;38(10):579–85.
4. International Society for Telemedicine and eHealth (ISfTeH): https://www.isfteh.org/, verified November 9, 2019.
5. American Telemedicine Association (ATA) and it's international Chapters (https://www.americantelemed.org/), verified November 9, 2019.
6. Swinfen Charitable Trust (SCT):http://swinfencharitabletrust.org/, verified November 9, 2019.
7. Doctors without Borders or Medecins Sans Frontieres (MSF): https://www.doctorswithoutborders.org/, verified November 9, 2019.
8. Asociacion Iberoamericana de Telesalud y Telemedicina (AITT) http://teleiberoamerica.com/index.html, verified November 9, 2019.
9. Night Hawk Radiology: https://www.nighthawkradiology.com/, verified November 9, 2019.
10. Emory International Critical Care program: http://www.news.emory.edu/stories/2018/05/buchman-hiddleson_eicu_perth_australia/index.html, verified November 9, 2019.

11. World Health Organization. Health-for-all policy for the twenty first century (Document EB101/INF. DOC./9). Geneva: WHO; 1998.
12. World Health Organization. WHA58.28 e-health. Geneva: WHO; 2005.
13. World Health Organization. Strategy 2004–2007. E-health for health care delivery. Geneva: WHO; 2004.
14. WHO Sustainable Development Goalshttps://sustainabledevelopment.un.org/sdgs, verified November 9, 2019
15. United Nations. Millennium Development Goals. Available at www.un.org/millenniumgoals/, verified November 9, 2019
16. Simmons S, Alverson DC, Poropatich R, D'Iorio J, DeVany M, Doarn CR. Applying telehealth in natural and anthropogenic disasters. Telemed e-Health. 2008;14(9):968–71.
17. Alverson DC, Edison K, Flournoy L, Korte B, Magruder C, Miller C. Telehealth tools for public health, emergency or disaster preparedness and response: a summary report. Telemed eHealth. 2010;16:112–4.
18. Arora S, Kalishman S, et al. Expanding access to hepatitis C virus treatment—Extension for Community Healthcare Outcomes (ECHO) project: disruptive innovation in specialty care. Hepatology. 2010;52(3):1124–33.
19. Arora S, Kalishman S, et al. Outcomes of treatment for hepatitis C virus infection by primary care providers. N Engl J Med. 2011;364(23):2199–207.
20. Arora S, et al. Academic health center management of chronic diseases through knowledge networks: project ECHO. Acad med. 2007;82:2.
21. Arora S, Thornton K, Jenkusky SM, Parish B, Scaletti JV. Project ECHO: linking university specialists with rural and prison-based clinicians to improve care for people with chronic hepatitis C in New Mexico. Public Health Rep. 2007;122(2):74–7.
22. Arora S, et al. Partnering urban academic medical centers and rural primary care clinicians to provide complex chronic disease care. Health Aff. 2011;30(6):1176–84.
23. Arora S, Kalishman S, Dion D, Thornton K, Murata G, Fassler C, et al. Knowledge networks for treating complex diseases in remote, rural, and underserved communities. In: Learning trajectories, innovation and identity for professional development. Cham: Springer; 2012. p. 47–70.
24. Child Ready Program: https://emed.unm.edu/pem/programs/child-ready-program/index.html, verified November 9, 2019.
25. Mowafi MY, Summers KL, Holten J, Greenfield JA, Sherstyuk A, Nickles D, Aalseth E, Takamiya W, Saiki S, Alverson D, Caudell TP. Distributed interactive virtual environments for collaborative medical education and training: Design and characterization. Stud Health Technol Inform. 2004;98:259–61.
26. Alverson DC, Saiki SM, Jacobs J, Saland L, Keep MF, Norenberg J, Baker R, Nakatsu C, Kalishman S, Lindberg M, Wax D, Mowafi M, Summers KL, Holten JIV, Greenfield J, Aalseth E, Nickles D, Sherstyuk A, Haines K, Caudell TP. Distributed interactive virtual environments for collaborative experiential learning and training independent of distance over Internet2. Stud Health Technol Inform. 2004;98:7–12.
27. Alverson DC, Saiki SM, Caudell TP. Telehealth in cyberspace-virtual reality for distance learning in health education & training, Chap. 24. In: Whitten P, Cook D, Jossey-Bass A, editors. Understanding health communication technologies: a case book approach. San Francisco: Wiley; 2004.
28. Alverson DC, Caudell TP, Goldsmith TE. Creating virtual reality medical simulations: a knowledge-based design and assessment approach, Chap. 31. In: Riley R, editor. Manual of Simulation in Healthcare. Oxford: Oxford University Press; 2008. p. 449–64.
29. Pierce J, Gutierrez F, Vergara V, Alverson DC, Qualls C, Saland L, Goldsmith T, Caudell TP. Comparative usability studies of full vs. partial immersive virtual reality simulation for medical education and training. Stud Health Technol Inform. 2008;132:372–7.
30. Alverson DC, Saiki SM Jr, Kalishman S, Lindberg M, Mennin S, Mines J, Serna L, Summers K, Jacobs J, Lozanoff S, Lozanoff B, Saland L, Mitchell S, Umland B, Greene G, Buchanan

HS, Keep M, Wilks D, Wax DS, Coulter R, Goldsmith TE, Caudell TP. Medical students learn over distance using virtual reality simulation. Sim Healthcare. 2008;3:10–5.
31. Alverson DC, Caudell TP, Goldsmith TE. Creating Virtual Reality Medical Simulations: A Knowledge-based Design and Assessment Approach, Chap. 30. In: Riley R, editor. Manual of simulation in healthcare. Oxford: Oxford University Press; 2016. p. 411–23.
32. Sable C, Roca T, Gold J, Gutierrez A, Gulotta E, Culpepper W. Live transmission of neonatal echocardiograms from underserved areas: accuracy, patient care, and cost. Telemed J. 1999;5:339–47.
33. Sable C. Telemedicine applications in pediatric cardiology. Minerva Pediatr. 2003;55:1–13.
34. Pearl PL, Sable C, Evans S, Knight K, Cunningham P, Lotrecchiano GR, Gropman A, Stuart S, Glass P, Anne Conway A, Ramadan I, Paiva T, Batshaw ML, Packer RJ. International telemedicine consultations for neurodevelopmental disabilities. Telemed e-Health. 2014;20(6):559–62.
35. Augusterfer EF, Mollica RF, Lavelle J. A review of telemental health in international and post-disaster settings. Int Rev Psychiatry. 2015;27(6):540–6. https://doi.org/10.3109/09540261.2015.1082985.
36. Jefee-Bahloul H, Moustafa MK, Shebl FM, Barkil-Oteo A. Pilot assessment and survey of Syrian refugees' psychological stress and openness to referral for telepsychiatry (PASSPORT Study). Telemed J E Health. 2014;20(10):977–9. https://doi.org/10.1089/tmj.2013.0373.
37. Branagan L, Chase LL.Organizational Implementation of Telemedicine Technology; Methodology and Field Experience. In 2012 IEEE Global Humanitarian Technology Conference. Seattle, Washington USA; 2012. p. 271–276.
38. Hidalgo R, Alverson DC, Cartagenova G, Maldonado L. Development of a Collaborative Telehealth Network in Ecuador: Programa Nacional de Telemedicina. American Telemedicine Association National Annual Meeting, Seattle, WA, April 6–9, 2008. Telemed e-Health. 2008;14(supp1):51.
39. Hopkins KS, Alverson DC, Hidalgo RO, Cartagenova G, Johnson-Moser S. Integrating cross-cultural indigenous and western healing with modern technology update. American Telemedicine Association National Annual Meeting, Seattle, WA, April 6–9, 2008. Telemed e-Health. 2008;14(Supp 1):52–3.
40. Akter S, Ray P. mHealth – an ultimate platform to serve the unserved. IMIA yearbook of medical informatics. 2010. p. 75–81, file:///C:/Users/Dale/AppData/Local/Packages/Microsoft.MicrosoftEdge_8wekyb3d8bbwe/TempState/Downloads/mHealth_An_Ultimate_Platform_to_Serve_th%20(3).pdf, verified November 16, 2019.
41. Diez-Canseco F, Zavala-Loayza JA, Beratarrechea A, Kanter R, Ramirez-Zea M, Rubinstein A, Martinez H, Miranda JJ. Design and multi-country validation of text messages for an mHealth intervention for primary prevention of progression to hypertension in Latin America. JMIR mHealth uHealth. 2015;3(1):e19.
42. Iribarren SJ, Sward A, Beck L, Thurston D, Chirico C. Qualitative evaluation of a text messaging intervention to support patients with active tuberculosis: implementation considerations. JMIR Mhealth Uhealth. 2015;3(1):e21.
43. Nhavoto JA, Grönlund A. Mobile technologies and geographic information systems to improve health care systems: a literature review. JMIR Mhealth Uhealth. 2014;2(2):e21.
44. Moghaddasi H, Amanzadeh M, Rahimi F, Hamedan M. (Iran). Ehealth equity: current perspectives. J Int Soc Telemed eHealth. 2017;5:e9.
45. Oliver-Williams C, Brown E, Devereux S, Fairhead C, Holeman I. Using Mobile phones to improve vaccination uptake in 21 lowand middle-income countries: systematic review. JMIR Mhealth Uhealth. 2017;5(10):e148.
46. Burney A, Abbas Z, Mahmood N, Q-ul A. (Pakistan). Prospects for Mobile health in Pakistan and other developing countries. Adv Internet Things. 2013;3:27–32. https://doi.org/10.4236/ait.2013.32A004.
47. Wootton R, Patil NG, Scott RE, Ho K. Tele-health in the developing world. London: Royal Society of Medicine Press, IDRC; 2009. ISBN 978-1-85315-784.

48. mHealth New horizons for health through mobile technologies: based on the findings of the second global survey on eHealth, Global Observatory for eHealth series – Vol. 3. WHO; 2011.
49. Pan American Health Organization. eHealth in the Region of the Americas: breaking down the barriers to implementation. Results of the World Health Organization's Third Global Survey on eHealth. Washington: PAHO; 2016.
50. Global diffusion of eHealth: making universal health coverage achievable. Report of the third global survey on eHealth. WHO 2016 technologies (ICTs) in support of health services in both developed and developing countries since the early 2000s.
51. WHO library cataloguing-in-publication data management of patient information: trends and challenges in Member States: based on the findings of the second global survey on eHealth. Global Observatory for eHealth Series, 6.
52. Randhawa G, Singh S. Telemedicine: integrating ICT and health care system. Dias Technol Rev. 2018;14(2)
53. Telemedicine: opportunities and developments in member states: report on the second global survey on eHealth 2009. WHO 2009
54. Ghani MKA, Mostafa SA, Mustapha A, Aman H, Mohamed MA, Jaber MM. Investigating telemedicine approaches: a 10-country comparison. Int J Eng Technol. 2018;7(3.20):451–60.
55. Internet of Medical Things (IOMT). https://www.mindinventory.com/blog/internet-of-medical-things-will-change-face-of-healthcare/, verified November 13, 2019.
56. mHealth in developing countries file:///C:/Users/Dale/AppData/Local/Packages/Microsoft.MicrosoftEdge_8wekyb3d8bbwe/TempState/Downloads/Strengthening_health_systems_in_mHealth%20(1).pdf, verified November 14, 2019.
57. Store and Forward Asynchronous Telehealth. https://www.cchpca.org/about/about-telehealth/store-and-forward-asynchronous, verified November 13, 2019.
58. Store and Forward. https://www.telehealth.org.nz/what-is-telehealth/store-and-forward/, verified November 13, 2109.
59. Remote Patient Monitoring. https://www.cchpca.org/about/about-telehealth/remote-patient-monitoring-rpm, verified November 13, 2019.
60. Remote Patient Monitoring. https://searchhealthit.techtarget.com/definition/remote-patient-monitoring-RPM, verified November 13, 2019,
61. Alverson DC. The role of telehealth in international humanitarian outreach in understanding telehealth. In: Rheuban KS, Krupinski EA, editors. Chap. 20. McGraw Hill Education; 2017. p. 251–266.
62. Helping Babies Breathe/Helping Babies Survive. https://www.aap.org/en-us/advocacy-and-policy/aap-health-initiatives/helping-babies-survive/Pages/Helping-Babies-Breathe.aspx, verified November 14, 2019.
63. Alverson DC, Holtz B, D'Iorio J, DeVany M, Simmons S, Poropatich R. One size Doesn't fit all; bringing Telehealth services to special populations. Telemed e-Health. 2008;14(9):957–63.
64. Creating a framework to support measure development for telehealth, NQF report. 2107. http://www.qualityforum.org/Publications/2017/08/Creating_a_Framework_to_Support_Measure_Development_for_Telehealth.aspx, verified November 13, 2019.
65. Bashur RL, Shannon GW. History of telemedicine: evolution, context, and transformation. New Rochelle: Mary Anne Liebert; 2009.
66. Wootton R, Craig J, Patterson V. Introduction to telemedicine. 2nd ed. Boston: Rittenhouse Book Distributors; 2006.
67. Achieving the millennium development goals in Africa. Recommendations of the MDG Africa Steering Group. 2008. http://www.mdgafrica.org/pdf/MDG%20Africa%20Steering%20Group%20Recommendations%20-%20English%20-%20LowRes.pdf. Accessed 4 July 2009.
68. United nations department of economic and social affairs, population division. World population prospects: the 2008 revision, highlights, working paper no. ESA/P/WP.210. 2009; 1–109.

69. Asturias EJ, Heinrichs G, Domek G, Brett J, Shick E, Cunningham M, Bull S, Celada M, Newman LS, Tenney L, Krisher L, Luna-Asturias C, McConnell K, Berman S. The Center for Human Development in Guatemala: an innovative model for global population health. Adv Pediatr. 2016;63:357–87.
70. Wootton R. Telemedicine support in the developing world. J Telemed Telecare. 2008;14:109–14.
71. DeVany M, Alverson D, D'Iorio J, Simmons S. Employing telehealth to enhance overall quality of life and health for families. Telemed e-Health. 2008;14(9):1003–7.

Technological Advances Making Telemedicine and Telepresence Possible

16

Charles R. Doarn

Historical Context

Technology has always played a role in healthcare. From antiquity to the present time, humans have interacted with one another through a variety of communication modalities to address healthcare needs. From cave paintings to smoke signals to papyrus to books to text messaging, we have adapted tools, technologies, and processes to meet our needs and to effectively understand and manage our health. Today of course, innovation has taken society to a whole new level. We communicate across the globe instantaneously. We watch movies on our smartphones or even our smart watches. We can add small devices to our smartphones that can make them medical devices such as spirometer or a mini microscope. The list goes on and on.

These advancements have been brought on by the technological revolution of the twentieth century and the early twenty-first century. Up until the time of Laennec (ca 1816) and Semmelweis (ca 1846), the concepts of medical care were much different than today. While not "Dark Ages"-like, there were still many unknowns in medicine at the time. No one really understood the etiology of disease or what bacteria or virus was. Medical education was not structured as it is today. Those who did practice medicine did so as gentlemen and were considered the individual who might have all the answers. They developed "standards of care," which were to be adhered to by all who called themselves physician. Figure 16.1 illustrates a nineteenth-century physician making house calls. The patient looks to the traveling physician with anticipation that he may perhaps help her alleviate her malady.

Standards of care began to be questioned in the early part of the nineteenth century. In 1816, a "standard of care" was for the physician to lay his head upon the

C. R. Doarn (✉)
Department of Environmental and Public Health Sciences, College of Medicine, University of Cincinnati, Cincinnati, OH, USA
e-mail: charles.doarn@uc.edu

© Springer Nature Switzerland AG 2021
R. Latifi et al. (eds.), *Telemedicine, Telehealth and Telepresence*,
https://doi.org/10.1007/978-3-030-56917-4_16

Fig. 16.1 Nineteenth-century physician making a house call

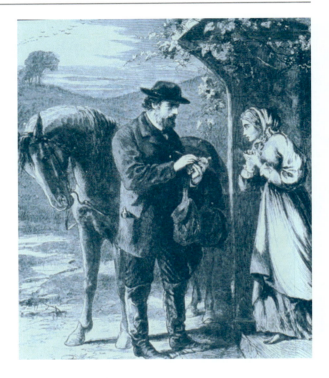

patient's chest to hear heart and lung sounds. The first female patient to refuse this procedure led her physician, Rene Theophile-Hyacinthe Laennec, to develop the monaural stethoscope [1]. It took nearly 100 years for the stethoscope to become commonplace in clinical practice.

A second vignette is one of handwashing and puerperal fever. Ignaz Semmelweis, a physician in Vienna, observed a significant number of maternal deaths after childbirth. Unbeknownst to him, his patients were being infected by bacteria being transferred from cadaveric remains. He was employed as physician at a teaching institution and went directly from the teaching anatomy lab to the delivery room without washing his hands. The midwives of Vienna did not have the same level of mortality due to this crucial step of handwashing. Semmelweis instituted handwashing in his hospital with soap and chlorine, and while he saw a decrease in patient death, his colleagues thought he was not stable – this was not the "standard of care" [2]. A physician colleague, Charles Meigs, even quipped "gentleman did not have dirty hands." Semmelweis was pushed out, eventually institutionalized, and died of sepsis. His idea of handwashing took several years to become standard practice.

In the late nineteenth century, there were those who thought everything that needed to be invented had already been invented and there was not much room for improvement. In fact, Heinrich Rudolf Hertz (Fig. 16.2), a German physicist, proved that electromagnetic waves existed but was not exactly sure of their utility. Hertz's experiments proved James Clerk Maxwell's theory about electromagnetic waves.

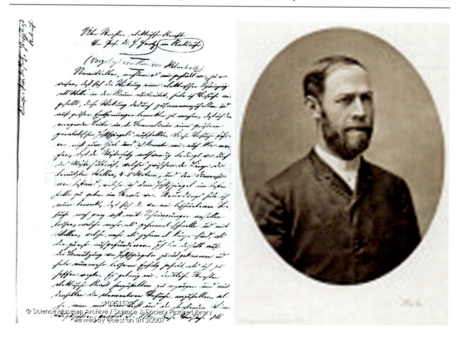

Fig. 16.2 Letter stating his concerns on his discovery, and photograph of Heinz Hertz

Hertz posited the following in 1880 "I do not think the wireless waves that I have discovered will have any practical application." We obviously use this concept every day in almost everything we do.

In 1901, Georg Kelling of Dresden, Germany, developed and tested what has become known as laparoscopy [3, 4]. But the wide adoption of it in surgical practice took nearly 90 years to become commonplace. Minimally invasive surgery took off in the mid-1990s, and that led to the development of robotic-assisted surgery with Computer Motion (Zeus) and Intuitive Surgical (da Vinci). Telemanipulation in surgery was even thought of in the 1920s (see Fig. 16.3).

While technology development rapidly increased during the post-World War II era and the ensuing Space Race and Cold War, teaching in medical schools was also changing, although perhaps not as fast [5]. William Osler, a founding physician of Johns Hopkins Hospital, worked in the early twentieth century to lead medicine into a new paradigm in education, training, and clinical practice [6].

Over the course of the nineteenth and twentieth century, innovation in computing power, image acquisition, photography, communications, informatics, and data storage has changed all of human life. These tools are critical in bringing the nineteenth-century physician to the twenty-first-century patient through seamless technologies. Telemedicine and telepresence are two disciplines that have benefited from this un-seemingly endless growth in technology and innovation.

By introducing telemedicine, telehealth, e-health, m-health, robotics, artificial intelligence (AI), etc. into public health practice and public health education,

Fig. 16.3 Cover of *Science and Invention* illustrates a physician and nurse with a distal patient (ca 1925)

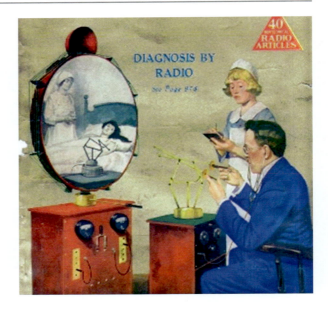

society and the healthcare systems have benefited. Bernhardt discusses the vital importance of science and communications in public health in his 2004 manuscript entitled "Communication at the Core of Effective Public Health" [7]. He goes on to state that Healthy People 2010 defined health communication as "…the art and technique of informing, influencing, and motivating individual, institutional, and public audiences about important health issue" [8].

Development of Telemedicine and Telepresence

Throughout history, the patient and physician or healthcare provider have not always been in the same place. Figure 16.4 is the front cover of technology-based publication from 1924. This photo captures the essences of healthcare delivery at a distance. What is interesting in this photo is that the fax machine on the right was invented in 1971 and the television (center) in 1939. "Maybe" is absolutely correct, as we do this all the time today.

Telemedicine of course did not really become a "thing" until the late 1950s into the 1960s. At the time, there were several government-funded initiatives with academia and of course the human spaceflight programs of the United States (US) and the Union of Soviet Socialist Republics (USSR). From a technological push, these two programs really drove the development of telemedicine, which was used to support humans in space and on the transit to the moon and back as well as monitor the astronauts during surface operations on the Moon [9]. Telemedicine has also been

Fig. 16.4 Cover of the 1924 issue of *Radio News*

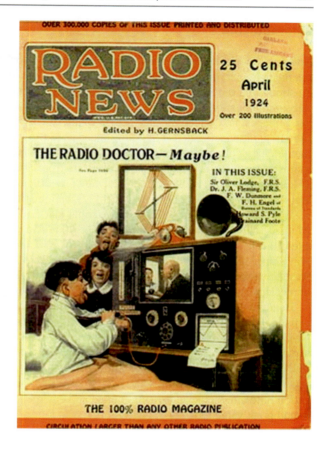

used in the military [10] and, as Bashshur et al. reports, in chronic diseases among almost every clinical practice [11–13].

The ability to operate a device wirelessly involves the concept of telepresence. This has evolved into a very useful tool in many other applications, including underwater operations, surgery, and unmanned aerial vehicles (UAVs) – also known as drones.

The development of much of this capability was done so in support of a need. Today, innovation less from government-funded initiatives and more from new startups, industry investment, and philanthropy play a much bigger role – consider SpaceX, Google, Microsoft, and Amazon, although, investment in technology remains at very high levels as evidenced by the continuous introduction of new technologies. Imagine your packages or pizza being delivered to your home by a drone!

Telemedicine

Some will posit that telemedicine has been around a long time. However, initially, telemedicine or the concept was applied in earnest with radio waves between Australia and the Antarctic in the mid-1920s and over these past 100 years or so; telecommunications and information systems have greatly enhanced our ability to send images, text, video, or data sets in many instances across great distance with little trepidation and often at lightning speed [14]. But it was not until the mid-1950s that telemedicine was applied in psychiatric cases in Nebraska [15], the space programs of the USA and USSR [9], in disasters from1985 until the present time [16, 17], in the operating room and surgical care [18–20], and from extreme and remote areas including alpine [21], high desert [22], and jungles [23, 24].

While there are thousands of manuscripts that have been published in the last 25 years, they cannot all be listed here. There are two premier specialty journals on telemedicine – the *Telemedicine and e-Health Journal*, published by Mary Ann Liebert Publishing, and the *Journal of Telemedicine and Telecare*, published by the Royal Academy Press. In addition, now that telemedicine and telehealth are in the mainstream of medicine, there are scientific papers in a wide variety of specialty clinical journals.

Beginning in the early 1990s, federal funding for telemedicine really began to expand through grant-funded research and technology development, driven in large part by new capabilities offered by the Internet, the World Wide Web, and computing power. Today, we can send a full CT scan across a 5G network in seconds. An individual, buried in the rubble of a collapsed building, can text their location, aiding first responders in their rescue. And as Latifi et al. have demonstrated, the application of telemedicine addressing trauma and emergency medicine has been shown to add great value [25–27].

Mobile Health

As smartphones have become widespread, they have also become powerful and extremely useful tools in not only our everyday lives but in how we manage our health. There are apps for almost everything. In healthcare, the future of medicine may be the smartphone. This was reported by Foster et al. in 2017 [28]. Of course the actual evidence is not quite there but the utility is certainly on the rise. A search of the term "smartphone apps in medicine" yielded 759 results which ranges in scope from mental health, cancer, pain management, menstruation tracking, to diabetes, to name a few.

The point is that each generation of smartphone that is made available to the consumer has more capabilities with concomitant increases in utility, utilization, and reliability – that is just since 2007. However, studies have shown that while utilization has increased, there is still little understanding of the motivating factors that foster sustainability [29].

Sensors

The human body has a vast array of sensing capabilities. Over the years, we have developed a wide variety of sensors that can detect a vast array of things, each helping us in some way. My favorite is the lane assist sensor on new cars – the one that tells you there is a car in the lane next to you. Today, sensors can be embedded in nearly everything we do. They are in our phones and appliances. They can be in our domicile telling us that there is too much carbon monoxide or carbon dioxide in the air. Many sensors can be integrated into the smartphone that can track our steps, monitor our blood sugar, and monitor our respiratory volume, gait, tremors, etc. While there are multiple examples, the work by Hsu et al. discusses wearable sensors in poststroke patients [30]. There is literally no limit to what can be sensed. Wearable devices and the Internet of Things have been integrated into telemedicine and telehealth, and this will further "digitize" medicine and healthcare [31, 32].

Robotics

The inset figure (Fig. 16.5) is rather far-fetched but is illustrative of where technology is pushing us. Manufacturing has used robotic systems for several decades now, but in medicine, the adoption has been a little slower. Robotics has been integrated into healthcare and in the surgical care. There are several companies that have developed robotic-assisted devices, and while they are mostly operated by humans, there are some that are sort of on their own. The Rumba comes to mind.

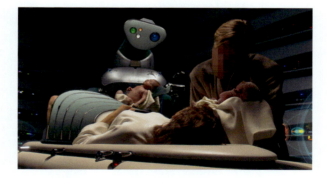

Fig. 16.5 A robotic labor and delivery physician (Star Wars)

In Healthcare

In the early 2000s, several companies developed remotely controlled devices that could be driven from one patient room to another (Fig. 16.6). These have been successfully deployed in military hospitals, hospitals, and nursing facilities. These

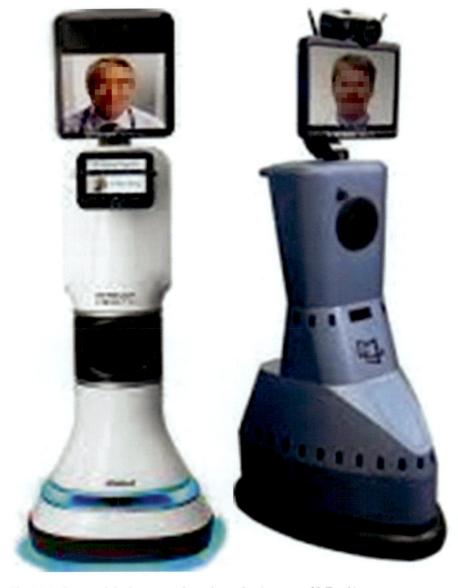

Fig. 16.6 Commercial robots currently on the market (courtesy of InTouch)

systems can check on the status of patients with the provider linked via a video teleconferencing system that permits the physician to remain at his/her location and monitor patients at a distant site [33].

Robotics in the Operating Room

During the 1990s, two companies battled for supremacy in surgical robotics that would support minimally invasive surgical procedures. Both company's foundations were based on technologies developed in part which were Computer Motion's "Zeus platform" and Intuitive Surgical's "da Vinci platform" [34].

The operating room as seen in Fig. 16.7 has changed significantly because of technology. First, there is electricity, and second, the windows do not open. Telemedicine has also found its way into the operating room [18]. AI and robotics have been integrated into the operating room for both surgical care and surgical education [35, 36].

Furthermore, Jell et al. report that as the new 5G cellular network roles out, it may be a significant adjunct to both telemedicine, telepresence, and of course surgery, minimizing latency and improving performance for command and control of imagery and clinical efforts [37].

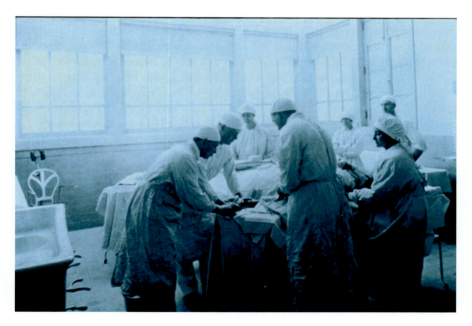

Fig. 16.7 Operating theater in the late nineteenth century

World Wide Web

We can only imagine how painful life might be today without the utility of the World Wide Web. The Web and all the associated capabilities provide enormous benefits and, as with any other technology, challenges. In1960, Joseph Licklider's paper, entitled "Man-Computer Symbiosis," wrote "....augment human intellect by freeing it from mundane tasks...." [38]. He discussed at great length the symbiotic relationship between humans and machines that perhaps might improve human thinking, including problem-solving. Several years later, he coauthored a paper with Welden Clark, entitled "On-Line Man Computer Communication," in which they describe a networked future [39].

These early concepts set the stage for the Advanced Research Projects Agency (ARPA) to develop ARPA net (ARPANET) in the late 1960s. ARPANET was created to permit multiple computers to communicate with a single network. In the 1970s, Transmission Control Protocol/Internet Protocol (TCP/IP) was developed by Robert E. Kahn and Vinton Cerf as a communication model for data transmission between multiple networks. Over the next two decades, a wide variety of government and commercial entities developed networks for scientist to share information.

Tim Berners-Lee, a British computer scientist, is credited with inventing the World Wide Web. In 1990, working at CERN in Switzerland, he developed the first Web browser – World Wide Web – later named Nexus. Berners-Lee's work led to the development of Mosaic – later known as Netscape at the National Center for Supercomputing Applications at the University of Illinois, Champaign). Today, of course we are all familiar with several well-known browsers on our computers and phones. This year (2020) marks the 30th anniversary of Berners-Lee invention.

While the Web has changed all of humanity and access to it continues to grow, there are, however, some key challenges that must be addressed for the Web to be truly worldwide in its reach and its potential. These include the following: (1) content gap, (2) technology gap, and (3) research gap [40]. Perhaps the Web will reach its potential in the coming decades as these challenges are ameliorated. We certainly could not function successfully and timely in American society without it. Just imagine going back to the days when you had to go to the library for information. Today, you can get it on your smart phone.

Artificial Intelligence

It has taken millennia for humans to understand and adapt to an ever-changing environment, to communicate and to survive in extreme environments, all with immense struggle and amazing reward. Since the beginning of the computer age, engineers, computer scientists, and researchers have been making computer systems smarter. This has been done in large part to support automation and making things easier for all of us. As these systems get smarter, they also can begin emulating or mimicking human behavior and thought. An AI system can add tremendous value in medicine and public health. AI will take in external data, analyze it, rationalize it, and act. A recent *New York Times* article (January 1, 2020) reports that AI can provide doctors a much faster and perhaps better diagnosis of breast cancer [41]. Yu et al. discuss breakthroughs in AI technology and how it is being used in biomedical applications [42].

AI capabilities are being embedded in everything we do: self-driving cars, banking, inventory control, etc. For healthcare, AI is seen as effective and transformative tool for communicating with patients, managing their healthcare, and teaching [42–45]. While the future is promising and unlimited for AI in healthcare, we must always be cognizant of security and reliability of these systems.

Electronic Health Records

Electronic health records (EHRs), electronic patient records (EPRs), and/or electronic medical records (EMRs) are relatively new additions to the healthcare industry. Each is different but can and does overlap. Data is collected through some kind of interface that is linked to a database where the data are stored in a secure environment. Access is via a credential that is unique to each user, usually a user ID and password. The stored data can be easily accessed and permits analytical tools to be applied with significant output that can improve outcomes in the management of an individual's health.

While adoption continues to march forward, usually at great expense, the value may be in question [46]. In addition, some have reported that the value is questionable [47], and yet there are those who have found tremendous value in their application [48]. Jensen et al. report that large data sets have proven to be very useful in both research applications and clinical care [49].

Regardless of your opinion on the utility of these tools, they are integral to our healthcare systems around the world. Many of the current systems continue to be refined, including interfacing with telemedicine, telehealth, and e-health technologies, which further enhance the record.

Education and Distance Learning

Sitting in a classroom or watching and learning from a teacher with sage advice and expertise are ways of learning. Utilizing new tools – the Web, smartphone apps, immersive environments such as virtual reality, etc. – provides a new and perhaps more effective pedagogical environment in which to learn new skills and competencies. Figure 16.8, Thomas Eakins painting of the Agnew Clinic in 1889, is illustrative of how we have taught for hundreds of years, perhaps even millennia. Another very effective way of training is on the job training.

Video technology permits easy access to the teaching arena or operative theater, the latter being one of startling isolation. A student can see exactly what the professor or preceptor sees, the same angle and the same vantage point. In medical education, Osler fundamentally changed how residents were taught [6]. Distance learning

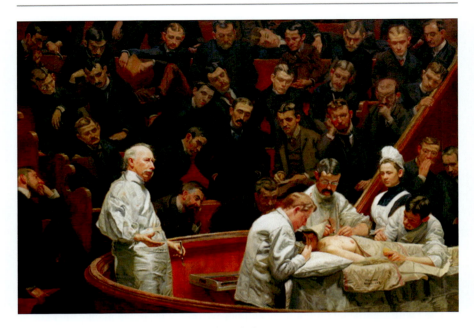

Fig. 16.8 Thomas Eakins – The Agnew Clinic 1889

and telementoring have ensconced themselves firmly in the educational paradigm and remain current in application in academia and in many other venues.

Gruson et al. describe an e-learning platform for training stakeholders in laboratory medicine [50]. Gleason et al. studied telementoring in geriatrics for nurses and social workers in skilled nursing facilities [51]. This type of continuing medical educational approach is of great importance in maintaining skills and learning new approaches or protocols for caring for patients. This approach also adds value for improving education of medical students through the use of telemedicine [52]. Telementoring has been used in a wide variety of applications from space exploration [53] to surgical procedures in austere environments [54].

Aside for Web-based training, Project Extension for Community Healthcare Outcomes (ECHO) has been an excellent adjunct for training and education. An expert panel was assembled in 2018 to review the evidence base on the utility and effectiveness of ECHO and ECHO-like models [55]. Project ECHO has been useful and successful in building capacity for managing complex clinical cases in rural and underserved areas [56].

Conclusion

Advances in technology have provided ample opportunity for change in healthcare. What was once the purview of the few (physicians and the like) is now readily and ubiquitously available for the masses. We can search the Web for information without physically setting foot in a library. We can ask sites like WebMD simple questions about our condition, and we receive detailed descriptions often accompanied by images and videos that further explain. This was not possible 2–3 generations ago, and it is readily available to anyone who has a computer and Internet access [57].

The application of telemedicine in education, clinical care [58], space, military, humanitarian crisis, and disasters [59] continues in earnest. While some have begun referring this discipline to e-health rather than telemedicine or telehealth [60], the state of telehealth continues onward [61]. Challenges will always be a part of change, but change prevails, and innovation makes the system, all systems, better [62].

References

1. Roguin A. Rene theophile hyacinthe laënnec (1781–1826): the man behind the stethoscope. Clin Med Res. 2006;4(3):230–5.
2. Vermeil T, Peters A, Kilpatrick C, Pires D, Allegranzi B, Pittet D. Hand hygiene in hospitals: an anatomy of a revolution. J Hosp Infect. 2019;101(4):383–92.
3. Vecchio R, MacFayden BV, Palazzo F. History of laparoscopic surgery. Panminerva Med. 2000;42(1):87–90.
4. Stellato TA. History of laparoscopic surgery. Surg Clin North Am. 1992;72(5):997–1002.
5. Doarn CR, Mohler SR. Physician training in aerospace medicine-an historical review in the United States. Aviat Space Environ Med. 2013;84(2):158–62.
6. Osler W. Evolution of modern medicine: DevCom; 1921.
7. Bernhardt JM. Communication at the core of effective public health. Am J Public Health. 2004;94(12):2051–3.
8. Healthy people 2010. 2nd ed. Washington: U.S. Department of Health and Human Services; 2000.
9. Doarn CR, Nicogossian AE, Merrell RC. Applications of telemedicine in the United States space program. Telemed J. 1998;4(1):19–30.
10. Rayman RB. Telemedicine: military applications. Aviat Space Environ Med. 1992;63(2):135–7.
11. Bashshur RL, Armstrong PA. Telemedicine: a new mode for the delivery of health care. Inquiry. 1976;13(3):233–44.
12. Bashshur RL, Reardon TG, Shannon GW. Telemedicine: a new health care delivery system. Annu Rev Public Health. 2000;21:613–37.
13. Bashshur RL, Shannon GW, Smith BR, Alverson DC, Antoniotti N, Barsan WG, Bashshur N, Brown EM, Coye MJ, Doarn CR, Ferguson S, Grigsby J, Krupinski EA, Kvedar JC, Linkous J, Merrell RC, Nesbitt T, Poropatich R, Rheuban KS, Sanders JH, Watson AR, Weinstein RS, Yellowlees P. The empirical foundations of telemedicine interventions for chronic disease management. Telemed J E Health. 2014;20(9):769–800.
14. Bashshur RL, Howell JD, Krupinski EA, Harms KM, Bashshur N, Doarn CR. The empirical foundations of telemedicine interventions in primary care. Telemed J E Health. 2016;22(5):342–75.
15. Park B. An introduction to telemedicine: interactive television for delivery of health services. ERIC. https://files.eric.ed.gov/fulltext/ED110028.pdf. Last accessed 14 Feb 2020.
16. Nicogossian AE, Doarn CR. Armenia 1988 earthquake and telemedicine: lessons learned and forgotten. Telemed J E Health. 2011;17(9):741–5.
17. Houtchens BA, Clemmer TP, Holloway HC, Kiselev AA, Logan JS, Merrell RC, Nicogossian AE, Nikogossian HA, Rayman RB, Sarkisian AE, Siegel JH. Telemedicine and international disaster response: medical consultation to Armenia and Russia via a Telemedicine Spacebridge. Prehosp Disaster Med. 1993;8(1):57–66.

18. Doarn CR. Telemedicine in tomorrow's operating room: a natural fit. Semin Laparosc Surg. 2003;10(3):121–6.
19. Hung AJ, Chen J, Shah A, Bill IS. Telementoring and telesurgery for minimally invasive procedures. J Urol. 2018;199(2):355–69.
20. Senapati S, Advincula AP. 2005. Telemedicine and robotics: paving the way to the globalization of surgery. Int J Gynecol Obstet. 2005;91(3):210–6.
21. Angood PB, Satava R, Doarn C, Merrell R, E3 Group. Telemedicine at the top of the world: the 1998 and 1999 Everest extreme expeditions. Telemed J E Health. 2000;6(3):315–25.
22. Lum MJ, Rosen J, King H, Friedman DC, Donlin G, Sankaranarayanan G, Harnett B, Huffman L, Doarn C, Broderick T, Hannaford B. Telesurgery via Unmanned Aerial Vehicle (UAV) with a field deployable surgical robot. Stud Health Technol Inform. 2007;125:313–5.
23. Rosser JC Jr, Bell RL, Harnett B, Rodas E, Murayama M, Merrell R. Use of mobile low-bandwith telemedical techniques for extreme telemedicine applications. J Am Coll Surg. 1999;189(4):397–404.
24. Latifi R, Stanonik Mde L, Merrell RC, Weinstein RS. Telemedicine in extreme conditions: supporting the Martin Strel Amazon Swim Expedition. Telemed J E Health. 2009;15(1):93–100.
25. Latifi R. Telepresence and telemedicine in trauma and emergency. Stud Health Technol Inform. 2008;131:275–80.
26. Latifi R, Hadeed GJ, Rhee P, O'Keeffe T, Friese RS, Wynne JL, Ziemba ML, Judkins D. Initial experiences and outcomes of telepresence in the management of trauma and emergency surgical patients. Am J Surg. 2009;198(6):905–10.
27. Latifi R, Weinstein RS, Porter JM, Ziemba M, Judkins D, Ridings D, Nassi R, Valenzuela T, Holcomb M, Leyva F. Telemedicine and telepresence for trauma and emergency care management. Scand J Surg. 2007;96(4):281–9.
28. Foster KR, Callans DJ. Smartphone apps meet evidence-based medicine: the future of medicine may (or may not) be in your smartphone. IEEE Pulse. 2017;8(6):34–9.
29. Birkoff SD, Smeltzer SC. Perceptions of smartphone user-centered mobile health tracking apps across various chronic illness populations: an integrative review. J Nurs Scholarsh. 2017;49(4):371–8.
30. Hsu WC, Chang CC, Lin YJ, Yang FC, Lin LF, Chou KN. The use of wearable sensors for the movement assessment on muscle contraction sequences in post-stroke patients during sit-to-stand. Sensors (Basel). 2019;19(3):E657.
31. Haghi M, Thurow K, Stoll R. Wearable devices in medical internet of things: scientific research and commercially available devices. Healthc Inform Res. 2017;23(1):4–15.
32. Bhavnani SP, Narula J, Sengupta PP. Mobile technology and the digitization of healthcare. Eur Heart J. 2016;37(18):1428–38.
33. Archibald MM, Barnard A. Futurism in nursing: technology, robotics and the fundamentals of care. J Clin Nurs. 2018;27(11–12):2473–80.
34. George EI, Brand TC, LaPorta A, Marescaux J, Satava RM. Origins of robotic surgery: from skepticism to standard of care. JSLS. 2018;22(4):e2018.
35. Andras I, Mazzone E, van Leeuwen FWB, De Naeyer G, van Oosterom MN, Beato S, Buckle T, O'Sullivan S, van Leeuwen PJ, Beulens A, Crisan N, D'Hondt F, Schatteman P, van Der Poel H, Dell'Oglio P, Mottrie A. Artificial intelligence and robotics: a combination that is changing the operating room. World J Urol. 2019;2019:1–18.
36. Huang EY, Knight S, Guetter CR, Davis CH, Moller M, Slama E, Crandall M. Telemedicine and telementoring in the surgical specialties: a narrative review. Am J Surg. 2019;218(4):760–6.
37. Jell A, Vogel T, Ostler D, Marahrens N, Wilhelm D, Samm N, Eichinger J, Weigel W, Feussner H, Friess H, Kranzfelder M. 5th-generation mobile communication: data highway for surgery 4.0. Surg Technol Int. 2019;35:36–42.
38. Licklider JCR. Man-computer symbiosis. HFE. 1960;1:4–11.
39. Licklider JCR, Clark WE. On-line man-computer communication. Proceedings of the May 1–3, 1962, spring joint computer conference. ACM; 1962. p. 113–128.
40. Summerfelt WT, Sulo S, Robinson A, Chess D, Catanzano K. Scalable hospital at home with virtual physician visits: pilot study. Am J Manag Care. 2015;21(10):675–84.

41. Grady D. A.I. is learning to read mammograms. New York Times. 2020. https://www.nytimes.com/2020/01/01/health/breast-cancer-mammogram-artificial-intelligence.html. Last accessed 18 Feb 2020.
42. Yu KH, Beam AL, Kohane IS. Artificial intelligence in healthcare. Nat Biomed Eng. 2018;2(10):719–31.
43. Butow P, Hoque E. Using artificial intelligence to analyse and teach communication in healthcare. Breast. 2020;50:49–55.
44. Alsuliman T, Humaidan D, Sliman L. Machine learning and artificial intelligence in the service of medicine: necessity or potentiality? Curr Res Transl Med. 2020;
45. Ahuja AS. The impact of artificial intelligence in medicine on the future role of the physician. PeerJ. 2019;7:e7702.
46. Jha AK, DesRoches CM, Campbell EG, Donelan K, Rao SR, Ferris TG, Shields A, Rosenbaum S, Blumenthal D. Use of electronic health records in US hospitals. N Engl J Med. 2009;360(16):1628–38.
47. Greenhalgh T, Potts HW, Wong G, Bark P, Swinglehurst D. Tensions and paradoxes in electronic patient record research: a systematic literature review using the meta-narrative method. Milbank Q. 2009;87(4):729–88.
48. Sidebottom AC, Johnson PJ, VanWormer JJ, Sillah A, Winden TJ, Boucher JL. Exploring electronic health records as a population health surveillance tool of cardiovascular disease risk factors. Popul Health Manag. 2015;18(2):79–85.
49. Jensen PB, Jensen LJ, Brunak S. Mining electronic health records: towards better research applications and clinical care. Nat Rev Genet. 2012;13(6):395–405.
50. Gruson D, Faure G, Gouget B, Haliassos A, Kisikuchin D, Reguengo H, Topic E, Blaton V. A position paper of the EFLM Committee on Education and Training and Working Group on Distance Education Programmes/E-Learning: developing an e-learning platform for the education of stakeholders in laboratory medicine. Clin Chem Lab Med. 2013;51(4):775–80.
51. Gleason LJ, Martinchek M, Long M, Rapier N, Hamlish T, Johnson D, Thompson K. An innovative model using telementoring to provide geriatrics education for nurses and social workers at skilled nursing facilities. Geriatr Nurs. 2019;40(5):517–21.
52. de Araújo Novaes M, Sá de Campos Filho A, Diniz PRB. Improving education of medical students through telehealth. Stud Health Technol Inform. 2019;264:1917–8.
53. Dawson DL. On the practicality of emergency surgery during long-duration space missions. Aviat Space Environ Med. 2008;79(7):712–3.
54. Prince SW, Kang C, Simonelli J, Lee YH, Gerber MJ, Lim C, Chu K, Dutson EP, Tsao TC. A robotic system for telementoring and training in laparoscopic surgery. Int J Med Robot. 2019;16(2):e2040.
55. Faherty LJ, Rose AJ, Chappel A, Taplin C, Martineau M, Fischer SH. Assessing and expanding the evidence base for project ECHO and ECHO-like models: findings of a technical expert panel. J Gen Intern Med. 2020;8:1–4.
56. Furlan AD, Pajer KA, Gardner W, MacLeod B. Project ECHO: building capacity to manage complex conditions in rural, remote and underserved areas. Can J Rural Med. 2019;24(4):115–20.
57. Sadah SA, Shahbazi M, Wiley MT, Hristidis V. Demographic-based content analysis of web-based health-related social media. J Med Internet Res. 2016;18(6):e148.
58. Weinstein RS, Krupinski EA, Doarn CR. Clinical examination component of telemedicine, telehealth, mhealth, and connected health medical practices. Med Clin North Am. 2018;102(3):533–44.
59. Doarn CR, Latifi R, Poropatich RK, Sokolovich N, Kosiak D, Hostiuc F, Zoicas C, Buciu A, Arafat R. Development and validation of telemedicine for disaster response: the North Atlantic treaty organization multinational system. Telemed J E Health. 2018;24(9):657–68.
60. Mea VD. What is e-health (2): the death of telemedicine. J Med Internet Res. 2001;3(2):e22.
61. Dorsey ER, Topol EJ. State of telehealth. N Engl J Med. 2016;375(2):154–61.
62. Ellimoottil C, An L, Moyer M, Sossong S, Hollander JE. Challenges and opportunities faced by large health systems implementing telehealth. Health Aff (Millwood). 2018;37(12):1955–9.

Part III

Outcomes Based Evidence Clinical Applications of Telemedicine

Survey of the Direct-to-Hospital (DTH) Telemedicine and Telehealth Service Industry (2014–2018)

17

Ronald S. Weinstein, Nicholas Rolig, Nancy Rowe, Gail P. Barker, Kristine A. Erps, Michael J. Holcomb, Rifat Latifi, and Elizabeth A. Krupinski

Introduction

The Arizona Telemedicine Program (ATP) was established in 1996, to improve the access to healthcare resources throughout rural Arizona. To do this the ATP designed and implemented:

1. A giant 160 site, 70 community telecommunication network, using asynchronous transfer mode methods on T1 carriers, an application service provider business model adapted from the software industry where it was commonly used in the 1980s.
2. The Arizona Telemedicine Council, to provide a consistent and direct line of communications between the ATP and the Arizona State Legislature.
3. An international award-winning state-of-the-art "e-classroom of the future" at its T-Health Institute in downtown Phoenix, AZ, in which to provide training for the healthcare industry on uses of telemedicine and telehealth in medical and nursing practice [1–4].

Since the successful rollout of its original broadband telecommunications network, the ATP has expanded its program goals in order to maintain and expand its telecommunication network, support telemedicine research and education, and

---

The original version of this chapter was revised. The correction to this chapter is available at https://doi.org/10.1007/978-3-030-56917-4_30.

R. S. Weinstein (✉) · N. Rolig · N. Rowe · G. P. Barker · K. A. Erps · M. J. Holcomb
Arizona Telemedicine Program, The University of Arizona's College of Medicine, Tucson, AZ, USA
e-mail: rweinstein@telemedicine.arizona.edu

R. Latifi
New York Medical College, School of Medicine, Valhalla, NY, USA

Department of Surgery, Westchester Medical Center Health, Valhalla, NY, USA

E. A. Krupinski
Department of Radiology, Emory University, Atlanta, GA, USA

© The Author(s) 2021, corrected publication 2021
R. Latifi et al. (eds.), *Telemedicine, Telehealth and Telepresence*,
https://doi.org/10.1007/978-3-030-56917-4_17

serve as the headquarters of the Southwest Telehealth Resource Center (SWTRC), a HRSA (Health Resources and Services Administration)-funded telemedicine resource center for its region [5–14].

In 2014, the Arizona Telemedicine Program created two new, complimentary programs, intended to promote the direct-to-hospital (DTH) telemedicine services industry and provide it with an academic home: (1) an annual national "Service Provider Showcase" (SPS) meeting and (2) the Telemedicine/Telehealth Service Provider Directory (SPD) [15]. The SPS and SPD were run in tandem for 4 years. The SPS was discontinued after 4 years, as planned, and the SPD would continue indefinitely. These two entities were envisioned as having reciprocal relationships and would link the evolving DTH telemedicine service industry with academic medicine and telemedicine research. Each would showcase aspects of the DTH industry and, hopefully, catalyze its growth. This was an ambitious undertaking since the plan was to create both programs, SPS and SPD, without increasing the size of the ATP staff, which consisted of 16 FTE employees at that time.

The SPS was a medical meeting for both the healthcare industry which focused on all aspects of the delivery of specialty care services into hospitals and clinics by outside telemedicine service vendors. The ATP was experienced in creating and managing professional meetings including the prior successful series of four correction telemedicine meetings, held in Arizona a decade before. The new series of SPS meetings and the SPD would be jointly marketed. Marketing of the SPS meetings to exhibitors was coupled with recruiting of telemedicine service provider companies to list their companies in the SPD which was for free. Furthermore, facets of the emerging DTH industry were topics for consideration at plenary lectures, panel discussions, and poster presentations. At the time SPS was created, no other professional conferences in the United States were dedicated exclusively to the DTH industry.

At the same time, rural Arizona hospitals were becoming increasingly interested in partnering with third party specialty telemedicine services from commercial telemedicine service vendors. Awareness of that option was being driven by the dramatic demonstration of successes of the tele-stroke option, a service requiring the diagnosis and treatment of ischemic stroke patients within a "golden hour" in order to prevent progression of the stroke process. That could be accomplished at rural hospitals using tele-stroke service vendors to provide a tele-neurologist to carry out a remote physical examination and a distant tele-neurovascular radiologists to render the CT diagnosis at a distance. Table 17.1 reflects the growth of the SPS industry over the timeframe that SPS meetings were held (2014–2018) (Table 17.1; Figs. 17.1 and 17.2).

As the popularity of the Telemedicine and Telehealth SPS grew, so did the growth of the online Service Provider Directory. Currently 168 companies are listed in the directory and we receive requests to be listed on a weekly basis.

"Advancing Telehealth Partnerships" was the tagline for SPS. Our initial goal was to assist healthcare organization to partner with a vendor service provider. Networking was a key to the partnership; our conference agenda was designed

Table 17.1 ATP/SWTRC-sponsored Service Provider Showcase (2014–2018)

Name	Location	Date	Attendees	Abstracts	Exhibitors	# SPD listings
Service Provider Showcase 2014	Hyatt regency, Phoenix, AZ	October 6–7 2014	243	-----	36	16
Service Provider Showcase 2016	Hyatt regency, Phoenix, AZ	June 21–22 2016	386	29	40	75
Service Provider Showcase 2017	Hyatt regency, Phoenix, AZ	October 2–3 2017	385	38	41	104
Service Provider Summit 2018[a]	Renaissance Hotel, Glendale, AZ	October 8–9 2018	393	35	45	122
--------	--------	Year 2020	--------	--------	--------	168

[a]Name changed in 2018

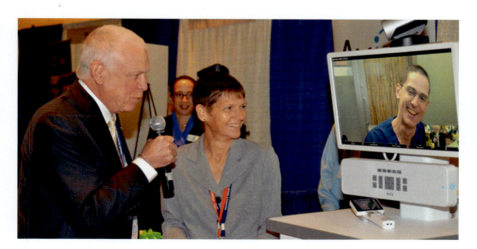

Fig. 17.1 Co-chairs of SPS, Dr. Dale Alverson (left) and Dr. Elizabeth Krupinski (middle), interviewing vendor Alan Pitt, chief medical officer of Avizia (right, video screen) during "lighting rounds" at the SPS meeting. They are in the expo hall, broadcasting their string of focused "what's new?" interviews back to the lecture hall during the SPS's "lighting rounds." These proved to be popular, and informative, events and an efficient way to introduce SPS conference attendees in the lecture hall to the 40 exhibitors at SPS 2017. SPS, Telemedicine and Telehealth Service Provider Showcase. (Image reprinted from [16])

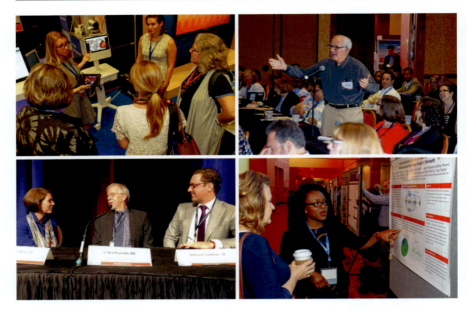

Fig. 17.2 2018 Telemedicine and Telehealth Service Provider Summit. Upper left: vendor in the exhibit hall demonstrating a new telemedicine cart. Upper right: former director of the Arizona Department of Health Services posing a question to a panel in the lecture hall. Lower left: panel members Alexis Gilroy, JD, H. Neal Reynolds, MD, and Nathaniel Lackman, JD, discussing a question from the audience. Lower right: poster presentation during a break in the program

around learning about this new industry. SPS certainly elevated this new industry. Not only did we see cultivation of networking between one healthcare organization and one service provider, but we saw healthcare organizations networking and partnering with multiple service providers. We even saw service providers networking with other service providers to help expand their reach.

The SPD was designed to provide healthcare system telemedicine service users critical information about DTH organizations at a single, reliable, web site.

In 2015, the SPD, a joint venture of the ATP and SWTRC, came online.

The SPD was established with the expressed purpose of providing rural and urban hospitals a resource for identifying and connecting with clinical commercial telemedicine service companies to which they could outsource specialty medicine consultations (Figs. 17.2 and 17.3). By 2018, it was estimated that the SPD represented a significant number of the commercial telemedicine/telehealth companies delivering specialty medical services to healthcare organizations. Some of these companies gradually offered direct-to-consumer (DTC) telemedicine service products but that segment of the telehealth industry was outside of the areas of interest of either the ATP or the SWTRC at the time (Figs. 17.2 and 17.3). Table 17.1 reflects the growth of the DTH telehealth industry over a 4-year period, from 2014 to 2018. Since then, there has been a dramatic increase in the market share of the DTC slice of the telemedicine and telehealth service industry.

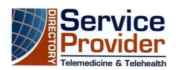

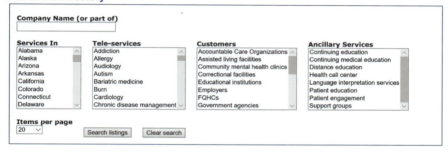

Fig. 17.3 Screenshot of the Service Provider Directory home page. Logos: upper left, Service Provider Directory; upper right, Logo for the Service Provider Summit; upper middle, Arizona Telemedicine Program (ATP) and Southwest Telehealth Resource Center (TRC). Bottom: "Search the Directory" with four columns (left to right): "Service In (location)," "Tele-services," "Customers," and "Ancillary Services" [13]

Introduction to the Service Provider Directory (SPD)

The SPD was designed to assist users in locating specific specialty medicine services and ancillary healthcare services [17]. In practice, a user could filter and sort through the SPD of companies using lists grossly describing 4 of the 87 variables gathered to characterize each company. The four variables are the state to which the service will be delivered, the specific teleservice being sought, customer base, and ancillary services. After selecting one or more of these variables, a list of companies is generated, all sharing the characteristics the SPD user had selected. From this list, the user can further investigate each company by opening their SPD profile, which shows all 87 variables that make up the directory. An instructional training video on how to use the SPD can be accessed from the SPD home page (Fig. 17.4).

Upper left, "Introduction-Service Provider Directory" video; upper right, word cloud representing the frequency of service offerings across 129 telemedicine service provider companies; lower left, criteria selection in four categories, "Services In" (location of the insourcing hospital or clinic), "Tele-services," "Customers," and "Ancillary." In this example, the user has selected "Arizona," "Telepsychiatry,"

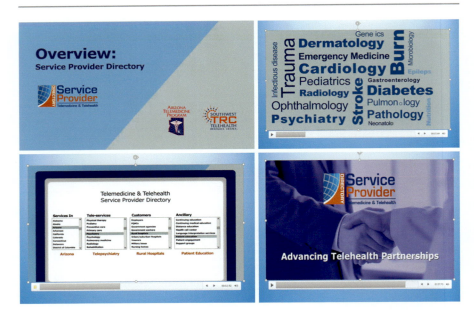

Fig. 17.4 Screenshots from an instructive video on the uses of the Service Provider Directory

"Rural hospitals," and "Patient education" as topics of interest. At the time of writing of the chapter (May 28, 2020), this search yields a set of 12 out of 163 companies for further assessment by the SPD user. Each company's web site can be immediately accessed by clicking on the company's listing in the SPD. Lower right: closing screen of the video "Overview: Service Provider Directory" video [15, 16, 18].

The primary aim of this chapter is to analyze the SPD's database to characterize the telemedicine/telemedicine direct-to-hospital service industry (Fig. 17.3). A limitation of the study is that accrual of data included in this survey ended on June 4, 2018, approximately 2 years ago. On the other hand, the study does provide a snapshot of the telemedicine/telehealth service industry as it existed before the recent COVID-19-related DTC telehealth surge in telemedicine, and telehealth clinical activity began to dominate the telemedicine service industry.

Methodology

Criteria for Inclusion of Companies in the Service Provider Directory

Since the primary reason for creating the SPD was to foster connections between telemedicine/telehealth clinical service providers and healthcare organizations in need of specific specialty services, telemedicine service companies are only listed if they meet four criteria. First, they must provide medical or clinical specialty services and/or ancillary services that "touch" the patient. Second, they serve, or be willing to serve, intermediary organizations such as hospitals. Third, they currently provide services in at least one US state. Fourth, they employ or contract with other service providers. Companies may also provide DTC telemedicine and telehealth services, in addition to organizations such as hospitals.

Solicitation of Companies

In late 2014, the ATP/SWTRC began identifying telemedicine/telehealth service provider companies, via email, phone, and in person, to start the directory. Once found, service providers were then solicited to be listed within the directory. Interested companies then used a 32-item SurveyMonkey form, to describe themselves and the services they provide. Until 2018, these efforts actively continued as part of daily business and networking of ATP/SWTRC after attending multiple telemedicine/telehealth conferences.

To maintain the directory, the ATP/SWTRC maintains contact with listed companies. Through this effort, companies can update their directory listing upon request. At least once per year, companies are solicited for updated information. This analysis was of the 129 telemedicine service companies listed in 2018. At the time of the writing of this chapter, in May 2020, there are currently 168 listed companies.

Directory Analysis

This analysis was conducted using 18 selected variables of the 2018 SPD's underlying database: company name, company type, payment model, targeted customers, teleservices, ancillary services, method of connection, EHR compliance, HIPAA compliance, headquarter address information (5 variables), states serving, provider's location (states), licenses (states), and planned expansion (states). Variables with complex observations, such as the list of teleservices offered per company, were disaggregated and collectively listed in two columns. For example, the variable "teleservices" listed company names in the first column and their respective services as individual observations in the second column. Variables with simple observations were formatted using the same two-column method. All lists were analyzed using Microsoft Excel's Pivot Table function and relevant statistical equations.

Geospatial Analysis

Latitude and longitude for headquarters for individual companies were found after aggregating each company's address information into one variable and running said variable through Geocode, a Google Sheets add-on. Latitude and longitude information were then exported to QGIS, where they were plotted on top of a US state map layer, obtained from www.gadm.org [17]. Major US cities from Esri's data and maps were then added [19] and used as visual reference points.

For variable geospatial association, companies were joined to the states in which they provided services to, using Microsoft Access's Simple Query function. The resulting query was made up of three columns: (1) company name, (2) state, and (3) variable. Each observation of these lists was then used as a metric, which we define as a service provision unit (SPU). SPUs can be conceptualized by imagining the following example: if company A offers two services to three states, in total the query would yield a list with six observations or SPUs. The purpose of using SPUs is to count the number of companies offering a service in a specific state. Once determined, SPUs for states' tele- and ancillary services were then associated with a graduated color scheme and then coupled with their respective geometry on the US state map layer [19].

Telemedicine/Telehealth Market Analysis

Gross Description of Companies

Using a multiple choice-multiple answer question in the SPD company listing form, companies were asked to describe themselves. Eighty-four percent of companies indicated they were medical specialty service providers to healthcare providers; and 57% were medical specialty service providers to non-healthcare systems, such as prisons. Nearly 25% of companies classified themselves as patient education/engagement service providers.

Focusing on the business characteristics of companies, 55% of companies reported using a fee for service payment model, while just over 10% reported using a subscription business model, and 1.5% reported using both.

These data indicated that most of the telemedicine/telehealth companies listed in the SPD supplement specialized services within larger healthcare systems.

Targeted Customers

The two most reported targets for marketing of telemedicine and telehealth services were rural hospitals and urban/suburban hospitals, accounting for more than 85% and 75% of companies listed within the SPD, respectively. The third most stated target market was private physician practices, at 65%. In addition, DTC telemedicine services were reported to be provided by 55% of SPD companies, a surprisingly high percentage in June 2018. This indicated that the DTC industry was already well developed by June 2018.

Considering the gross description of companies (above), this makes sense and supports the idea that most telemedicine/telehealth companies support the provision of specialty services both within larger organizations as well as DTC telehealth.

Teleservices

Of the 70 services surveyed in the directory listing form, the lowest number of services offered by a company was 1, while the maximum was 69. On average, companies were found to provide 9 to 10 telemedicine and /or telehealth services. The most popular services, psychiatry and mental health, were provided by 44% and 41% of companies, respectively. Remote patient monitoring and mobile health (mHealth) were reported to be offered by 30% of companies. Services associated with chronic diseases, such as diabetes, neurology, and cardiology, were reported being offered by 25–27% of companies. Specialties under the general practice umbrella, including pediatrics, primary care, urgent care, integrated care, and internal medicine were reported being provided by 18–26% of companies.

Collectively, these data indicate the presence of a strong association between telemedicine/telehealth and mental health, primary care, and subspecialties of primary care related to chronic diseases.

Ancillary Services

Ancillary services are defined as services that support the provision of telemedicine and telehealth. Using the SPD data entry form, eight ancillary services were surveyed. In total, 58% of SPD companies reported providing ancillary services. The top three ancillary services were patient education, offered by more than 41% of companies; patient engagement, provided by more than 37% of companies; and distance education, offered by more than 25% of companies.

Language Services

Of the 129 companies listed in the SPD in June 2018, 4 companies reported they focused exclusively on language interpretation, which is classified as an ancillary service in SPD. Some language interpretation services were offered by a total of 15% of companies.

Telemedicine Systems Used to Connect to Customers

In aggregate, companies reported using 57 specific telemedicine systems to connect with customers. An average company used only one or two platforms. Of these systems, nearly 19% of companies reported their systems were proprietary, while 17% reported their systems were platform agnostic. Vidyo, Cisco, and Polycom were the top three third-party specific telemedicine systems, used by 16%, 13%, and 10% of the telemedicine service companies, respectively.

It is noteworthy that 72% of companies reported their telemedicine services can be incorporated into an electronic health record, of which 41% were certified by the

Office of the National Coordinator (ONC). Nearly all telemedicine service companies (93%) listed in SPD claimed that their patient information system complies with Health Insurance Portability and Accountability Act (HIPAA) and Health Information Technology for Economic and Clinical Health (HITECH) Act.

Comprehensive List of Teleservices and Ancillary Services

Although thousands of telemedicine and telehealth academic articles have been published, none describe a comprehensive list of services. It is for this reason that we utilized the SPD database to derive such a list.

In the SPD listing form, companies are surveyed about which services they offer, using a multiple choice-multiple answer list of 70 teleservices and 8 ancillary services. Open text space was also provided for telemedicine and telehealth service companies to report additional telemedicine and telehealth services they currently provide.

Upon analyzing company details, it was found that all the healthcare services ATP and SWTRC included in the multiple choice-multiple answer question were offered by at least one company. Furthermore, upon review of the "other teleservices" companies stated they offer, no services were found that were not included in the SPD listing.

Tables 17.2 and 17.3 detail the comprehensive lists of teleservices and ancillary services, listed in SPD as of June 2018.

Table 17.2 A comprehensive list of teleservices offered in June 2018

Addiction	Allergy	Audiology	Bariatric medicine	Burn
Cardiology	Chronic disease management	Dementia	Dentistry	Dermatology
Diabetes	Emergency medicine	Endocrinology	Epilepsy	Gastroenterology
Genetics/genetic counseling	Geriatrics	Gynecology	Hematology	Hepatology
Homecare	Hospice	Hospitalist	ICU (intensive care unit)	Infectious disease
Integrated care	Internal medicine	Long-term care	Maternal care	Menopause care
Mental health	Microbiology	Mobile health (mHealth)	Neonatology	Nephrology
Neurology	Neuropsychological testing	Nursing	Nutrition	Obstetrics
Occupational therapy	Ophthalmology	Orthopedic surgery	Otorhinolaryngology (ENT)	Pain management
Pathology	Patient monitoring (remote)	Pediatrics	Pharmacy	Physical therapy
Podiatry	Preventive care	Primary care	Psychiatry	Psychology
Pulmonary medicine	Radiology	Rehabilitation	Rheumatology	Sleep medicine
Sonography	Speech language pathology	Stroke	Surgery	Toxicology
Trauma	Urgent care	Urology	Weight control	Wound care

Table 17.3 List of ancillary services offered in June 2018

Patient education	Patient engagement	Distance education	Language interpretation service
Support groups	Continuing medical education	Health call center	Continuing education

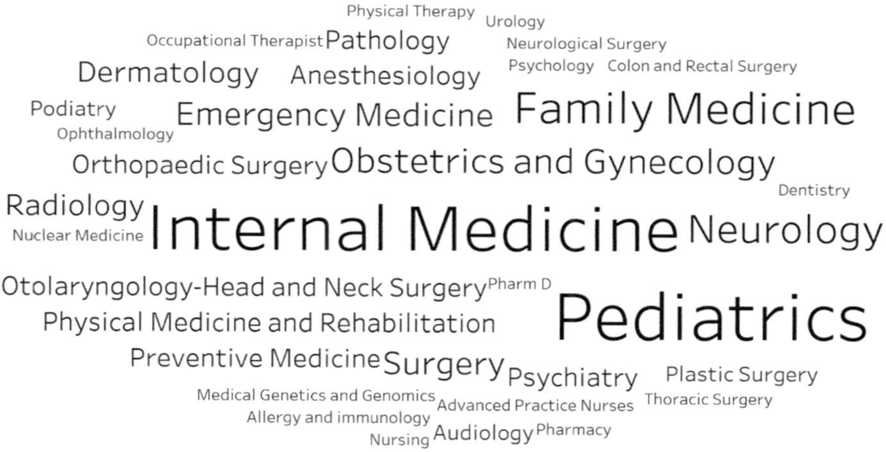

Fig. 17.5 Specialties of users of telemedicine and telehealth services. This word cloud is based on pooled numbers of services per board

Cross-Referencing Teleservices with the American Board of Medical Specialties

During the analysis of the SPD directory, two questions were posed: first, what specialty would a clinician be classified as if they offered a given service? Second, what specialty boards are associated with the provision of care using tele- and ancillary services?

To better understand the teleservice and ancillary service provision among medical specialties, each service was cross-referenced with the American Board of Medical Specialties [20] or select allied health fields. The number of services were pooled per board and used to create the word cloud seen in Fig. 17.5.

Through this analysis, it was found that providers who belong to general practice specialty boards, internal medicine, gynecology, pediatrics, and family medicine, are the greatest users of telemedicine services.

Geospatial Processing

Headquarter Distribution

After vectorizing companies' headquarters on a map, a nearest neighbor vector analysis was run. It was found that headquarters were significantly clustered, with a nearest neighbor index of 0.382 and z-score of −13.43. Based on visual inspection, referencing Esri's city coordinates [17, 19], multiple companies were found to be located around Seattle, San Francisco, Los Angeles, Phoenix, Dallas, Houston, Atlanta, Miami, Jacksonville, DC, and Minneapolis.

This may suggest the location of companies' headquarters, and their respective service footprint may be determined by population density, indicative of case volume, and/or telemedicine policies.

Teleservices and Ancillary Services

The primary finding of geospatial analysis was that nearly all 70 teleservices and 8 ancillary services were found to be available in all 50 states, provided by at least one company, tele-addiction not being provided by any service provider in Utah, Vermont, or Washington.

Analyzing this further, we used SPUs to determine the presence of tele- and ancillary service pooling. The resulting maps are seen in Figs. 17.6 and 17.7.

Like the clustering of companies' headquarters, service pooling may be a result of population density, case volume, and/or telemedicine legislative policies. Furthermore, these maps illustrate telemedicine/telehealth service disparities.

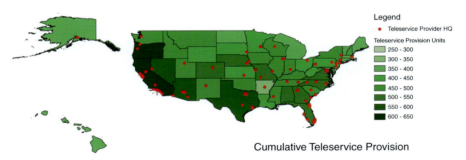

Fig. 17.6 Cumulative teleservice provision, measured using service provision units

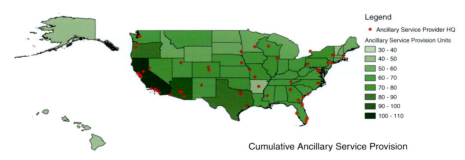

Fig. 17.7 Cumulative ancillary service provision, measured using service provision units

States Served, Provider Location, Licenses, and Planned Expansion

Comparing the lists of states which companies provide services to and the lists of states in which providers are located, it was found that 35% of companies offer services in the states where their providers reside. Thirteen percent of companies provide services to less states than where their providers are physically located. And, 53% of companies provide services beyond the states in which their telehealth service providers reside.

Focusing on the list of states in which companies have providers licensed, 43% of companies practice in the same number of states as they are licensed. Thirty-four percent of companies have more state licenses than what they reported practicing in.

By independently comparing the states of planned extension to currently served, service provider locations, and licensed, it was found that 7% of companies plan to expand to states where they hold unused licenses.

Collectively, these data imply an association between medical licensure and the growth of telemedicine/telehealth service provision.

Summary

As an innovative leader in telemedicine, the Arizona Telemedicine Program and Southwest Regional Training Center created the Service Provider Directory (SPD), an online directory used to foster connections between healthcare administrators and commercial telemedicine/telehealth service providers. With its continued curation and sustained expansion, it serves as one of the most comprehensive resources for seeking commercial teleservices. In 2018, the directory was estimated to include approximately 25% of the commercial telemedicine/telehealth service provider companies. It is for this reason we believe that the directory was an accurate representation of the telemedicine/telehealth market, contained enough data to be statistically significant, and used to identify market trends through a standalone analysis. Prior to the aggregation and analysis of these data, basic market trends and statistics were largely only known by service provider companies themselves and the experience of industry leaders.

Findings

According to our analysis of the SPD, an average company was fee for service and indicated targeting 10 customer types on a multiple choice-multiple answer list, the most frequent being medical specialty service provider to healthcare providers and non-healthcare systems. On average, a company offered 9–10 teleservices, with the most frequently provided services being psychiatry, mental health, and remote patient monitoring. Relatedly, an average company also provided 1–2 ancillary services, patient education and patient engagement being the most popular. Companies provided services to an average of 18 states. States with the most service provision units were California, Arizona, and Texas. Service delivery was reported to be done using two connection methods, on average. Nearly all companies reported their services could be integrated into an electronic health record and are HIPAA and HITECH compliant. Only 41% of companies said they use an EHR that is ONC certified.

Tables 17.1 and 17.2 list the 70 teleservices and 8 ancillary services, used to survey companies during the company listing process. These services were used as answers on a multiple choice-multiple answer question, surveying what services each company provides. All found to be provided by at least one company.

When all 70 teleservices were cross-referenced with the specialties and subspecialties of the American Board of Medical Specialties, it was found that more teleservices were related to the boards of pediatrics, internal medicine, and family medicine than any other, as can be seen in Fig. 17.5. This may indicate a significant number of providers that use telemedicine are related to general practice.

The two most significant findings of this chapter are related to the geospatial analysis of the SPD. First is the discovery that nearly all 70 services and all 8 ancillary services were available in all 50 states, the only shortfall being that tele-addiction not being specifically available in Utah, Vermont, or Washington. However, due to addiction medicine being a subspecialty under preventive medicine [6], which is available in all 50 states, we feel confident that the provision of care, under one service or another, is available across the United States.

Second is the creation and application of a methodology that identifies telehealth/telemedicine service disparities. This methodology used service provision units (SPUs), which we defined as a service provided within a specific state by a single company. Using SPUs as a unit of measure, we aggregated all SPUs for every tele- and ancillary service to create Figs. 17.6 and 17.7. The darker green the state, the more teleservices and companies providing those services within the state. Furthermore, these maps can be disaggregated by a selected service to determine the number of companies providing said service per state. In practice, this can be used as a metric within public health or a means for business planning.

Implications of Findings

The implications of the findings described in this chapter can be summarized in three points. First, in 2018, telemedicine/telehealth was transitioning from an independent niche market; second, the directory was an accurate representation of the market; and third, medical licensing was a significant challenge for service providers.

Although the average commercial telemedicine/telehealth company was found to provide 9–10 teleservices and 1–2 ancillary services to 18 states, these statistics do not paint a completely accurate picture of the market. Rather, the market was polarized. For example, only 28% of the companies in the SPD offer ten or more services, while 59% offer five or less, with 25% offering only one. Similarly, 41% of companies do not offer any ancillary services, and 54% of companies provide services to eight or less states. We chose not to exclude companies with larger telemedicine footprints from this analysis, because they accounted for a significant portion of the directory, and we predict companies will continue to grow in this way. Startup companies, capitalizing on niche markets, are getting acquired, partnered, or merged by larger companies. An interesting example of this can be seen when looking back at a 2017 snapshot of the directory, when InTouch, a large company, acquired a smaller company C30 Telemedicine, which provided acute teleneurology, tele-stroke, distance education, and patient engagement to six states [21]. Since 2018, four of the companies within the SPD have also been involved in acquisitions, InDemand Interpreting being acquired by Stratus, Aligned Telehealth being acquired by American Well, and InSight Telepsychiatry merging with Regroup Telehealth [22–25]. Considering this collectively we think that the years surrounding 2018 were a transitional period for telemedicine, from independent niche to supply and demand.

As stated on the home page of the SPD, its purpose is to serve as a resource for hospital and healthcare administrators to expand and improve their institution's healthcare services [15]. With 129 commercial companies listed in 2018, which collectively provide 70 teleservices and 8 ancillary services to all 50 states, we argue it fulfills its objective quite well. The question then arises, "does the SPD only represent the commercial clinical telemedicine/telehealth market, or does it represent the clinical market as a whole?" The main difference between included and excluded clinical provision-based companies is companies that provided services in tandem with larger organizations were listed and companies that operated independently for the sole purpose of DTC telemedicine were not. The most obvious answer to the earlier question is that the clinical commercial market was based on the inclusion-exclusion criteria. However, after reviewing the 21 companies of GoodRx's Telehealth Marketplace, a directory which connects patients with DTC telehealth service providers, we found their listings are comparable to the larger companies that have historically acquired, partnered, or merged with niche companies [26]. Examples of this include HealthTap acquiring Docphin, MDLive acquiring Breakthrough Behavioral, and Teladoc acquiring both TelaDietitian and MedecinDirect [27–30]. From these examples and the cross listing of two companies between GoodRx Telehealth and the SPD, which now offer both clinical commercial services (also called "direct-to-hospital" telemedicine and telehealth) and DTC services, despite its exclusion-inclusion criteria, we think the SPD serves as an accurate snapshot of the entire 2018 telemedicine/telehealth "clinical market," illustrating the transition from clinical commercial (direct-to-hospital) to DTC telemedicine and telehealth as the largest segment of the telemedicine/telehealth industry [31, 32]. Significant growth of DTC telemedicine companies was observed to the extent that it warranted a formal definition within a recent Frequently Asked Question section in a telemedicine/telehealth industry-related congressional report [33, 34].

In a separate 2016 congressional report, it was suggested that one of the greatest policy challenges for the growth of telemedicine/telehealth is medical licensure, the report specifically stating "…state licensure requirements may be inhibiting broader use of telehealth, with as many as 4 out of 5 states requiring out-of-state clinicians providing telehealth services to be medical licensed in the state where the patients reside" [35]. Given that our data indicate 7% of companies planned to expand to states for which their providers already have medical licenses, we agree. Later in the document, the authors state that the Federation of State Medical Boards drafted an interstate licensure compact, which would solve this problem [35]. To date, the Interstate Medical Licensure Compact (IMLC) includes 29 states [36]. As participation in the IMLC expands, we think telemedicine companies' service footprints will grow, and the telehealth disparities among states, illustrated by a lack of ubiquity in Figs. 17.2 and 17.3, could be mitigated.

Currently, the ATP's and SWTRC's SPD is listed at both the Center for Medicare and Medicaid Services (CMS) and the Health and Human Services (HHS) web sites as telehealth and telemedicine resources [37, 38].

Acknowledgments SWTRC activity is supported by grants from the Office of Advancement of Telehealth, Federal Office of Rural Health Policy, Health Resources and Services Administration, and Department of Health and Human Services.

References

1. McNeill KM, Weinstein RS, Holcomb MJ. Arizona telemedicine program: implementing a statewide health care network. J Am Inform Assoc. 1998;5:441–7.
2. Krupinski E, Webster P, Dolliver M, Weinstein RS, Lopez AM. Efficiency analysis of a multispecialty telemedicine service. Telemed J. 1999;5:265–71.
3. McNeill KM, Barker G, McElroy J. Experience using an ASP model to expand a state-initiated telemedicine program. Comput Ass Radiol Surg. 2001;1230:824–9.
4. Weinstein RS, Barker G, Beinar S, Holcomb M, Krupinski EA, Lopez AM, Hughes A, McNeely RA. Policy and the origins of the Arizona statewide telemedicine program. In: Whitten P, Cook D, editors. Understanding health communications technologies. San Francisco: Jossey-Bass; 2004. p. 299–309.
5. Barker GP, Krupinski EA, Schellenberg B, Weinstein RS. Expense comparison of a telemedicine practice versus a traditional clinical practice. Telemed J e-Health. 2004;10:376–80.
6. Barker GP, Krupinski EA, McNeely RA, Holcomb MJ, Krupinski EA, Lopez AM, Weinstein RS. The Arizona telemedicine program business model. J Telemed Telecare. 2005;11:397–402.
7. Latifi R, Weinstein RS, Porter JM, Ziemba M, Judkins D, Ridings D, Nassi R, Valenzuela T, Holcomb M, Leyva F. Telemedicine and telepresence for trauma and emergency care management. Scand J Surg. 2007;96:281–9.
8. Weinstein RS, Lopez AM, Krupinski EA, Beinar SJ, Holcomb M, Barker G. Integrating telemedicine and telehealth: putting it all together. In: Latifi R, editor. Current principles and practices of telemedicine and e-health. Washington, DC: IOS Press; 2008. p. 23–38.
9. Krupinski EA, Weinstein RS. Telemedicine in an academic center—the Arizona telemedicine program. Telemed e-Health. 2013;19:349–56.
10. Weinstein RS, Lopez AM, Joseph BA, Erps KA, Holcomb M, Barker GP, Krupinski EA. Telemedicine, telehealth, and mobile health applications that work: opportunities and barriers. Am J Med. 2014;127:183–7.

11. Weinstein RS, Lopez AM, Barker GP, Krupinski EA, Beinar SJ, Major J, Skinner T, Holcomb MJ, McNeely RA. Arizona telemedicine program interprofessional learning center: facility design and curriculum development. J Interprofessional Care. 2007;21(SI):51–63.
12. Weinstein RS, McNeely RA, Holcomb MJ, Sotelo MJ, Lopez AM, Erps KA, Martin CJ, Krupinski EA, Graham AR, Barker GP. Technologies in interprofessional education. The interprofessional education distributed "e-Classroom-of-the-future". J Applied Health. 2010;39(3 pt 2):238–45.
13. Southwest Telehealth Resource Center. https://southwesttrc.org/. Last accessed 29 May 2020.
14. "Goals". The University of Arizona, Arizona Telemedicine Program. 2020. https://telemedicine.arizona.edu/about-us/goals. Last accessed 19 May 2020.
15. "Service Provider Directory." The University of Arizona, Arizona Telemedicine Program. 2020. https://telemedicine.arizona.edu/servicedirectory
16. Alverson DC, Krupinski EA, Erps KA, Rowe NS, Weinstein RS. The Third National Telemedicine & Telehealth Service Provider Showcase Conference: Advancing Telehealth Partnerships. Telemedicine and e-Health. 2019.332-40. https://doi.org/10.1089/tmj.2018.0096.
17. "Administrative Boundaries (GADM)" https://www.arcgis.com/home/item.html?id=5372763e5f9f4cb29e6a696523cad557. Last accessed 19 May 2020.
18. "Information: Service Provider Directory" https://swtrc.wistia.com/medias/2n51626yug. Last accessed 29 May 2020.
19. "ArcMap City" https://desktop.arcgis.com/en/arcmap/10.3/manage-data/editing-fundamentals/exercise-1a-creating-new-points.htm. Last accessed 19 May 2020.
20. "Specialty and Subspecialty Certificates." American Board of Medical Specialties. 2020. https://www.abms.org/member-boards/specialty-subspecialty-certificates/
21. "InTouch Health Acquires C30 Medical Corporation." InTouchHealth. 2017. https://intouchhealth.com/acquires-c30-medical-corporation/. Last accessed 19 May 2020.
22. Eddy N. Stratus video buys InDemand interpreting to expand healthcare services. HealthcareITNews. 2019. https://www.healthcareitnews.com/news/stratus-video-buys-indemand-interpreting-expand-healthcare-services. Last accessed 19 May 2020.
23. Muoio D. American Well acquires Aligned Telehealth to flesh out its behavioral health, telepsychiatry capabilities. mobi health news. 2019.
24. https://www.mobihealthnews.com/news/north-america/american-well-acquires-aligned-telehealth-flesh-out-its-behavioral-health. Last accessed 19 May 2020.
25. Muoio D. InSight Telepsychiatry, Regroup Telehealth merge to create US' largest telepsychiatry provider. mobi health news. 2019. https://www.mobihealthnews.com/news/insight-telepsychiatry-regroup-telehealth-merge-create-us-largest-telepsychiatry-provider. Last accessed 19 May 2020.
26. "GoodRx/Online Doctors" GoodRx. https://www.goodrx.com/treatment. Last accessed 19 May 2020.
27. Hall G. Telehealth platform HealthTap buys Docphin to expand online education for doctors. 2016. Silicon Valley Business Journal. https://www.bizjournals.com/sanjose/blog/techflash/2016/07/telehealth-platform-healthtap-buys-docphin-to.html. Last accessed 19 May 2020.
28. Pai A. MDLive acquires virtual therapy visits provider Breakthrough Behavioral. mobi health news. 2014. https://www.mobihealthnews.com/38116/mdlive-acquires-virtual-therapy-visits-provider-breakthrough-behavioral. Last accessed 19 May 2020.
29. Muoio D. Scoop: a 2018 acquisition paved the way for Teladoc Health's new nutrition offering. mobi health news. 2019. https://www.mobihealthnews.com/news/north-america/scoop-2018-acquisition-paved-way-teladoc-healths-new-nutrition-offering. Last accessed 19 May 2020.
30. Comstock J. Teladoc Health acquires MédecinDirect to secure French foothold. mobi health news. 2019. https://www.mobihealthnews.com/content/teladoc-health-acquires-médecindirect-secure-french-foothold. Last accessed 19 May 2020.
31. "dr. on demand" Doctor on Demand Professionals. https://www.doctorondemand.com. Last accessed 19 May 2020.
32. "MDLIVE" MDLIVE Medical Group. https://www.mdlive.com. Last accessed 19 May 2020.

33. Elliot T, Yopes MC. Direct-to-consumer telemedicine. Curr Allergy Asthma Rep. 2019;19(1) https://doi.org/10.1007/s11882-019-0837-7. Last accessed 19 May 2020.
34. Elliot VL. Telehealth and telemedicine: frequently asked questions. Congressional Research Service https://fas.org/sgp/crs/misc/R46239.pdf. Last accessed 19 May 2020.
35. Office of Health Policy, Office of the Assistant Secretary for Planning and Evaluation. August 12, 2016 Report to Congress: E-health and Telemedicine. U.S. Department of Health and Human Services. 2016. https://aspe.hhs.gov/system/files/pdf/206751/TelemedicineE-HealthReport.pdf Last accessed 19 May 2020.
36. "A Faster Pathway to Physician Licensure." Interstate Medical Licensure Compact. https://www.imlcc.org/a-faster-pathway-to-physician-licensure/. Last accessed 19 May 2020.
37. "CMS General Provider Telehealth and Telemedicine Toolkit" https://www.cms.gov/files/document/general-telemedicine-toolkit.pdf
38. "Telemedicine Service Provider Directory" https://telehealth.hhs.gov/providers/getting-started/

Open Access This chapter is licensed under the terms of the Creative Commons Attribution 4.0 International License (http://creativecommons.org/licenses/by/4.0/), which permits use, sharing, adaptation, distribution and reproduction in any medium or format, as long as you give appropriate credit to the original author(s) and the source, provide a link to the Creative Commons license and indicate if changes were made.

The images or other third party material in this chapter are included in the chapter's Creative Commons license, unless indicated otherwise in a credit line to the material. If material is not included in the chapter's Creative Commons license and your intended use is not permitted by statutory regulation or exceeds the permitted use, you will need to obtain permission directly from the copyright holder.

Telemedicine for Trauma and Emergency Care Management

18

Rifat Latifi

Introduction

Telemedicine for trauma and emergency or teletrauma care (TCC) has been in use for decades. It can be difficult to keep up with its developments. The telepresence of an expert can save the patient's life, restore the healthcare teams' confidence, and save the day. The initial experiences with teletrauma in caring for the critically ill and injured trauma patients and in reducing the overall cost of trauma care have been rewarding and successful [1]. The acceptance of teletrauma by trauma surgeons, referring physicians, nurses, and other providers, as well as by patients, has been excellent. The telepresence of trauma surgeons through the teletrauma system provides the missing segment of care in rural hospitals. Furthermore, during teletrauma sessions, experts can often identify significant knowledge gaps and the need for instituting new outreach educational programs in such hospitals. As technology becomes friendlier and cheaper, the concepts of teletrauma, telepresence, and teleresuscitation continue to evolve and to become more integrated into the modern care of trauma and surgical patients.

While telemedicine has been advocated for and used during all three phases of disaster management (pre-disaster phase, acute post-disaster phase, and post-disaster phase) [2], in this chapter we will concentrate only on trauma, burns, and emergency medicine.

R. Latifi (✉)
New York Medical College, School of Medicine, Valhalla, NY, USA

Department of Surgery, Westchester Medical Center Health, Valhalla, NY, USA
e-mail: Rifat.Latifi@wmchealth.org; Rifat_Latifi@nymc.edu

© Springer Nature Switzerland AG 2021
R. Latifi et al. (eds.), *Telemedicine, Telehealth and Telepresence*,
https://doi.org/10.1007/978-3-030-56917-4_18

A Case for Telemedicine for Trauma: Disparity in Trauma Care

Most hospitals around the world that provide care to injured patients are not "dedicated" trauma centers. Worse, most trauma centers are concentrated in major urban settings, while the rural world has little or no tools and support to provide advanced trauma care. This means that much of the population is not immediately covered by specialized trauma systems and thus is vulnerable to trauma, emergencies, and disasters. Most trauma systems are located in the cities and regions with the greatest population densities [3]. Branas et al. [4] noted that 190 level I, 255 level II, and 258 level III trauma centers are located throughout the United States (i.e., 1.5 level I and II and 2.4 level I, II, and III trauma centers per million population). Those numbers may appear impressive and certainly cover most Americans, yet 46.7 million Americans still do not have access to a trauma center within the first hour of an emergency [4]. Those uncovered Americans live mostly in rural areas and are more likely to die or become severely disabled as compared to their urban counterparts [5]. Other researchers have also reported that the more trauma centers are clustered together, fatality rates are lower. Moreover, in this study, counties without a trauma center had higher population density than counties with a trauma center (5.7% versus 1.2%, $p < 0.01$) [3].

The southwestern region of the United States has the lowest number of trauma centers. In Arizona, trauma accounts for 66% of all deaths reported in the state. Furthermore, of the 24,000 Arizonans who are severely injured each year, 40% do not reach a designated trauma center within the "golden first hour" [1]. Clearly, in rural areas, trauma access is limited; the nearest trauma center is often more than a hundred miles away. Most rural communities without specialized trauma systems have much higher morbidity and mortality rates. For example, although only 23–25% of the US population lives in rural America, 56.9% of deaths caused by motor vehicle crashes (MVCs) occur in the rural population [6]. As a result, rural patients are at a greater risk of traumatic death than urban patients [7]. In fact, patients involved in MVCs in rural America have twice the mortality rate as urban patients with the same injury severity score [7, 8]. This mortality rate represents the serious disparity in trauma care provision.

A systematic review and random effects meta-analysis of 35 studies demonstrated that uninsured patients were more likely to die than privately insured patients. Furthermore, these authors demonstrated that the African-American population was associated with higher odds of death when compared with the Caucasian population. But disparity in providing trauma care is much more pronounced in low- and middle-income countries. In a recent study, patients with geographic disparities and low-income level increased in-hospital mortality for patients with major torso trauma even in a system of healthcare insurance [9].

Many factors have been identified for this disparity in trauma care between rural and urban America. First, rural emergency rooms with low-volume trauma care often have limited experience with major trauma, lack of adequately trained personnel, and limited requirements for continuing medical education, all of which may lead to serious management errors [10–13]. Second, trauma patients in remote locations lack immediate access to subspecialty care (such as trauma surgeons, neurosurgeons, and orthopedic, vascular, or cardiac surgeons). Creating sophisticated and advanced trauma systems to cover the entire country, while desirable, is impossible and impractical.

This major disparity between urban and rural trauma care must be eliminated. If we have a sophisticated and advanced trauma teletrauma program, its applications could cover the entire spectrum of care, from the site of injury (prehospital care), to the site where the patient is seen first (the rural hospital), to the tertiary hospital or dedicated trauma center (definitive care).

Decision on the Fly and with No Data

Currently, trauma surgeons and trauma centers provide consultation over the telephone for patients in rural or community hospitals. Often, however, such advice is based on limited, if not outright wrong, information. No one knows better than trauma surgeons what we hear on a daily basis when we are consulted for a trauma patient. Of course, this depends on the training and the experience of the referring staff. Often, as receiving consultants attempt to assess the situation over the telephone with scant information, they recommend the minimum diagnostic test and transfers to trauma centers, only to find out that the description from the referring hospital was not as "advertised" or that the injuries were minor. My most memorable story was when a referring staff told one of my partners that the Glasgow Coma Scale (GCS) of a trauma patient with head trauma was 2.

Furthermore, the inability even to recognize injuries or the lack thereof often results, understandably, in their simply "playing it safe" by transferring injured patients. As a result, patients might receive no care at all at first, or preliminary poor care, before being subjected to a sometimes unnecessary and almost always expensive transport to another facility.

When teletrauma services are in place, the consultant(s) have the ability to see the patient directly, perform or witness the primary and secondary survey of the patient, view the vital signs and other medical records, and assess radiologic images when indicated. Together with the referring physician and/or other healthcare providers, telephone consultants can make the appropriate treatment decisions. However, such success can be accomplished only if small emergency rooms or other centers in rural areas have access to major trauma centers and trauma surgeons 24/7.

What Is Expected from Telemedicine for Trauma

Telemedicine for trauma and emergency *is* expected to facilitate the basic resuscitation, airway, transfusion, and other essential trauma-related procedures that ensure safe transportation of patients [2]. The initial goal of virtual management is to ensure brain protection (in cases of head injury), secure the airway, and maintain blood pressure (in all critically injured patients). While these seemingly simple procedures may be taken for granted in major trauma centers, they will prevent major morbidities and mortality. Many rural hospitals often are ill-staffed and clearly unable to care for the sickest and most injured patients. Yet, they often undergo major workups, only to be transferred to the tertiary hospitals and trauma centers. Only the most important diagnostic tests such as chest XR and pelvis XR should be done in unstable patients. Other diagnostic studies can be done based on the ability of referring centers but not in the centers where the results of these test will not change patient care in the local hospital. Above all, teletrauma helps prevent unnecessary and highly costly transportation of certain patients, lessening the economic impacts on patients, their families, and the entire healthcare system. Teletrauma supports the basic elements of safe treatment and initial evaluation. One has to realize though that for critically ill trauma patients, use of telemedicine does not decrease transfer rate [14]. Of the 9281 trauma patients, 2837 were treated in an emergency department (ED); telemedicine use did not reduce interhospital transfer. This is never the sole or main mission of telemedicine though. Those who do not need to be transferred should remain in the small hospitals. Such a finding was recently reported by our group [15].

Prehospital Telemedicine

Previously, we have described how the wireless telemedicine system that linked moving ambulances with trauma and emergency centers would facilitate and advance the care of critical trauma patients. Such a model would also help dispatch emergency resources for incident command, accident management, medical triage, and mechanical assessment of the scene for the trauma team [16]. While, this system is no longer in place, mostly due to changes in leadership and telemedicine champions, it is worth reviewing here, as it was the first system of mobile telemedicine from fire department ambulances.

The city of Tucson, the Tucson Fire Department, and the University of Arizona Medical Center trauma center deployed the ER (emergency room)-Link system that allowed physicians to be virtually present at the scene and/or in the ambulance, while a patient was being transported to the hospital ER [17]. The system provided emergency dispatchers and responders with a view of the incident scene(s), so that they could assign additional emergency resources for incident management. It ensures near-constant two-way audio-video and medical data transmissions between the attending paramedic in the ambulance and the trauma and ER medical personnel. Communication was accomplished via the regional traffic control and city communications infrastructure based on wireless technology. Telepresence at the incident scene(s) was possible by cameras mounted externally on the emergency vehicle. Those cameras, in conjunction with existing highway cameras operating along the freeway or at intersections, provide command and control video to the regional E-911 centers and emergency department. The video images facilitate the dispatch and management of emergency resources.

The key components of the ER-Link system in Tucson were the robustness of the network and the reliability of its connectivity. However, it was very complex and required constant technical support. While the program in Tucson is no longer active, we learned a great deal during this project. We were ahead of our time which is a great place to be.

Technological advances, and particularly the spread of Internet, have made it possible to connect ambulances with hospital in many countries and regions [18]. These authors conducted a retrospective analysis of all primary emergency missions with telemedicine consultations to 11 mobile ambulances and demonstrated that it is safe and technically feasible. Only 6 of 6265 patients experienced adverse events, but none were due to teleconsultations. Technical malfunctions during two-way voice communications occurred in 1.9% during two-way real-time vital data transmissions. These are exceptionally good results. Furthermore, this group reported that a total of 6.43% presented a life-threatening condition, and the majority of patients (69.08%) was treated on-site by the tele-emergency medical services (EMS) physician and subsequently transferred to a hospital. However, almost 8% (489/6265) were neither treated on-site nor transferred to the hospital. The superb results the authors report may be due to robust technical support and significant educational and checklist use [19].

The technical aspect of using cellular networks for 3G/4G networks has been greatly improved with setups that allow to increase the available bandwidth and redundancy [20]. A recent systematic review of prehospital telehealth utilization concluded despite positive trends; telehealth utilization in prehospital emergency care is fairly limited given the sheer number of EMS agencies worldwide [21].

Earlier Teletrauma Experience

The first attempt to simulate the use of telemedicine in real-time trauma resuscitation was in 1978 by Dr. R. Adams Cowley, who staged a disaster exercise at Friendship Airport in Baltimore, in an aged DC-6 aircraft, using old and cumbersome satellite technology [2].

Years later, Rogers et al. reported their use of a teletrauma service in rural Vermont where 68% of that state's population lives in rural areas [22]. Their initial experience with 41 teletrauma consultations was very encouraging. Of 41 patients seen via the teletrauma system, 31 were transferred to a tertiary care center. For 59% of the patients, transfer was recommended immediately, because of their critical condition; 41% of transfers were accomplished by helicopter. In three patients, teletrauma consultation was considered lifesaving. The most common recommendations from the teletrauma consultant concerned patient disposition; for example, for 15% of the patients, the consultant recommended keeping them at the referring facility. Other recommendations included suggestions for diagnostics (such as obtaining or foregoing a computed tomography scan) and for additional therapeutics (such as placement of a nasogastric tube, placement of a chest tube, or transfusion of blood).

Other investigators have described various applications of teletrauma in rural settings, such as the management of orthopedic injuries, including the evaluation and treatment of extremity and pelvic injuries [23–28] . In one study, 68 of 100 patients referred for teletrauma were able to remain in the rural community hospital with pelvic fractures. That outcome certainly has major cost implications, minimizing the number of costly transfers to major medical centers, increasing the use of local healthcare facilities, and avoiding the array of social and financial issues involved with treating patients away from their families [1, 29–32]. The clinical accuracy of teletrauma has also been affirmed.

Of our own first 59 patients evaluated [1], 50 (85%) came from the program's first hospital (Douglas, Arizona). Overall, 35 (59%) of the patients were treated for trauma and 24 (41%) for general surgery. Of the 35 trauma patients, 32 (91%) suffered blunt injuries; 3 (9%) suffered penetrating injuries. The most common injuries were, overwhelmingly, either orthopedic injuries or closed head injuries; several intra-abdominal and thoracic injuries also occurred.

In our series, of the 27 trauma patients transferred to the University of Arizona, 8 (30%) underwent surgery, and 19 (70%) received nonoperative care. For transferred patients, the average injury severity score was 10 (range, 1–41); the average patient age was 34.3 years (range, 1.5–80). Of the 27 transferred trauma patients, 18 (67%) were discharged home directly from the trauma room. Of the 9 (33%) admitted for inpatient treatment, 6 were discharged to long-term care facilities. The average length of stay for transferred trauma patients was 5.5 days (range, 1–30).

The telepresence of the trauma surgeon was considered lifesaving in 6 of our patients: 5 (14%) of the 35 trauma patients and 1 (4%) of the 24 general surgery patients (that 1 patient had a necrotizing soft tissue infection). A total of 17 patients (29%) were kept in the rural hospitals (8 trauma patients and 9 who underwent general surgery). Treating patients in the rural hospitals avoided transfers, saving an average of $19,698 per air transport or $2055 per ground transport. The most memorable case of teletrauma was my first case [16].

An 18-month-old girl was the only survivor of a severe car crash with three fatalities in Agua Prieta, Sonora, Mexico [16]. She was brought to Douglas Hospital in Arizona, 3 hours after the car crash, in critical condition. She was hypotensive; her oxygen saturation was at 70%; she had a Glasgow Coma Scale score of 7, multiple visible injuries to the head, and bilateral lower extremity fractures with no intravenous access. The physician on call in Douglas intubated the patient successfully, but once she was intubated, the saturation was not coming up as expected. Worse still, with each bagging, her systolic blood pressure would get lower, and her saturations would get lower as well. The chest radiography clearly demonstrated that the endotracheal tube was deep in right lower lobe. Pulling the endotracheal tube back solved the problem of saturations. Her grossly dilated stomach was decompressed with a nasogastric tube.

Getting intravenous access in shocked patients is always difficult as all the veins are collapsed. The only choice is accessing central veins, such as femoral, jugular, subclavian vein, or osseous access. In a shocked patient, femoral access is the fastest and the safest. However, this was the physician's first "femoral stick" in a child.

Using telemedicine, I guided her successfully through femoral line placement. Once she gained access, we were able to transfuse the patient with packed RBC. The arterial blood gas analysis showed severe acidosis (base deficit 10, from acute blood losses, hemoglobin 5.8 gr/dL). After the patient was placed on the helicopter for a 150 km ride, the joyful but exhausted and pale-looking physician turned to the camera, her face filling the screen, and said: "Thank you so much for being with us here today. Without you, this child would have died." I thanked her, then congratulated her and her nursing staff and all others that were involved in saving this child's life and told her that she had done great and heroic work. To this day, I remember her face and the hope in her eyes. A couple of years ago, I learned that my patient is a happy teenager now.

The University of Mississippi Medical Center reported its experience using telemedicine and the impact on trauma care. Over 5 years at that center, 814 traumatically injured patients were grouped as follows: 351 in the pre-teletrauma era and 463 in the teletrauma era. In the pre-teletrauma era, those 351 patients were transferred directly from the local community hospital for definitive care to a trauma center. In the teletrauma era, those 463 patients were the focus of virtual consultations, and 51 of them were triaged to the trauma center. The implementation of teletrauma in rural hospitals shortened patients' length of stay in local hospitals and dramatically decreased local hospitals' costs. Moreover, teletrauma significantly improved rural hospitals' evaluation and care of trauma patients. More severely injured trauma patients were identified and more rapidly transferred to the trauma center [32]. At the University of Mississippi study, 83% of the referring doctors and 61% of the trauma surgeons thought that the teletrauma consultations improved patient care. In addition, 67% of all the doctors thought that the consultations could not have been performed as well by telephone. That study demonstrated the effective use of teletrauma for consultations, for delivery of expert opinions, and for determining the need to transfer patients to the trauma center. Both patients and the referring doctors in those rural communities benefited greatly from the expertise that teletrauma made possible at a distance

Most Recent Teletrauma Results

The largest trauma telemedicine study was reported by Mohr et al. [14]. Between 2008 and 2014, authors reported a total of 9281 trauma patients seen in North Dakota Critical Access Health (CAH) EDs, of which 31% ($n = 2837$) were seen in hospitals that had an active telemedicine connection. Of those, 11% ($n = 301$) of patients had the telemedicine provider consulted by the local CAH for help with patient management or arranging interhospital transfer. Patients seen by telemedicine were transferred more (13.1% vs. 8.5%, difference = 4.6%, 95% CI = 2.3% to 6.9%). As expected, transferred patients when compared to those non-transferred had significantly more severe injuries (mean ISS = 7.8 vs. 3.7) and had more head injuries (19.2% vs. 11.4%), chest injuries (12.2% vs. 7.7%), difference = 4.5%, 95% CI = 2.2% to 6.7%, and required more resuscitative interventions (e.g., endotracheal intubation [7.6% vs. 1.1%]) and chest tube placement [1.9% vs. 0.6%]. Two most common types of injuries transferred were penetrating trauma and burn patients, which reflect the human capacities in rural North Dakota.

Another major French study, with a total of 23,710 patients, had telemedicine consultations in the region; 36% had head or spinal injuries, while 30% were used for stroke [33]. These authors report that the number of patients examined by telemedicine and admitted for head or spinal injuries also increased over the 13-year period (12% vs. 21%), while interhospital transfers were halved for both pathologies. Telemedicine networks facilitate acute-phase neurological assessment and prevent unnecessary secondary interhospital transfers. This was demonstrated by our group as well [15, 34]. A case series study of patients [34] with isolated head and spine injuries was conducted at the Department of Neurosurgery at the National Trauma Center of Tirana, in Albania, between January 2014 and December 2016 that serves the entire country via a telemedicine network. Patient demographics, associated diagnostic testing, mechanism of injury, whether the patient was transferred or was maintained for further observation in the referring hospital, length of hospital stay, and operative management and discharge status of those transferred to trauma center were included. In addition, the referring hospital, recommendations by consulting team, and the mode of teleconsultation synchronous (i.e., live), asynchronous (i.e., store and forward), or a combination of the two (i.e., live and store and forward used) were reported, as well as the date and time of each teleconsultation. In this study, the asynchronous technology (store and forward) accounted for the majority of the teleconsultations (84%), while the live plus store-and-forward technique was employed in 15% of the cases. Sixty-six percent of patients did not require transfer to the tertiary hospital. Four patients who were advised to stay in the regional hospital by the teleconsultation service were transferred to the tertiary hospital.

As in most traumas, 70% of patients who underwent teleneurotrauma consultations were males and the mean age was 43.8 years old. Nearly 32% were 60 years or older, and 16% were 15 years or younger. Nearly 88% of the patients were taken to the hospital by ground emergency medical services. Of patients transferred to the University Hospital of Trauma (tertiary hospital), 12% were transported by helicopter or emergency medical service ambulance. Of the patients seen in the regional hospitals, 76% had brain injuries and 23% had spinal injuries. Nearly 97% were blunt trauma. The most common mechanism of injury was fall from height (47%) followed by motor vehicle crashes (38%). Eleven percent of patients suffered intentional injuries. Sixty-three percent of the injuries occurred in motor vehicles, 32% at home, and 5% at the workplace. No illness other than injuries at the time of admission was reported in 97%. Of those transferred to the tertiary hospital, 71% had brain injuries and 29% had spinal injuries. Nearly 88% were blunt injuries, of which 48% were caused by fall from heights and 34% by motor vehicle crashes. Interestingly, the majority of transferred patients (91%) to tertiary trauma center underwent nonoperative treatments at the regional hospital. Of those who underwent surgery, the majority of patients (56%) were operated for fractures in 9%, thoracic injuries in 3%, craniectomy in 6%, and craniotomy in 18%. The median length of stay in the intensive care unit was 1 (0–8) day, and in the hospital, it was 2 (1–39) days.

A subsequent follow-up study (15) combined with our initial report of 146 patients reported (34), of 590 teleconsultations for neurotrauma, most patients (76%) did not require a transfer to the tertiary center, and 187 were transferred and treated locally by non-neurosurgeons [15]. Analysis by diagnosis indicated that most cases of low severity were not transferred, whereas higher severity cases were twice as likely to be transferred (P < 0.05). The mean age of patients was 43.31 years with a median of 46.5 years (range, 1–93 years); 449 patients (76.23%) were male, and 140 patients (23.77%) were female. In one patient, the sex was not recorded. A number of interesting elements came to light during the analysis of these patients.

1. *Telemedicine for trauma does not burden the trauma center.* The average number of teleconsultations was 12.5 cases per month (monthly average range, 8.5–16). Following a gradual increase during the first 2 years, the number of consultations taking place each month is now stable at 14–16 cases per month. This steady rate is indicative of the maturity and stability of the teleneurotrauma program. The maximum number of teleconsultations in a day was four cases.
2. *Most traumas happen during the daytime and does not overload the night team on call.* Of 590 teleconsultations, 417 patients were seen during regular business hours (8:00 AM–4:30 PM), and only 173 patients were seen at night and on weekends.
3. *Most suspected head and spine injury patients can be treated at local hospitals without a neurosurgeon.* Of the 590 patients with isolated head and spine injuries, only 187 were transferred to the tertiary facility (31.69%), whereas 403 were treated in the local hospital (68.31%). The mean age of transferred patients was 45.12 years, whereas the mean age of patients treated locally was 42.47 years ($P < 0.05$).

Moreover, analysis by diagnosis demonstrated that most cases with low severity (ICD-10 codes S00, S01, and S02) were not transferred (<20% referral rate), whereas cases with higher severity (in particular, S06, S07, and S09) were twice as likely to be transferred (almost 40% referral rate) ($P < 0.05$); based on these studies, we can conclude that structured and coordinated telemedicine for neurotrauma increases access to care for neurosurgery patients in countries that do not have widespread neurosurgery services.

Sustainability of Teletrauma Programs

We have previously published the requirement for a successful teletrauma program. While technology has changed dramatically, it still requires careful planning, a highly sophisticated telemedicine network, and technical support on a 24-hour basis. In addition, buy-in from each member of the multidisciplinary team is mandatory, because it represents a new paradigm for providing services.

Ongoing education on the use of any teletrauma system is extremely important. It is imperative that the staff at both the University of Arizona and the rural hospitals are trained continuously through interactive training sessions, online training modules, on-site training manuals, and a 24/7 help line. The software's design should be as intuitive as possible.

Establishing a teletrauma system has other benefits that are difficult to scientifically measure. Local physicians and nurses take comfort in knowing that they can have a trauma surgeon "present" on a moment's notice. One of the most important elements of sustaining a teletrauma program is continuous education of healthcare providers. Hands-on education of physicians and nurses in providing trauma care is a substantive advantage; everyone can learn different approaches from patient to patient. In a rural setting, such education becomes difficult, because of the high turnover in staff members. A myriad of educational programs can be done "virtually," but nothing substitutes for face-to-face interaction.

The first case in any new teletrauma program is the most important; efforts should be made to ensure it goes smoothly. As the local physicians gain experience and interact repeatedly with trauma surgeons, they master an advanced decision-making process that is directed toward endpoint resuscitation and modern techniques.

Establishing a teletrauma program is a complex process, but for injured and critically ill patients, it can potentially reduce mortality, morbidity, and cost. However, for such a program to become a sustainable part of the clinical fabric and of everyday practice, we have learned that certain requirements are essential.

The user interface of a teletrauma system needs to be addressed upfront. Nurses and physicians may find the system intimidating, even avoiding it because of its perceived complexity. A two-step training program should be developed to first introduce the basic usage of the system and then move on to its advanced features. Training should be available anytime at the request of the rural hospital and should include the information technology (IT) department at each hospital. Involving the IT department is of paramount significance for basic assistance as well as for help with troubleshooting.

In addition to solving technical difficulties, attending to several human factors is key to the success and use of a teletrauma system. First, complete buy-in from all parties involved is critical, including the doctors, nurses, and IT staff in the rural hospitals. Without this buy-in, the program will face many obstacles and challenges and much resistance. Second, a champion for teletrauma must be identified in the rural hospital, someone to act as a catalyst and a pivotal stakeholder for the system's use and implementation. Third, support and training for each site must be plentiful, positive, and continuous, allowing all staff members to be confident in their use of the system. In the training program we implemented, any of the sites could request a training session for the staff, anytime, which helped overcome the inherent fear of a new technology.

Once established, a successful teletrauma program will become an integral part of trauma care. In addition to providing state-of-the-art care to trauma patients on a moment's notice, it will mean significant cost savings for the entire medical system.

If the program is genuinely accepted by the participating hospitals, caregivers, and insurance companies, the quality of trauma patient care will be considerably enhanced. The trauma surgeons at the central location must feel fully comfortable and confident in their ability to supervise and manage trauma resuscitation in a remote site; likewise, the referring healthcare providers at the remote site must feel valued and respected as essential, well-trained members of the team. Finally, sustainability of teletrauma programs should not be left to individuals, but rather should be institutional and truly sustainable. With departing of local champions, the next leader of the trauma program or hospital may neglect it, completely.

Conclusion

Teletrauma is a major tool in trauma care and has significantly increased access to care and trauma education. Trauma resuscitation can be performed successfully and safely using telemedicine principles, when guided by and under the direct supervision of a trauma surgeon. Furthermore, major trauma centers can render direct help in primary resuscitation of trauma victims to small hospitals that do not have trauma specialists—potentially reducing costs, preventing unnecessary transfers, and promoting early transfers, when indicated, to a level I trauma center. Investments in effective technology and creation of substantial networks are needed, along with ongoing creativity and cooperation among trauma surgeons, emergency medicine physicians, and other healthcare workers striving to save and enhance the lives of trauma patients.

Finally, we can conclude that low-cost telemedicine solutions to provide structured and coordinated telemedicine for trauma are an excellent approach to ensure access to care for neurosurgery in countries that do not have widespread neurosurgery. Nearly 70% of patients do not require transfer to trauma centers and can be managed by local physicians.

References

1. Latifi R, Hadeed GJ, Rhee P, et al. Initial experiences and outcomes of telepresence in the management of trauma and emergency surgical patients. Am J Surg. 2009;198(6):905–10.
2. Latifi R, editor. Telemedicine for trauma, emergencies, and disaster management. Boston: Artech House; 2011.
3. Brown JB, Rosengart MR, Billiar TR, Peitzman AB, Sperry JL. Geographic distribution of trauma centers and injury-related mortality in the United States. J Trauma Acute Care Surg. 2016;80(1):42–9; discussion 49–50.
4. Branas CC, MacKenzie EJ, Williams JC, et al. Access to trauma centers in the United States. JAMA. 2005;293(21):2626–33.
5. Rural americans at higher risk of death from five leading causes. CDC Web site. Published January 12, 2017. Updated 2017.
6. Murdock D. Trauma: when there's no time to count. AORN J. 2008;87(2):322–8.
7. Jarman MP, Castillo RC, Carlini AR, Kodadek LM, Haider AH. Rural risk: geographic disparities in trauma mortality. Surgery. 2016;160(6):1551–9.

8. Voelker R. Access to trauma care. JAMA. 2000;284(16):2048.
9. Kuo LW, Fu CY, Liao CA, et al. Inequality of trauma care under a single-payer universal coverage system in Taiwan: a nationwide cohort study from the national health insurance research database. BMJ Open. 2019;9(11):e032062-2019-032062.
10. Ricci MA, Caputo M, Amour J, et al. Telemedicine reduces discrepancies in rural trauma care. Telemed J E Health. 2003;9(1):3–11.
11. Baker SP, Whitfield RA, O'Neill B. Geographic variations in mortality from motor vehicle crashes. N Engl J Med. 1987;316(22):1384–7.
12. Flowe KM, Cunningham PR, Foil MB. Rural trauma. Systems in evolution. Surg Annu. 1995;27:29–39.
13. Rogers FB, Ricci M, Caputo M, et al. The use of telemedicine for real-time video consultation between trauma center and community hospital in a rural setting improves early trauma care: preliminary results. J Trauma. 2001;51(6):1037–41.
14. Mohr NM, Harland KK, Chrischilles EA, Bell A, Shane DM, Ward MM. Emergency department telemedicine is used for more severely injured rural trauma patients, but does not decrease transfer: a cohort study. Acad Emerg Med. 2017;24(2):177–85.
15. Olldashi F, Latifi R, Parsikia A, et al. Telemedicine for neurotrauma prevents unnecessary transfers: an update from a nationwide program in Albania and analysis of 590 patients. World Neurosurg. 2019;128:e340–6.
16. Latifi R, Weinstein RS, Porter JM, et al. Telemedicine and telepresence for trauma and emergency care management. Scand J Surg. 2007;96(4):281–9.
17. Latifi R, Peck K, Porter J, Poropatich R, Geare T III, Nassi R. Telepresence and telementoring in trauma and emergency care management. In: Establishing telemedicine in developing countries: from inception to implementation. Amsterdam: IOS Press; 2004. p. 193–9.
18. Felzen M, Beckers SK, Kork F, et al. Utilization, safety, and technical performance of a telemedicine system for prehospital emergency care: observational study. J Med Internet Res. 2019;21(10):e14907.
19. Kerner T, Schmidbauer W, Tietz M, Marung H, Genzwuerker HV. Use of checklists improves the quality and safety of prehospital emergency care. Eur J Emerg Med. 2017;24(2):114–9.
20. Johansson A, Esbjornsson M, Nordqvist P, et al. Dataset on multichannel connectivity and video transmission carried on commercial 3G/4G networks in southern Sweden. Data Brief. 2019;25:104192.
21. Winburn AS, Brixey JJ, Langabeer J 2nd, Champagne-Langabeer T. A systematic review of prehospital telehealth utilization. J Telemed Telecare. 2018;24(7):473–81.
22. Rogers FB, Shackford SR, Osler TM, Vane DW, Davis JH. Rural trauma: the challenge for the next decade. J Trauma. 1999;47(4):802–21.
23. Aucar J, Granchi T, Liscum K, Wall M, Mattox K. Is regionalization of trauma care using telemedicine feasible and desirable? Am J Surg. 2000;180(6):535–9.
24. Corr P, Couper I, Beningfield SJ, Mars M. A simple telemedicine system using a digital camera. J Telemed Telecare. 2000;6(4):233–6.
25. Lambrecht CJ. Telemedicine in trauma care: description of 100 trauma teleconsults. Telemed J. 1997;3(4):265–8.
26. Tachakra S, Lynch M, Newson R, et al. A comparison of telemedicine with face-to-face consultations for trauma management. J Telemed Telecare. 2000;6 Suppl 1:S178–81.
27. Wirthlin DJ, Buradagunta S, Edwards RA, et al. Telemedicine in vascular surgery: feasibility of digital imaging for remote management of wounds. J Vasc Surg. 1998;27(6):1089–99; discussion 1099–100.
28. Tachakra S, Jaye P, Bak J, Hayes J, Sivakumar A. Supervising trauma life support by telemedicine. J Telemed Telecare. 2000;6 Suppl 1:S7–11.
29. Boulanger B, Kearney P, Ochoa J, Tsuei B, Sands F. Telemedicine: a solution to the followup of rural trauma patients? J Am Coll Surg. 2001;192(4):447–52.
30. Smith RS. Telemedicine and trauma care. South Med J. 2001;94(8):825–9.
31. Redlick F, Roston B, Gomez M, Fish JS. An initial experience with telemedicine in follow-up burn care. J Burn Care Rehabil. 2002;23(2):110–5.

32. Duchesne JC, Kyle A, Simmons J, et al. Impact of telemedicine upon rural trauma care. J Trauma. 2008;64(1):92–7; discussion 97–8.
33. Medeiros de Bustos E, Berthier E, Chavot D, Bouamra B, Moulin T. Evaluation of a french regional telemedicine network dedicated to neurological emergencies: a 14-year study. Telemed J E Health. 2018;24(2):155–60.
34. Latifi R, Olldashi F, Dogjani A, Dasho E, Boci A, El-Menyar A. Telemedicine for neurotrauma in Albania: initial results from case series of 146 patients. World Neurosurg. 2018;112:e747–53.

Telemedicine for Burn Care: The Commonsense Telemedicine

Dylan Stewart, Joseph R. Turkowski, and Rifat Latifi

Introduction

The use of telemedicine for burn care seems simply intuitive. Burn assessment has a highly visual component, providers with burn expertise are highly concentrated, and technological capability is expanding. No other surgical discipline would seem more amenable to the use of telemedicine than modern burn care. Through telemedicine, burn surgeons should be able to make a relatively accurate assessment of burn size and depth and help guide decisions regarding referral to a burn center and utilization of costly transport resources. Surgeons can also assist remotely with the acute phase of burn critical care management. The postoperative management of major burns and the chronic wound management of less serious, nonoperative burns also can have a highly efficient telemedicine component. In this chapter we will concentrate on the current status of telemedicine in burn management.

Burns continue to be a major cause of mortality and morbidity worldwide, particularly in developing countries. According to the World Health Organization (WHO), almost 200,000 thermal injury-related deaths occur each year worldwide [1]. An astounding 96% of the deaths resulting from fire occur in low-income and low middle-income countries (LIC and LMIC) [1–4]. In addition to the mortalities, millions of people suffer from nonfatal burn injuries with significant morbidity that

---

D. Stewart (✉)
Westchester Medical Center and Maria Fareri Children's Hospital, Valhalla, NY, USA

New York Medical College, School of Medicine, Valhalla, NY, USA
e-mail: Dylan.Stewart@wmchealth.org

J. R. Turkowski
Department of Surgery, Westchester Medical Center Health, Valhalla, NY, USA

R. Latifi
Department of Surgery, Westchester Medical Center Health, Valhalla, NY, USA

New York Medical College, School of Medicine, Valhalla, NY, USA

© Springer Nature Switzerland AG 2021
R. Latifi et al. (eds.), *Telemedicine, Telehealth and Telepresence*,
https://doi.org/10.1007/978-3-030-56917-4_19

often are devastating [1]. For example, in India, over one million people are moderately or severely burned every year. In Bangladesh, 173,000 children are moderately or severely burned every year. Furthermore, in Bangladesh, Colombia, Egypt, and Pakistan, 17% of children with burns have a temporary disability, and 18% have a permanent disability. Burns are the second most common injury in rural Nepal, accounting for 5% of disabilities [1]. Burns are not only a problem in developing countries. In 2011, over 486,000 burn injuries occurred in the United States (US) with approximately 40,000 requiring hospitalization [2].

Not only do burns have high morbidity and mortality rates, but they also inflict high economic damage. In the USA alone, estimated medical costs associated with burn care approximated $1.5 billion in 2010 [3]. Indirect costs, such as days lost at work, totaled another $5 billion [3]. These lost wages, coupled with commitment of family resources and extended wound care burden, contribute to the devastating impact that burns have on the lives of individuals. The WHO has created the burn prevention and services report that documents several prevention and rehabilitation strategies that can be used to circumvent the problems associated with burn care [4]. One specific problem with the treatment of burns is providing adequate wound management in LIC and LMIC [1]. An individual who has suffered from a moderate and survivable burn is at much higher risk in a LIC or LMIC. An individual in a high-income country with the same sort of burn would receive adequate post-injury treatment. This problem is due to inadequate resources to provide burn care in remote and/or poor regions and has great potential for improvement with telemedicine.

Even in the USA, geography can be challenging. Although the number of yearly burns in the USA has declined significantly since the 1970s, the number of burn centers has declined as well [2]. This has created serious geographical gaps in providing access to burn care. Only 69% of the US population lives within 4 hours from a verified burn center [5]. For the geographical area, encompassing much of upstate New York and eastern Pennsylvania, there are only three burn centers that are hundreds of miles away from one another. This disparity of burns centers leaves large portions of the rural population in New York with no immediate access to burn care. In remote and poor environments, without telemedicine, the intensive management and monitoring that burn care requires are not possible. Telemedicine provides a unique opportunity to monitor and provide teleconsultation for wound and burn management. The goal of this chapter is to discuss current successful telemedicine initiatives for burn care and to provide practical guidance for establishing successful burn and wound care telemedicine programs.

Opportunities for Telemedicine in Burn Care

Greatly improved survival and enhanced outcomes for patients treated at modern highly specialized burn centers are undisputed. With the impressive success of improving prevention strategies and public awareness, burn incidence in general has steadily declined in many countries, triggering a decrease in the number of active burn centers.

Subsequently, the expertise needed to obtain favorable outcomes has become increasingly centralized within a diminishing number of centers of excellence. Burn centers are covering ever-larger referral areas. They are routinely running at or near capacity and are facing mounting financial challenges [6]. In parallel, access to specialized burn care has become more difficult, being restricted by distance and resources for many people known to suffer increased risks of burn injuries and mortality and living in poverty or in rural medically underserved communities [7, 8].

Whenever a burn patient reaches a local hospital, physicians on-site may have limited familiarity with burn treatment. Under such circumstances, assessment and treatment in consultation with a remote burn specialist using telemedicine technology become highly valuable [6, 7].

Instant visual communication together with electronic exchange of interactive video, digital photography, medical information, and electronic health records extends the expertise of burn centers to peripheral hospitals with limited or no access to specialized burn care [6, 7]. Assessment of transmitted digital images by a specialist may lead to significantly different courses of burn care, including appropriately deferring intubation, significantly changing fluid resuscitation rates, changing the route and timing of referral, and avoiding over-triage and unnecessary transfer of patients over long distances [7].

Telemedicine for burns has made it possible for the patients to access specialists and receive healthcare services even when there is a limited financial resource; therefore, by this technology, distance loses its importance [8].

The use of telemedicine for wound and burn care, while prevalent to an extent, has not been used as extensively as it has for other areas of medicine, such as intensive care; however many studies have documented the usefulness of telemedicine in burn and wound care [9–11]. For example, Saffle et al. [10] conducted a comparison trial of burn patients, 80 of whom used telemedicine services and 28 of whom used traditional services, and found that telemedicine was an effective way to treat burn patients. With the rapid increase in technological advances, it is important to ensure that digital images are accurate and provide a clear representation of the actual wound. Ong has provided a list of recommended methods for remote wound assessment using digital images [12].

As the utility of telemedicine continues to gain adherence and acceptance, several aspects of its use specifically to the care of burn patients deserve special attention.

Burn Size and Severity Assessment

A number of studies revealed a significant difference between the experienced and inexperienced physicians when estimating the burn size [13–15]. Incorrect assessment may lead to invalid decisions that increase healthcare expenses and decrease the quality of healthcare services [9, 13, 16]. Unnecessary fluid resuscitation [9], unnecessary endotracheal intubation, and both under- and over-triage decisions about transferring the patient to specialized burn centers are among inappropriate decisions that are caused by inaccurate assessment and diagnosis [17].

According to a study conducted in the USA, the estimation of the burn size made by the referring physicians was about 6% more than the burn size assessment by the specialists. Estimation of the burn size according to the total body surface area (TBSA) index was higher in 30% of the cases and lower than normal in 13% of the cases [9]. Moreover, up to 29% of patient transfers were found unnecessary, and their referral was found to waste valuable resources [16]. Due to the visual nature of burn injuries and the possibility of external observations, it is possible to use imaging techniques to assess and diagnose burn injuries [14, 18]. Numerous studies demonstrated that the results of burn size estimation and assessment through imaging techniques and telemedicine are very close to the results of the face-to-face assessments and diagnosis [19, 20]. Various findings indicated that using telemedicine to assess and diagnose burn injuries results in saving time and money, increasing productivity, reducing unnecessary referrals, and choosing the right and most efficient method for patient transfer.

Consequently, it can improve the overall quality of healthcare services and patient care management [14, 16–18, 21]. Roa et al. performed a study to evaluate the quality and density of burn patients' digital images to use it in telemedicine applications. They reported that digital images are economical and easily transferable, and obtaining these images did not cause tension nor anxiety in the patients. They also demonstrated that diagnoses made based on these images were highly valid and that digital photography could be used as an efficient and appropriate method to diagnose burn injuries [19, 22].

Numerous imaging tools have been introduced for burn clinical diagnosis; however, the use of these tools outside the specialized burn centers is limited due to their cost [14]. As a result, low-cost tools such as mobile phones are preferable. To have a preliminary assessment and diagnosis of burns, Shokrollahi et al. evaluated the use of mobile phones for digital photography in telemedicine [14]. The results of this study revealed that the low cost, lack of need for specific infrastructure or training, and transferring images without losing quality were among the benefits of using this device. The usability of this method has been proven for minor burn injuries. However, the screen resolution of mobile phones is as important as its camera quality. In addition, privacy concerns and medicolegal aspects are other issues that must be taken into account when using mobile phones [14, 19].

Other methods for transferring digital images include e-mail, instant photo sharing using the Internet infrastructure, and videoconferencing [16]. Simons noted that the main difficulties of digital imaging in telemedicine technology are related to a lack of access to the thickness, flexibility, and swelling of the wounds [23]. The high likelihood of telemedicine inaccessibility during natural or man-made disasters is another problem of this technology [18]. It is worth mentioning that despite the weaknesses noted above, the use of telemedicine for different purposes is increasing in the specialized burn centers [21], and it has been suggested that wound digital imaging would be a substantial part of telemedicine in the future.

Over- and Under-Triage

Unfortunately, errors in estimation of burn size and severity, particularly by nonspecialist inexperienced clinicians, are commonplace; patients are often transferred to burn centers with overestimation of burn size or severity, excessive or inadequate fluid resuscitation, and airway support that at times is deemed inappropriate [10, 24–27]. Evaluation is becoming even more difficult with the decreasing familiarity of most physicians with burn treatment and the widening gap in expertise between burn centers and many smaller, particularly rural, hospitals. Telemedicine for initial burn assessment, one of the most important factors determining the path of burn care, has been demonstrated to improve accuracy of triage as well as initial fluid resuscitation, allowing correct evaluation of burn victims by determining the urgency and need for transfer to a specialized burn center and avoiding unnecessary costs [17, 25, 28–32].

At present, fewer and fewer local physicians have any familiarity with burn care and out of caution may needlessly send minor burns to specialized centers for care [10, 31]. Most burns, however, can be treated at local general hospitals, while few require the highly specialized care of a burn center [31]. With fewer burn centers servicing larger catchment areas, unnecessary referrals might not only overwhelm system resources but are also time and resource demanding [13, 31]. Even though collaboration between a burn center and a rural primary care trauma center is a controversial concept and may seem to flout the dogma of providing burn care only at specialized centers, telemedicine may allow less-experienced surgeons to treat and follow-up those patients more appropriately [28, 29, 33].

By reducing the incidence of over-triage and transporting only those patients who truly require specialized care, resources can be better spent and used when truly needed, which may also reduce costs [13, 31, 34]. Cost analysis studies have also demonstrated savings by decreasing the likelihood of inconvenient and prolonged unnecessary referrals, particularly when aeromedical transport is required. However, economic benefits in smaller nations and for centers with small catchment areas are less clear [10, 13, 28, 29, 31, 33].

Adequacy of Virtual Examination of Burn Injuries at a Distance

Extent and depth of the burn injury are mainly assessed by visual inspection. These factors are very important for selecting the most appropriate type of emergency treatment required, as well as the place and method for the patient's disposition [11, 22]. In the absence of a skilled burn specialist, a transmitted picture of the injury is worth a thousand words. Technological advances from analogue to digital images have rendered documentation of the visible external nature of burn injuries appropriate and extremely reliable [11].

Transmission of digital images for the remote diagnosis of burn injuries has been advocated as early as 1999 [11]. Since that time, visual communications with digital technology has progressed tremendously. Today, digital images, whether static or in motion, form a major part of a great variety of modern communication systems. Since digital technology allows near instantaneous transmission of images through an information network from a referring hospital to a remote specialized tertiary center, telemedicine has emerged as a modality of particular value in conditions for which assessment is primarily a visual skill [18, 20, 22]. To expedite clinical decision-making without reliance on oral descriptions given over the phone, digital images are well suited for evaluation by either synchronous ("interactive") video-conferencing or asynchronous (store and forward,) imagery, with much greater confidence [16, 25, 31]. Images can be stored, reviewed, and accessed from any computer terminal allowing senior input to be obtained for immediate advice on management.

Avoiding Unnecessary Intubations

With the emphasis on the airway, breathing, and circulation (ABC) in advanced trauma life support and the advanced burn life support recommendation to have a low threshold for intubation of patients with facial burns, there has been an increase in the number of patients arriving to burn units intubated.

In contrast, previously, patients had a lower rate of intubation: in a study of 740 patients admitted to a single burn unit between 1972 and 1975, no patient arrived intubated [24]. Thirty-six patients in this study required intubation on arrival at the burn center. In contrast, a study conducted at a regional burn center between 2000 and 2003 revealed that 26% arrived intubated [34]. Although the concerns about airway edema and losing the ability to intubate a patient with burns are real, intubation is not a risk-free procedure. Risks of intubation include difficulty or inability to intubate, accidental extubation, atelectasis, pneumothorax, nosocomial infection, tracheal injury, and death.

Most of the decisions on whether burn patient should be intubated are often made before the patient arrives at the burn center and in some cases before the patient arrives at a non-burn center hospital. Often the people making these decisions have little training in burns and limited experience in making critical airway decisions in burn patients. The removal of mandatory burn training from surgery residency programs only serves to compound the problem. We as a burn community need to provide guidance to these pre-burn center caregivers to minimize unnecessary intubations, while protecting patients who legitimately need early intubation to protect their airway.

A study of 111 patients who were intubated and transported more than 90 miles to a regional burn center found that 53.1% of patients were able to be extubated in the first 24 hours and 64.8% were extubated by hospital day 2 [35].

Romanowski et al. hypothesized that many intubations performed before burn center transport are unnecessary. They conducted a retrospective review of all adults who were intubated before burn transfer and survived to discharge from August 2003 to June 2013. Intubations that had 2 or fewer ventilator days (i.e., potentially unnecessary intubations) were compared with those lasting longer than 2 days. Data collected included age, ventilator days, length of stay, % TBSA burn, % second degree, % third degree, % second-degree face burn, % third-degree face burn, and origin of burns. A total of 416 patient met inclusion criteria. Of these, 129 patients (31.0%) were intubated less than or equal to 1 day, and a total of 171 (40.1%) patients remained intubated for less than or equal to 2 days [36]. The authors concluded that many unnecessary intubations could expose burn patients to serious complications, and they proposed guidelines for intubation in the pre-burn center setting. It is incumbent for burn physicians to guide these decisions with the goal of keeping patients safe, while avoiding unnecessary intubations. Although there is no current published data, it seems extremely likely that with the guidance afforded by telemedicine, it would be possible to significantly lower the number of unnecessary intubations.

Overusage of Aeromedical Transport

In recent years, widespread support for regional trauma systems has led to increased use of aeromedical transport of patients. However, the real benefits of air transport for trauma and burn patients remain poorly defined. Saffle et al. reviewed all burn patients transported by air during 2000 to 2001 [13]. Each patient was classified as being most appropriate for air, ground, or family transport. In addition, a decision was made regarding whether telemedicine evaluation of the patient before transport could have significantly altered initial treatment decisions. In the study, 225 acutely burned patients were transferred from referring hospitals in 9 states, at a mean distance of 246 air miles. Mean burn size calculated by burn center physicians was 19.7% total body surface area, whereas referring physicians' mean estimate was 29% total body surface area. In 92 cases, over- or underestimation of burn size by referring physicians of as much as 560% or decisions regarding performance of endotracheal intubation suggested that telemedicine evaluation before transport might have significantly altered transport decisions or care. Air transport charges exceeded hospital charges in 21 cases. The authors concluded that frequent discrepancies in burn assessment contribute to overuse of air transport. The ability to evaluate burn patients by telemedicine may have the potential to assist decisions regarding transfer, avoid errors in initial care, and reduce costs [13].

Roman et al. conducted a 5-year retrospective analysis of patients transported by helicopter EMS (HEMS) and ground transport (EMS). They found that within the cohort transported by HEMS, 53% of patients suffered smaller burns, compared with 73% transported by EMS, and that 1/4 of those transported via HEMS with smaller burns were discharged from the ED after burn consultation, debridement, and dressing. The average cost per helicopter transport was US$29 K. They concluded that accurate triage and burn center consultation before scene transport or hospital transfer could help identify patients not benefiting from HEMS yet safely transferrable by ground, or better served by early clinic follow-up, which would reduce cost without compromising care in this cohort [37].

Telemedicine for Pediatric Burn Care

Centers adept and capable for providing pediatric burn care are even more scarce, despite the high disease burden of burn in the pediatric population, especially children under 5 years of age [2]. The costs associated with pediatric burn care are high [38], and the avoidance of unnecessary admission could have significant cost savings and more efficient use of burn center resources. Though costs associated with inpatient pediatric burn care are high, outpatient care comes with significant costs as well. Nearly 90% of children with burns are treated as outpatients [2], but this treatment may involve multiple visits for dressing changes, with the potential need for long distance travel and the burden of missed days of both school and work. Telemedicine for pediatric burn care would be expected to have all the same advantages as for adult burn care, with perhaps an even greater opportunity to prevent over-triage and provide cost savings. Despite these possible advantages, there is a paucity of literature examining the deployment of telemedicine in this setting. McWilliams et al. describe extensive experience with a pediatric telehealth program in rural Western Australia [39]. A retrospective examination of their data over a period from 2005 to 2013 showed that with over 4000 telehealth burn reviews, 364 transfers to the regional pediatric burn center were avoided, 4905 hospital days were saved, and in 1 year alone over AUD 1.8 million was saved. An important addition to the authors clinical burn review was a regional education program for rural providers, offered over the same telehealth network [39]. Integration of both clinical and educational programs seems to be a very novel idea with excellent potential for both sustaining and improving a telemedicine burn effort.

Another excellent initiative in pediatric burn telemedicine was reported by Garcia et al. [40]. They formed a multidisciplinary team to create a smartphone application that was offered to parents at the first emergency department or clinical visit. Smartphone savvy parents were then able to communicate in almost real time with pediatric burn experts, without the lag time associated with weekly or biweekly clinic visits, which allowed the study to document faster wound healing times. The authors also suggest that given the ubiquitous nature of smartphones, using this technology rather than a "hub and spoke" model of telemedicine will have more widespread applicability [40].

Pediatric burn telemedicine is likely to continue to expand, given many of its obvious advantages. Burn center with combined adult and pediatric populations should design their telemedicine programs to fit the needs of both patient cohorts.

Outpatient Burn Telemedicine

In the outpatient long-term follow-up and burn rehabilitation phase, telemedicine consultation service using digital imaging provides cost-effective valuable advice which is especially valuable for patients who live great distances from the burn center, as telemedicine eliminates the inconvenience and costs of frequent and difficult journeys by the patient to the specialized center. It may also be used for consultation and advice about limited burn injuries [21, 25, 30, 33]. Yoder et al. found that patients were satisfied with the use of videophone technology for follow-up burn care treatment [41]. Yoder's study utilized commercial-off-the-shelf (COTS) technology that worked in conjunction with the home phone lines of patients. This is one example of an inexpensive and convenient way to use telemedicine, in areas that provide land telephone line service. In areas where landlines are not available, mobile technology may be more convenient. For example, Knoblich et al. describe using a Nokia cell phone to obtain images of a burn victims wounds for follow-up treatment [11].

Global Efforts for Burn Telemedicine

Whereas telemedicine may have the greatest potential for improving the lives of people in developing countries, it is in this setting that the greatest challenges are encountered. The major difficulty in providing effective wound care in LICs and LMICs is that many of these countries do not often have the infrastructure to provide videophone or even mobile phone services; however, many of these countries are beginning to acquire access to these technologies. The World Health Organization has worked with many of its member states to create the infrastructure that is needed to provide effective telemedicine options [42]. The implementation of successful telemedicine programs is an ongoing global effort.

The Grossman Burn Foundation established the first telemedicine burn treatment center in Indonesia [43]. This treatment center is located in Kusuri, Indonesia, a LMIC with a gross national income per capita of $3420 [44]. Women in Southeast Asia have the highest rate of burn deaths in the world, accounting for 27% of global burn deaths [4]. They have the highest rates of burn deaths in the region, accounting for 70% of burn deaths [4]. The Grossman Foundation has collaborated with several international partners to provide effective solutions for burn and wound management. These solutions include telemedicine. The Grossman Foundation telemedicine center in Indonesia trained local doctors to use the equipment which will be housed at the facility in Indonesia and serves as a prime example of a successful effort in a challenged locale.

Principles for Establishing a Burn Telemedicine Program

The ideal teleburn unit should be an integral part of a modern burn center. The American Telemedicine Association (ATA) has published guidelines for telemedicine in burns. These guidelines include in-depth coverage of every aspect of a teleburn center, including administrative requirements for telemedicine networks; human resources management; privacy and confidentiality; federal, state, and other credentialing and regulatory agency requirements; fiscal management; ownership of patient records; patient rights and responsibilities; documentation protocols; network security; equipment use; and research protocols [45].

Policies and Protocols/Agreement Required

With each policy and protocol, all personnel, contractors, and members of a clinical medicine group will need to complete appropriate credentialing that includes security policies, personnel policies, and technical policies that ensure the confidentiality and integrity of data are maintained. Inclusion of local legal policies is necessary in these agreements.

Technical Requirements

The ATA has published a list of technical standards as well [46]. While live consultations are very important, store and forward can be very useful in burn management. For live consultations, technical requirements include high-quality network communications. Data communication networks can include local area networks (LAN) that interconnects hosts in small areas such as a building; small office/home office (SOHO) networks, which is similar to a LAN but has less hosts; metropolitan area network (MAN) which connects multiple sites; or a wide area network (WAN), which interconnects multiple sites over long distances [47]. Another form of connectivity is that of T-carrier lines. T-carrier lines are high-speed digital network transport services that support both voice and data transmission. Recent advances in satellite technology allow for portable satellite applications. Broadband global area network (BGAN) is one example of portable satellite applications. It uses a compact, portable satellite terminal that is easy to set up and use. The International Telecommunication Union (ITU) has also defined several standards for videoconferencing equipment [48, 49]. Videoconferencing can be used for educational purposes, consultation following surgery, surgical telementoring, trauma and emergency medicine situations, and discussion among multidisciplinary teams.

How to Perform Teleconsultations

Most burn centers receive patients from the medical centers of the area or region. Some of these centers take patients from across the international borders as well.

Having in place protocols and agreements regarding how to conduct consultation for burns is an important aspect for a smooth and coordinated care. As we have described in the previous chapters, there are guidelines in place for any staff members performing teleconsultation [50]. First, privacy and confidentiality should be taken into account; therefore, the location should be in a small room dedicated to providing teleconsultation services. Privacy must be ensured by either locking the door or placing a "Do Not Disturb" notice on the door. While the normal teleconsultation office may be set up much like a standard clinical space, telemedicine for burns may be done from the trauma and resuscitation units in the emergency department or on occasion from the scene itself. Nonetheless, care should be provided to ensure privacy both for the referring physicians and patients during the consultation process. ATA clinical guidelines to provide telemedicine for burn have been designed to cover every aspect of burn, and the recommendations are categorized by the character of the burn injury [45]:

1. Acute burns – major systems with a high burn percentage.
2. Acute burns – small single burn with low-percentage coverage.
3. Follow-up visits.

Other aspects of the teleburn guidelines include technical guidelines and communication, image acquisition, videoconference, data storage, and others elements. While principles of telemedicine for burns remain unchanged, some of these technical aspects of practice evolve with technical development.

Referring the Patient for Consultation

As alluded above, protocols and agreements detailing how and when to conduct consultation for burns are an important aspect for a smooth and coordinated care. Ideally, verified burn centers will maintain written agreements with hospitals that refer patients for further treatment to a burn center regarding the usage of a telemedicine consult.

Billing and Documentation

The rules for billing for services apply to all telemedicine consultations and should be regulated between the institutions, providers, and insurance companies. Documentation must be solid and should become a permanent part of the medical records as in all telemedicine consultations.

Saving the Data

Data security and accessibility are essential to a successful telemedicine program [24]. Several protocols should be established for saving and use of data. These protocols include authentication, encryption, access control, integrity, confidentiality, auditing and accounting system, and security policy. User control has to be established for every stage of access to the system. Encryption, or scrambling transmission of data, should be carried out using a "behind the scenes" algorithm or program. A policy that is strictly adhered to that incorporates effective procedures to maintain confidentiality, data integrity, and security should be established.

Reporting the Data

When reporting the data, all rules regarding confidentiality and security of the data are paramount.

Summary and Recommendation

The implementation of successful telemedicine programs for burn care has been slow [6]. The use of store-and-forward programs to transmit digital images for wound and burn monitoring [23] has been shown to be effective. The use of videophones [9] has also been shown to be effective for monitoring of burn and wound patients. Even a web-based wound-monitoring program has been established to provide a platform to assess multiple data [24]. However, establishing these sorts of programs in LICs and LMICs, where effective tele-wound care is needed for populations living in remote or high-poverty areas, will be more difficult. With the help of the World Health Organization and foundations such as International Virtual e-Hospital [25] and the Grossman Burn Foundation [4], establishing successful tele-wound programs is more likely to occur in developing countries. The ATA provides clear guidelines to help burn centers develop this exciting resource.

References

1. World Health Organization Burns Fact Sheet [Internet]. [cited Accessed on February 6 2014]. Available from: http://www.who.int/mediacentre/factsheets/fs365/en/index.html.
2. Burn Incidence Fact Sheet [Internet]. [cited Accessed 20 march 2020]. Available from: http://ameriburn.org/who-we-are/media/burn-incidence-fact-sheet/.
3. Burn-Related Hospital Inpatient Stays and Emergency Department Visits, 2013 [Internet]. [cited 20 March 2020]. Available from: https://www.hcup-us.ahrq.gov/reports/statbriefs/sb217-Burn-Hospital-Stays-ED-Visits-2013.pdf.
4. World Health Organization. A WHO Plan for Burn Prevention and Care [Internet]. [cited February 6, 2014]. Available from: http://whqlibdoc.who.int/publications/2008/9789241596299_eng.pdf?ua=1.
5. Klein MB, Kramer CB, Nelson J, Rivara FP, Gibran NS, Concannon T. Geographic access to burn center hospitals. JAMA. 2009;302(16):1774–81.
6. Duchesne JC, Kyle A, Simmons J, Islam S, Schmieg RE, Olivier J, et al. Impact of telemedicine upon rural trauma care. J Trauma. 2008;64(1):92–8.
7. Hoseini F, Ayatollahi H, Salehi SH. systematized review of telemedicine applications in treating burn patients. Med J Islam Repub Iran. 2016;30:459.
8. Nguyen LT, Massman NJ, Franzen BJ, Ahrenholz DH, Sorensen NW, Mohr WJ, et al. Telemedicine follow-up of burns: lessons learned from the first thousand visits. J Burn Care Rehabil. 2004;25(6):485–90.

9. Massman NJ, Dodge JD, Fortman KK, Schwartz KJ, Solem LD. Burns follow-up: an innovative application of telemedicine. J Telemed Telecare. 1999;5 Suppl 1:52.
10. Saffle JR. Telemedicine for acute burn treatment: the time has come. J Telemed Telecare. 2006;12(1):1–3.
11. Knobloch K, Rennekampff H, Vogt PM. Cell-phone based multimedia messaging service (MMS) and burn injuries. Burns. 2009;35(8):1191–3.
12. Ong CA. Telemedicine and wound care. Stud Health Technol Inform. 2008;131:211–25.
13. Saffle JR, Edelman L, Morris SE. Regional air transport of burn patients: a case for telemedicine? J Trauma. 2004;57(1):57,64; discussion 64.
14. Shokrollahi K, Sayed M, Dickson W, Potokar T. Mobile phones for the assessment of burns: we have the technology. Emerg Med J. 2007;24(11):753–5.
15. Onyekwelu O, Dheansa B. Response to the systematic review of the evidence for telemedicine in burn care: with a UK perspective. Burns. 2013;39(3):532–3.
16. Jones OC, Wilson DI, Andrews S. The reliability of digital images when used to assess burn wounds. J Telemed Telecare. 2003;9 Suppl 1:22.
17. Smith AC, Kimble R, Mill J, Bailey D, O'Rourke P, Wootton R. Diagnostic accuracy of and patient satisfaction with telemedicine for the follow-up of paediatric burns patients. J Telemed Telecare. 2004;10(4):193–8.
18. Gardiner S, Hartzell TL. Telemedicine and plastic surgery: a review of its applications, limitations and legal pitfalls. J Plast Reconstr Aesthet Surg. 2012;65(3):47.
19. Neild TO, Davey RB. Skin colour in digital images. Burns. 2001;27(3):297–8.
20. Wallace DL, Jones SM, Milroy C, Pickford MA. Telemedicine for acute plastic surgical trauma and burns. J Plast Reconstr Aesthet Surg. 2008;61(1):31–6.
21. Redlick F, Roston B, Gomez M, Fish JS. An initial experience with telemedicine in follow-up burn care. J Burn Care Rehabil. 2002;23(2):110–5.
22. Roa L, Gómez-Cía T, Acha B, Serrano C. Digital imaging in remote diagnosis of burns. Burns. 1999;25(7):617–23.
23. Simons M, Tyack Z. Health professionals' and consumers' opinion: what is considered important when rating burn scars from photographs? J Burn Care Res. 2011;32(2):275–85.
24. Saffle JR, Edelman L, Theurer L, Morris SE, Cochran A. Telemedicine evaluation of acute burns is accurate and cost-effective. J Trauma. 2009;67(2):358–65.
25. Holt B, Faraklas I, Theurer L, Cochran A, Saffle JR. Telemedicine use among burn centers in the United States: a survey. J Burn Care Res. 2012 Jan-Feb;33(1):157–62.
26. Collis N, Smith G, Fenton OM. Accuracy of burn size estimation and subsequent fluid resuscitation prior to arrival at the Yorkshire Regional Burns Unit. A three year retrospective study. Burns. 1999;25(4):345–51.
27. Atiyeh BS, Gunn SW, Hayek SN. State of the art in burn treatment. World J Surg. 2005;29(2):131–48.
28. Dunne JA, Rawlins JM. A systematic review of telemedicine in burn care [Internet]. [cited 20 March 2020]. Available from: http://www.cdesign.com.au/anzba2013/posters/anzba2013asm1final00038.pdf.
29. Turk E, Karagulle E, Aydogan C, Oguz H, Tarim A, Karakayali H, et al. Use of telemedicine and telephone consultation in decision-making and follow-up of burn patients: initial experience from two burn units. Burns. 2011;37(3):415–9.
30. Wallace DL, Hussain A, Khan N, Wilson YT. A systematic review of the evidence for telemedicine in burn care: with a UK perspective. Burns. 2012;38(4):465–80.
31. Reiband HK, Lundin K, Alsbjørn B, Sørensen AM, Rasmussen LS. Optimization of burn referrals. Burns. 2014;40(3):397–401.
32. Atiyeh B, Gunn SWA, Dibo S. Primary triage of mass burn casualties with associated severe traumatic injuries. Ann Burns Fire Disasters. 2013;26(1):48–52.
33. Smith AC, Youngberry K, Mill J, Kimble R, Wootton R. A review of three years experience using email and videoconferencing for the delivery of post-acute burns care to children in Queensland. Burns. 2004;30(3):248–52.

34. Fuzaylov G, Knittel J, Driscoll DN. Use of telemedicine to improve burn care in Ukraine. J Burn Care Res. 2013;34(4):232.
35. Klein MB, Nathens AB, Emerson D, Heimbach DM, Gibran NS. An analysis of the long-distance transport of burn patients to a regional burn center. J Burn Care Res. 2007;28(1):49–55.
36. Romanowski KS, Palmieri TL, Sen S, Greenhalgh DG. More than one third of intubations in patients transferred to burn centers are unnecessary: proposed guidelines for appropriate intubation of the burn patient. J Burn Care Res. 2016;37(5):409.
37. Roman J, Shank W, Demirjian J, Tang A, Vercruysse GA. Overutilization of Helicopter Transport in the Minimally Burned-A Healthcare System Problem That Should Be Corrected. J Burn Care Res. 2020;41(1):15–22.
38. Klein MB, Hollingworth W, Rivara FP, Kramer CB, Askay SW, Heimbach DM, et al. Hospital costs associated with pediatric burn injury. J Burn Care Res. 2008;29(4):632–7.
39. McWilliams T, Hendricks J, Twigg D, Wood F, Giles M. Telehealth for paediatric burn patients in rural areas: a retrospective audit of activity and cost savings. Burns. 2016;42(7):1487–93.
40. Garcia DI, Howard HR, Cina RA, Patel S, Ruggiero K, Treiber FA, et al. Expert Outpatient Burn Care in the Home Through Mobile Health Technology. J Burn Care Res. 2018;39(5):680–4.
41. Yoder LH, McFall DC, Cancio LC. Use of the videophone to collect quality of life data from burn patients. Int J Burns Trauma. 2012;2(3):135–44.
42. World Health Organization Global Observatory for e-Health Vol. 2 [Internet]. [cited 6 February 2014]. Available from: http://www.who.int/goe/publications/goe_telemedicine_2010.pdf.
43. Grossman Burn Foundation Establishes First-Ever Telemedicine Based Burn Treatment Center [Internet]. [cited 6 February 2014]. Available from: http://www.grossmanburnfoundation.org/telemedicine_burn_center.html.
44. World Bank Indonesia Profile [Internet]. [cited 6 February 2014]. Available from: http://data.worldbank.org/country/indonesia.
45. Practical Guidelines for Teleburn Care 2016 [Internet]. [cited 20 March 2020]. Available from: https://www.americantelemed.org/wp-content/themes/ata-custom/download.php?id=1557.
46. Augestad KM, Lindsetmo RO. Videoconferencing as a clinical tool for surgeons. Norwood, MA, Artech House; 2011.
47. 25. Australian National Government Department of Health [Internet]. [cited 28 January 2014]. Available from: http://www.mbsonline.gov.au/internet/mbsonline/publishing.nsf/Content/connectinghealthservices-clinicalpract.
48. Graschew G, Roelofs TA, Rakowsky S, Schlag PM. Telemedicine for trauma, emergencies, and disaster management. R. Latifi (Ed.). Artech House: Norwood, MA; 2011.
49. Wirthlin DJ, Buradagunta S, Edwards RA, Brewster DC, Cambria RP, Gertler JP, et al. Telemedicine in vascular surgery: feasibility of digital imaging for remote management of wounds. J Vasc Surg. 1998;27(6):1089–100.
50. Baer CA, Williams CM, Vickers L, Kvedar JC. A pilot study of specialized nursing care for home health patients. J Telemed Telecare. 2004;10(6):342–5.

Telemedicine for Intensive Care

Rifat Latifi and Kalterina Osmani

Introduction

The management of critically ill patients has transformed incredibly over the last few decades. Part of this transformation has been our increased knowledge of managing the most critically ill patients. The most important transformation has been technological advances which make it possible to manage the most critically ill patients such as sustaining life while waiting for transplants and remote monitoring and intervention in situations where ICU staff is limited.

According to the 2015 American Hospital Association annual survey, in the USA, there were 4862 acute care registered hospitals and 5229 ICUs with 94,837 ICU beds (14.3% of ICU beds/total beds). Of these ICU beds, 46,490 are medical-surgical beds in 2644 units; 14,731 are cardiac beds in 976 units; 6588 are other beds in 379 units; 4698 are pediatric beds in 307 units; and 22,330 are neonatal beds in 920 units. The median number of beds in medical-surgical, cardiac, and other units was 12, with 10 beds in pediatrics and 18 in neonatal. Fifty-two percent of hospitals had 1 unit, 24% had 2 units, and 24% had 3 or more units [1].

The establishment of ICU and technological advances, while associated with significantly reduced mortality (a 35% relative decrease in mortality for ICU admissions from 1988 to 2012), is associated with serious cost. According to the Society of Critical Care Medicine (SCCM) website data, the annual cost of critical care between 2000 and 2010 has increased by 92% (from $56.6 billion to $108 billion). The 2010 costs represent 13.2% of hospital costs, 4.1% of national health

---

R. Latifi (✉)
New York Medical College, School of Medicine, Valhalla, NY, USA

Department of Surgery, Westchester Medical Center Health, Valhalla, NY, USA
e-mail: Rifat.Latifi@wmchealth.org; Rifat_Latifi@nymc.edu

K. Osmani
Department of Surgery, Westchester Medical Center Health, Valhalla, NY, USA

© Springer Nature Switzerland AG 2021
R. Latifi et al. (eds.), *Telemedicine, Telehealth and Telepresence*,
https://doi.org/10.1007/978-3-030-56917-4_20

expenditures, and 0.72% of gross domestic product. Intensive care unit (ICU) costs per day in 2010 were estimated to be $4300 per day, a 61% increase from the 2000 cost per day of $2669 [1].

Overall, there has been a dramatic change in modern hospitals [2]. Most care required, even surgical care, is done in ambulatory fashion so that only truly critically ill patients are hospitalized. In US ICUs, five million patients are admitted annually. 20–40% of US ICU admissions require mechanical ventilation support [1], and it is expected that the number of patients requiring ICU admission will continue to grow, particularly with the growing elderly population as elderly patients who undergo major surgeries require postoperative intensive care.

According to a report [1] from the US Centers for Medicare and Medicaid Services Healthcare Cost Report Information System (HCRIS), the number of critical care beds in the USA increased by 17.8% from 2000 to 2010. The majority of the growth in critical care bed supply is occurring in a small number of US regions that have large populations, fewer baseline ICUs per 100,000 capita, higher baseline ICU occupancy, and increased market competition. Additionally, between 2000 and 2010, the greatest percentage of ICU beds increased in the neonatal sector (29%), followed by adult beds (26%). Of the 103,900 ICU beds in 2010, 83,417 (80.3%) were adult, 1917 (1.8%) were pediatric, and 18,567 (17.9%) were neonatal.

According to the study of Wallace DJ et al. that included 4457 hospitals, the majority of intensive care bed growth occurred in teaching hospitals (net, +13,471 beds; 72.1% of total growth), hospitals with 250 or more beds (net, +18,327 beds; 91.8% of total growth), and hospitals in the highest quartile of occupancy (net, +10,157 beds; 54.0% of total growth) [3]. The greatest odds of increasing ICU beds were in hospitals with 500 or more beds in the highest quartile of occupancy (adjusted odds ratio, 18.9; 95% CI, 14.0–25.5; $p < 0.01$) and large teaching hospitals in the highest quartile of occupancy (adjusted odds ratio, 7.3; 95% CI, 5.3–9.9; $p < 0.01$).

In other words, only major hospitals around the world can afford to find intensivists that provide quality intensive care due to the shortage of physicians in certain specialties (i.e., intensivists, neurologists).

While there is a large number of ICU beds in the USA, there is a misdistribution of ICU beds. Of the 2814 acute care hospitals studied, by Halpern et al., 1469 (52%) had intensivists, while 1345 (48%) had no intensivists [4]. Compared with hospitals without intensivists, hospitals with privileged intensivists were primarily located in metropolitan areas (91% vs 50%; $p < 0.001$) and at the aggregate level had nearly 3 times the number of hospital beds (403,522 [75%] versus 137,146 [25%]), 3.6 times the number of ICU beds (74,222 [78%] vs 20,615 [22%]), and almost 2 times as many ICUs (3383 [65%] vs 1846 [35%]).

The above information clearly set the stage for new solutions providing lifesaving critical care through telemedicine and telepresence of intensivists both as primary caregivers or as an additional set of eyes on the patients.

Telemedicine for Intensive Care Units

Telemedicine has increased access to care everywhere, but particularly in low- and middle-income countries and in specialized care sectors [5–11]. Tele-ICU has proven to be the most beneficial of all fields of clinical telemedicine in reducing mortality and morbidity. Telemedicine for intensive care units has become popular, in particular in organized major health systems. As the elderly population grows, so will the demand of intensive care and the need for intensivists. However, there is a major shortage of intensivists caring for these patients, and thus telemedicine for ICU has been promoted [12] and subsequently demonstrated [13] as a solution to advancing critical care and access to intensivists. With the help of tele-ICU, intensivists can manage a number of patients, often in different geographical areas, at the same time.

A tele-ICU offers the expertise of specialists and intensivists through a dedicated secure network system comprised of one central location hub that provides support for several off-site ICUs. Patients are remotely monitored by physicians or nurses. Accordingly, the primary benefit of telemedicine is the ability to provide high-end, structured, evidence-based guidelines that allow for directed medical care at multiple sites from a distance [13–22]. Patients are monitored live from a command and control center using audio and video connectivity [23–25], assisted by evidence-based medicine guidelines and protocols and created by the telemedicine industry which were based on major societies and association guidelines. According to the official website, over 4.25 million patients have been monitored by tele-ICU programs across the USA [26]. A recent update from the Tele-ICU Committee of the Society of Critical Care concluded that tele-ICU care is an established mechanism to leverage critical care expertise to ICUs and beyond, but systematic research comparing different models, approaches, and technologies is still needed [27].

Moreover, tele-ICU is mostly driven by clinical decision support systems (CDSS), applications of machine learning (ML) algorithms to critical care, and opportunities to integrate ML with tele-ICU CDSS. The enormous quantities of data generated by tele-ICU systems is a major opportunity for data-driven research [28]. While machine learning and artificial intelligence will continue to play a major role in the future, the role of clinical expertise at the bedside is irreplaceable at this moment and will continue to be so [29].

Prevalence of Tele-ICU and Models of Operations

Tele-ICU is becoming more and more prevalent, although the exact number of tele-ICU beds is unknown. Despite tele-ICU adoption and growth, only a minority of critically ill patients in the USA are taken care of through tele-ICU [30].

A 2014 study examined tele-ICU deployments between 2002 and 2010 using data from the Centers for Medicare and Medicaid Services and has demonstrated that the number of hospitals adopting tele-ICUs increased from 16 (0.4%) to 213 (4.6%), while covered beds increased from 598 (0.9%) to 5799 (7.9%) [31]. In 2014, formal ICU telemedicine programs supported around 11% of nonfederal hospital critically ill adult patients [13].

The tele-ICU database on more than 200 hospitals and over 139,000 ICU patients across the USA with wide-ranging clinical data and diagnoses was studied by Essay et al. [32]. Most commonly, tele-ICU is used for mixed medical-surgical ICU, followed by patients with cardiovascular conditions (>20%) and patients with neurological or respiratory illness (>15%).

The Benefits and Effectiveness of Tele-ICU in Reducing Mortality and Morbidity

The published literature has demonstrated a number of benefits on the use of tele-ICU including decreased mortality and length of ICU stay [33], particularly in mortality rates among the sickest population although there is a lack of randomized, controlled, blinded studies.

While a number of papers have reported improved outcomes, I agree with Yoo et al. that the best results from the use of tele-ICU are achieved in select situations [34]. These authors found that the best cost-efficiency results were achieved when tele-ICU was applied to 30–40% of highest risk patients. Other authors have reported significant savings in a large healthcare network [35]. Yet, measuring tele-ICU impact and how it affects outcomes in critically ill patients is not an easy task. It requires taking into consideration that there are multiple factors affecting the overall outcomes of critically ill patients [36]. For one, the impact tele-ICU has on mortality is variable, but tele-ICU enhances the compliance with bundle care [37] and may affect the system-wide centralization of the intensive care [38].

Chen J et al. studied 19 studies about the pooled effects and demonstrated that tele-ICU programs were associated with reductions in ICU mortality (15 studies; risk ratio [RR], 0.83; 95% confidence interval [CI], 0.72 to 0.96; $P = 0.01$), hospital mortality (13 studies; RR, 0.74; 95% CI, 0.58 to 0.96; $P = 0.02$), and ICU length of stay (9 studies; mean difference [MD], −0.63; 95% CI, −0.28 to 0.17; $P = 0.007$). Interestingly these authors did not find any significant association between the reduction in hospital length of stay and tele-ICU programs.

One early meta-analysis showed that telemedicine, compared with standard of care, is associated with lower ICU mortality and hospital mortality [39]. Moreover, these authors concluded that continuous patient-data monitoring, with or without alerts, reduced ICU mortality versus those with remote intensivist consultation only but effects were statistically similar (interaction $P = 0.74$). Effects were also similar in higher- (RR, 0.83; 95% CI, 0.68 to 1.02) versus lower-quality (RR, 0.69; 95% CI, 0.40 to 1.19; interaction, $P = 0.53$) studies. Reductions in ICU and hospital length of stay were statistically significant (weighted mean difference [telemedicine-control], −0.62 days; 95% CI, −1.21 to −0.04 days and −1.26 days; 95% CI, −2.49 to −0.03 days, respectively; I2 >90% for both).

A retrospective, single-center study by Ramakrishnan et al. revealed that the addition of a nighttime intensivist via tele-ICU did not lead to a statistically significant improvement in mortality (hospital and ICU) and length of stay (hospital and ICU) [40].

Lilly et al. reported the effects of nonrandomized ICU telemedicine interventions on crude and adjusted mortality and length of stay (LOS) [41]. This study included 118,990 adult patients from 56 ICUs in 32 hospitals from 19 US healthcare systems. Lilly et al. found that after adjustment, hospital and ICU mortality in the ICU telemedicine intervention group, and hospital LOS and adjusted ICU LOS was reduced by 1.1 days among those who stayed in the ICU for ≥ 7, ≥ 14, and ≥ 30 days, respectively. The authors reported that timely review of patients, with timely use of performance data, practice of ICU best practices, and (4) quicker alert response times were factors affecting mortality rate and LOS.

There is a need for multi-institutional randomized clinical trials in this evolving field, as optimal tailoring of tele-ICU programs still remains unclear. For ICUs with intensivists, do we need every patient to be monitored by both staff at the bedside and tele-ICU? Should only certain severity scores trigger the need for additional tele-ICU assistance? Or perhaps, tele-ICU should be used only where there is no intensivist present in the unit. Furthermore, there is a need for structured study in order to definitively understand and quantify the benefits of tele-ICU [42].

Challenges and Barriers Implementing Tele-ICU

As with any other telemedicine service implementation, tele-ICU has its own challenges and barriers. These can be structured into cost, human factors (staffing acceptance), and reporting and selecting the patients and setting that will most benefit from tele-ICU care. In the following pages, I will discuss these three issues.

Cost of Tele-ICU

Some argue against the cost-effectiveness of tele-ICU programs [43]. These authors reviewed the cost per bed for patients before and after the implementation of a tele-ICU in five hospitals within a large nonprofit group. The cost per bed for patients included software and hardware implementation. Costs per patient increased 28%. Hospital costs per case increased 43%. Because the sickest of the patients had lower mortality and length of stay, these authors suggest cautious implementation of tele-ICU programs and possibly for the sickest of patients only [43]. Specifically, the best benefit-to-cost ratio has not been defined. Others have suggested further financial analysis [44].

It has been reported that initial cost is approximately $50,000 to $100,000 per tele-ICU bed [45]. These authors concluded that tele-ICU approaches may reduce the ICU and hospital mortality, shorten the ICU length of stay, but have no significant effect on hospital LOS. Implementation of tele-ICU programs' initial costs and long-term cost-effectiveness is still unclear.

In a study simulation analyses among four types of ICU in urban tertiary (primary analysis), urban community, rural tertiary, and rural community, Yoo et al. found a U-shaped relationship between the economic efficiency and selected tele-ICU use among all four hospital types [34]. Optimal cost-effectiveness was achieved when tele-ICU was applied to the 30–40% highest-risk patients among all ICU patients (incremental cost-effectiveness ratio = $25,392 [2014 US dollars] per extending a quality-adjusted life year) in urban tertiary hospitals (primary analysis). Their further break-even analyses indicated that cost saving was more feasible when reducing ICU medical care cost, rather than lowering the cost to operate telemedicine alone. This is in line with the author's previous study which concluded that telemedicine in the ICU is cost-effective in most cases and cost saving in some cases [46].

Staff Perception and Building the Bedside and Tele-ICU Team

Intensive care units are staffed by the best and brightest critical care physicians, nurses, and physician's assistants (PAs). Adding a new set of eyes to existing ICU staffed by intensivist and critical care nurses may be helpful but may also potentially cause problems. As in any other form of telemedicine, the concept and syndrome of "Big Brother watching" can have serious consequences and will affect the trust among the team members and make the adaptation process of tele-ICU difficult. Involving both teams (tele-ICU and bedside team) to work together for the good of the patients into one integrated team is a difficult process and has to be done professionally, with mutual collaboration.

We at Westchester Medical Center have a robust e-ICU covering over 100 ICU bed over 3 campuses 24/7. This is additional service provided to our patients and clinical staff at the bedside. However, in order to better integrate the tele-ICU with clinical staff (physician and nurses), we have started handoffs between the team at the bedside and tele-ICU, as well as other initiatives, such as having the intensivist rotate through the surgical and medical intensive care units for week at a time. This improves greatly the relationship required for optimal work between the teams. Moreover, there is a need for leadership of clinical services to work together with tele-ICU teams and agree on the workflow, particularly in busy services such as trauma and surgical intensive care units. As others have pointed out in the early days of e-ICU, there was a process of acceptance of staff of e-ICU, and there is an ongoing need for education, coordination, and developing interpersonal relationships and systems. If these processes are not taken care of, the tele-ICU will not have major effects on patients care and will not be accepted by ICU staff at the bedside.

Numerous studies have been conducted on staff perception, usability, and satisfaction with tele-intensive care units. For example, physicians expressed that they were extremely satisfied [47]. Others found that there was an increase in satisfaction among nursing team members, particularly during nighttime hours [48]. Physicians felt they could better manage critically ill patients, were more equipped to communicate with bedside care teams, and were better able to provide reassurance to families [49]. The change from traditional face-to-face nursing to the use of telehealth calls for local agreements and further discussions among professionals on how this change will be accepted and implemented into practice [50] in order to improve nursing perceptions of working conditions and communications.

Overall, the majority of studies that included quantitative and qualitative data provides support for the use of telemedicine in intensive care settings, although one earlier study found that some nurses felt that the transition from bedside caregiver to information manager can be difficult [51]. Fewer studies that provide evidence for patient satisfaction are available. Evidence suggests that patients report higher satisfaction with tele-ICUs; however, vigilance of staff and nurses in the use of these services plays a role in patient satisfaction [36, 52].

Other Challenges of Implementation of ICU

While implementation of tele-ICU has expanded dramatically, there are a number of challenges to implement tele-ICU, both in developing countries and developed countries. These challenges include financial, legislative, attitudinal, and cultural. Despite these barriers, with the advancing of technological option and as technology becomes cheaper, the use of tele-ICU will also grow. These challenges include financial, legislative, attitudinal, business plans, distance and geographical, and cultural. While the benefits of tele-ICU programs outweigh the risks associated with them, the barriers need to be overcome to allow for successful establishment and integration of tele-ICU services.

Policies and Protocols and Patient (Setting) Selection

Tele-ICU protocols and procedures are based on the institutional policies and the setup. Most practices require 12–24 hours of telepresence of critical care specialist. Providers such as physician's assistants, nurse practitioners, or residents are usually involved in the site where patients are present, in addition to bedside critical care nurses. Scheduled bedside rounds and rounds on demand are done. The main point is the fact that critical care specialist has access to both visual and audio and all the data and medical records. In addition, most of the tele-ICU models use guidelines, protocols, and algorithms to manage certain critical conditions. Many authors have suggested that only the sickest and most critically ill patients will benefit from being tele-ICU patients. I fully agree with this notion but want to note that ICUs without in-person intensivists could also greatly benefit from tele-ICU.

Few places use telemedicine for ICU as a "second set of eyes" and do not bill for tele-ICU services. While there is difficult justification for the long-term sustainability of such practices, if tele-ICU improves outcomes, then this is truly justifiable.

Major academic institutions that have a number of satellite-type hospitals with ICUs but without intensivists or that are short-staffed or have mid-level coverage are most likely the best examples of the necessity of remote tele-ICU services.

Summary

Tele-ICU has dramatically improved the access to ICU patients remotely by intensivists. Although it is not clear which patient population will be best served by tele-ICU, I agree with the authors who suggest that only the sickest patients should be attended by tele-ICU. There is no question that tele-ICU is a must-have for hospitals that do not have 24/7 ICU in-person coverage such as smaller and community hospitals. The tele-ICU team should take full charge and responsibility for ICU patients and should not simply serve to write an admit note or wait for alarms to go off. While the initial cost may be prohibitive for many hospitals, technology is rapidly advancing and becoming less expensive. The most common finding among all studies reviewed was a reduction in mortality rates and LOS. These are the goals to keep in mind when establishing a successful tele-ICU program.

In their provocative review of the current status of tele-ICU entitled "When Will Telemedicine Appear in the ICU?," Avdalovic and Marcin concluded that although the clinical footprint of telemedicine in ICU has grown over the past 20 years, there has been a relative slowing of implementation of telemedicine for ICU [53].

I believe, however, that the future of tele-ICU is bright. Tele-ICU practices must be incorporated on a day-to-day basis, and we must display creativity in reaching for integrative approaches with bedside teams in order to make the practice truly functional and useful. The focus should not only be on integrating artificial intelligence and advanced technologies but on being truly present, reviewing the patients often, and caring for them as though their life depends on us. Because depend it does.

References

1. Critical care statistics. Society of Critical Care Medicine Web site. https://www.sccm.org/Communications/Critical-Care-Statistics. Updated 2019. Accessed 18 Jan 2020.
2. Latifi R, editor. The modern hospital: patient-centered and science based: Patient centered, disease based, research oriented, technology driven. 1st ed: Springer; 2019.
3. Wallace DJ, Seymour CW, Kahn JM. Hospital-level changes in adult ICU bed supply in the United States. Crit Care Med. 2017;45(1):e67–76.
4. Halpern NA, Tan KS, DeWitt M, Pastores SM. Intensivists in U.S. acute care hospitals. Crit Care Med. 2019;47(4):517–25.
5. Latifi R, Dasho E, Shatri Z, et al. Telemedicine as an innovative model for rebuilding medical systems in developing countries through multipartnership collaboration: the case of Albania. Telemed J E Health. 2015;21(6):503–9.
6. Latifi R, Dasho E, Merrell RC, et al. Cabo verde telemedicine program: initial results of nationwide implementation. Telemed J E Health. 2014;20(11):1027–34.

7. Olldashi F, Latifi R, Parsikia A, et al. Telemedicine for neurotrauma prevents unnecessary transfers: an update from a nationwide program in Albania and analysis of 590 patients. World Neurosurg. 2019;128:e340–6.
8. Latifi R, Parsikia A, Boci A, Doarn CR, Merrell RC. Increases access to care through telemedicine in Albania: an analysis of 2,724 patients. Telemed J E Health. 2020;26:164–75.
9. Latifi R, Olldashi F, Dogjani A, Dasho E, Boci A, El-Menyar A. Telemedicine for neurotrauma in Albania: initial results from case series of 146 patients. World Neurosurg. 2018;112:e747–53.
10. Latifi R, Gunn JK, Stroster JA, et al. The readiness of emergency and trauma care in low- and middle-income countries: a cross-sectional descriptive study of 42 public hospitals in Albania. Int J Emerg Med. 2016;9(1):26-016-0124-5. Epub 2016 Oct 7.
11. Latifi R, Gunn JK, Bakiu E, et al. Access to specialized care through telemedicine in limited-resource country: initial 1,065 teleconsultations in Albania. Telemed J E Health. 2016;22(12):1024–31.
12. Breslow MJ, Rosenfeld BA, Doerfler M, et al. Effect of a multiple-site intensive care unit telemedicine program on clinical and economic outcomes: an alternative paradigm for intensivist staffing. Crit Care Med. 2004;32(1):31–8.
13. Lilly CM, Zubrow MT, Kempner KM, et al. Critical care telemedicine: evolution and state of the art. Crit Care Med. 2014;42(11):2429–36.
14. Latifi R, Peck K, Satava R, Anvari M. Telepresence and telementoring in surgery. In: Latifi R, editor. Establishing telemedicine in developing countries: from inception to implementation. Amsterdam: IOS Press; 2004. p. 201–6.
15. Reynolds HN, Rogove H, Bander J, McCambridge M, Cowboy E, Niemeier M. A working lexicon for the tele-intensive care unit: we need to define tele-intensive care unit to grow and understand it. Telemed J E Health. 2011;17(10):773–83.
16. Rosenfeld BA, Dorman T, Breslow MJ, et al. Intensive care unit telemedicine: Alternate paradigm for providing continuous intensivist care. Crit Care Med. 2000;28(12):3925–31.
17. Thomas EJ, Lucke JF, Wueste L, Weavind L, Patel B. Association of telemedicine for remote monitoring of intensive care patients with mortality, complications, and length of stay. JAMA. 2009;302(24):2671–8.
18. Lilly CM, Thomas EJ. Tele-ICU: Experience to date. J Intensive Care Med. 2010;25(1):16–22.
19. Zawada ET Jr, Herr P, Larson D, Fromm R, Kapaska D, Erickson D. Impact of an intensive care unit telemedicine program on a rural health care system. Postgrad Med. 2009;121(3):160–70.
20. Willmitch B, Golembeski S, Kim SS, Nelson LD, Gidel L. Clinical outcomes after telemedicine intensive care unit implementation. Crit Care Med. 2012;40(2):450–4.
21. Reynolds EM, Grujovski A, Wright T, Foster M, Reynolds HN. Utilization of robotic "remote presence" technology within north american intensive care units. Telemed J E Health. 2012;18(7):507–15.
22. Fortis S, Weinert C, Bushinski R, Koehler AG, Beilman G. A health system-based critical care program with a novel tele-ICU: implementation, cost, and structure details. J Am Coll Surg. 2014;219(4):676–83.
23. Kumar S, Merchant S, Reynolds R. Tele-ICU: efficacy and cost-effectiveness approach of remotely managing the critical care. Open Med Inform J. 2013;7:24–9.
24. Ramnath VR, Ho L, Maggio LA, Khazeni N. Centralized monitoring and virtual consultant models of tele-ICU care: a systematic review. Telemed J E Health. 2014;20(10):936–61.
25. Ramnath VR, Khazeni N. Centralized monitoring and virtual consultant models of tele-ICU care: a side-by-side review. Telemed J E Health. 2014;20(10):962–71.
26. Philips ICU telemedicine program. Philips Web site. https://www.usa.philips.com/healthcare/resources/landing/teleicu. Updated 2017. Accessed 05 Jan 2019.
27. Subramanian S, Pamplin JC, Hravnak M, et al. Tele-critical care: an update from the society of critical care medicine tele-ICU committee. Crit Care Med. 2020;48(4):553–61.
28. Kindle RD, Badawi O, Celi LA, Sturland S. Intensive care unit telemedicine in the era of big data, artificial intelligence, and computer clinical decision support systems. Crit Care Clin. 2019;35(3):483–95.

29. Al-Mufti F, Kim M, Dodson V, et al. Machine learning and artificial intelligence in neurocritical care: a specialty-wide disruptive transformation or a strategy for success. Curr Neurol Neurosci Rep. 2019;19(11):89-019-0998-8.
30. Udeh C, Udeh B, Rahman N, Canfield C, Campbell J, Hata JS. Telemedicine/virtual ICU: where are we and where are we going? Methodist Debakey Cardiovasc J. 2018;14(2):126–33.
31. Kahn JM, Cicero BD, Wallace DJ, Iwashyna TJ. Adoption of ICU telemedicine in the United States. Crit Care Med. 2014;42(2):362–8.
32. Essay P, Shahin TB, Balkan B, Mosier J, Subbian V. The connected intensive care unit patient: exploratory analyses and cohort discovery from a critical care telemedicine database. JMIR Med Inform. 2019;7(1):e13006.
33. Coustasse A, Deslich S, Bailey D, Hairston A, Paul D. A business case for tele-intensive care units. Perm J. 2014;18(4):76–84.
34. Yoo BK, Kim M, Sasaki T, Hoch JS, Marcin JP. Selected use of telemedicine in intensive care units based on severity of illness improves cost-effectiveness. Telemed J E Health. 2018;24(1):21–36.
35. Lilly CM, Motzkus C, Rincon T, et al. ICU telemedicine program financial outcomes. Chest. 2017;151(2):286–97.
36. Goran SF. Measuring tele-ICU impact: does it optimize quality outcomes for the critically ill patient? J Nurs Manag. 2012;20(3):414–28.
37. Venkataraman R, Ramakrishnan N. Outcomes related to telemedicine in the intensive care unit: what we know and would like to know. Crit Care Clin. 2015;31(2):225–37.
38. Kopec IC. Impact of intensive care unit telemedicine on outcomes. Crit Care Clin. 2019;35(3):439–49.
39. Wilcox ME, Adhikari NK. The effect of telemedicine in critically ill patients: systematic review and meta-analysis. Crit Care. 2012;16(4):R127.
40. Ramakrishnan M, Taduru SS, Patel P, Younis M, Hamarshi M. External intensivists versus in-house intensivists: analysis of outcomes of nighttime coverage of ICUs by external on-call and in-house on-call intensivists. Mo Med. 2019;116(4):331–5.
41. Lilly CM, McLaughlin JM, Zhao H, et al. A multicenter study of ICU telemedicine reengineering of adult critical care. Chest. 2014;145(3):500–7.
42. Rak KJ, Kuza CC, Ashcraft LE, et al. Identifying strategies for effective telemedicine use in intensive care units: the ConnECCT study protocol. Int J Qual Methods. 2017;16(1):10.1177/1609406917733387. Epub 2017 Oct 6.
43. Franzini L, Sail KR, Thomas EJ, Wueste L. Costs and cost-effectiveness of a telemedicine intensive care unit program in 6 intensive care units in a large health care system. J Crit Care. 2011;26(3):329.e1–6.
44. Sadaka F, Palagiri A, Trottier S, et al. Telemedicine intervention improves ICU outcomes. Crit Care Res Pract. 2013;2013:456389.
45. Chen J, Sun D, Yang W, et al. Clinical and economic outcomes of telemedicine programs in the intensive care unit: a systematic review and meta-analysis. J Intensive Care Med. 2018;33(7):383–93.
46. Yoo BK, Kim M, Sasaki T, Melnikow J, Marcin JP. Economic evaluation of telemedicine for patients in ICUs. Crit Care Med. 2016;44(2):265–74.
47. Rogove H, Atkins C, Kramer J. Enhanced access to neurointensivists through a telemedicine program. Crit Care Med. 2009;37(Suppl):A1.
48. Rincon T, Seiver A, Farrell W, Daly M. Increased documentation of ICD-9-CM codes 995.92 and 785.52 with template-oriented monitoring and screen- ing by a tele-ICU. Crit Care Med. 2009;37(Suppl):A4.
49. Yager P, Whalen M, Cummings B, Noviski N. Use of telemedicine to provide enhanced communication between at-home attendings and bedside personnel in a pediatric intensive care unit. Crit Care Med. 2010;38:U28.
50. Koivunen M, Saranto K. Nursing professionals' experiences of the facilitators and barriers to the use of telehealth applications: a systematic review of qualitative studies. Scand J Caring Sci. 2018;32(1):24–44.

51. Hoonakker PL, Carayon P, McGuire K, et al. Motivation and job satisfaction of tele-ICU nurses. J Crit Care. 2013;28(3):315.e13–21.
52. Young LB, Chan PS, Cram P. Staff acceptance of tele-ICU coverage: a systematic review. Chest. 2011;139(2):279–88.
53. Avdalovic MV, Marcin JP. When will telemedicine appear in the ICU? J Intensive Care Med. 2019;34(4):271–6.

Telehealth in Pediatric Care

21

Jennifer L. Rosenthal, Jamie L. Mouzoon, and James P. Marcin

Introduction

Telehealth is increasingly utilized and becoming a common standard in the delivery of care for pediatric patients. Over the past two decades, the use of telehealth has developed and spread from small pilots to its current use which includes a broad variety of models of care [1]. Its use is also expected to continue to increase as technologies improve and costs of equipment and hardware become more affordable. Telehealth applications are a practical means of delivering or augmenting pediatric-focused care to remote locations that is convenient for patients and families or where providers may not otherwise be available [2–6]. The use of telehealth allows providers the ability to be "virtually present" in remote clinics, hospitals, and homes as if they were physically present. The technology allows virtual access to high-definition patient views, treating providers, family, as well as remote patient monitoring of medical equipment and devices. In addition, with the availability of home devices, mobile health, eHealth, and telehealth technologies are providing the means to more proactively and nonintrusively monitor infants, children, and adolescents in the era of "remote patient monitoring."

While telehealth is becoming a part of the solution to increase convenience of care and decrease disparities in access to primary and specialty care providers, it is not meant to always replace in-person care or obviate the need to have children treated in regionalized centers. Instead, numerous clinical programs across the country are leveraging telehealth and remote monitoring technologies to augment and better care for children in a variety of clinical scenarios [3]. In this chapter, we will review and discuss evidence of how telehealth can be used across the spectrum

J. L. Rosenthal (✉) · J. L. Mouzoon · J. P. Marcin
Department of Pediatrics, University of California Davis, Sacramento, CA, USA
e-mail: rosenthal@ucdavis.edu

of pediatric care. Specifically, we will review how telehealth can be used for ambulatory care, behavioral and mental health, school-based health, hospital-based care (including labor and delivery and newborn care as well as emergency care services), and finally, direct to consumer models of care.

Telehealth in Pediatric Ambulatory Care

The application of telehealth to deliver outpatient subspecialty consultations to children living in rural communities was among the first use cases in pediatric care. These "provider-to-provider" telehealth consultations connect a patient visiting their primary care provider to a distant specialist over live video. Ambulatory telehealth consultations have been successfully used in pediatric specialties most amenable to video such as psychiatry and behavioral health, developmental pediatrics, neurology, and endocrinology [7]. Other ambulatory applications that are amenable to store-and-forward telehealth applications, including dermatology and cardiology, have also been used as a convenient way of providing provider-to-provider consultations [7].

Many published articles on the use of telehealth in the ambulatory setting report strong patient, caregiver, and provider satisfaction [8–10]. Obvious advantages that have been documented in the literature include reductions in patient and physician travel time and out of pocket expenses for patients and families. Telehealth in pediatric ambulatory care has also been shown to sometimes reduce the costs of healthcare, by simultaneously bringing together the primary care provider and the specialist so that diagnostic and therapeutic plans can be agreed upon in a more efficient manner [11]. In some cases, the use of telehealth in the ambulatory setting has reduced the need for additional office visits and has mitigated the need for urgent care and emergency department encounters [12].

Because care can be delivered in a more convenient manner, the use of telehealth can enhance access to subspecialty care for children with special healthcare needs, particularly those living in rural underserved communities [13]. Pediatric subspecialists are largely concentrated in urban areas, and certain pediatric subspecialists are particularly limited. In standard practice, the referral process to connect a patient with a subspecialist involves numerous steps, whereby any breakdowns in a single step in the series can impede care access and care quality. Lost referral placements, long appointment wait times, long travel distances for families, and poor communication and handoffs between providers are some of the many barriers. Telehealth can mitigate these challenges by virtually bringing the subspecialist into the local primary care clinic [14]. The geographic access and utilization disparities are dampened with the application of telehealth in this context. In fact, pediatric telehealth programs have extensive geographic reaches that span across states, multistate regions, and even nationwide [7].

In addition to improved access and utilization, research published in peer-reviewed journals has shown that telehealth consultations in the ambulatory setting can facilitate more rapid diagnoses and treatment plans and improve clinical outcomes. As an example, pediatric tele-neurology consultations are a specific telehealth application that has been shown to have significant patient benefits. Many pediatric neurological conditions require rapid diagnosis and treatment initiation, but the geographic and socioeconomic disparities impede the ability of many children to have timely access to a pediatric neurologist. Pediatric tele-neurology has been shown to improve patient outcomes for diagnoses including epilepsy, traumatic brain injury, and behavioral disorders [15].

Store-and-forward is a type of telehealth application that is applicable when synchronous video-based telehealth visits are not feasible or necessary. Store-and-forward telehealth ambulatory visits are an asynchronous telehealth application, whereby electronic communication, such as messages or images, is transmitted between the primary care provider and subspecialists. A primary care physician can upload and securely send a consultation question with associated case description and images [16]. In this way, store-and-forward telehealth can replace initial consultations or subsequent visits with subspecialists. Since these ambulatory visits are not live, this type of subspecialty use of telehealth can be more feasible by permitting flexibility in when the electronic material is reviewed and managed [14].

Tele-dermatology is another widely used application of store-and-forward. The most common pediatric tele-dermatology diagnoses include atopic dermatitis, rash, benign nevi, and acne [17]. Tele-dermatology is particularly valuable to children given the pronounced lack of access to pediatric dermatologic services due to both a shortage of pediatric dermatologists and insurance-based disparities in access. The use of tele-dermatology to obtain dermatologic subspecialist consultation has been shown to not only reduce barriers to access but also yield high rates of diagnostic concordance [11, 17].

Another model of care that uses telehealth in the ambulatory setting is specifically focused on primary care provider education and case reviews as opposed to direct patient care. Project ECHO (Extension for Community Healthcare Outcomes) was formed to employ telehealth more broadly to enhance chronic disease management in rural New Mexico [18]. This model uses telehealth telecommunication to link expert specialist teams at typically academic hubs with community primary care clinicians. Frequent ECHO educational encounters using a provider-focused curriculum that sometimes combine patient case presentations result in a mentoring and educational model to elevate the level of expertise and care provided in remote areas. While Project ECHO was originally described in the care of patients with hepatitis C, it has expanded to allow primary care providers and specialists to work collaboratively as a team to address a variety of chronic conditions [19]. A variety of ECHO models are supported throughout the country, including specific programs sponsored by the American Academy of Pediatrics [20].

Telehealth in Pediatric Behavioral and Mental Health

It is estimated that nearly 20% of children and adolescents in the United States ages 9–17 report some degree of mental and/or behavioral health problems. Unfortunately, these health issues are frequently not recognized and underappreciated. It is well documented that primary care providers identify only a small proportion or these children and young adults [21, 22]. Even for these patients that are identified, significant barriers exist in the referral process, including lack of available specialists, insurance restrictions, appointment delays, and stigma [23]. These obstacles are even more troublesome in rural areas where access to child and adolescent psychiatric, behavioral, and psychological services is exceedingly poor. The dearth of resources for these children and adolescents with mental health concerns places a significant burden on primary care providers and the family members of the afflicted patient to identify and access behavioral and mental health specialists.

The use of telehealth to provide behavioral and mental health treatment can address some of the access issues. This modality has been well validated as feasible for mental health diagnosis, assessment, and treatment for children and adolescents [24–26]. Telehealth for behavioral and mental health has been used to diagnose and treat a variety of disorders in children and adolescents, including attention deficit hyperactivity disorder, autism spectrum disorder, depression, obsessive-compulsive disorder, and substance abuse, including opioid addiction [24, 25, 27]. And because of the modality, these services increase access because they can be delivered to a variety of settings, including community health outpatient settings, primary care settings, schools, day care centers, juvenile justice, and child welfare settings [24, 28]. Simultaneously, telehealth facilitates improved collaboration with increased frequency between pediatric mental health providers and other professionals, including school staff and primary care physicians [29].

There have been several published reviews on the use of telehealth in the treatment of children and adolescents in need of behavioral and mental health consultations [30–32]. These reviews discuss the utility of telehealth in both clinical mental health emergencies and scheduled outpatient encounters. The published data on nonurgent consultations note that the use of telehealth requires several changes to practice compared to adult models of care, cultural values, rapport-building, pharmacotherapy, and psychotherapy. Particular to scheduled behavioral and mental health visits, infrastructure accommodations at the patient site including space and staffing to conduct developmentally appropriate evaluations and treatment planning with parents and community services are important. For urgent and emergency behavioral and mental health consultations, again, the literature is generally supportive of the quality and timing of telehealth consultations even suggesting that consultations over telehealth can be more cost-effective and efficient than the current standard of care with in-person visits [32]. For recommendations on operations, the American Telemedicine Association has produced practice guidelines for the use of telehealth for behavioral and mental health encounters among children and adolescents [33].

School-Based Telehealth

School-based health centers have provided healthcare in school settings since the late 1960s. With the identification of new models of care to further expand comprehensive services to children, the application of telehealth to school-based health centers emerged in the late 1990s [34]. Subsequently, the use of school-based telehealth has more than doubled in the past 20 years [35]. Data from the 2016–2017 National School-Based Health Care Census identified that 267 of the 2317 school-based health centers were exclusively telehealth-based. In comparison, 2013–2014 census data identified four school-based health centers that were exclusively telehealth-based [35].

School-based telehealth was initially implemented to address the lack in access to and often fragmented care that many children face in rural and underserved areas. Children living in underserved communities are at higher risk of not having regular health maintenance visits and typically receive care from multiple settings including schools, medical offices, family planning centers, mental health clinics, and emergency departments [36, 37]. This fragmented care model creates a lack in the continuity of care, is time-consuming, and puts children at higher risk from being chronically absent from school, experiencing suspension, or dropping out of school [38, 39].

School-based telehealth is an appropriate response to meet these needs. Services offered through school-based telehealth typically include primary care, mental healthcare, social services, oral healthcare, reproductive health, nutrition education, and vision services [35]. Providing these services helps to reduce many barriers that families in underserved communities face such as transportation, time, costs, and lack of continuity of care [35].

School-based telehealth has been associated with improved health outcomes including preventive screening for oral health, vision, substance use, and nutrition; increased vaccinations; increased access to and use of mental and behavioral health services; decreased high-risk behaviors; and decreased emergency department use [40, 41]. School-based telehealth has also been shown to show promise in improving health benefits among children with asthma on Medicaid [42]. The presence or use of the centers is also associated with improved student achievement outcomes and improved feelings of connectedness to the learning environment for students, parents, and school personnel [43, 44].

Future opportunities for school-based telehealth services can include novel models of care delivery. For example, one such model is using school-based telehealth for directly observed therapy to ensure patient adherence to treatment. Most studies on telehealth directly observed therapy have involved management of adult; however, asynchronous or synchronous telehealth directly observed therapy could be used for children during school hours [41]. Such application of telehealth would simultaneously decrease the resources required by health departments and increase the convenience for families.

Importantly, school-based telehealth applications pose unique and special considerations. Given that telehealth delivery involves contracts between school systems and healthcare providers, specific policies for these services need to be developed to ensure that both Family Educational Rights and Privacy Act (FERPA) and Health Insurance Portability and Accountability Act (HIPAA) regulations are met [45].

Telehealth for Labor and Delivery and Newborn Settings

Telehealth is recently becoming integrated into labor and delivery and newborn settings for a variety of clinical applications [46]. Pediatricians and pediatric subspecialists like neonatologists, genomic medicine experts, and pediatric surgeons can become involved in providing consultations to obstetricians and during labor and delivery if there are anticipated congenital, metabolic, or other abnormalities such as malformations [47]. Some of the uses include consultation during labor when complications or the need for transfer are anticipated as well as during the newborn period such as for neonatal resuscitation assistance, tele-echocardiography consultations, tele-ophthalmology consultations, or discharge/transfer assistance and family involvement [48–55]. The ability to access neonatologists and expert neonatal care contributes to improvements in outcomes. Given that neonatal expertise is regionalized, telehealth is an appealing modality for reducing healthcare disparities, particularly for rural and underserved communities.

Because newborn nurseries and/or hospitals providing level I and level II newborn care are less equipped for children needing a higher level of care, there tends to be the approach of transferring newborns if there is any concern. This "err on the side of caution" approach is safe but results in over-triage and many newborns being transferred than may be necessary. If telehealth is used under these circumstances, one might suspect that costs and transfer rates could be significantly decreased with the use of telehealth for newborn consultations. Indeed, some research has shown that the use of synchronous telehealth for video-assisted consultations was associated with a 20–30% reduction in a newborn's risk of being transferred [56, 57]. As expected, because of the reduction in transfers, the use of telehealth resulted in significant cost savings [56, 57].

In addition to having a positive impact on otherwise healthy newborns, telehealth is used on newborns in need of emergent care and consultation. Providers at rural and community hospitals often do not have as much opportunity for practice of their resuscitation skills as providers at larger centers and are, therefore, often unable to provide the high level of care needed in an emergency. Education through telehealth can bring additional training opportunities to these rural sites in a low-resource model in order to better prepare them for advanced neonatal resuscitation [58]. Telehealth also offers the opportunity to immediately bring a more experienced team to newborns to provide support or even lead the resuscitation. Telehealth can also be used to train and assist in the performance of emergent procedures occasionally required during a neonatal resuscitation including airway management, needle thoracentesis, and umbilical line placement [59]. Telehealth can provide unique opportunities to significantly increase the quality of neonatal resuscitation and stabilization in rural or community hospitals.

A new wave of telehealth technologies for neonatal support is emerging through home-based programs utilizing videoconferencing and mobile health technologies. Home-based programs allow for families to care for their babies, most commonly preterm babies who otherwise would require NICU hospitalization. While at home, families are able to manage care such as tube feeding, breastfeeding, and bottle establishment with the support of NICU nurses and physicians through a telehealth app or videoconferencing [60]. These types of programs have unique benefits in not only reducing the length of stay within hospitals but increasing family-centered care providing tools that strengthen the parent-child relationship and increased confidence in the caregivers' decision-making [60].

Pediatric Emergency Telehealth Services

The majority of children seeking emergency care is seen in EDs with a pediatric volume of fewer than 15 children per day [61]. These EDs are, at times, inadequately equipped to care for pediatric emergencies, with physicians, nurses, pharmacists, and support staff that are often less experienced in caring for critically ill children [62–65]. The relative lack of equipment, infrastructure, and personnel experienced in delivering specialty care to children may result in delayed or incorrect diagnoses and suboptimal therapies and medical management [66–68]. As a consequence, children often receive lower quality of care than children presenting to EDs in regionalized children's hospitals [69–72]. In fact, children presenting to EDs with lower level of readiness to care for pediatric emergencies are associated with increased odds of mortality [73]. Moreover, children are at high risk of over-triage, whereby they are unnecessarily transferred to a subsequent hospital. Upward of 39% of pediatric transfers is avoidable [74–78]. This over-triage imposes distress and burden to patients, families, and providers. Furthermore, under-triage can also occur and impose significant patient safety risks.

Fortunately, the use of telehealth in emergency settings has produced positive outcomes, demonstrating the ability of telehealth use to overcome some of these recognized pediatric emergency challenges. Research suggests that the use of telehealth to virtually bring the consulting physician to the ED bedside can improve the consulting physician's ability to remotely assess the patient's illness severity and medical needs, thereby facilitating improved patient, family, and utilization outcomes [79–81]. Research demonstrates that telehealth consultations, in comparison to standard telephone consultations, result in patients receiving higher overall quality of care [2, 82]. Telehealth pediatric emergency consultations have been shown to result in lower rates of medication errors when compared to both telephone consultations and no consultations [83]. Finally, among critically ill children requiring transfer to another hospital for definitive care, data suggest that the use of telehealth can help patients arrive more stable to the accepting pediatric ICU compared to when pre-transfer care is made over the telephone [84].

There is also evidence that pediatric emergency telehealth use can address the considerable transfer triage problems. Research supports that when pediatric critical care physicians provide telehealth consultations to seriously ill children in remote and rural EDs, the initial care and management of these patients will not only be higher but also inappropriate transfers will be reduced. Specifically, the use of telehealth has shown to reduce the overall rates of transfer of children, particularly those with very low measures of severity of illness, by approximately 20% [85]. Increased adoption of pediatric emergency telehealth applications will allow for more children to be treated in their local EDs rather than unnecessarily transferred to a children's hospital. By reducing unnecessary transfers, telehealth helps to reduce the associated excessive stress, burdens, and safety risks.

Telehealth application in the emergency setting can also directly improve the patient and family experience. Research suggests that telehealth use for pediatric emergencies can lessen family stress [86, 87]. The virtual presence of the consulting physician at the patient's bedside permits enhanced family-centeredness of care through improved information sharing, shared decision-making, and coordination [88]. Telehealth allows for the family to participate in conversations between the ED and consulting physician, which allows for increased family understanding, reassurance, and trust. As such, research has shown that parents of children in the ED are more satisfied when telehealth is used for consultations compared to the telephone [2]. In fact, pediatric emergency telehealth applications have been reported as feasible and well liked among not only patients and parents but also remote providers and specialists [2, 89].

Regarding the adoption of pediatric emergency telehealth services, the majority of EDs that receive these telehealth services is EDs not staffed by board-certified pediatric emergency medicine physicians or pediatricians [90]. Therefore, telehealth is largely used in the EDs with limited access to pediatric expertise. Pediatric emergency telehealth users most frequently report using telehealth for patient placement and transfer coordination (80%); other frequent uses include assistance with treatment and assistance with diagnosis of conditions [90].

Direct to Consumer Telehealth

One of the most rapidly emerging uses of telehealth in pediatric care is "direct to consumer" or "direct to patient" telehealth. This type of telehealth connects a provider over video directly to the patient/family when the patient is not located in an originating site, such as a clinic or hospital. Patients can be located at home, at work, at school, or elsewhere [54, 91, 92]. For the encounter, a telehealth application directly connects the provider to the patient on their personal computer, tablet, or smart phone. As one can imagine, the convenience for this type of visit is significant but can be limiting given the fact that many aspects of an office visit may not be readily available given infrastructure limitations, including vital signs and assistance with a local provider during the physical exam.

Direct to consumer pediatric telehealth has been increasing as it has been shown to result in high patient/parent satisfaction given the convenience of care. There is also some evidence that the care provided using this model can result in more efficient and appropriate care. For example, during an acute illness, there is some evidence that these encounters can obviate the need to an urgent care facility or emergency department [93, 94]. Also, these visits have been shown to be very appropriate for follow-up from ambulatory encounters, medication change follow-ups, post-surgical checks, or post-discharge follow-up, particularly for patients and families that live in faraway rural communities.

However, direct to consumer telehealth care must be delivered directly to families within the context and inside the medical home. That is, care must be patient-centered, comprehensive, team-based, coordinated, accessible, and focused on quality and safety. This can only be accomplished if the direct to consumer model of care includes some connection to the primary care team. Ideally, the providers would be familiar with the patient and have access to their medical record [95]. Some research has found that when direct to consumer telehealth visits are provided outside of the medical home and exclude the primary care provider, children are more likely to inappropriately receive therapies such as antibiotics and less likely to receive guideline-concordant management compared to children treated in person [96, 97]. There is even some evidence that these visits, when conducted outside of the medical home, result in more utilization and higher costs of care [94, 96].

Although stand-alone episodic care offered to families using telehealth is appealing to some payers and tech-savvy patients for convenience and affordability, the loss of continuity, variable quality, and limited data on safety are substantial [94, 98–101]. Care models, as outlined by the American Academy of Pediatrics, need to support the patient-centered medical home to avoid these potentially negative consequences [95, 102]. When provided within the medical home, these models of care can contribute to safe, patient-centered, timely, effective, efficient, and equitable care.

Conclusion

Application of telehealth to pediatric care services is feasible and effective. Pediatric telehealth can significantly improve provider satisfaction, patient and family experience, quality of care, patient safety, and costs of care. As technology advances and telehealth services become increasingly ubiquitous, expansion of telehealth applications and increased adoption of various telehealth models of care have the potential to drastically improve pediatric healthcare access and care quality. Importantly, telehealth can overcome many of the geographical and socioeconomic disparities that exist and prevent children from receiving optimal comprehensive healthcare.

Telehealth will increasingly become a standard part of the healthcare system. As the telehealth landscape evolves, health providers must incorporate into their telehealth practices the up-to-date practice guidelines, position statements, and recommendations from professional organizations such as the American Telemedicine

Association [45]. As pediatric telehealth applications expand, continued rigorous research is needed to evaluate these care models in order to optimize their implementation and effectiveness.

References

1. Dorsey ER, Topol EJ. State of telehealth. N Engl J Med. 2016;375(2):154–61.
2. Dharmar M, Romano PS, Kuppermann N, Nesbitt TS, Cole SL, Andrada ER, et al. Impact of critical care telemedicine consultations on children in rural emergency departments. Crit Care Med. 2013;41(10):2388–95.
3. Uscher-Pines L, Kahn JM. Barriers and facilitators to pediatric emergency telemedicine in the United States. Telemed J E Health. 2014;20(11):990–6.
4. Rogers FB, Ricci M, Caputo M, Shackford S, Sartorelli K, Callas P, et al. The use of telemedicine for real-time video consultation between trauma center and community hospital in a rural setting improves early trauma care: preliminary results. J Trauma. 2001;51(6):1037–41.
5. Brennan JA, Kealy JA, Gerardi LH, Shih R, Allegra J, Sannipoli L, et al. A randomized controlled trial of telemedicine in an emergency department. J Telemed Telecare. 1998;4 Suppl 1:18–20.
6. Brennan JA, Kealy JA, Gerardi LH, Shih R, Allegra J, Sannipoli L, et al. Telemedicine in the emergency department: a randomized controlled trial. J Telemed Telecare. 1999;5(1):18–22.
7. Olson CA, McSwain SD, Curfman AL, Chuo J. The current pediatric telehealth landscape. Pediatrics. 2018;141(3):e20172334.
8. Marcin JP, Shaikh U, Steinhorn RH. Addressing health disparities in rural communities using telehealth. Pediatr Res. 2015;79(1–2):169–76.
9. Gustke KA, Golladay GJ, Roche MW, Jerry GJ, Elson LC, Anderson CR. Increased satisfaction after total knee replacement using sensor-guided technology. Bone Joint J. 2014;96-B(10):1333–8.
10. Saleh S, Larsen JP, Bergsaker-Aspoy J, Grundt H. Re-admissions to hospital and patient satisfaction among patients with chronic obstructive pulmonary disease after telemedicine video consultation – a retrospective pilot study. Multidiscip Respir Med. 2014;9(1):6.
11. Marcin JP, Nesbitt TS, Cole SL, Knuttel RM, Hilty DM, Prescott PT, et al. Changes in diagnosis, treatment, and clinical improvement among patients receiving telemedicine consultations. Telemed J E Health. 2005;11(1):36–43.
12. Dayal P, Chang CH, Benko WS, Pollock BH, Crossen SS, Kissee J, et al. Hospital utilization among rural children served by pediatric neurology telemedicine clinics. JAMA Netw Open. 2019;2(8):e199364.
13. Dayal P, Chang CH, Benko WS, Ulmer AM, Crossen SS, Pollock BH, et al. Appointment completion in pediatric neurology telemedicine clinics serving underserved patients. Neurol Clin Pract. 2019;9(4):314–21.
14. Ray KN, Kahn JM. Connected subspecialty care: applying telehealth strategies to specific referral barriers. Acad Pediatr. 2020;20(1):16–22.
15. Patel UK, Malik P, DeMasi M, Lunagariya A, Jani VB. Multidisciplinary approach and outcomes of tele-neurology: a review. Cureus. 2019;11(4)
16. Olson CA, Thomas JF. Telehealth: no longer an idea for the future. Adv Pediatr. 2017;64(1):347–70.
17. Naka F, Makkar H, Lu J. Teledermatology: kids are not just little people. Clin Dermatol. 2017;35(6):594–600.
18. Komaromy M, Duhigg D, Metcalf A, Carlson C, Kalishman S, Hayes L, et al. Project ECHO (Extension for Community Healthcare Outcomes): a new model for educating primary care providers about treatment of substance use disorders. Subst Abus. 2016;37(1):20–4.

19. Zhou C, Crawford A, Serhal E, Kurdyak P, Sockalingam S. The impact of project ECHO on participant and patient outcomes: a systematic review. Acad Med. 2016;91(10):1439–61.
20. American Academy of Pediatrics (AAP) ECHO 2020. Available from: https://www.aap.org/en-us/professional-resources/practice-transformation/echo/Pages/default.aspx.
21. Centers for Disease Control and Prevention. Mental health surveillance among children — United States, 2005–2011. Morbidity and Mortality Weekly Report (MMWR) Surveill Summ. 2013;62:1–35.
22. Rhew IC, David Hawkins J, Oesterle S. Drug use and risk among youth in different rural contexts. Health Place. 2011;17(3):775–83.
23. American Academy of Child and Adolescent Psychiatry (AACAP) Committee on Telepsychiatry and AACAP Committee on Quality Issues. Clinical update: telepsychiatry with children and adolescents. J Am Acad Child Adolesc Psychiatry. 2017;56(10):875–93.
24. Nelson EL, Sharp S. A review of pediatric telemental health. Pediatr Clin N Am. 2016;63(5):913–31.
25. Archangeli C, Marti FA, Wobga-Pasiah EA, Zima B. Mobile health interventions for psychiatric conditions in children: a scoping review. Child Adolesc Psychiatr Clin N Am. 2017;26(1):13–31.
26. Van Allen J, Davis AM, Lassen S. The use of telemedicine in pediatric psychology: research review and current applications. Child Adolesc Psychiatr Clin N Am. 2011;20(1):55–66.
27. LaBelle B, Franklyn AM, Pkh Nguyen V, Anderson KE, Eibl JK, Marsh DC. Characterizing the use of telepsychiatry for patients with opioid use disorder and cooccurring mental health disorders in Ontario. Can Int J Telemed Appl. 2018;2018:7937610.
28. Keilman P. Telepsychiatry with child welfare families referred to a family service agency. Telemed J E Health. 2005;11(1):98–101.
29. Roth DE, Ramtekkar U, Zeković-Roth S. Telepsychiatry: a new treatment venue for pediatric depression. Child Adoles Psychiatr Clin. 2019;28(3):377–95.
30. Gloff NE, LeNoue SR, Novins DK, Myers K. Telemental health for children and adolescents. Int Rev Psychiatry. 2015;27(6):513–24.
31. Ellington E, McGuinness TM. Telepsychiatry for children and adolescents. J Psychosoc Nurs Ment Health Serv. 2011;49(2):19–22.
32. Thomas JF, Novins DK, Hosokawa PW, Olson CA, Hunter D, Brent AS, et al. The use of telepsychiatry to provide cost-efficient care during pediatric mental health emergencies. Psychiatr Serv. 2018;69(2):161–8.
33. Myers K, Nelson EL, Rabinowitz T, Hilty D, Baker D, Barnwell SS, et al. American telemedicine association practice guidelines for telemental health with children and adolescents. Telemed J E Health. 2017;23(10):779–804.
34. Lessard JA, Rn RK. Telehealth in a rural school-based health center. J Sch Nurs. 2000;16(2):38–41.
35. Love HE, Schlitt J, Soleimanpour S, Panchal N, Behr C. Twenty years of school-based health care growth and expansion. Health Aff (Millwood). 2019;38(5):755–64.
36. Irwin CE Jr, Adams SH, Park MJ, Newacheck PW. Preventive care for adolescents: few get visits and fewer get services. Pediatrics. 2009;123(4):e565–72.
37. Lawrence RS, Appleton Gootman J, Sim LJ, editors. Adolescent health services: missing opportunities. Washington, DC; 2009.
38. Basch CE. Healthier students are better learners: a missing link in school reforms to close the achievement gap. J Sch Health. 2011;81(10):593–8.
39. Council On School Health. School-based health centers and pediatric practice. Pediatrics. 2012;129(2):387–93.
40. Knopf JA, Finnie RK, Peng Y, Hahn RA, Truman BI, Vernon-Smiley M, et al. School-based health centers to advance health equity: a community guide systematic review. Am J Prev Med. 2016;51(1):114–26.
41. Tomines A. Pediatric telehealth: approaches by specialty and implications for general pediatric care. Adv Pediatr. 2019;66:55.

42. Bian J, Cristaldi KK, Summer AP, Su Z, Marsden J, Mauldin PD, et al. Association of a School-Based, Asthma-Focused Telehealth Program With Emergency Department Visits Among Children Enrolled in South Carolina Medicaid. JAMA Pediatr. 2019;73(11):1041–8.
43. Keeton V, Soleimanpour S, Brindis CD. School-based health centers in an era of health care reform: building on history. Curr Probl Pediatr Adolesc Health Care. 2012;42(6):132–56; discussion 57–8.
44. Strolin-Goltzman J, Sisselman A, Melekis K, Auerbach C. Understanding the relationship between school-based health center use, school connection, and academic performance. Health Soc Work. 2014;39(2):83–91.
45. American Academy of Pediatrics. Operating procedures for pediatric telehealth. Pediatrics. 2017;140(2):e20171756.
46. Alves DS, Times VC, da Silva EMA, Melo PSA, Novaes MA. Advances in obstetric tele-monitoring: a systematic review. Int J Med Inform. 2020;134:104004.
47. Weissman SM, Zellmer K, Gill N, Wham D. Implementing a virtual health telemedicine program in a community setting. J Genet Couns. 2018;27(2):323–5.
48. Makkar A, McCoy M, Hallford G, Foulks A, Anderson M, Milam J, et al. Evaluation of neonatal services provided in a level II NICU utilizing hybrid telemedicine: a prospective study. Telemed J E Health. 2020;26(2):176–83.
49. Wenger TL, Gerdes J, Taub K, Swarr DT, Deardorff MA, Abend NS. Telemedicine for genetic and neurologic evaluation in the neonatal intensive care unit. J Perinatol: official journal of the California Perinatal Association. 2014;34(3):234–40.
50. Fang JL, Collura CA, Johnson RV, Asay GF, Carey WA, Derleth DP, et al. Emergency video telemedicine consultation for newborn resuscitations: the Mayo Clinic experience. Mayo Clin Proc. 2016;91(12):1735–43.
51. Moser L, Diogenes T, Mourato FA, Mattos S. Learning echocardiography and changing realities through telemedicine. Med Educ. 2014;48(11):1125–6.
52. Wang SK, Callaway NF, Wallenstein MB, Henderson MT, Leng T, Moshfeghi DM. SUNDROP: six years of screening for retinopathy of prematurity with telemedicine. Can J Ophthalmol. 2015;50(2):101–6.
53. Jain A, Agarwal R, Chawla D, Paul V, Deorari A. Tele-education vs classroom training of neonatal resuscitation: a randomized trial. J Perinatol. 2010;30(12):773–9.
54. Willard A, Brown E, Masten M, Brant M, Pouppirt N, Moran K, et al. Complex surgical infants benefit from postdischarge telemedicine visits. Adv Neonatal Care. 2018;18(1):22–30.
55. Gray J, Jones PC, Phillips M, Gertman P, Veroff D, Safran C. Telematics in the neonatal ICU and beyond: improving care for high-risk newborns and their families. Proc AMIA Annu Fall Symp. 1997:413–7.
56. Haynes SC, Dharmar M, Hill BC, Hoffman KR, Donohue LT, Kuhn-Riordon KM, et al. The impact of telemedicine on transfer rates of newborns at rural community hospitals. Acad Pediatr. 2020;20(5):636–41.
57. Albritton J, Maddox L, Dalto J, Ridout E, Minton S. The effect of a newborn telehealth program on transfers avoided: a multiple-baseline study. Health Aff. 2018;37(12):1990–6.
58. Donohue LT, Hoffman KR, Marcin JP. Use of Telemedicine to Improve Neonatal Resuscitation. Children (Basel). 2019;6(4)
59. Sauers-Ford HS, Marcin JP, Underwood MA, Kim JH, Nicolau Y, Uy C, et al. The use of telemedicine to address disparities in access to specialist care for neonates. Telemed J E Health. 2019;25(9):775–80.
60. Garne Holm K, Brodsgaard A, Zachariassen G, Smith AC, Clemensen J. Parent perspectives of neonatal tele-homecare: a qualitative study. J Telemed Telecare. 2019;25(4):221–9.
61. Gausche-Hill M, Ely M, Schmuhl P, Telford R, Remick KE, Edgerton EA, et al. A national assessment of pediatric readiness of emergency departments. JAMA Pediatr. 2015;169(6):527–34.
62. Remick K, Kaji AH, Olson L, Ely M, Schmuhl P, McGrath N, et al. Pediatric readiness and facility verification. Ann Emerg Med. 2016;67(3):320–8. e1

63. Middleton KR, Burt CW. Availability of pediatric services and equipment in emergency departments: United States, 2002–03. Adv Data. 2006;367:1–16.
64. Gausche-Hill M, Schmitz C, Lewis RJ. Pediatric preparedness of US emergency departments: a 2003 survey. Pediatrics. 2007;120(6):1229–37.
65. Bourgeois FT, Shannon MW. Emergency care for children in pediatric and general emergency departments. Pediatr Emerg Care. 2007;23(2):94–102.
66. Phibbs CS, Bronstein JM, Buxton E, Phibbs RH. The effects of patient volume and level of care at the hospital of birth on neonatal mortality. JAMA. 1996;276(13):1054–9.
67. Pollack MM, Alexander SR, Clarke N, Ruttimann UE, Tesselaar HM, Bachulis AC. Improved outcomes from tertiary center pediatric intensive care: a statewide comparison of tertiary and nontertiary care facilities. Crit Care Med. 1991;19(2):150–9.
68. Tilford JM, Roberson PK, Lensing S, Fiser DH. Improvement in pediatric critical care outcomes. Crit Care Med. 2000;28(2):601–3.
69. Dharmar M, Marcin JP, Romano PS, Andrada ER, Overly F, Valente JH, et al. Quality of care of children in the emergency department: association with hospital setting and physician training. J Pediatr. 2008;153(6):783–9.
70. Seidel JS, Hornbein M, Yoshiyama K, Kuznets D, Finklestein JZ, St Geme JW Jr. Emergency medical services and the pediatric patient: are the needs being met? Pediatrics. 1984;73(6):769–72.
71. Seidel JS, Henderson DP, Ward P, Wayland BW, Ness B. Pediatric prehospital care in urban and rural areas. Pediatrics. 1991;88(4):681–90.
72. Durch JS, Lohr KN. From the Institute of Medicine. JAMA. 1993;270(8):929.
73. Ames SG, Davis BS, Marin JR, Fink EL, Olson LM, Gausche-Hill M, et al. Emergency department pediatric readiness and mortality in critically ill children. Pediatrics. 2019;144(3):e20190568.
74. Mohr NM, Harland KK, Shane DM, Miller SL, Torner JC. Potentially avoidable pediatric interfacility transfer is a costly burden for rural families: a cohort study. Acad Emerg Med. 2016;23(8):885–94.
75. Li J, Monuteaux MC, Bachur RG. Interfacility transfers of noncritically III children to academic pediatric emergency departments. Pediatrics. 2012:peds. 2011-1819.
76. Gattu RK, Teshome G, Cai L, Wright C, Lichenstein R. Interhospital pediatric patient transfers—factors influencing rapid disposition after transfer. Pediatr Emerg Care. 2014;30(1):26–30.
77. Peebles ER, Miller MR, Lynch TP, Tijssen JA. Factors associated with discharge home after transfer to a pediatric emergency department. Pediatr Emerg Care. 2018;34(9):650–5.
78. Ray KN, Marin JR, Li J, Davis BS, Kahn JM. Referring hospital characteristics associated with potentially avoidable emergency department transfers. Acad Emerg Med. 2019;26(2):205–16.
79. Desai S, Williams ML, Smith AC. Teleconsultation from a secondary hospital for paediatric emergencies occurring at rural hospitals in Queensland. J Telemed Telecare. 2013;19(7):405–10.
80. Tachakra S, Uche CU, Stinson A. Four years' experience of telemedicine support of a minor accident and treatment service. J Telemed Telecare. 2002;8(2 suppl):87–9.
81. Marcin JP, Nesbitt TS, Struve S, Traugott C, Dimand RJ. Financial benefits of a pediatric intensive care unit-based telemedicine program to a rural adult intensive care unit: impact of keeping acutely ill and injured children in their local community. Telemed J e-Health. 2004;10(Supplement 2):S-1–5.
82. Dharmar M, Marcin JP, Kuppermann N, Andrada ER, Cole S, Harvey DJ, et al. A new implicit review instrument for measuring quality of care delivered to pediatric patients in the emergency department. BMC Emerg Med. 2007;7:13.
83. Dharmar M, Kuppermann N, Romano PS, Yang NH, Nesbitt TS, Phan J, et al. Telemedicine consultations and medication errors in rural emergency departments. Pediatrics. 2013;132(6):1090–7.

84. Dayal P, Hojman NM, Kissee JL, Evans J, Natale JE, Huang Y, et al. Impact of telemedicine on severity of illness and outcomes among children transferred from referring emergency departments to a children's hospital PICU. Pediatr Critical Care Med. 2016;17(6):516–21.
85. Yang NH, Dharmar M, Kuppermann N, Romano PS, Nesbitt TS, Hojman NM, et al. Appropriateness of disposition following telemedicine consultations in rural emergency departments. Pediatr Crit Care Med. 2015;16(3):e59–64.
86. Rosenthal JL, Li S-TT, Hernandez L, Alvarez M, Rehm RS, Okumura MJ. Familial caregiver and physician perceptions of the family-physician interactions during interfacility transfers. Hosp Pediatr. 2017;7(6):344–51.
87. Sauers-Ford HS, Hamline MY, Gosdin MM, Kair LR, Weinberg GM, Marcin JP, et al. Acceptability, usability, and effectiveness: a qualitative study evaluating a pediatric telemedicine program. Acad Emerg Med. 2019;26(9):1022–33.
88. Byczkowski TL, Gillespie GL, Kennebeck SS, Fitzgerald MR, Downing KA, Alessandrini EA. Family-centered pediatric emergency care: a framework for measuring what parents want and value. Acad Pediatr. 2016;16(4):327–35.
89. Heath B, Salerno R, Hopkins A, Hertzig J, Caputo M. Pediatric critical care telemedicine in rural underserved emergency departments. Pediatr Crit Care Med. 2009;10(5):588–91.
90. Brova M, Boggs KM, Zachrison KS, Freid RD, Sullivan AF, Espinola JA, et al. Pediatric Telemedicine Use in United States Emergency Departments. Acad Emerg Med. 2018;25(12):1427–32.
91. Choi YS, Berry-Caban C, Nance J. Telemedicine in paediatric patients with poorly controlled type 1 diabetes. J Telemed Telecare. 2013;19(4):219–21.
92. Lindgren S, Wacker D, Suess A, Schieltz K, Pelzel K, Kopelman T, et al. Telehealth and autism: treating challenging behavior at lower cost. Pediatrics. 2016;137 Suppl 2:S167–75.
93. Foster CB, Martinez KA, Sabella C, Weaver GP, Rothberg MB. Patient satisfaction and antibiotic prescribing for respiratory infections by telemedicine. Pediatrics. 2019;144(3)
94. Ashwood JS, Mehrotra A, Cowling D, Uscher-Pines L. Direct-to-consumer telehealth may increase access to care but does not decrease spending. Health Aff (Millwood). 2017;36(3):485–91.
95. Basco WT, Rimsza ME, Committee on Pediatric W, American Academy of P. Pediatrician workforce policy statement. Pediatrics. 2013;132(2):390–7.
96. Ray KN, Shi Z, Gidengil CA, Poon SJ, Uscher-Pines L, Mehrotra A. Antibiotic Prescribing During Pediatric Direct-to-Consumer Telemedicine Visits. Pediatrics. 2019;143(5)
97. Martinez KA, Rood M, Jhangiani N, Boissy A, Rothberg MB. Antibiotic prescribing for respiratory tract infections and encounter length: an observational study of telemedicine. Ann Intern Med. 2019;170(4):275–7.
98. Mehrotra A, Paone S, Martich GD, Albert SM, Shevchik GJ. Characteristics of patients who seek care via eVisits instead of office visits. Telemed J e-Health. 2013;19(7):515–9.
99. Mehrotra A, Paone S, Martich GD, Albert SM, Shevchik GJ. A comparison of care at e-visits and physician office visits for sinusitis and urinary tract infection. JAMA Intern Med. 2013;173(1):72–4.
100. Hickson R, Talbert J, Thornbury WC, Perin NR, Goodin AJ. Online medical care: the current state of "eVisits" in acute primary care delivery. Telemed J e-Health. 2015;21(2):90–6.
101. Martinez KA, Rood M, Jhangiani N, Kou L, Boissy A, Rothberg MB. Association between antibiotic prescribing for respiratory tract infections and patient satisfaction in direct-to-consumer telemedicine. JAMA Intern Med. 2018;178(11):1558–60.
102. Price J, Brandt ML, Hudak ML, American Academy of Pediatrics, Committee on Child Health Financing. Principles of financing the medical home for children. Pediatrics. 2020;145(1):e20193451.

Overview of Child Telebehavioral Interventions Using Real-Time Videoconferencing

22

Alexandra D. Monzon, E. Zhang, Arwen M. Marker, and Eve-Lynn Nelson

Introduction

Many children and adolescents with behavioral health concerns do not receive any intervention, let alone evidence-based treatments delivered by behavioral health specialists [1]. Pediatric behavioral telehealth interventions have steadily increased the opportunity for youth and their families to receive services not previously accessible. This is particularly true for families living in rural areas, underserved communities, families that do not have access to adequate mental health insurance, and families with limited transportation options [2]. Further, behavioral telehealth interventions provide the opportunity for increased attendance to sessions by diminishing the financial and temporal barriers of travel and time from work as well as offering access to a therapist outside of the community via health clinics and schools, which may be less stigmatizing than traditional mental health settings. Ultimately, telehealth services have increased the supply of psychotherapy or behavioral approaches to support children and their families in coping with a range of challenges. Similarly, pediatric tele-psychopharmacology has a growing evidence base [5], with results described in other chapters.

With adults, the research base regarding behavioral telehealth interventions has exponentially grown over the past few decades. Child providers draw lessons from this information as well as a growing child research base. The authors first summarize research to date related to interventions using videoconferencing to address (1) psychopathology in general clinical child cases, (2) issues in pediatric psychology, and (3) Applied Behavior Analysis (ABA) and developmental concerns. Similar to previous search criteria [3], studies were included if they (1) consisted of

A. D. Monzon · A. M. Marker
Clinical Child Psychology, University of Kansas, Lawrence, KS, USA

E. Zhang · E.-L. Nelson (✉)
Pediatrics, University of Kansas Medical Center, Kansas City, KS, USA
e-mail: enelson2@kumc.edu

© Springer Nature Switzerland AG 2021
R. Latifi et al. (eds.), *Telemedicine, Telehealth and Telepresence*,
https://doi.org/10.1007/978-3-030-56917-4_22

videoconferencing applications across the child and adolescent age range; (2) included individual psychotherapy, pediatric psychology interventions, or a developmental concern; (3) included videoconferencing as the method of intervention; and (4) consisted of real-time videoconferencing across devices regardless of setting. Studies were excluded if they (1) used web-based or eHealth interventions as a primary method for service delivery, and/or (2) focused solely on education/training or population description. Telebehavioral studies informing diagnostic accuracy and on assessment are very important areas in telehealth but are beyond the scope of the chapter.

Clinical Child Therapy

The studies that have addressed clinical child interventions using videoconferencing are summarized in Table 22.1. While interest in child telebehavioral health services has grown over the last 5 years, there are a limited number of additional clinical child studies from previous reviews [4]. Overall, the evidence continues to support the use of videoconferencing-delivered therapies across child externalizing and internalizing disorders, within the context of consensus-based child telemental health guidelines [5] and best practices [6].

There is also emerging literature about the use of videoconferencing to deliver the empirically supported Parent–Child Interaction Therapy (PCIT) [7]. Comer et al. [8] suggested that videoconferencing may be a good fit for PCIT because the PCIT therapist is not in the same room as the family for most of the intervention and is monitoring from another room and providing real-time feedback to the parent(s) through a bug-in-the-ear device. They randomized 40 young children with disruptive behavior disorders to two conditions—PCIT delivered through videoconferencing to the home and PCIT delivered onsite in the clinic. After treatment, the intent-to-treatment analyses found that 70% of children treated with the telebehavioral intervention showed treatment response, and at 6-month follow-up, over half continued to show treatment response. Limitations were noted around the need for a larger sample size and noninferiority designs. With these positive results, there is growing national and international interest in PCIT over videoconferencing, including PCIT delivered to the school setting [9]. Similarly, Dadds et al. [10] completed two randomized controlled trials with children exhibiting conduct problems. They found that the effects of the therapist-assisted online parenting interventions (that included videoconferencing) were similar to the onsite clinic-based interventions, with positive outcomes across outcome and process measures and promising effect sizes.

Early telebehavioral work suggests positive outcomes for teletherapy interventions for children with Attention-Deficit Hyperactivity Disorder (ADHD) [4]. As part of a large randomized trial for children with ADHD (CATTS; [11]), Tse et al. [12] reported findings from a subsample of 37 children. All families received pharmacotherapy through videoconferencing. Twelve families received caregiver training over videoconferencing and 25 received the intervention in-person. They found

Table 22.1 Clinical child therapy using videoconferencing

Study	Population	Sample description & sample size	Study design	Findings
Carpenter et al. (2018) [22]	Anxiety	$N = 14$ youth Mean age: 9.85 years	VC feasibility	Family-based CBT for child anxiety delivered to the home setting via VC. The intervention was feasible and acceptable. Treatment gains were largely maintained at 3-month follow-up evaluation
Comer et al. (2017) [15]	OCD	$N = 22$ youth Mean age: 6.5 years	RCT, VC vs. F2F	Family-based CBT for OCD; outcomes similar for VC and F2F at posttreatment and follow-up
Comer et al. (2017) [8]	Disruptive behaviors	$N = 40$ youth Ages: 3–5 years	RCT, VC vs. F2F	Similar outcomes for in-person PCIT vs. i-PCIT at posttreatment and follow-up
Dadds et al., 2019 [10]	ODD, Conduct Disorder	Study 1: $N = 133$ families (rural) Ages = 3–9 years Study 2: $N = 73$ families (urban) Ages = 3–14 years	RCT, VC vs. F2F	Study 1: VC group attended more treatment sessions than F2F. Study 1 & 2: Significant reduction in child clinical disruptive behavior disorder, child oppositional behavior, and mother internalizing symptoms pre–post for both VC and F2F groups. No significant differences between groups. Study 2: VC group reported higher treatment satisfaction that F2F
Fox et al. (2008) [23]	Juvenile offenders	$N = 190$ youth Ages: 12–19 years	VC pre–post	Youth increased goal achievement in areas of health, family, and social skills
Himle et al. (2012) [24]	Tic disorders	$N = 18$ youth Ages: 8–17 years	RCT, VC vs. F2F	Across groups, significant improvements in tic behaviors and strong ratings for acceptability and therapist–client alliance. No differences between treatment groups
Kirkman et al. (2016) [25]	ODD and Conduct Disorder	$N = 47$ youth Ages: 3–12 years	VC vs. F2F pre–post	At posttreatment, parent who had received either intervention reported a significant reduction in oppositional behaviors and ADHD symptoms. Effects were maintained at 3 months

(continued)

Table 22.1 (continued)

Study	Population	Sample description & sample size	Study design	Findings
Myers et al. (2013) [26]	ADHD	$N = 223$ youth Ages: 5–12 years	Feasibility of RCT	The trial demonstrated the feasibility of conducting an RCT. The treatment included an individual therapy component in which the child psychologist used VC to supervise local therapists
Myers et al. (2015) [11]	ADHD	$N = 223$ youth Ages: 5–12 years	RCT, VC vs. F2F	Children in both service models improved; however, children assigned to the VC service model improved significantly more
Nelson et al. (2003) [27]	Depression	$N = 28$ youth Ages: 8–14 years $M = 10.3$ years	RCT, VC vs. F2F	VC and in-person CBT-based intervention demonstrated a comparable reduction in depressive symptoms
Nelson et al. (2006) [17]	Depression	$N = 28$ youth $M = 10.3$ years	RCT, VC vs. F2F	Treatment yielded significant improvement for depression in both conditions, with no between group differences
Nelson et al. (2012) [28]	ADHD	$N = 22$ youth $M = 9.3$ years	VC feasibility	No factor inherent to the VC delivery mechanism impeded adherence to national ADHD guidelines
Reese et al. (2012) [29]	ADHD	$N = 8$ youth $M = 7.6$ years	VC pre–post	Using Group Triple P Positive Parenting Program over VC, families reported improved child behavior and decreased parent distress
Sayal et al. (2019) [18]	Depression, self-harm	$N = 22$ youth Ages: 16–30 years	RCT, VC vs. usual care	Study found to not be feasible ($N = 4$ completed VC intervention) due to recruitment/retention barriers with high risk, severely depressed population
Sibley et al. (2017) [13]	ADHD	$N = 20$ youth Ages: 11–16 years	VC Feasibility	Families reported high satisfaction, and treatment integrity and fidelity were acceptable. Parents and teachers reported reductions in ADHD symptoms and organization, time management, and planning problems from baseline to posttreatment

(continued)

Table 22.1 (continued)

Study	Population	Sample description & sample size	Study design	Findings
Stewart et al. (2017) [21]	Trauma	$N = 15$ youth Ages: 7–16 years	VC Feasibility	Trauma-focused cognitive–behavioral therapy (TF-CBT) delivered to underserved trauma-exposed youth via VC. Results demonstrated clinically meaningful symptom change posttreatment
Storch et al. (2011) [30]	OCD	$N = 31$ youth Ages: 7–16 years $M = 11.1$ years	Waitlist control, VC vs. F2F	VC was superior to F2F on all primary outcome measures, with a significantly higher percent of individuals in the VC group meeting remission criteria than the F2F group
Tse et al. (2015) [12]	ADHD	$N = 22$ youth Ages: 5.5–12 years	RCT, VC vs. F2F	Caregivers in both conditions reported comparable outcomes for their children's ADHD-related behaviors and functioning, but caregivers in the VC group did not report improvement in their own distress
Xie et al. (2013) [31]	ADHD	$N = 22$ parents children $M = 10.4$ years	RCT, VC vs. F2F	Parent training via VC showed same degree of improvement in disciplinary practices, ADHD symptoms, and overall functioning as F2F.

Note: *VC* Videoconferencing, *F2F* Face-to-Face, *RCT* Randomized Controlled Trial, *M* Mean

similar outcomes across measures of attendance, satisfaction, and their children's ADHD-related behaviors and functioning. Sibley et al. [13] reported similar promising results in a preliminary unrandomized investigation of delivering parent–teen therapy for ADHD through videoconferencing to 20 adolescents with ADHD and their parents. The Supporting Teens' Autonomy Daily (STAND) intervention, ten 60-minute manualized family therapy sessions, was delivered via videoconferencing. They summarize their findings as follows:

1. Most families completed a full course of treatment and intervention fidelity and integrity was acceptable.
2. Delivering the intervention was feasible, with minor technological difficulties.
3. Therapeutic alliance was acceptable.
4. Key mechanisms of change appeared to be engaged.
5. ADHD symptoms changed at a rate similar to face-to-face trials; and families were satisfied with treatment.

The adolescent-focused therapy is particularly promising given the negative outcomes often associated with ADHD in adolescence and adulthood [14] and the barriers to onsite treatment with this age group.

Innovative research is also emerging concerning home-based telemedicine for pediatric OCD. Comer et al. [15] found promising results from the first controlled trial evaluating videoconferencing to deliver real-time treatment for early-onset OCD. The family-based CBT intervention showed strong engagement and satisfaction, with over 90% of youth in the intervention completing the full course of treatment. The empirical findings suggest high therapeutic alliance and very high satisfaction. At treatment conclusion, approximately three-fourths of the telebehavioral intervention group showed an "excellent response." Response rates in the intervention group were similar to those found in previous work evaluating the clinic-based OCD intervention. While the authors acknowledge limitations with the sample size in the pilot RCT, findings support the overall feasibility and acceptability of the intervention.

In relation to videoconferencing interventions for childhood depression, much comes from an extrapolation for effective use of similar empirically supported depression therapies (e.g., Cognitive behavioral therapy (CBT)) with adults [16]. An early pilot randomized trial suggested an eight-session CBT intervention for childhood depression was equally effective in the videoconferencing and the control conditions [17]. Sayal et al. [18] noted overall barriers to trials with severe depression and self-harm span onsite and videoconferencing interventions. Luxton et al. [5] outline safety best practices in telepractice, including with children and young adults.

Similarly, guidance concerning videoconferencing interventions related to anxiety disorders [19] and to trauma [20] often comes from adult telebehavioral literature. Stewart et al. [21] presented a promising pilot study of trauma-focused cognitive–behavioral therapy (TF-CBT) delivered using videoconferencing with 15 trauma-exposed youth. They found treatment effects comparable with TF-CBT delivered in an in-person, office-based setting.

Pediatric Psychology Interventions

The authors summarize pediatric psychology interventions using videoconferencing in Table 22.2. Telehealth interventions for pediatric populations have increased over the last decade and a growing number of families report a preference for telehealth-based treatment services [32]. Telehealth services provide an ideal opportunity for families of youth with chronic conditions to receive continuing education or intervention because these services are low burden and more accessible. In a study by Tschamper and Jakobsen [33], families of youth with epilepsy indicated they preferred videoconferencing as opposed to face-to-face meeting, for exchanging information and reducing the frequency of misunderstanding between medical providers and the families. Further, medical providers can assess health outcomes more frequently and facilitate near real-time monitoring and feedback for patients who are unable to attend recurrent clinic visits. Telehealth approaches can aid the

Table 22.2 Pediatric psychology intervention using videoconferencing

Study	Population	Sample description & sample size	Study design	Findings
Anderson et al. (2017) [37]	Anorexia nervosa	$N = 10$ Ages: 13–18	VC feasibility	Recruitment and retention of participants for VC was acceptable. Participant weight increased significantly from pre- to postintervention. Comorbid psychological symptoms (i.e., depression, self-esteem) showed significant improvements at the 6-month follow-up
Bensink, et al. (2008) [34]	Pediatric cancer	$N = 8$ youths Not reported	VC feasibility	Using VC over videophone to families with a child diagnosed with cancer, the study noted technical feasibility and high parental satisfaction
Clawson et al. (2008) [38]	Pediatric feeding Disorders	$N = 15$ youths Ages: 8 months to 10 years	VC feasibility	VC was feasible with the pediatric feeding disorder population and resulted in cost savings
Davis et al. (2013) [39]	Pediatric obesity	$N = 58$ youths Age: 5–11 years $M = 8.6$ years	RCT, VC vs. F2F physician visits	Both groups showed improvements in BMI, nutrition, and physical activity, and the groups did not differ significantly on primary outcomes
Freeman et al. (2013) [40]	Diabetes adherence	$N = 71$ youths VC $M = 15.2$ years F2F $M = 14.9$ years	RCT, VC vs. F2F	No differences were found in therapeutic alliance between the groups
Glueckauf et al. (2002) [41]	Pediatric epilepsy	$N = 22$ youths $M = 15.4$ years	RCT, VC, F2F, and telephone	All groups improved in psychosocial problem severity and frequency and child prosocial behavior, with no significant differences across groups. No differences in adherence between the groups were noted
Hommel et al. (2013) [36]	IBD, adherence	$N = 9$ youths $M = 13.7$ years	VC pre–post	The VC approach resulted in improved adherence and cost savings across patients
Lipana et al. (2013) [42]	Pediatric obesity	$N = 243$ youths $M = 11$ years	Pre–post, VC, and F2F	Using a nonrandomized design, the VC group demonstrated more improvement than the F2F group in enhancing nutrition, increasing activity, and decreasing screen time

(continued)

Table 22.2 (continued)

Study	Population	Sample description & sample size	Study design	Findings
Marker et al. (2019) [43]	Type 1 diabetes	N = 43 families Ages: 1–6 years	VC feasibility	High attendance, low attrition, and high parent-reported satisfaction with group-based telemedicine intervention to reduce fear of hypoglycemia
McCrossan et al. (2007) [44]	Congenital heart disease	N = 66 Ages: 15–542 days	RCT, VC vs. phone vs. F2F	VC was technically feasible and is safe for families of children with congenital heart disease. Clinical assessment of the patient was rated as at least adequate in 94% consultations in the VC group compared with 64% in the telephone group.
Morgan, et al. (2008) [45]	Congenital heart disease	N = 27 parents Child ages: 0–25 months	RCT, VC, and telephone	The VC approach decreased parent anxiety significantly more than phone, and resulted in significantly greater clinical information
Mulgrew et al. (2011) [46]	Pediatric obesity	n = 25 youth Age: 4–11 years	VC feasibility	No significant difference in parent satisfaction between consultations for weight management delivered by VC or F2F
Patton et al. (2020) [35]	Type 1 diabetes	N = 43 families M_{child} = 4.4 years; M_{parent} = 35.2 years	RCT, VC pre–post, 3-month follow-up vs. waitlist	Significant reduction in hypoglycemia fear, trend toward reduction in parent stress frequency compared to waitlist (pre–post). Significant reduction in hypoglycemia fear, parenting stress frequency and difficulty (3-month follow-up). Significant reduction in hemoglobin A1c pre–post for children who entered trial above target range
Shaikh, et al. (2008) [47]	Pediatric obesity	N = 99 youth Ages: 1–17 years	VC pre–post	VC consultations resulted in substantial changes/additions to diagnoses. For a subset of patients, repeated VC consultations led to improved health behaviors, weight maintenance, and/or weight loss

(continued)

Table 22.2 (continued)

Study	Population	Sample description & sample size	Study design	Findings
Tschamper et al. (2019) [33]	Epilepsy	N = 5 Ages: 5–12 years	Qualitative review	VC communication with multidisciplinary team preferred vs. F2F
Wilkinson et al. (2008) [48]	Cystic fibrosis	N = 16 youth Not reported	RCT, videophone vs. F2F	No significant differences in quality of life, anxiety levels, depression levels, admissions to hospital or clinic attendances, general practitioner calls or intravenous antibiotic use between the two groups
Witmans et al. (2008) [49]	Sleep disorders	N = 89 Ages: 1–18 years	VC feasibility	Patients were very satisfied with the delivery of multidisciplinary pediatric sleep medicine services over VC

Note: VC Videoconferencing, F2F Face-to-Face, RCT Randomized Controlled Trial, M Mean

medical team in extending care to patients and their families without requiring them to stay at or near the hospital. Bensink and colleagues [34] discussed how videoconferencing modalities aid in providing additional support regarding referral, scheduling upcoming appointments, and collecting certain data in families of pediatric oncology patients recently discharged. The studies included in Table 22.2 spanned a wide range of chronic and acute childhood illnesses (e.g., oncology, type 1 diabetes, pediatric obesity, epilepsy, cystic fibrosis, and pediatric sleep disorders) and used multiple pediatric psychology interventions, such as cognitive–behavioral strategies to promote coping and strategies to enhance treatment adherence [35]. As with clinical child interventions, findings were overall positive for feasibility, satisfaction, and outcome, although definitive statements are difficult in light of the limited number of studies, small sample sizes, and limited replication.

In addition to consultation services, pediatric psychology interventions delivered via telemedicine are increasingly being tested to promote self-care adherence in patients with different chronic illnesses (i.e., inflammatory bowel disease, type 1 diabetes, obesity). In one study, a tailored multicomponent nonadherence intervention provided preliminary efficacy to improve medication adherence in adolescents with inflammatory bowel disease [36]. These telehealth interventions have the potential to reach a larger patient population and patients who otherwise might be unable to access in-clinic interventions (e.g., rural or medically underserved families). Efficacy trials are beginning to demonstrate that these interventions are just as efficacious as face-to-face interventions in clinic. Interestingly, the interventions summarized in Table 22.2 primarily targeted one to two specific treatment goals, or address issues as they came up through a consultation model. The tailored nature of these studies likely adds to the growing evidence toward efficacy due to specific behavioral outcomes and increased attendance rates among youth and their families. Large-scale efficacy trials will be necessary to determine the full impact of these interventions on medication adherence, treatment adherence, and health outcomes.

Developmental Pediatric Interventions

The authors summarize developmental pediatric interventions using videoconferencing in Table 22.3. The use of videoconferencing-based telehealth to provide developmental pediatric diagnosis and intervention has increased in recent years. Studies confirming this trend were conducted largely with children with autism spectrum disorders (ASD) (see previous systematic reviews [50–52]). ASD is a neurodevelopmental disorder characterized by impairments in social communication and restrictions in behaviors or thought patterns [53]. Early diagnosis and early intervention are both critical in the prognosis for children with ASD and other developmental delays [54, 55]. Early diagnosis can potentially lead to early intervention, which should involve evidence-based practices (EBP) (e.g., Functional Analysis (FA), Functional Communication Training (FCT), naturalistic teaching, discrete trial teaching) that are based on principles of applied behavior analysis (ABA). However, there are many barriers impeding both early diagnosis and access to early intervention, resulting in delayed diagnosis [56] and delayed or no EBP-based intervention after a diagnosis of ASD [57]. One common barrier is the lack of appropriately trained professionals who can provide the diagnosis and/or EBP; this scarcity of qualified providers is greatly exacerbated in rural areas [58, 59].

The majority of the studies of ASD and videoconferencing-based telehealth has focused on behavioral assessment and intervention-based research. One study explored providing cognitive–behavioral intervention via telehealth to treat anxiety experienced by youth with ASD, a common comorbid condition for ASD [60]. The rest of the studies examined provided behavior analytic interventions/EBPs to treat the core symptoms of ASD via telehealth videoconferencing. Training and utilizing parents and other professionals to implement EBPs via telehealth is an important and effective way of addressing the lack of qualified providers and increasing access to services. In particular, training parents as therapists in behavioral intervention has been widely accepted as a parent-mediated intervention option that dates back to the mid-20th century. Parents as therapists are particularly meaningful for the treatment of ASD and are considered an EBP. ASD is considered to be a lifelong disability that may require different levels of support [61]. Additionally, empowering parents of children with ASD with the knowledge and skills to support their children at home and in the community can have a positive impact on the generality and maintenance of the intervention effects [62, 63].

There are two major types of outcomes associated with the behavior analytic intervention studies. One is the interventionist (parent/professional) outcome and the other is the child outcome associated with children with ASD. Interventionist outcome measures often included one or multiple of these components: fidelity of implemented EBP skills, knowledge acquisition, social validity on usability,

Table 22.3 Developmental pediatric interventions using videoconferencing

Study	Population	Sample description & sample size	Study design	Findings
Heitzman Powell et al. (2013) [70]	Autism	N = 7 parents Youth age not reported	VC pre–post	Parents increased their knowledge and self-reported implementation of Applied Behavior Analysis (ABA) strategies
Hepburn et al. (2016) [60]	Autism and anxiety	N = 33 youth ages: 7–19 years	VC vs. waitlist control	Families reported high acceptability of the VC intervention, however issues with the technology impeded some sessions. Families reported improvements in anxiety and parents reported more competence posttreatment
Ingersoll et al. (2016) [71]	Autism	N = 28 families Ages: 1–6 years	VC vs. control	The VC group parents reported increases in their positive perceptions of their child, in their child meeting language targets, in their child's social skills
Lindgren, et al. (2016) [72]	Autism and developmental disabilities	N = 94 Ages: 1–7 years	In-home therapy vs. clinic-based VC vs. and home-based VC	Each intervention significantly reduced problem behaviors from pre- to posttreatment in all 3 groups, and treatment acceptability based on parent ratings was high for all groups. Total costs for implementing treatment were lowest for home VC, but both VC models were significantly less costly than in-home therapy
Monlux et al. (2019) [73]	Fragile X	N = 8 youth Ages: 3–10 years	VC pre–post	Rate of problem behaviors decreased pre–post; high parent-reported acceptability and treatment integrity
Reese et al. (2013) [74]	Autism	N = 21 youth Ages: 3–5 years	VC vs. F2F diagnostic evaluation	VC similar to in-person evaluations in reliability, diagnostic accuracy, reported symptoms, and satisfaction
Simacek et al. (2017) [75]	Autism and Rett syndrome	N = 3 Ages: 3–4 years	VC feasibility	All the children acquired the targeted communication responses. The findings support the efficacy of telehealth as a service delivery model to coach parents on intervention strategies for their children's early communication skills

(continued)

Table 22.3 (continued)

Study	Population	Sample description & sample size	Study design	Findings
Suess et al. (2016) [76]	Autism	N = 5 Ages: 2–7 years	VC feasibility Ppre–post	Across participants, problem behaviors reduced by approximately 65.1% and independent task completion increased by approximately 34.3%
Vismara et al. (2013) [77]	Autism	N = 8 Ages: 18–45 months	VC feasibility single-subject, multiple-baseline design	Parents rated VC with therapists as highly important for understanding how to use the intervention in their daily life. Parents reported having a better understanding and appreciation for helping their child learn new skills at home
Wacker et al. (2013) [78]	Autism	N = 20 Ages: 2–6 years	VC feasibility	The capacity to identify social functions of problem behavior and the length of assessment in VC were comparable to direct service delivery in children's homes. The VC delivery model provided a cost-effective alternative strategy for delivering behavioral services

Note: *VC* Videoconferencing, *F2F* Face-to-Face, *RCT* Randomized Controlled Trial, *M* Mean

acceptability, engagement, and/or satisfaction, and secondary measures such as parental stress and depressive symptoms. Child outcome measures often included parent-reported child behavior measures such as the Vineland Adaptive Behavior Checklists and observational data on targeted skill deficits (e.g., increased child demands or requesting) or problem behavior (e.g., decrease in self-injurious behavior).

All studies reported positive outcomes in at least one of their outcome measures, showing that delivering EBPs via videoconferencing is a promising treatment delivery option. However, it is worth noting that the quality of the studies, group design, and single subject design was in general weak, using the *Evaluative Method for Evaluating and Determining Evidence-Based Practices in Autism* [64, 65]. It is imperative that future research employs more rigorous evaluation methodologies and procedures, for both group design and single subject design studies. In addition, it is important for future research to examine the long-term effects of both interventionists' skill maintenance and child outcome measures with longitudinal studies.

Future developmental behavioral pediatric research should also expand the age range and targeted skills and challenges of participating children with ASD, considering most of the studies focused on early intervention of children under 6 years old.

As young children with ASD age, they often face more challenges due to increased social and behavioral expectations and decreased resources and support [66, 67]. They need more support in developing skills such as social skills, self-management skills, and independent living skills [68]; they also need more support in coping with comorbid conditions such as anxiety, depression, and ADHD as they are at a much higher risk of developing these conditions [69].

Conclusion

The growing evidence base in child behavioral interventions goes hand-in-hand with innovative delivery systems such as telebehavioral health services delivered through videoconferencing. As digital natives, children and adolescents offer a promising population for telehealth interventions. Overall, the studies presented are promising across process measures and patient outcome measures, and across clinical child, pediatric psychology, and applied behavior analysis/developmental studies. Overall, the studies note use of readily available, secure technologies with limited technical difficulties. Most studies also translated an intervention validated in the onsite clinical setting to the outreach telebehavioral setting. Interventions were informed by child telebehavioral health best practices and guidelines [5], including safety best practices. Many studies noted the unique advantages of the telehealth system in allowing the child and/or parent to engage in the intervention in their lived environment, with the goal that this may assist in lasting behavior change.

Because of the nature of telebehavioral health services to rural/underserved areas, sample size continues to be a limitation noted by many of the studies reviewed in the chapter. The rapidly evolving technologies and models of health care delivery (e.g., medical homes, Affordable Care Organizations, etc.) are further challenges and opportunities for telebehavioral research. Emerging implementation and dissemination models that explore factors that inform which intervention works under what conditions may be a particularly useful avenue for future research, such as work exploring the facilitators and barriers to the adoption of ADHD guidelines [28]. Such implementation research may be especially helpful in teasing apart what telehealth setting (e.g., home, school, primary care, community mental health center, etc.) may be the most effective service with different diagnoses and patient/family needs.

Other areas of emerging work are group interventions, including support group interventions as well as group therapy interventions. For example, Patton et al. [35] developed a group-based parent intervention for parents of young children with type 1 diabetes, which may inform group-based telebehavioral interventions with other chronic illnesses and child clinical concerns. Future studies may also explore the impact of multiple technologies on intervention effectiveness, such as use of both synchronous videoconferencing and asynchronous online materials [21].

The elephant in the telemedicine room is the worsening workforce shortages across behavioral specialists. The telebehavioral interventions described have the potential to increase access, but much need remains. Pairing these emerging telebehavioral interventions with innovative workforce strategies, including telementoring/Project ECHO (Extension for Community Healthcare Outcomes), is another avenue for future evaluation. Finally, the federally funded Telehealth Resource Centers (telehealthresourcecenter.org) and the related Telebehavioral Health Center of Excellence (tbhcoe.org) offer many opportunities to share lessons learned from child telebehavioral health studies with healthcare audiences, child-serving systems, diverse communities, and consumers.

References

1. Merikangas KR, He J, Burstein M, Swendsen J, Avenevoli S, Case B, et al. Service utilization for lifetime mental disorders in US adolescents: results of the National Comorbidity Survey–Adolescent Supplement (NCS-A). J Am Acad Child Adolesc Psychiatry. 2011;50:32–45.
2. Smalley KB, Rainer J. Rural mental health: issues, policies, and best practices. Cham: Springer Publishing Company; 2012.
3. Van Allen J, Davis AM, Lassen S. The use of telemedicine in pediatric psychology: research review and current applications. Child Adolesc Psychiatr Clin. 2011;20:55–66.
4. Nelson E-L, Patton S. Using videoconferencing to deliver individual therapy and pediatric psychology interventions with children and adolescents. J Child Adolesc Psychopharmacol. 2016;26:212–20.
5. Myers K, Nelson EL, Rabinowitz T, Hilty D, Baker D, Barnwell SS, et al. American telemedicine association practice guidelines for telemental health with children and adolescents. Telemed J E Health. 2017;23(10):779–804.
6. Luxton DD, Nelson E-L, Maheu MM. A practitioner's guide to telemental health: ow to conduct legal, ethical, and evidence-based telepractice. Arlington: American Psychological Association; 2016.
7. Eyberg SM, Funderburk B. PCIT: parent-child interaction therapy protocol: 2011. PCIT International, Incorporated; 2011.
8. Comer JS, Furr JM, Miguel EM, Cooper-Vince CE, Carpenter AL, Elkins RM, et al. Remotely delivering real-time parent training to the home: an initial randomized trial of internet-delivered parent-child interaction therapy (I-PCIT). J Consult Clin Psychol. 2017;85:909–17.
9. Bellinger S, Nelson E-L. Telehealth ROCKS: telemedicine approaches for improving rural access to behavioral care. Natl Assoc Rural Ment Heal. 2018;
10. Dadds MR, Thai C, Diaz AM, Broderick J, Moul C, Tully LA, et al. Therapist-assisted online treatment for child conduct problems in rural and urban families: two randomized controlled trials. J Consult Clin Psychol. 2019;87:706–19.
11. Myers K, Vander Stoep A, Zhou C, McCarty CA, Katon W. Effectiveness of a telehealth service delivery model for treating attention-deficit/hyperactivity disorder: a community-based randomized controlled trial. J Am Acad Child Adolesc Psychiatry. 2015;54:263–74.
12. Tse YJ, McCarty CA, Vander SA, Myers KM. Teletherapy delivery of caregiver behavior training for children with attention-deficit hyperactivity disorder. Telemed e-Health. 2015;21:451–8.
13. Sibley MH, Comer JS, Gonzalez J. Delivering parent-teen therapy for ADHD through videoconferencing: a preliminary investigation. J Psychopathol Behav Assess. 2017;39:467–85.
14. Barkley RA, Murphy KR, Fischer M. ADHD in adults: what the science says. New York: Guilford Press; 2010.
15. Comer JS, Furr JM, Kerns CE, Miguel E, Coxe S, Meredith Elkins R, et al. Internet-delivered, family-based treatment for early-onset OCD: a pilot randomized trial. J Consult Clin Psychol. 2017;85:178–86.
16. Berryhill MB, Culmer N, Williams N, Halli-Tierney A, Betancourt A, Roberts H, et al. Videoconferencing psychotherapy and depression: a systematic review. Telemed e-Health. 2019;25:435–46.

17. Nelson E-L, Barnard M, Cain S. Feasibility of telemedicine intervention for childhood depression. Couns Psychother Res. 2006;6:191–5.
18. Sayal K, Roe J, Ball H, Atha C, Kaylor-Hughes C, Guo B, et al. Feasibility of a randomised controlled trial of remotely delivered problem-solving cognitive behaviour therapy versus usual care for young people with depression and repeat self-harm: lessons learnt (e-DASH). BMC Psychiatry. 2019;19:1–12.
19. Berryhill MB, Halli-Tierney A, Culmer N, Williams N, Betancourt A, King M, et al. Videoconferencing psychological therapy and anxiety: a systematic review. Fam Pract. 2018;36:53–63.
20. Acierno R, Gros DF, Ruggiero KJ, Hernandez-Tejada MA, Knapp RG, Lejuez CW, et al. Behavioral activation and therapeutic exposure for posttraumatic stress disorder: a noninferiority trial of treatment delivered in person versus home-based telehealth. Depress Anxiety. 2016;33:415–23.
21. Stewart RW, Orengo-Aguayo RE, Cohen JA, Mannarino AP, de Arellano MA. A pilot study of trauma-focused cognitive–behavioral therapy delivered via telehealth technology. Child Maltreat. 2017;22:324–33.
22. Carpenter AL, Pincus DB, Furr JM, Comer JS. Working from home: an initial pilot examination of videoconferencing-based cognitive behavioral therapy for anxious youth delivered to the home setting. Behav Ther. 2018;49:917–30. Available from: https://www.dropbox.com/sh/4gv3jc5q6ok4nsg/AACNwJkt-DMrbeAmY2NJ4UvPa/Clinical Child/Carpenter (2018) VC Anxiety.pdf?dl=0.
23. Fox KC, Connor P, McCullers E, Waters T. Effect of a behavioural health and specialty care telemedicine programme on goal attainment for youths in juvenile detention. J Telemed Telecare. 2008;14:227–30.
24. Himle MB, Freitag M, Walther M, Franklin SA, Ely L, Woods DW. A randomized pilot trial comparing videoconference versus face-to-face delivery of behavior therapy for childhood tic disorders. Behav Res Ther. 2012;50:565–70. https://doi.org/10.1016/j.brat.2012.05.009.
25. Kirkman JJL, Hawes DJ, Dadds MR. An open trial for an E-health treatment for child behavior disorders II: outcomes and clinical implications. Evidence-Based Pract Child Adolesc Ment Heal. 2016;1:213–29. https://doi.org/10.1080/23794925.2016.1230482.
26. Myers K, Vander SA, Lobdell C. Feasibility of conducting a randomized controlled trial of telemental health with children diagnosed with attention-deficit/hyperactivity disorder in underserved communities. J Child Adolesc Psychopharmacol. 2013;23:372–8.
27. Nelson EL, Barnard M, Cain S. Treating childhood depression over videoconferencing. Telemed J e-Health. 2003;9:49–55.
28. Nelson EL, Duncan AB, Peacock G, Bui T. Telemedicine and adherence to national guidelines for ADHD evaluation: a case study. Psychol Serv. 2012;9:293–7.
29. Reese RJ, Slone NC, Soares N, Sprang R. Telehealth for underserved families: an evidence-based parenting program. Psychol Serv. 2012;9:320–2.
30. Storch EA, Caporino NE, Morgan JR, Lewin AB, Rojas A, Brauer L, et al. Preliminary investigation of web-camera delivered cognitive-behavioral therapy for youth with obsessive-compulsive disorder. Psychiatry Res. 2011;189:407–12. https://doi.org/10.1016/j.psychres.2011.05.047.
31. Xie Y, Dixon JF, Yee OM, Zhang J, Chen YA, Deangelo S, et al. A study on the effectiveness of videoconferencing on teaching parent training skills to parents of children with ADHD. Telemed e-Health. 2013;19:192–9.
32. Shivji S, Metcalfe P, Khan A, Bratu I. Pediatric surgery telehealth: patient and clinician satisfaction. Pediatr Surg Int. 2011;27:523–6.
33. Tschamper MK, Jakobsen R. Parents' experiences of videoconference as a tool for multidisciplinary information exchange for children with epilepsy and disability. J Clin Nurs. 2019;28:1506–16.
34. Bensink M, Armfield N, Irving H, Hallahan A, Theodoros D, Russell T, et al. A pilot study of videotelephone-based support for newly diagnosed paediatric oncology patients and their families. J Telemed Telecare. 2008;14:315–21.

35. Patton SR, Clements MA, Marker AM, Nelson E. Intervention to reduce hypoglycemia fear in parents of young kids using video-based telehealth (REDCHiP). Pediatr Diabetes. 2020;21:112–9.
36. Hommel KA, Hente E, Herzer M, Ingerski LM, Denson LA. Telehealth behavioral treatment for medication nonadherence: a pilot and feasibility study. Eur J Gastroenterol Hepatol. 2013;25:469–73.
37. Anderson KE, Byrne CE, Crosby RD, Le Grange D. Utilizing Telehealth to deliver family-based treatment for adolescent anorexia nervosa. Int J Eat Disord. 2017;50:1235–8.
38. Clawson B, Selden M, Lacks M, Deaton AV, Hall B, Bach R. Complex pediatric feeding disorders: using teleconferencing technology to improve access to a treatment program. Pediatr Nurs. 2008;34:213–6.
39. Davis AMG, Sampilo M, Gallagher KS, Landrum Y, Malone B. Treating rural pediatric obesity through telemedicine: outcomes from a small randomized controlled trial. J Pediatr Psychol. 2013;38:932–43.
40. Freeman KA, Duke DC, Harris MA. Behavioral health care for adolescents with poorly controlled diabetes via Skype: does working alliance remain intact? J Diabetes Sci Technol. 2013;7:727–35. Available from: www.journalofdst.org.
41. Glueckauf RL, Fritz SP, Ecklund-Johnson EP, Liss HJ, Dages P, Carney P. Videoconferencing-based family counseling for rural teenagers with epilepsy: phase 1 findings. Rehabil Psychol. 2002;47:49–72.
42. Lipana LS, Bindal D, Nettiksimmons J, Shaikh U. Telemedicine and face-to-face care for pediatric obesity. Telemed e-Health. 2013;19(10):806–8.
43. Marker AM, Monzon AD, Nelson E-L, Clements MA, Patton S. An intervention to reduce hypoglycemia fear in parents of young kids with type 1 diabetes via video-based telemedicine (REDCHIP): trial design, feasibility, and acceptability. Diabetes Technol Ther. 2020;22:25–33.
44. McCrossan B, Morgan G, Grant B, Sands A, Craig B, Casey F. Assisting the transition from hospital to home for children with major congenital heart disease by telemedicine: a feasibility study and initial results. Med Inform Internet Med. 2007;32:297–304.
45. Morgan GJ, Craig B, Grant B, Sands A, Doherty N, Casey F. Home videoconferencing for patients with severe congenital heart disease following discharge. Congenit Heart Dis. 2008;3:317–24.
46. Mulgrew KW, Shaikh U, Nettiksimmons J. Comparison of parent satisfaction with care for childhood obesity delivered face-to-face and by telemedicine. Telemed e-Health. 2011;17:383–7.
47. Shaikh U, Cole SL, Marcin JP, Nesbitt TS. Clinical management and patient outcomes among children and adolescents receiving telemedicine consultations for obesity. Telemed e-Health. 2008;14:434–40.
48. Wilkinson OM, Duncan-Skingle F, Pryor JA, Hodson ME. A feasibility study of home telemedicine for patients with cystic fibrosis awaiting transplantation. J Telemed Telecare. 2008;14:182–5.
49. Witmans MB, Dick B, Good J, Schoepp G, Dosman C, Hawkins ME, et al. Delivery of pediatric sleep services via telehealth: the Alberta experience and lessons learned. Behav Sleep Med. 2008;6:207–19.
50. Knutsen J, Wolfe A, Burke BL, Hepburn S, Lindgren S, Coury D. A systematic review of telemedicine in autism spectrum disorders. Rev J Autism Dev Disord. 2016;3:330–44.
51. Neely L, Rispoli M, Gerow S, Hong ER, Hagan-Burke S. Fidelity outcomes for autism-focused interventionists coached via telepractice: a systematic literature review. J Dev Phys Disabil. 2017;29:849–74.
52. Parsons D, Cordier R, Vaz S, Lee HC. Parent-mediated intervention training delivered remotely for children with autism spectrum disorder living outside of urban areas: systematic review. J Med Internet Res. 2017;e198:19.
53. Association AP. Diagnostic and statistical manual of mental disorders (DSM-5®). Arlington: American Psychiatric Association; 2013.

54. Dawson G, Jones EJH, Merkle K, Venema K, Lowy R, Faja S, et al. Early behavioral intervention is associated with normalized brain activity in young children with autism. J Am Acad Child Adolesc Psychiatry. 2012;51:1150–9.
55. Estes A, Munson J, Rogers SJ, Greenson J, Winter J, Dawson G. Long-term outcomes of early intervention in 6-year-old children with autism spectrum disorder. J Am Acad Child Adolesc Psychiatry. 2015;54:580–7.
56. Wiggins LD, Baio JON, Rice C. Examination of the time between first evaluation and first autism spectrum diagnosis in a population-based sample. J Dev Behav Pediatr. 2006;27:S79–87.
57. Yingling ME, Hock RM, Bell BA. Time-lag between diagnosis of autism spectrum disorder and onset of publicly-funded early intensive behavioral intervention: do race–ethnicity and neighborhood matter. J Autism Dev Disord. 2018;48:561–71.
58. Elder JH, Brasher S, Alexander B. Identifying the barriers to early diagnosis and treatment in underserved individuals with autism spectrum disorders (ASD) and their families: a qualitative study. Issues Ment Health Nurs. 2016;37:412–20.
59. Antezana L, Scarpa A, Valdespino A, Albright J, Richey JA. Rural trends in diagnosis and services for autism spectrum disorder. Front Psychol. 2017;8:590.
60. Hepburn SL, Blakeley-Smith A, Wolff B, Reaven JA. Telehealth delivery of cognitive-behavioral intervention to youth with autism spectrum disorder and anxiety: a pilot study. Autism. 2016;20:207–18.
61. Barrett B. Substantial lifelong cost of autism spectrum disorder. J Pediatr. 2014;165:1068–9.
62. Kashinath S, Woods J, Goldstein H. Enhancing generalized teaching strategy use in daily routines by parents of children with autism. J Speech Lang Hear Res. 2006;49(3):466–85.
63. Crockett JL, Fleming RK, Doepke KJ, Stevens JS. Parent training: acquisition and generalization of discrete trials teaching skills with parents of children with autism. Res Dev Disabil. 2007;28:23–36.
64. Reichow B, Doehring P, Cicchetti D V, Volkmar FR. comprar evidence-based practices and treatments for children with autism. In: Reichow B. Evidence-Based Pract Treat Child with Autism-9781441969736-14646000000, 9781441969736|Springer. Springer; 2011
65. Reichow B, Volkmar FR, Cicchetti DV. Development of the evaluative method for evaluating and determining evidence-based practices in autism. J Autism Dev Disord. 2008;38:1311–9.
66. Volkmar FR, Jackson SLJ, Hart L. Transition issues and challenges for youth with autism spectrum disorders. Pediatr Ann. 2017;46:e219–23.
67. Wood JJ, Gadow KD. Exploring the nature and function of anxiety in youth with autism spectrum disorders. Clin Psychol Sci Pract. 2010;17:281–92.
68. Hampshire PK, Allred KW. A parent-implemented, technology-mediated approach to increasing self-management homework skills in middle school students with autism. Exceptionality. 2018;26:119–36.
69. Joshi G, Petty C, Wozniak J, Henin A, Fried R, Galdo M, et al. The heavy burden of psychiatric comorbidity in youth with autism spectrum disorders: a large comparative study of a psychiatrically referred population. J Autism Dev Disord. 2010;40:1361–70.
70. Heitzman-Powell LS, Buzhardt J, Rusinko LC, Miller TM. Formative evaluation of an ABA outreach training program for parents of children with autism in remote areas. Focus Autism Other Dev Disabl. 2014;29:23–38.
71. Ingersoll B, Wainer AL, Berger NI, Pickard KE, Bonter N. Comparison of a self-directed and therapist-assisted telehealth parent-mediated intervention for children with ASD: a pilot RCT. J Autism Dev Disord. 2016;46:2275–84.
72. Lindgren S, Wacker D, Suess A, Schieltz K, Pelzel K, Kopelman T, et al. Telehealth and autism: treating challenging behavior at lower cost. Pediatrics. 2016;137:S167–75.
73. Monlux KD, Pollard JS, Bujanda Rodriguez AY, Hall SS. Telehealth delivery of function-based behavioral treatment for problem behaviors exhibited by boys with fragile X syndrome. J Autism Dev Disord. 2019;49(6):2461–75.
74. Reese RM, Jamison R, Wendland M, Fleming K, Braun MJ, Schuttler JO, et al. Evaluating interactive videoconferencing for assessing symptoms of autism. Telemed e-Health. 2013;19:671–7.

75. Simacek J, Dimian AF, McComas JJ. Communication intervention for young children with severe neurodevelopmental disabilities via telehealth. J Autism Dev Disord. 2017;47:744–67.
76. Suess AN, Wacker DP, Schwartz JE, Lustig N, Detrick J. Preliminary evidence on the use of telehealth in an outpatient behavior clinic. J Appl Behav Anal. 2016;49:686–92.
77. Vismara LA, McCormick C, Young GS, Nadhan A, Monlux K. Preliminary findings of a telehealth approach to parent training in autism. J Autism Dev Disord. 2013;43:2953–69.
78. Wacker DP, Lee JF, Dalmau YCP, Kopelman TG, Lindgren SD, Kuhle J, et al. Conducting functional analyses of problem behavior via telehealth. J Appl Behav Anal. 2013;46:31–46.

Telemedicine for Psychiatry and Mental Health

23

Matthew Garofalo, Sarah Vaithilingam, and Stephen Ferrando

Introduction

Telepsychiatry refers to provision of psychiatric care services with telecommunications technology. Synchronous telepsychiatry (STP) or a live, two-way videoconferencing model has become synonymous with telepsychiatry, but multiple models using various technologies have also been used and studied. As psychiatric assessments primarily rely on a verbal history and audiovisual mental status exam, STP is a theoretically valid assessment tool. Additionally, the shortage of psychiatrists in the United States, especially certain subspecialists, and their concentration in high-resource regions, places telepsychiatry in a position to mitigate regional gaps and limit transportation costs.

Despite growing popularity, need, implementation, and models, the practice of telepsychiatry has not been standardized and suffers from a relative lack of high-quality research. In the United States, the most significant barrier to implementation remains reimbursement, as there are gaps in Medicare coverage and Medicaid coverage varies between states. Lack of interstate coverage standards is particularly challenging here because many large health systems may be delivering remote psychiatric care across state lines. Additionally, telepsychiatry only becomes sustainable after a certain patient volume [1], limiting expansion to smaller systems. The Veteran's Affairs (VA) telepsychiatry system is the exception that proves the rule; as a singular reimbursement system and large-scale implementation has enabled it to become sustainable and standardized [2–4]. Despite an incompletely developed system, telepsychiatry has significantly increased mental healthcare access in the United States [1].

M. Garofalo · S. Vaithilingam · S. Ferrando (✉)
Department of Psychiatry, Westchester Medical Center Health System, New York Medical College, Valhalla, NY, USA
e-mail: Stephen.ferrando@wmchealth.org

This chapter will provide a broad overview of telepsychiatry and cover the (1) history, (2) technology and methods, (3) models and settings, (4) effectiveness, (5) practice guidelines and training, (6) legal and ethical concerns, and (7) digital health interventions.

The discussion will be largely limited to the United States, but some relevant foreign studies will be referenced. Although the initial literature review was limited to 2002, earlier literature will also be included here.

History

The first documented use of clinical telepsychiatry was from the University of Nebraska and emerged from a one-way, closed circuit television used for medical education in the 1950s [5]. With funding from the National Institute of Mental Health (NIMH), the program expanded later to include interactive audio between the Nebraska Psychiatric Institute and other regional hospitals so that lecturers could answer questions. In 1959, an interactive audiovisual system was created, which was used in 1964 to link the Nebraska Psychiatric Institute with Norfolk State Hospital. By the late 1960s this same model linked Veteran's Administration hospitals to the network. The NIMH funded a similar audiovisual telepsychiatry project at Dartmouth Medical School in 1968 [5].

Concurrently in 1968, Massachusetts General Hospital used a bidirectional television transmission system to deliver psychiatric services to Logan International Airport [6]. This system enabled the psychiatrist to tilt, zoom, and pan the remote camera. The paper describing it [6] contains the first known usage of the term "telepsychiatry" [7]. Another early published telepsychiatry project was from Mount Sinai School of Medicine to a child clinic in East Harlem [8]. These programs were closed when federal funding dried up in the 1970s [5], and telepsychiatry programs did not receive much attention clinically or in the literature until the growth of the Internet and associated audiovisual technologies in the 1990s.

Since that time telepsychiatry has expanded in scope and practice both in the United States and abroad. With increased appreciation of the discrepancy between need and availability of psychiatric care, particularly in underserved and rural areas, interest in telepsychiatry continues to grow.

Technology, Setup, and Technique

On each side of the typical videoconferencing system, there will one or two display screens, one microphone, speakers and/or headsets, a video camera, and a coder–decoder (codec) for compression/decompression and audiovisual synchronization. Remote camera control is recommended [9] so that the operator can pan, tilt, and zoom the camera on the patient. Internet Protocol (IP) networks have generally replaced point-to-point connections (fraction T-1 or ISDN) [10], but satellite networks are also used in some remote sites [9]. Consistent with Health Insurance Portability and Accountability Act of 1996 (HIPAA) requirements, 128-bit encryption must be provided. Unless otherwise specified, STP programs described here transmit data at a minimum bandwidth of 384 Kbps. This bandwidth is the recommended minimum specified by the American Telemedicine Association (ATA), and has been shown to be significantly more acceptable to users than 128 Kbps and more cost effective than 768 Kbps [9]. Geriatric assessments are more sensitive to bandwidth due to common patient sensory deficits and cognitive assessment tools with written visual components such as the Mini Mental Status Exam [2].

The physical space is important to facilitate a therapeutic encounter and ensure privacy. Audio is ideally transmitted between soft, "quiet" rooms with carpeting, draperies, sound panels, etc. [7, 9]. The ATA specifies minimum lighting of 150-foot candles and recommends a spectrum close to daylight [9]. Blue backdrops may be used [9]. The clinician and patient's locations are both considered examination rooms and subject to the same privacy standards [9]. As such, all present parties on each side must be identified prior to examination [9]. All participating parties must be accommodated in the camera view [7, 9], including parents and caregivers [7].

Videoconferencing techniques will vary according to patient demographics and conditions [2, 7, 9, 11]. One universal barrier to rapport and assessment is the impossibility of maintaining mutual eye contact because the camera is always placed above or below the monitor [7]. By alternating gaze from the camera to the monitor, the clinician can facilitate rapport, but may have to formally inquire about the patient's ability to initiate or maintain eye contact if it is unclear [7].

For more technical requirements and recommendations, refer to the ATA's 2010 policy guidelines [9] and the American Academy of Child and Adolescent Psychiatry's (AACAP) 2017 telepsychiatry clinical update [7].

Models and Settings

Telepsychiatry in the United States exists in many settings, including (1) outpatient, (2) inpatient, (3) consultation–liaison (C–L), (4) emergency, (5) schools, (6) corrections, (7) home-based, and (8) nursing homes. Electronic delivery models extend beyond STP and include asynchronous telepsychiatry (ATP) and "curbside" consultations [12]. Novel digital interfaces such as mobile applications [13–16] will be discussed in the *digital health interventions* section. Due to lack of a standardized database, the overall prevalence of United States telepsychiatry programs is unknown, as is the percentage breakdown for settings and populations.

Outpatient

The primary outpatient telepsychiatry model is direct care interactive videoconferencing. Patients in this model are evaluated and treated by a psychiatrist. The providers operate from a central location and patients present to regional offices. Providers directly write prescriptions and patients follow-up with the same program and clinical findings are documented in the central electronic medical record (EMR).

This direct care model is appropriate for higher need and more complicated psychiatric patients who are already connected with the psychiatric system. However, as the vast majority of psychiatric assessments and treatments occur in the primary care setting, telepsychiatry can, and does, provide a valuable resource for expert consultation, follow-up as needed, and training [12, 11]. In these models, the primary care physician (PCP) utilizes psychiatrists to aid assessments, guide interventions, and provide medical education. This "task sharing" approach, with technology functioning to leverage psychiatric services, has been implemented and studied in rural areas in the United States [11].

The most evidence-based model in the United States is the collaborative care model [12]. Collaborative care functions by connecting patients, PCPs, and psychiatrists through behavioral health care managers. STP can be used for the initial consult and follow-up as needed for patients with high and middle psychiatric needs. The psychiatrist communicates with the PCP via telephone and/or email to communicate diagnostic findings and treatment recommendations. High need patients can continue to be followed by consulting psychiatrists via STP, while middle needs psychiatric patients may be followed with more STP or asynchronous telepsychiatry (ATP). ATP involves a video-recorded primary care encounter which is reviewed by the psychiatrist for assessment and treatment recommendations. Both STP and ATP have been shown to improve outcomes and provide educational benefits for PCPs [12]. ATP is more cost effective and is evidence-based for middle needs psychiatric patients [12].

Lower-needs psychiatric patients can benefit from informal "curbside" consults in which a PCP remotely discusses a case with a psychiatrist who provides guidance for diagnosis and management [12]. Roughly 33% of PCP's psychiatric needs can be met with this system and it does improve patient care and PCP skills [12].

Stepped care systems in which more intensive psychiatric interventions are implemented according to patient needs have been studied abroad, but the evidence base for telepsychiatry is limited to one study [12].

Consultation–Liaison

Although remote medical–surgical hospitals have limited access to inpatient psychiatric consultation, literature on C–L telepsychiatry is limited [17]. The University of Pittsburgh Medical Center has been using telepsychiatry (mainly synchronous videoconferencing) to cover C–L consults at a remote satellite hospital and retrospectively (2014–2016) studied patient demographics, reasons for consult, diagnoses, recommendations, longitudinal volume of requested consultations, and follow-up [17].

The most commons consultation questions were altered mental status, mood, and decisional capacity. The most common primary diagnoses were delirium, dementia, and mood disorders, but 12 diagnostic categories were utilized as either primary or secondary diagnoses. Most recommendations were for studies or medication initiation, changes, or discontinuation. Two patients were referred for inpatient psychiatric care and nearly half for outpatient follow-up. Volume of consultation requests increased throughout the study period, perhaps indicating a positive response from inpatient physicians. Of note, this telepsychiatry program was grant funded, as managed care does not reimburse telepsychiatry in Pennsylvania [17].

Emergency

Emergency departments (EDs) in the United States are increasingly burdened by patients with primary psychiatric complaints [18] and have become the frontline access points for many psychiatric patients [19]. EDs in rural and underserved areas often lack on-call psychiatrists and behaviorally trained staff, leading to substandard care, substandard follow-up, increased costs, pressure to admit for psychiatric complaints, and decreased ability to address medical emergencies [18, 19]. By improving access, telepsychiatry may mitigate the above issues, but the literature base is sparse [20].

Emergency telepsychiatry operates as a consulting service delivered via STP, usually from a central hub [18–22]. The evaluating psychiatrist provides a diagnostic impression and recommendations for disposition, discharge medications, social services, and follow-up.

In 2009 South Carolina implemented an emergency telepsychiatry program and studied outpatient follow-up, rate of hospitalization after ED assessment, length of stay if admitted, inpatient costs if admitted, and total health care costs [18]. Over 7000 telepsychiatry recipients were matched with and compared to controls who did not receive telepsychiatric services. The only metric without statistically significant difference was the 30-day total health care cost. Differences between groups in 30- and 90-day outpatient follow-up remarkably demonstrated favorable results for the telepsychiatry group (46% versus 16% and 54% versus 20%, respectively), while decreases in hospitalization rate and inpatient length of stay for the telepsychiatry group were modest [18].

The need for emergency child and adolescent telepsychiatry may be even more pronounced, as child and adolescent psychiatric emergency presentations, hospitalizations, and suicidal/self-injurious behaviors have significantly increased in the United States during this century [23]. Pediatric EDs also suffer from lack of behavioral resources and there is a massive shortage of child and adolescent specialists. As a result, psychiatric care in traditional pediatric EDs can be unsafe, and low reimbursement for child and adolescent psychiatric emergency evaluations all but precludes specialized programs. Institutions with psychiatric emergency programs, such as a Comprehensive Psychiatric Emergency Program (CPEP), are primarily designed for adults and can be unsafe and ill-suited for the child and adolescent population [23].

The limited available data from the United States and Canada support emergency child and adolescent psychiatry as a way to decrease ED length of stay and cost while also increasing patient and family satisfaction [23]. Data on safety and other clinical outcomes is limited, but one prospective Canadian study [21] on 60 assessments of primarily Aboriginal children showed a statistically improvement in patient satisfaction compared to a face-to-face control population. There was no significant difference in other clinical outcomes. This study suffered from significant demographic and diagnostic differences between the control and study groups [21].

Schools

More children receive mental health care in schools than in outpatient clinics [7], but access to psychiatrists in schools is limited. Telepsychiatry has been successfully used to close this gap, but confidentiality issues and prescribing protocols represent significant hurdles [7].

Corrections

In 2016 it was estimated that upwards of 350,000 people with severe psychiatric illness were in state prisons or jails at a given time, a number far exceeding all psychiatric inpatients at a given time [24–26] and creating a massive need for psychiatric care in the correctional setting. Telepsychiatry has been used in adult [27] and child [7] corrections.

Data on correctional systems telepsychiatry is limited. One literature review [27], which included five randomized controlled trials (RCTs), was only able to identify 345 subjects in efficacy studies and found that the studies were rife with methodological issues, such as poor controls. Nevertheless, patient and provider acceptance were generally high [27]. To mitigate sometimes unavoidable confidentiality issues, the article suggests that telepsychiatry via telephone should be compared head-to-head with interactive videoconferencing [27].

Home-Based

Patients with mobility issues, difficulty tolerating in-person care, or frequent physical relocation may benefit from home-based STP [7, 2, 28]. Specific care must be taken to avoid or mitigate high-risk situations and patients with a history of severe adverse reactions to therapy are not appropriate [28]. However, this model has been studied in child and adolescent [7], geriatric [2], and general adult [28] populations, although data on efficacy and safety is scarce. Privacy issues provide a barrier for the child and adolescent population [7], while some geriatric patients find home-based telepsychiatry to be more private [2].

Nursing Homes

Although literature on nursing home telepsychiatry is mostly limited to descriptive studies, data does suggest that this model may have be clinically feasible, cost-effective, efficient, and acceptable to patients [2]. Initial concerns about geriatric patients' familiarity with technology, cognitive impairment, and sensory deficits (auditory and visual) are generally alleviated with high bandwidth connections and standardized scales for cognitive impairment, depression, and psychosis have been reliably applied [2].

Effectiveness

There have been over one hundred published studies on telepsychiatry's clinical effectiveness, particularly STP [1, 29, 30]. Despite the impressive number of studies, the vast majority are small, descriptive, or retrospective studies. Prospective studies, including RCTs, are less common. The prospective studies performed generally utilize equivalency methods and/or noninferiority methods to compare telepsychiatry to care as usual (primary care or waitlists) or face-to-face assessments [3]. Endpoints studied include patient and/or provider satisfaction, diagnostic reliability/validity, symptom reduction, rehospitalization rates, and medication compliance [1, 30, 31].

Many populations have been studied including, but not limited to, child and adolescent [7], geriatric [2], correctional [27], ethnic [1], and developmentally disabled [32]. In addition to assessments and medication management, studies also exist on psychotherapy outcomes and include systematic reviews and meta-analyses [33, 34]. Although most effectiveness data are on STP, effectiveness of ATP and other telecommunications delivered care (mobile apps) have also been studied [14–16, 1].

Results thus far for all of the above metrics and populations have generally supported the hypothesis that telepsychiatry is at least comparable to face-to-face assessment and superior to treatment as usual [1, 3]. Some disorders, such as autism spectrum disorder, may be more suited for telepsychiatry than face-to-face, although more study is needed [1]. Intriguingly, patients have been more satisfied and accepting toward telepsychiatry than providers, as providers have expressed concern over therapeutic rapport [3]. It is also likely that some patients may only have experience with telepsychiatry, while providers are more experienced with face-to-face.

Although telepsychiatry has been shown to meet minimum standards of broad acceptability as well as favorable treatment outcomes and diagnostic reliability, Hubley et al. [3] express concerns over the literature, particularly reliance on self-report, selection biases, insufficient blinding and small sample sizes. Nevertheless, the overwhelmingly favorable evidence warrants more nuanced studies that guide implementation by quantifying the types of assessments and interventions suited for specific conditions and settings [3]. Hilty et al. [1] point out the need for more high-quality prospective and condition specific studies. To conclude, telepsychiatry clearly meets acceptability standards for patient satisfaction, diagnostic reliability and validity, and basic treatment outcomes for multiple populations and settings, but data is insufficient to establish evidence-based telepsychiatry specific standards of care.

Practice Guidelines and Training

Although, for the above reasons, telepsychiatry clinical standards of care follow face-to-face standards, practice guidelines have been proposed by the ATA [9] and American Academy of Child and Adolescent Psychiatry (AACAP) [7]. This section will cover administrative, population specific, treatment, safety, and training guidelines for STP.

Before initiating a telepsychiatry program, a needs assessment must be conducted, and appropriate sites identified [7, 9]. General office support staff must be available to facilitate encounters and institutional administrative processes and protocols formally established and followed [7, 9]. Specific topics include, but are not limited to, infection control, credentialing, training, quality improvement, prescribing, documentation, billing/coding, and confidentiality. The system must include redundant technology. Safety is a legitimate concern and institutional safety protocols, including for psychiatric and medical emergencies, must be established and should follow procedures for any face-to-face system with additional communication systems readily available and known. Vaithilingam's unpublished account [35] of a telepsychiatric emergency involving a concealed weapon outlines these issues. Note that recommendations only specify that institutional administrative policies and protocols be established, as no specific national guidelines are available.

There are no specific contraindications to telepsychiatric assessments and treatments [7, 9] and services may be requested and/or performed at the discretion of the psychiatrist and/or consulting physician. As specified earlier, diverse populations and illnesses with specific needs receive telepsychiatry services. Psychotherapy and medication management services should follow general psychiatric standards of care [9].

Geriatric patients may have sensory issues and/or be unfamiliar with technology. Therefore, they will benefit from a bandwidth of at least 384 Kbps and, possibly, enhanced audiovisual definition [9, 2]. All populations receiving remote cognitive testing must have access to qualified ancillary staff to administer tests [9].

As telepsychiatrists may reside and originate from areas dramatically different from served patient populations, it is recommended that cultural/ethnic differences are considered [9]. Firearm ownership and safety is a specific, sensitive issue that telepsychiatrists must be prepared to discuss [9]. Community-based mental health outreach workers can breach the gap between telepsychiatrists and patients and educate the provider [11].

Guidelines for children and adolescents largely follow those for the general population, but it is recommended that those patients are provided larger rooms, toys, and a table to promote comfort, accommodate parents, and enable observation of play and motor skills [9]. Setting specific issues, such as knowledge of schools and correctional facilities, and appropriate communication with them, as well as potentially hostile/abusive family settings must be considered [7]. Some developmentally disabled populations may not be able to tolerate the interactive platform and require face-to-face services [7].

Given the expanding role of telepsychiatry in providing access to care, it is evident that there is need for telepsychiatry education in Graduate Psychiatry Residency Training programs; however, the consensus within the literature is that programs are lagging behind the evolving standard of care. Further, telepsychiatry training is not well established or standardized [7, 9, 10, 36]. Training in telepsychiatry is not a requirement for psychiatry residents in the United States and the Accreditation Council for Graduate Medical Education (ACGME) competencies for technology are limited to the use of the EMR [10]. There is concern that without formal preparation, psychiatrists may be reluctant to take up an unfamiliar practice that requires specific clinical skills [37]. Despite the absence of any streamlined education for early psychiatrists, professional guidelines for telemedicine and telepsychiatry do exist [10].

A Canadian team identified three barriers to telepsychiatry training in Graduate education:

1. Competencies are not well defined.
2. Teaching methods for training in tele psychiatry are undetermined.
3. There is no clear vision for how telepsychiatry training should be integrated into existing curricula and rotations [37].

One way to mitigate this problem is by introducing an "elective" which would allow residents to gain experience in telepsychiatry. A group in East Carolina recommended that electives be reserved for senior residents so that the primary focus is on learning the challenges and unique aspects of using technology, once basic interviewing and psychotherapeutic and pharmacology practice have been mastered [10]. They went on to suggest that training should also involve associated readings that includes medical–legal issues, ethical concerns, logistic challenges, and guidelines on the industry standards [10].

In another residency program, trainees were required to complete a six-month outpatient telepsychiatry rotation in their second year. Their model was unique in that it included a mix of in-person and instant messaging supervision by an attending [38]. Residents preferred this method of communicating with their supervisors because it gave them a sense of autonomy [38]. At the same time, they were able to discuss treatment decisions without interrupting the session. This protocol also allowed residents and attendings to communicate efficiently and handle difficult clinical situations in real time [38].

At our training program in Westchester County, New York, telepsychiatry training is integrated into the third-year outpatient curriculum. Telepsychiatry practice is considered integral and on par with face-to-face contact and residents flow freely back and forth between modalities. Supervision is focused on identifying the similarities, differences, and clinical challenges inherent in both frameworks. Residents report that they appreciate the autonomy and relative equivalence of both treatments, and appreciate the advantages of access to remote patient populations, but can feel unprepared for the complexities of telepsychiatry early in their outpatient year, particularly with more challenging patients. This requires vigilance by supervisory staff, who are always available to intervene in person when the resident is challenged with an individual encounter. As an educational tool, the residency program is developing telepsychiatry mock scenarios in order to help prepare residents for their clinical encounters, which focuses on practice with the technology, establishing rapport with this medium, and collaborating with remote "hub" staff in managing difficult crisis situations, such as suicidality and aggression. Furthermore, telepsychiatry education is integrated into the lecture-based curriculum.

Overall, few telepsychiatry training experiences for residents have been evaluated, thus, it is difficult to determine which approaches are the most effective in educating trainees [37]. It has been speculated that the use of telepsychiatry to treat marginalized and underserved populations during residency can promote a sense of responsibility and interest post residency [10]. Furthermore, the Department of Veterans Affairs suggest that residents that participated in this type of experience continued with the Department of Veterans Affairs after graduating, and thus telepsychiatry experience was a useful recruitment tool [39].

Legal and Regulatory

There are significant legal and regulatory issues that relate to the practice of telepsychiatry. Primary among these are the issues of informed consent, privacy, and civil commitment for individuals who require but do not agree to acute inpatient hospitalization. Informed consent should be obtained prior to any telepsychiatry encounter, and many state regulatory bodies mandate various forms of informed consent. Informed consent should include presentation of the benefits and limitations of the telepsychiatry encounter, including but not limited to options to see a provider in person when available as well as the important issue of maintaining privacy. In our health system, for instance, patients sign consent for telepsychiatry interventions upon entering relevant emergency departments, acute care, and outpatient programs where telepsychiatry is utilized. However, prior to or at the beginning of each encounter, the patient's consent to continue is affirmed. There are cases in which the patient is unable to provide informed consent, particularly where the patient has an acute psychotic or manic disorder, is grossly paranoid, or when they have significant neurocognitive impairment. In those instances, if telepsychiatric consultation is the only modality available, it may be used on an emergency basis. However, when possible, the patient should have a face-to-face encounter with a clinician at the next available opportunity. Occasionally, patients refuse telepsychiatry (<1% in our experience), in which case every effort is made to allow them to see a provider face-to-face, which will inevitably increase waiting time.

States vary widely in their laws governing involuntary commitment [40]. Generally, states require the presence of acute dangerousness to self or others, and some allow "grave disability" (or inability to care for oneself) as a requirement to hold an individual for safety and/or treatment against their will. The ability to involuntarily commit an individual via telepsychiatry is not universally articulated across state jurisdictions and we were unable to find a review of this issue. In New York State, a practitioner who is conducting a telepsychiatry consultation in the emergency setting is, with the exception of a small number of pilot programs, not permitted to fill out legal forms or sign for involuntary commitment. Thus, psychiatric consultation conducted by telepsychiatry can only be utilized as a recommendation to appropriately designated, onsite practitioners to fill out the legal commitment forms. Anecdotally, pilot projects that allow the telepsychiatrist to fill out and sign legal commitment forms for New York State have not encountered major hurdles; however, this practice has not received formal approval.

Digital Health Interventions

Digital health interventions (DHIs) such as computer programs, mobile applications, clinician-to-patient remote messaging, and Internet forums have been promoted as means to improve mental health access, utilization, compliance, patient comfort, monitoring, efficiency, cost-effectiveness, and personalization [13, 15, 29, 41]. Programs have been created to target conditions such as anxiety disorders, depression, psychosis, eating disorders, attention deficit hyperactivity disorder (ADHD), autism spectrum disorders, neurocognitive disorders, and post-traumatic stress disorder (PTSD) [15, 29]. Target populations include general adults, geriatrics, caregivers, and child and adolescents. Despite the theoretical benefits and number of programs, a robust evidence base has been precluded by the dynamic nature of these programs, their heterogeneity, and low-quality research.

DHIs targeting the child and adolescent population have been studied in the most depth [37, 41] and a 2016 systematic and meta-review [15] identified and studied 147 distinct DHIs. The article aimed to study the evidence base for treatment effects, cost-effectiveness, usability, access, acceptability, and compliance. Programs were divided based on symptom targets, including anxiety and depression, eating disorders, ADHD, autism, PTSD, and psychosis. Programs ranged from sit-down computer programs to mobile applications. Games, computerized cognitive behavioral therapy (cCBT), remote monitoring, and conference were some of the studied modalities.

Anxiety and depression DHIs hold a majority market share for child and adolescent patients and have the most robust evidence base [37]. The most clinically effective programs involved cCBT with face-to-face augmentation and therapist-facilitated support. Studies on depression generally targeted patients subthreshold for diagnosis and/or mild-moderate symptomatology, while some anxiety studies included patients carrying an anxiety disorder diagnosis. Consistently positive treatment outcomes were not found for the other diseases.

Across the board, cost-effectiveness has not been established for the child and adolescent population, although qualitative evidence suggests both direct and indirect return on investment benefits [37]. Acceptability, compliance, and usability have not been consistently established either [15]. However, the rapid increase in programs, heterogeneity, poor study quality, and lack of standard taxonomy has complicated our understanding of DHIs.

Increasing access to psychosocial interventions for psychosis is an area of interest, as acute pharmacological management alone is insufficient to prevent relapse and facilitate functional recovery [38]. Unfortunately, multiple barriers have hindered access to these interventions. DHIs provide some promise for closing this gap.

An Australian systematic review on user-led DHIs targeting psychosis [13] studied 12 appropriate articles from a pool of 38 potentials. Areas of interest were acceptability, usability and feasibility, and treatment effects. In controlled environments, web-based psycho-education and CBT were acceptable and feasible for most schizophrenic patients, as was real-world psycho-education with social media. Favorable treatment effects were supported for web-based CBT targeting positive symptoms and online therapy, peer/expert support, and social networking for depression and social connectedness. Digital monitoring may help to prevent relapse and hospitalizations and a personalized SMS-based program may improve positive symptom severity and social networking. Positive results for functional outcomes were not supported [42]. Most studies were found to be poor quality. One intriguing program enables psychotic patients to create and modify an avatar in order to reduce distress associated with auditory hallucinations [13].

References

1. Hilty DM, et al. The effectiveness of telemental health: a 2013 review. Telemed e-Health. 2013;19(6):444–54.
2. Gentry MT, Lapid MI, Rummans TA. Geriatric telepsychiatry: systematic review and policy considerations. Am J Geriatr Psychiatry. 2019;27(2):109–27.
3. Hubley, et al. Review of key telepsychiatry outcomes. World J Psychiatry. 2016;6(2):269–82.
4. Godleski L. A comprehensive national telemental health training program. Acad Psychiatry. 2012;36(5):408–10.
5. Smith HA, Allison RA. Telemental health: delivering mental health care at a distance. Rockville: U.S. Department of Health and Human Services. Substance Abuse and Mental Health Services Administration Center for Mental Health Services Health Resources and Services Administration Office for the Advancement of Telehealth; 1998. http://nebhands.nebraska.edu/files/telemental%20health%20systems.pdf.
6. Dwyer TF. Telepsychiatry: psychiatric consultation by interactive television. Am J Psychiatry. 1973;130(8):865–9.
7. American Academy of Child and Adolescent Psychiatry (AACAP) Committee on Telepsychiatry and AACAP Committee on Quality Issues. Clinical update: telepsychiatry with children and adolescents. J Am Acad Child Adolesc Psychiatry. 2017;56(10):875–93.
8. Straker N, Mostyn P, Marshall C. The use of two-way TV in bringing mental health services to the inner city. Am J Psychiatry. 1976;133(10):1202–5.

9. Yellowlees P, Shore J, Roberts L, American Telemedicine Association. Practice guidelines for videoconferencing-based telemental health – October 2009. Telemed J E Health. 2010;16(10):1074–89.
10. Saeed SA, Johnson TL, Bagga M, Glass O. Training residents in the use of telepsychiatry: review of the literature and a proposed elective. Psychiatry Q. 2017;88(2):271–83.
11. Hoeft TJ, et al. Task-sharing approaches to improve mental health care in rural and other low-resource settinvgs: a systematic review. J Rural Health. 2018;34(1):48–62.
12. Hilty DM, et al. An update on telepsychiatry and how it can leverage collaborative, stepped, and integrated services to primary care. Psychosomatics. 2018;59(3):227–50.
13. Powell AC, Chen M, Thammachart C. The economic benefits of mobile apps for mental health and telepsychiatry services when used by adolescents. Child Adolesc Psychiatric Clin N AM. 2017;26(1):125–33.
14. Alvarez-Jimenez A, et al. Online, social media and mobile technologies for psychosis treatment: a systematic review on novel user-led interventions. J Can Acad Child Adolesc Psychiatry. 2016;25(2):80–6.
15. Hollis C, et al. Annual research review: digital health interventions for children and young people with mental health problems – a systematic and meta-review. J Child Psychol Psychiatry. 2017;58(4):474–503.
16. Massoudi B, et al. The effectiveness and cost-effectiveness of e-health interventions for depression and anxiety in primary care: a systematic review and meta-analysis. J Affect Disord. 2019;245:728–43.
17. Graziane JA, Gopalan P, Cahalane J. Telepsychiatry consultation for medical and surgical inpatient units. Psychosomatics. 2018;59(1):62–6.
18. Narasimhan M, et al. Impact of a telepsychiatry program at emergency departments statewide on the quality, utilization, and costs of mental health services. Psychiatr Serv. 2015;66(11):1167–72.
19. Southard EP, Neufeld JD, Laws S. Telemental health evaluations enhance access and efficiency in a critical access hospital emergency department. Telemed J E Health. 2014;20(7):664–8.
20. Reinhardt I, Gouzoulis-Mayfrank E, Zielasek J. Use of telepsychiatry in emergency and crisis intervention: current evidence. Curr Psychiatry Rep. 2019;21(8):63.
21. Roberts N, et al. Child and adolescent emergency and urgent mental health delivery through telepsychiatry: 12-month prospective study. Telemed J E Health. 2017;23(10):842–6.
22. Saurman E, et al. A transferable telepsychiatry model for improving access to emergency mental health care. J Telemed Telecare. 2014;20(7):391–9.
23. Mroczkowski MM, Havens J. The state of emergency child and adolescent psychiatry: raising the bar. Child Adolesc Psychiatr Clin N Am. 2018;27(3):357–65.
24. Treatment Advocacy Center. A background paper from the Office of Research and Public Affairs: Serious Mental Illness (SMI) Prevalence in Jails and Prisons. 2016. https://www.treatmentadvocacycenter.org/storage/documents/backgrounders/smi-in-jails-and-prisons.pdf.
25. Torrey EF, Zdanowicz MT, Kennard AD, Lamb HR, Eslinger DF, Biasotti MI, Fuller DA. The treatment of persons with mental illness in prisons and jails: a state survey. Arlington: Treatment Advocacy Center; 2014.
26. Torrey EF, Kennard AD, Eslinger DF, Lamb HR, Pavle J. More mentally ill persons are in jails and prisons than hospitals: a survey of the states. Arlington: Treatment Advocacy Center; 2010.
27. Antonacci DJ, et al. Empirical evidence on the use and effectiveness of telepsychiatry via videoconferencing: implications for forensic and correctional psychiatry. Behav Sci Law. 2008;26(3):253–69.
28. Luxton DD, et al. Home-based telemental healthcare safety planning: what you need to know. Telemed J E Health. 2012;18(8):629–33.
29. Hilty D, Yellowlees PM, Parish MB, Chan S. Telepsychiatry: effective, evidence-based, and at a tipping point in health care delivery? Psychiatr Clin North Am. 2015;38(3):559–92.
30. O'Reilly R, et al. Is telepsychiatry equivalent to face-to-face psychiatry? Results from a randomized controlled equivalence trial. Psychiatr Serv. 2007;58(6):836–43.

31. Malas N, et al. Exploring the telepsychiatry experience: primary care provider perception of the Michigan Child Collaborative Care (MC3) program. Psychosomatics. 2019;60(2):179–89.
32. Szeftel R, et al. Improved access to mental health evaluation for patients with developmental disabilities using telepsychiatry. J Telemed Telecare. 2012;18(6):317–21.
33. Rees CS, Maclaine E. A systematic review of videoconference-delivered psychological treatment for anxiety disorders. Aust Psychol. 2015;50(4):259–64.
34. Jenkins-Guarnieri MA, et al. Patient perceptions of telemental health: systematic review of direct comparisons to in-person psychotherapeutic treatments. Telemed J E Health. 2015;21(8):652–60.
35. Vaithilingam S, Abdullah H, Vaithilingam D. A question of safety in telepsychiatry. Unpublished manuscript. 2019.
36. Hoffman P, Kane JM. Telepsychiatry education and curriculum development in residency training. Acad Psychiatry. 2015;39(1):108–9.
37. Sunderji N, Crawford A, Jovanovic M. Telepsychiatry in graduate medical education: a narrative review. Acad Psychiatry. 2015;39(1):55–62.
38. DeGaetano N, Greene CJ, Dearaujo N, Lindley SE. A pilot program in telepsychiatry for residents: initial outcomes and program development. Acad Psychiatry. 2015;39(1):114–8.
39. Glover JA, Williams E, Hazlett LJ, Campbell N. Connecting to the future: telepsychiatry in postgraduate medical education. Telemed J E Health. 2013;19(6):474–9.
40. Hedman LC, Petrilla J, Fisher WH, et al. State laws on emergency holds for mental health stabilization. Psychiatr Serv. 2106;67(5):529–35. https://doi.org/10.1176/appi.ps.201500205.
41. Alvarez-Jimenez M, Alcazar-Corcoles MA, González-Blanch C, Bendall S, McGorry PD, Gleeson JF. Online, social media and mobile technologies for psychosis treatment: a systematic review on novel user-led interventions. Schizophr Res. 2014;156(1):96–106.
42. Gottlieb JD, Gidugu V, Maru M, Tepper MC, Davis MJ, Greenwold J, Barron RA, Chiko BP, Mueser KT. Randomized controlled trial of an internet cognitive behavioral skills-based program for auditory hallucinations in persons with psychosis. Psychiatr Rehabil J. 2017;40(3):283–92.

Telecardiology

24

Milena Soriano Marcolino, Maria Beatriz Moreira Alkmim, Maira Viana Rego Souza e Silva, Renato Minelli Figueira, Raissa Eda de Resende, Letícia Baião Silva, and Antonio Luiz Ribeiro

Telecardiology

In this chapter, we aimed to make an overview of recent applications of telecardiology in primary and specialized care, as well as to give examples of our practice in telecardiology. Our group is part of a Brazilian public telehealth network, the Telehealth Network of Minas Gerais, a partnership among seven public universities, with broad experience in cardiology. Since 2005, more than 4.9 million tele-electrocardiograms have already been analyzed, as well as 3693 Holter, 655 ambulatory blood pressure monitoring, and 133,284 teleconsultations. We have been working on different clinical decision support systems and short message service (SMS) programs.

Telecardiology in Primary Care

In primary care, teleconsultations, tele-diagnosis, and tele-education, applied in an integrated manner, possibly associated with tools such as decision support systems (DSS), may improve the quality of care for cardiovascular diseases, especially hypertension, atrial fibrillation, heart failure, and acute myocardial infarction. In remote municipalities with few inhabitants, primary care is often the only level of local healthcare and may receive patients with acute cardiovascular disease in an outpatient setting, especially in large countries with less integrated systems with difficult patients' removal to a more complex healthcare unit. Thus, telecardiology

M. S. Marcolino (✉) · M. B. M. Alkmim · M. V. R. Souza e Silva · R. M. Figueira · R. E. de Resende · L. B. Silva · A. L. Ribeiro
Telehealth Center, University Hospital, Universidade Federal de Minas Gerais;
Telehealth Network of Minas Gerais, Belo Horizonte, Brazil
e-mail: milenamarc@ufmg.br

© Springer Nature Switzerland AG 2021
R. Latifi et al. (eds.), *Telemedicine, Telehealth and Telepresence*,
https://doi.org/10.1007/978-3-030-56917-4_24

in primary care may improve the quality of care not only for chronic diseases, but also may support the emergency care for acute coronary diseases and arrhythmias.

Tele-regulation may support primary care to qualify access to specialized care. The applications of telecardiology in primary care will be briefly reviewed.

Health Promotion and Prevention

In cardiology, health promotion actions for primary and secondary prevention of cardiovascular diseases have an outstanding impact in morbimortality, and may be associated with significant cost reduction in healthcare expenses due to the decrease in specialized consultations, hospitalizations, and emergency hospital admissions [1]. Telemedicine may be useful in controlling risk factors for coronary artery disease, such as improving blood pressure (BP) control [2–5], reducing glycohemoglobin in diabetic patients [6–8], and improving lipid profile [9, 10]. Furthermore, it may help to reduce weight, body mass index (BMI), and waist circumference in obese or overweight patients [5, 11–13] as well as increasing the success of smoking cessation programs [14].

Several modalities of telemedicine can assist in this regard, such as mobile phone text or audio messaging systems, which have shown positive results in medication adherence, change in eating habits, and physical activity in patients with hypertension, diabetes, obesity, or patients who had an acute myocardial infarction (AMI) [13, 15]. Twenty-four-hour monitoring services are becoming more frequent through the development of pieces of equipment which are linked to telemedicine systems, such as a stethoscope, balance, digital thermometer, BP monitors, remote monitoring of vital signs, and implantable electronic devices [16, 17]. Even simple watches have been transformed into monitoring systems with technology to report heart rate, presence of arrhythmias, stress level (analyzing humidity and skin temperature), optical BP monitoring, and physical activity [18, 19]. There are several applications which are now available for the guidance of healthcare professionals, patients, or even for self-care [16].

Decision Support Systems

Decision Support Systems (DSS) add knowledge and information of specific patients for physicians, other healthcare professionals, or patients themselves to improve the quality of the treatment and patient outcomes (www.healthit.gov/topic/safety/clinical decision support). The Community Preventive Services Task Force recommends using these systems in the prevention of cardiovascular diseases. Such recommendation is based on low-to-moderate quality of evidence, which show an increase in cardiovascular risk factors screening; antiplatelet therapy prescription for primary prevention; and also, healthy diet, physical activity, and smoking cessation counseling [20]. It may have wide application in primary healthcare, but results are still inconsistent when considering its clinical impact, with few isolated studies demonstrating an increase in smoking abstinence, adherence to drug treatment, and physical activity engagement, and a slight reduction in BMI (mean reduction = −0.10) [21].

Regarding emergency room (ER) admissions, hospitalizations, and cardiovascular events, studies have shown no consistent impact so far, but further studies are required. In one study, which assessed an educational strategy for health professionals associated with DSS alerts compared to an isolated educational strategy, lower mortality rates were observed in the intervention group [22].

Teleconsultation

Teleconsultation can be defined as a second opinion system that allows information exchange between distant healthcare professionals and local healthcare professionals to discuss a clinical case when a specialist is not locally available (Fig. 24.1) [23]. They can be synchronous/real-time (with simultaneous interaction; by video, web conference, telephone, or toll-free telephone number) or asynchronous/store-and-forward, in a time-independent basis (Fig. 24.1).

Teleconsultations may have great applications in primary care to support healthcare professionals in remote and resource-constrained areas, including timely access to correct medical information, quality improvement of the diagnosis and treatment process, increased physician trust, and significant improvement in the total quality of healthcare [24]. As a tool with potential to increase primary care resolution, it may be incorporated into the workflow of primary care units as a part of the

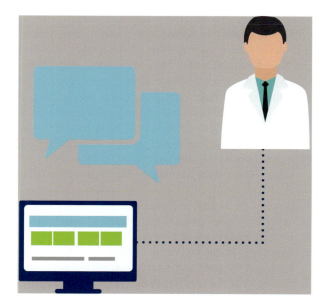

Fig. 24.1 Representation of the teleconsultation service

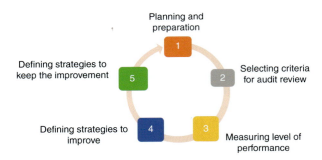

Fig. 24.2 The audit cycle. (Adapted from Benjamin A, 2008)

regulatory process of the municipality. Thus, it represents an efficient way to reduce waiting times for a face-to-face appointment with a cardiologist.

There are still few studies on the impact of teleconsultations on hard outcomes, such as mortality. A systematic review by Liddy et al. [25] cited a randomized study comparing patients who had had teleconsultation to those who had been offered a traditional referral. The authors assessed the impact on death, myocardial infarction, catheterization or emergency angioplasty, and ER visits. The teleconsultation group was more likely to have an appointment with the cardiologist and fewer ER admissions.

Continued education and professional qualification are other benefits of the teleconsultations, as well as a reduced sense of isolation, for the professionals who work in remote areas.

Overall, patients and medical professionals appear to be satisfied with teleconsultation services [26–28]. However, the quality of the service should be assessed periodically using predetermined criteria to ensure sustained positive effects (Fig. 24.2) [29]. Our group recently published a paper describing a methodology to analyze the quality of teleconsultations [24].

The methodology started with a literature review to analyze methodologies that had already been used to evaluate the quality of asynchronous teleconsultations in the following databases: Medline, Lilacs, and Scielo. In Medline, the following descriptors were used: telemedicine, remote consultation, medical audit; and terms: teleconsultation, audit, quality. In Lilacs and Scielo corresponding terms were used. Due to the lack of studies analyzing teleconsultation in the literature, it was necessary to develop our methodology. With this purpose, specialists from our group were consulted and an initial version was developed, tested, and improved over time, resulting in the criteria showed in Table 24.1.

We established five domains which represented important items to be assessed:

1. Quality: Technical and scientific knowledge based on the best online available evidence, point-of-care information summaries, and guidelines from the Brazilian Ministry of Health.
2. Objective: Focus and details which are required for an answer to be complete.
3. Ethics: If the teleconsultant has an ethical behavior.
4. Courtesy: If the teleconsultant is polite when answering a query.
5. Grammar: Adequacy of grammar and vocabulary basic rules).

Table 24.1 Criteria developed by our team as a methodology for teleconsultations audits

Criteria for teleconsultations audits

Domains	Score		
	3 Points	2 Points	1 Point
Quality	The answer is based on the best available evidence	The answer is outdated, but evidence based. *and/or*	The answer is based uniquely on common sense (nonexpert knowledge). *and/or*
			The teleconsultant wasn't able to answer the question (when there is available evidence). *and/or*
		The answer is evidence based, but it doesn't completely respond to the solicitor's question	The answer covers exclusively the knowledge acquired by the professional on his daily practice when there is available evidence. *and/or*
			The response is evidence-based, but doesn't answer the solicitor's question at all. *and/or*
			The answer's content is different from what is described on the best available evidence
Objectivity	The answer is focused on the question asked. *and*	The answer is brief, focused, but incomplete and/or wrong. *and/or*	The answer is long, doesn't focus on the solicitor's question, and doesn't cover enough of the requested topic (doesn't answer the question). *and/or*
	The answer is complete and has all the necessary details	The answer is not focused, but it answers all the questions asked	The answer is long, has no focus, and consists of a faithful reproduction of public material
Ethics	The answer responds to teleconsultations of patients registered on the National Health System (SUS). *and*		The answer criticizes the conduct of other professionals. *and/or*
	The answer's content is consistent with the solicitor's professional duties. *and*		The answer quotes inappropriate names. *and/or*
			The answer responds to a personal teleconsultation. *and/or*
			The answer's content is incompatible with the solicitor's professional duties (e.g. pharmacotherapy for non-prescribing professionals. *and/or*
	The answer responds to procedures in accordance with the flow of care established by the Minas Gerais State Health Secretariat (SES-MG)		The answer responds to procedures in disagreement with the flow of care established by the State Department of Education of Minas Gerais (SES-MG)

(continued)

Table 24.1 (continued)

Criteria for teleconsultations audits

Domains	Score		
	3 Points	2 Points	1 Point
Courtesy	The answer has two greetings - one at the beginning and another one at the end of the text	The answer has only one greeting - greeting or farewell. *and/or*	The teleconsultant is rude or impolite. *and/or*
		The answer uses only vocative, without greetings to the teleconsultant	There are no greetings at all. *and/or*
			The solicitor's name is misspelled
Grammar	The answer is in accordance to the norms of the Portuguese language. *and*	The answer is unstructured, but it is not prejudicial to understanding. *and/or*	The answer contains incomprehensible sentences. *and/or*
			The answer has no gender agreement between the greeting and the vocative (solicitor's name). *and/or*
		The answer contains only one mistake related to singular/plural or gender agreement (except if this mistake is on the greeting). *and/or*	The answer is unstructured in a way that undermines understanding. *and/or*
	The answer has no structural errors (e.g. changing the line in the middle of the sentence)	The answer contains only one grammatical mistake. *and/or*	The answer contains two or more mistakes in singular/plural or gender agreement. *and/or*
			The answer contains two or more grammatical mistakes. *and/or*
		The answer contains a moderate amount of typos, but they do not impair understanding	There is a great amount of typos that hinder understanding

Each category received a score from 1 to 3 from the lowest to the highest grade.

This methodology has been used for feedback of the teleconsultation team and continued improvement of our service (Fig. 24.2). It can be easily replicated in other services worldwide to guarantee high quality of periodic auditing and may have positive impact to the quality of services provided by large-scale telemedicine services.

Tele-Regulation

The demand for specialist referrals is growing worldwide, surpassing what most services can offer in terms of specialists' consultation, and thus waiting lists are becoming increasingly longer [30]. Telehealth interventions, especially when involving tele-regulation, have shown a great impact in reducing waiting times, qualifying demands to avoid unnecessary referrals [31–33]. By using guiding protocols, tele-regulation enables to classify the demand for specialized care according to a risk classification, and the final decision regarding referrals' priority is a joint decision between both the attending and the tele-regulator physician [30–33].

Telediagnosis

Tele-electrocardiography is a very popular modality in telecardiology, as it is a simple exam and requires low-cost technology for transmitting files easily, even with slow Internet connections (Fig. 24.3). It can be easily incorporated into the primary care routine, due to its great utility and technology suitability for places with basic infrastructure in poor and remote areas [34, 35]. Twenty-four-hour Holter monitoring and ambulatory blood pressure monitoring (ABPM) are other exams which have been analyzed by telecardiology services.

Recently, Artificial Intelligence (AI) has helped large electrocardiogram databases to facilitate the execution of the exam reports, as well as to increase their accuracy. Decision support systems qualify care, with the potential to improve the

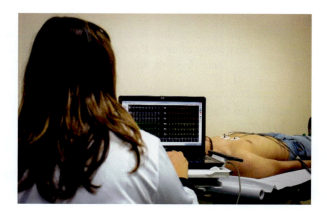

Fig. 24.3 Telediagnosis service in the primary care units in Brazil

management of patients with cardiovascular diseases, such as hypertension, atrial fibrillation, and heart failure.

Tele-echocardiography has also shown to be a promising strategy to enable access to initial cardiology investigation, early diagnosis, prioritization of referrals, and organization of waiting lines in healthcare systems. Initial evidence for its use comes from population-based screening studies, such as in rural India, where more than 1000 echocardiograms were performed in about 11 hours and sent to the cloud computing with good agreement between preliminary field diagnosis and expert reports ($k = 0.85$) and an alarming 16% rate of significant abnormalities (including 32.9% of heart valve abnormalities) [36]. Evidence also suggests that even in high-income regions such as the United Kingdom, population-based echocardiographic screening in primary care by non-specialists proved to be an attractive strategy, with clinically significant (moderate-to-severe) valve disease observed in 6.4% of asymptomatic population aged ≥65 years, with prevalence associated with socioeconomic factors [37]. The strategy may be especially useful in low-income countries, where presumably there is a high burden of undiagnosed cardiovascular disease and limitations in the provision of specialized care, including conventional echocardiography. The tele-echocardiography strategy was initially tested in Brazil in a rheumatic heart disease screening program (study PROVAR: Rheumatic Valve Disease Screening Program), which established a research protocol acquisition routine at the research level simplified with portable and ultraportable devices by paramedics (nurses and technologists), uploaded to dedicated cloud computing system for expert storage and remote interpretation [38, 39]. In addition to remote diagnostics, telemedicine was also used for training health professionals on basic principles of echocardiography through interactive online modules. The effectiveness of online training has been demonstrated even by the accuracy of these professionals for the basic diagnosis of rheumatic heart disease [38]. In this project, there was a high prevalence of subclinical rheumatic heart disease (4.2%), a significant finding considering the impact of the disease on public health [40].

Telediagnosis exams should be submitted to periodic audits, to guarantee the quality of the services (Fig. 24.2).

Tele-Education

Remote educational activities in cardiology for healthcare professionals may help improving the quality of care. Patient-focused educational activities should also be encouraged for their empowerment.

Specialized Care

Heart Failure

There is extensive literature on the use of telemedicine strategies to monitor patients with heart failure (HF), aiming to reduce hospitalizations, which are associated with increased morbidity, mortality, and costs. Additionally, there is evidence it may increase the patients' empowerment. Interventions range from using traditional technologies, such as structured telephone support, telemonitoring using innovative technologies with implantable or wearable devices, DSS, and machine learning to predict complications [41–43]. Although evidence is variable, overall there is a positive impact. However, the application of these strategies in clinical practice is still very limited by regulatory, logistical, and financial restraints [44].

Telemonitoring can be either invasive or noninvasive. Sensors are tools which are increasingly embedded in smartphones and other mobile devices, and are capable of detecting, recording, and responding to specific data, for instance, patients' vital signs. Sensor's logging can generate large data sets that can be transmitted in real time to healthcare professionals [45]. As many multi-professional intervention programs often have geographical, economic, and bureaucratic barriers, telemonitoring may be a solution to promote better care for patients with HF [41].

Evidence about structured telephone support and noninvasive telemonitoring in HF patients was summarized in a Cochrane systematic review, which included 41 studies. Structured telephone support has shown to reduce all-cause mortality (RR 0.87, 95% CI 0.77–0.98; $n = 9222$) and HF-related hospitalizations (RR 0.85, 95% CI 0.77–0.93; $n = 7030$), both with moderate quality of evidence. As for telemonitoring, it also reduced all-cause mortality (RR 0.80, 95% CI 0.68–0.94; $n = 3740$) and HF-related hospitalizations (RR 0.71, 95% CI 0.60–0.83; $n = 2148$), both with moderate quality of evidence [45].

In another meta-analysis [46], which assessed 26 studies, 2506 patients were followed by telemonitoring, including the transmission of vital signs, a time-dependent effect was observed. Short-term follow-up (up to 180 days) demonstrated better results in hard outcomes, including mortality, which were not achieved with a follow-up for a period longer than 1 year. On the other hand, telemonitoring has not shown to reduce hospitalization, regardless of the follow-up time. An increase in ER visits was observed in the telemonitoring group, thus, it raises the question of how an intervention that does not reduce hospitalization can impact on mortality. Perhaps early detection of decompensating sign encourages patients to seek medical attention, which can be promptly treated with diuretics and vasodilators without the need for intensive therapy.

The evidence regarding length of hospital stay is even more controversial as among seven structured telephone support and nine telemonitoring studies, only one study of each intervention observed a significant reduction in length of hospital stay. However, a much more noteworthy number of studies, 9 of 11 structured telephone support and 5 of 11 telemonitoring, reported significant improvements in quality of life and welfare. Three of nine structured telephone support studies and one of six cost-monitoring telemonitoring studies noted a reduction in cost, and two telemonitoring studies reported cost increases due to the cost of the intervention and increased medical management. Seven of the nine studies that assessed knowledge about HF and self-care behaviors observed significant improvements. Although acceptability among participants was observed between 76% and 97%, a decrease in participants' adherence over time can be challenging. In this review, adherence rates varied between 55.1% and 65.8% for structured telephone support and 75% and 98.5% for telemonitoring [45].

The benefit of telemonitoring in HF was recently confirmed by the publication of "The Interventional Telemedical Management in Heart Failure II (TIM-HF2)" study. This was a prospective, randomized, and multicenter clinical trial in which 1571 HF patients with New York Heart Association (NYHA) functional classification II or III or those who had been hospitalized for heart failure within 12 months prior to randomization and with ejection fraction (LVEF) of 45% or less were randomly assigned to remote management or just usual care lasting up to 393 days [47]. Patients assigned to remote patient care lost an average of 17.8 days per year due to unplanned cardiovascular hospital admissions compared to 24.2 days per year for patients assigned to usual care. All-cause mortality had a hazard ratio (HR) 0.70, 95% (CI 0.50–0.96; $p = 0.0280$) in favor of telemonitoring, but cardiovascular mortality was not significantly different between the two groups (HR 0.671, 95% CI 0.45–1.01; $p = 0.0560$) [47].

New devices which monitor intracardiac pressures have the most compelling evidence for the use of telemonitoring and are related to the use of more advanced technologies. CardioMEMS is a device implanted percutaneously in the pulmonary artery that transmits central pressure values to a platform. When pulmonary artery pressure levels reach values above a certain threshold, the physician receives an alert and a trend statement indicating pulmonary congestion or low cardiac output. Other devices for right ventricular implantation are already in experimental use. The "CardioMEMS Heart Sensor Allows Monitoring of Pressure to Improve Outcomes in NYHA Class III Heart Failure Patients (CHAMPION)" study [48] evaluated HF patients with NYHA function capacity III in 64 United States centers, who were randomized to use an electronic central unit that receives hemodynamic data from CardioMEMS or for control group treatment. In the monitored group, doctors used daily data from pulmonary artery pressure measurements to guide treatment. At the mean follow-up of 15 months, there was a 37% reduction in the rate of HF-related hospitalizations compared to the control group [49].

Hypertension

Telemonitoring strategies can also be applied to control BP. They are frequently confused with the self-monitoring BP approach. Studies which evaluated antihypertensive medication titration using self-monitoring present contradictory results; moreover, the precise role of telemonitoring on self-monitoring is unclear.

Several studies have demonstrated that hypertension telemonitoring strategies with clinical pharmacist involvement have a beneficial short- and medium-term impact on BP control. Margolis et al. [50] evaluated the effect of this intervention after a 54-month follow-up in a randomized cluster study of 16 primary care centers, which involved 450 patients (228 in telemonitoring and 222 in usual care). The intensive telemonitoring intervention has shown sustained effects on BP control for up to 24 months (12 months after the end of the intervention), losing longer-term efficacy [50].

The INTERACT study was a randomized controlled trial in which 303 patients using oral antihypertensive and/or hypolipidemic medication were allocated to receive or not SMS text messages. The group receiving text messages improved adherence to the prescribed medication at 6 months compared to the patients who did not receive any messages. Overall, there was a 16% improvement in medication adherence [50, 51].

In the TASMINH4 study, 1182 patients were randomly allocated (1:1:1) for antihypertensive titration by the attending physician who used clinical readings (usual care group), performing monitoring alone (self-monitoring group), or using telemonitoring self-monitoring (telemonitoring group). It has been observed that the use of BP self-monitoring to support antihypertensive therapy in the treatment of individuals with poorly controlled hypertension in primary care results in lower systolic BP without increasing the workload of the healthcare team. After 1 year, patients whose medication was adjusted using self-monitoring, with or without telemonitoring, had significantly lower systolic blood pressure than those who received office-adjusted BP treatment. Blood pressure in the telemonitoring group for medication titration has a faster decrease (at 6 months than the control group), an effect that is likely to reduce cardiovascular events even further and may improve management [52, 53].

A Cochrane systematic review [54] aimed to establish the effectiveness of mobile phone interventions to improve medication adherence for primary prevention of cardiovascular disease in adults. Participants were recruited from primary care units or outpatient clinics in high-income countries (Canada, Spain) and middle- and high-income countries (South Africa, China), but interventions received varied widely. One trial evaluated an intervention focused on adherence to blood pressure medication, provided exclusively through the SMS, whereas a different intervention involved blood pressure monitoring combined with feedback provided via smartphone. The authors judged the body of evidence for the efficacy of mobile phone–based interventions as poor quality with regards to objective outcomes (blood pressure and cholesterol). Considering two studies which evaluated medication adherence along with lifestyle modifications, one reported a slight improvement in lowering low-density lipoprotein cholesterol (LDL-c), while the other found no benefit whatsoever. A study (1372 participants) of a text-based intervention for adherence showed little effect in systolic blood pressure reduction for the intervention group which received informational-only text messages, and uncertain evidence of benefit about the second intervention model which provided additional interactivity with participants. One study examined the effect of blood pressure monitoring combined with a mobile phone text-messaging system and reported moderate benefits on systolic and diastolic blood pressure. There was conflicting evidence from two trials aimed at adherence to medication along with lifestyle advice using multicomponent interventions. While the former found great benefits on blood pressure levels, the latter showed no such effect. The authors concluded that there is poor quality evidence regarding the effects of mobile phone interventions to increase adherence to prescription drugs for primary prevention. In conclusion, there is currently uncertainty about the effectiveness of such interventions based on this review.

Emergency Services

Telemedicine has different applications in emergency services, including electrocardiogram transmission, which can be associated with synchronous teleconsultation, to assist the early diagnosis and management of acute coronary syndrome (ACS) cases (Fig. 24.4) [55].

Decision support systems could also to aid in the diagnosis, management, and prediction of cardiac complications in patients with ACS [56], prehospital bedside ultrasound image transmission, [57] and image transmission and support in the

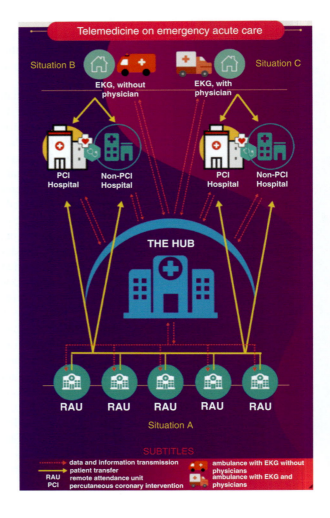

Fig. 24.4 Schematic representation of telemedicine for emergency acute care. Treatment strategies using telemedicine are shown for Acute Coronary Syndrome (ACS). EKG: surface electrocardiogram. Situation A: The patient goes to the nearest RAU for own means, or calls the prehospital care service and is taken to the RAU for a basic ambulance without electrocardiograph. Situation B: The patient calls the prehospital care service and an ambulance without a doctor, but with an electrocardiograph provides the care. Situation C: The patient calls the prehospital care service and an ambulance with a doctor and an electrocardiograph provides the care

diagnosis and management of patients with stroke [58]. The use of DSS could increase adherence to ACS patient management guidelines recommendations, but evidence on its impact on clinical outcomes is still lacking [58].

Telecardiology on Myocardial Infarction Systems of Care

Myocardial infarction systems of care aim to integrate prehospital, hospital, and hemodynamic services where patients with acute myocardial infarction (AMI) are managed in a given region to optimize their management. This system is proposed to better delineate these patients' care, involving early diagnosis, prehospital care, initial treatment, thrombolytic use, referral to a specialized hospital and post-event follow-up. It aims for high quality, effective, and safe care for patients with AMI, optimizing resources and reducing disparities in access to care [56, 59].

Telemedicine services play a crucial role in AMI systems of care as they facilitate communication from the physician in a low-complexity emergency unit or hospital and prehospital healthcare professional with cardiologists at a hub or hemodynamic center hospital that will receive the patient. Cardiologists may assist in the following:

1. Analyzing and interpreting the electrocardiogram in order to obtain an accurate and early diagnosis of ST-segment elevation myocardial infarction [54, 60]
2. Guidance on the best management, helping to decide if there is indication of thrombolytic use and other medications by using synchronous teleconsultations [55, 60]
3. Monitoring the patient's clinical condition through telemonitoring, with synchronous data transmission [60]

In patients submitted to primary PCI, prehospital electrocardiogram, and transmission to PCI center can decrease treatment time, by direct admission of the patient in the catheterization laboratory, bypassing the ER [55].

A typical telemedicine system of care consists of a specialized center (hub) and multiple remote care units distributed within a geographic region (spoke centers), connected bidirectionally with the help of a communication channel (Fig. 24.4). The specialized center can be a cardiology referral hospital, an ambulance regulation service, or a telemedicine center. Some AMI systems of care are comprised of more than one specialized center, each with certain remote units with regional coverage [61].

In recent years, the use of telemedicine tools in AMI has soared worldwide. A recent meta-analysis included studies in Europe (11), North America (8), South America (5), Asia (9), and Australia (2) with 16,960 patients. There was a moderate quality of evidence that the use of telemedicine strategies plus usual care reduces in-hospital mortality by 37% (relative risk [RR] 0.63 [95% CI 0.55–0.72]), with a number needed to treat (NNT) of 29 (confidence interval [CI] 95% 23–40), when compared to usual care without telemedicine. This analysis also showed poor quality of evidence that this intervention reduces door-to-balloon time (mean difference

28 (95% CI −35, −20) minutes), 30-day mortality (RR 0.62 [95% CI 0.43–0.85]) as well as long-term mortality (RR 0.61 [95% CI 0.40–0.92]) [55].

Management of Oral Anticoagulant Users

Self-management strategies have been associated with a significantly lower risk of ischemic stroke compared with treatment with direct oral anticoagulants, while no significant differences were observed for major bleeding or mortality. However, decreased vigilance is a potential problem in detecting patients who are unable to take care of their treatment. A structured education program is required for all stakeholders (patients, their caregivers, and healthcare professionals), as well as an increased quality control system [62–64].

Cardiac Rehabilitation

Guidelines recommend cardiac rehabilitation for patients after myocardial infarction, percutaneous coronary intervention (PCI), or coronary artery bypass graft (CABG) surgery. However, it is still underused, with only 14–31% of participants among all eligible patients. Difficulties in patient access to attend face-to-face sessions and high costs are important barriers [65]. In this sense, telehealth interventions using information and communication technologies to enable remote rehabilitation programs can overcome barriers to access while preserving clinical supervision and individualized exercise prescription [66].

In a systematic review that included 11 studies, the type of intervention proposed was highly variable and included the use of mobile or desktop applications, biosensors, and interventions using fixed-line phone calls. The interventions involved prescription and/or performance monitoring and adherence. All interventions included feedback, education, psychosocial support, and/or change behavior via fixed-line phone calls, mobile messaging, email, website, online tutorials, or online chat [67].

It was observed that the level of physical activity was higher in the intervention group compared to usual care. As for face-to-face rehabilitation, telehealth interventions were more effective for physical activity improvement, exercise adherence, in lowering diastolic blood pressure and LDL-c levels, with low to moderate quality of evidence. The telehealth rehabilitation was similar to face-to-face rehabilitation with regards to aerobic exercise levels and other modifiable cardiovascular risk factors [67].

The Telehab III study was a prospective multicenter randomized controlled clinical trial with cardiac rehabilitation patients. There were 140 patients randomly allocated to a 24-week tele-rehabilitation together with usual rehabilitation group and a usual rehabilitation group only. The additional intervention which involved tele-rehabilitation contributed even further to improvements in physical activity and quality of life and may induce persistent health benefits [68].

In a Chinese clinical trial, 98 NYHA classes I to III HF patients were randomized to either a home exercise training program via teleconsultation for 8 weeks or usual outpatient follow-up. Significant statistically improvements were observed in the experimental group regarding quality of life and 6-minute test compared to the control group. The results corroborate that physical training programs via teleconsultation is an effective alternative method for cardiac rehabilitation [69].

The REMOTE-CR is a non-inferiority randomized controlled trial which tested costs and effects of a real-time teleconsultation cardiac rehabilitation in 162 HF patients and demonstrated that it is a cost-effective alternative to increase the scope of rehabilitation [70].

Home cardiac rehabilitation may be an alternative to increase patient engagement in the program by offering greater flexibility and options for activities. Therefore, it is a reasonable choice which can suit the patient's values and preferences, and can be implemented in their daily routine [71]. The association of tele-rehabilitation with conventional rehabilitation was more effective and efficient when compared to the conventional rehabilitation program only, promoting a reduction in readmissions rate due to cardiovascular causes and increasing quality of life [68, 72].

Remote Monitoring Using Implantable Devices

Pacemaker telemonitoring showed no significant improvement in the quality of life and number of cardiovascular events; however, events were detected and treated earlier, thus reducing hospitalization and hospital visits (routine and emergency). Moreover, it was cheaper than the in-hospital follow-up [73].

Another form of implantable monitoring can be performed using implantable cardiac defibrillators (ICDs) or resynchronization devices. Some of these devices may have multiparameter monitoring software such as thoracic impedance and right ventricular filling pressure measurements captured by the electrode on the right ventricle. A groundbreaking 2008 study suggested that the use of such devices had clinical benefit in 92 NYHA class III patients [74]. Later, the IN-TIME study tested a similar strategy using multiparameter monitoring devices (ICDs and resynchronization devices). In this study, the parameters studied were events such as ventricular and atrial tachyarrhythmia, a low percentage of biventricular pacing, increased frequency of ventricular premature beats, decreased patient activity, and intracardiac electrogram abnormalities. If these parameters had any abnormalities, the system triggered phone calls to a specific contact. The group allocated for remote monitoring showed a significant reduction in combined clinical outcome and total mortality [75].

Other similar studies also demonstrated a reduction in combined clinical outcomes, often related to a decreased need for face-to-face visits [76]. Results from an unselected population cohort study also indicate benefits of using information obtained from remote monitoring with ICD/cardiac resynchronization therapy (CRT) on mortality [77]. However, a meta-analysis with 11 randomized trials evaluating 5703 patients showed no consistent results on clinical outcomes. In this meta-analysis, telemonitoring devices were associated with a reduction in the total number of visits (planned, unplanned, and ER) (RR 0.56; 95% CI 0.43–0.73, $P < 0.001$); however, hospitalization rates from cardiac causes (RR 0.96; 95% CI 0.82–1.12, $P = 0.60$) and the composite endpoints of ER, unplanned hospital visits, or hospitalizations (RR 0.99; 95% CI 0.68–1.43, $P = 0.96$) was similar between the groups. Total and cardiac mortality were also similar between groups [78].

Telecardiology Monitoring and Management

Cost and quality in a telecardiology service are strictly related to the monitoring and management of the process. To have adequate control of cost and quality it is necessary to establish the management framework based on Key Performance Indicators (KPI). Monitoring KPI variations, corrective actions are taken to reach the established goals.

There are two types of KPIs: those related to the final goals or objectives of the whole process (high-level KPIs) and those related to the subprocesses or activities necessary to achieve those goals (low-level KPIs). Initially, high-level indicators and respective goals must be defined based on the objective to be reached. In a second step, those KPIs are deployed according to the subprocesses to have control of every step along the main process. The deployment level has to compromise monitoring cost and amount of information: A very deep deployment results in detailed information but has a high monitoring cost.

To demonstrate the use of KPIs in telecardiology, it will be considered as an example a Tele-Electrocardiogram Service: ECG signal is collected in remote sites and sent to a diagnostic center to be analyzed by a cardiologist. Then a diagnostic report is sent back to requesting doctor. The main objective of such service is to produce a precise diagnostic report rapidly at low cost. The subprocesses involved to reach such objectives are ECG data collection and transfer, medical analysis, and report delivery. Based on these premises it is possible to establish the high-level KPIs and to deploy them in subprocess KPIs.

High-Level KPIs for a Tele-ECG Service

Based on the main objective of the tele-ECG service to produce a precise diagnostic report rapidly at low cost, it is possible to establish the following KPIs:

1. Production: The number of diagnostic reports made in a specific time interval, usually by month, and the accumulated number of reports. These KPI allows evaluation of the acceptance of the service and to scale future needs of labor and infrastructure.
2. Response time: Defined as the time interval between the ECG data, it is introduced in the system and the diagnostic report is available to the requesting

doctor. To reduce this KPI it is necessary to control each time step between these two events.
3. Report precision: This KPI depends on how precision evaluation is measured. In a specific quality control system, different cardiologists reevaluate a predetermined number of reports. The percentage of discordances can be used as KPI precision measurement.
4. Unitary report cost: Corresponds to the total expenditure in a specific time interval, usually in a month, divided by the total number of reports produced in the same time interval. A precise control of this KPI requires its deployment in each type of cost and activity. This KPI is usually compared to the savings concerning the face-to-face exam cost.

Deployment of High-Level KPIs for a Tele-ECG Service (Low-Level KPIs)

Once the high-level KPIs and their goals are established, it is necessary to obtain more detailed information regarding the subprocesses leading to main goals. The deployment of those high-level KPIs has to consider the following factors affecting the KPI:

1. Production: Depends on the number of remote sites implemented and the number of exams per site. The deployment of this KPI results in the following KPIs, for example:
   a. Percentage of service coverage defined as the number of implemented sites divided by the number of viable sites in a geographic area to be implemented
   b. The number of exams per site
   c. Percentage of service utilization defined as the number of sites using the service divided by the number of implemented sites
2. Response Time: The response time depends on the following subprocess time KPIs:
   a. Sending time defined as time interval between EGC data sent by remote site and acceptance by the system (it measures the quality of Internet infrastructure)
   b. Waiting time for report defined as the time interval between ECG data acceptance by the system and ECG data file opening by the cardiologist
   c. Report time corresponding to the time between data file opening and report availability
   d. Visualization time by the requesting doctor after report availability
3. Report precision: The quality of the report mainly depends on the cardiologist and the report time. Consequently, the KPI percent of discordances can be deployed:
   a. Percent of discordances by cardiologist
   b. Percent of discordances by report time (usually those below a specific report time)

4. Unitary report cost: Cost has different sources such as labor, equipment maintenance, utilities, depreciation, etc. The unitary report cost KPI can be deployed as:
   a. Unitary labor cost
   b. Unitary maintenance cost and etc.

These different categories permit to implement a cost follow-up to find the reason of cost increase or reduction in order to implement corrective actions to reduce cost or to implement good practices in case of cost reduction.

Splitting fixed and variable cost KPIs

   c. *Unitary fixed cost*
   d. *Unitary variable cost*
   allow to evaluate cost fluctuations due to exam demand variation.

Some of these KPIs, in a specific situation, demand a deeper deployment. For instance, a long waiting time for report can be caused by mismatch between demand and report production. In this case, deploying this KPI in an hourly demand KPI and comparing it to the hourly report production KPI, permit to adjust doctor's availability to exam demand.

In summary, KPIs are an important tool for management of any process and for a Tele ECG Service it would not be different, as it has been demonstrated by actual application of this method by the authors. Monthly, sometimes weekly or daily, follow-up of the KPIs results a strict control of the service, allowing correction of eventual deviations from established goals. Similarly, the method can be applied to other telecardiology applications.

References

1. Bashshur RL, Howell JD, Krupinski EA, Harms KM, Bashshur N, Doarn CR. The empirical foundations of telemedicine interventions in primary care. Telemed e-Health. 2016;22(5):342–75.
2. McKinstry B, Hanley J, Wild S, Pagliari C, Paterson M, Lewis S, et al. Telemonitoring based service redesign for the management of uncontrolled hypertension: multicentre randomised controlled trial. BMJ. 2013;346:f3030.
3. McManus RJ, Mant J, Bray EP, Holder R, Jones MI, Greenfield S, et al. Telemonitoring and self-management in the control of hypertension (TASMINH2): a randomised controlled trial. Lancet. 2010;376(9736):163–72.
4. Nilsson M, Rasmark U, Nordgren H, Hallberg P, Skönevik J, Westman G, et al. The physician at a distance: the use of videoconferencing in the treatment of patients with hypertension. J Telemed Telecare. 2009;15(8):397–403.
5. Park M-J, Kim H-S, Kim K-S. Cellular phone and internet-based individual intervention on blood pressure and obesity in obese patients with hypertension. Int J Med Inform. 2009;78(10):704–10.
6. Charpentier G, Benhamou P-Y, Dardari D, Clergeot A, Franc S, Schaepelynck-Belicar P, et al. The Diabeo software enabling individualized insulin dose adjustments combined with telemedicine support improves HbA1c in poorly controlled type 1 diabetic patients: a 6-month, randomized, open-label, parallel-group, multicenter trial (TeleDiab 1 Study). Diabetes Care. 2011;34(3):533–9.

7. Marcolino MS, Maia JX, Alkmim MBM, Boersma E, Ribeiro AL. Telemedicine application in the care of diabetes patients: systematic review and meta-analysis. PLoS One. 2013;8(11):e79246.
8. Ralston JD, Hirsch IB, Hoath J, Mullen M, Cheadle A, Goldberg HI. Web-based collaborative care for type 2 diabetes: a pilot randomized trial. Diabetes Care. 2009;32(2):234–9.
9. Goulis D, Giaglis G, Boren S, Lekka I, Bontis E, Balas EA, et al. Effectiveness of home-centered care through telemedicine applications for overweight and obese patients: a randomized controlled trial. Int J Obes. 2004;28(11):1391.
10. Rodriguez-Idigoras MI, Sepulveda-Munoz J, Sanchez-Garrido-Escudero R, Martinez-Gonzalez JL, Escolar-Castelló JL, Paniagua-Gomez IM, et al. Telemedicine influence on the follow-up of type 2 diabetes patients. Diabetes Technol Ther. 2009;11(7):431–7.
11. Appel LJ, Clark JM, Yeh H-C, Wang N-Y, Coughlin JW, Daumit G, et al. Comparative effectiveness of weight-loss interventions in clinical practice. N Engl J Med. 2011;365(21):1959–68.
12. Muñiz J, Gómez-Doblas JJ, Santiago-Pérez MI, Lekuona-Goya I, Murga-Eizagaetxebarría N, Cruz-Fernández JM, et al. The effect of post-discharge educational intervention on patients in achieving objectives in modifiable risk factors six months after discharge following an episode of acute coronary syndrome,(CAM-2 Project): a randomized controlled trial. Health Qual Life Outcomes. 2010;8(1):137.
13. Gusmão LL, Ribeiro AL, Souza-Silva MVR, Gomes PR, Beleigoli AM, Cardoso CS, et al. Implementation of a text message intervention to promote behavioural change and weight loss among overweight and obese Brazilian primary care patients. J Telemed Telecare. 2018;25(8):476–83.
14. Marcolino MS, Oliveira JAQ, D'Agostino M, Ribeiro AL, Alkmim MBM, Novillo-Ortiz D. The impact of mHealth interventions: systematic review of systematic reviews. JMIR Mhealth Uhealth. 2018;6(1):e23.
15. Chow CK, Redfern J, Hillis GS, Thakkar J, Santo K, Hackett ML, et al. Effect of lifestyle-focused text messaging on risk factor modification in patients with coronary heart disease: a randomized clinical trial. JAMA. 2015;314(12):1255–63.
16. Thangada ND, Garg N, Pandey A, Kumar N. The emerging role of mobile-health applications in the management of hypertension. Curr Cardiol Rep. 2018;20(9):78.
17. McConnell MV, Turakhia MP, Harrington RA, King AC, Ashley EA. Mobile health advances in physical activity, fitness, and atrial fibrillation: moving hearts. J Am Coll Cardiol. 2018;71(23):2691–701.
18. Kumari P, Mathew L, Syal P. Increasing trend of wearables and multimodal interface for human activity monitoring: a review. Biosens Bioelectron. 2017;90:298–307.
19. Riffenburg KM, Spartano NL. Physical activity and weight maintenance: the utility of wearable devices and mobile health technology in research and clinical settings. Curr Opin Endocrinol Diabetes Obes. 2018;25(5):310–4.
20. Hopkins D. Community preventive services task F. clinical decision support systems recommended to prevent cardiovascular disease. Am J Prev Med. 2015;49(5):796–9.
21. Njie GJ, Proia KK, Thota AB, Finnie RK, Hopkins DP, Banks SM, et al. Clinical decision support systems and prevention: a community guide cardiovascular disease systematic review. Am J Prev Med. 2015;49(5):784–95.
22. Roumie CL, Elasy TA, Greevy R, Griffin MR, Liu X, Stone WJ, et al. Improving blood pressure control through provider education, provider alerts, and patient education: a cluster randomized trial. Ann Intern Med. 2006;145(3):165–75.
23. Nerlich M, Balas EA, Schall T, Stieglitz S-P, Filzmaier R, Asbach P, et al. Teleconsultation practice guidelines: report from G8 global health applications subproject 4. Telemed J E Health. 2002;8(4):411–8.
24. Marcolino MS, Alkmim MB, Pessoa CG, Maia JX, Cardoso CS. Development and implementation of a methodology for quality assessment of asynchronous teleconsultations. Telemed e-Health. 2019;26(5):651–8.
25. Liddy C, Moroz I, Mihan A, Nawar N, Keely E. A systematic review of asynchronous, provider-to-provider, electronic consultation services to improve access to specialty care available worldwide. Telemed J e-Health. 2019;25(3):184–98.

26. Thijssing L, Tensen E, Jaspers MW, editors. Patient's perspective on quality of teleconsultation services. MIE; 2016.
27. Petcu R, Kimble C, Ologeanu-Taddei R, Bourdon I, Giraudeau N. Assessing patient's perception of oral teleconsultation. Int J Technol Assess Health Care. 2017;33(2):147–54.
28. Soriano Marcolino M, Minelli Figueira R, Pereira Afonso dos Santos J, Silva Cardoso C, Luiz Ribeiro A, Alkmim MB. The experience of a sustainable large-scale Brazilian telehealth network. Telemed e-Health. 2016;22(11):899–908.
29. Benjamin A. Audit: how to do it in practice. BMJ. 2008;336(7655):1241–5.
30. Olayiwola JN, Anderson D, Jepeal N, Aseltine R, Pickett C, Yan J, et al. Electronic consultations to improve the primary care-specialty care interface for cardiology in the medically underserved: a cluster-randomized controlled trial. Ann Family Med. 2016;14(2):133–40.
31. Caffery LJ, Farjian M, Smith AC. Telehealth interventions for reducing waiting lists and waiting times for specialist outpatient services: a scoping review. J Telemed Telecare. 2016;22(8):504–12.
32. Maeyama MA, Calvo MCM. A Integração do Telessaúde nas Centrais de Regulação: a Teleconsultoria como Mediadora entre a Atenção Básica e a Atenção Especializada. Revista Brasileira de Educação Médica. 2018;42(2):63–72.
33. Pfeil JN. Avaliação da regulação de consultas médicas especializadas baseada em Protocolo+ Teleconsultoria. 2018.
34. Ribeiro ALP, Alkmim MB, Cardoso CS, Carvalho GGR, Caiaffa WT, Andrade MV, et al. Implementation of a telecardiology system in the state of Minas Gerais: the Minas Telecardio Project. Arq Bras Cardiol. 2010;95(1):70–8.
35. Sparenberg A, Russomano T, de Azevedo D, editors. Transmission of digital electrocardiogram (ECG) via modem connection in Southern Brazil. The 26th Annual International Conference of the IEEE Engineering in Medicine and Biology Society; 2004: IEEE.
36. Singh S, Bansal M, Maheshwari P, Adams D, Sengupta SP, Price R, et al. American society of echocardiography: remote echocardiography with web-based assessments for referrals at a distance (ASE-REWARD) study. J Am Soc Echocardiogr. 2013;26(3):221–33.
37. d'Arcy JL, Coffey S, Loudon MA, Kennedy A, Pearson-Stuttard J, Birks J, et al. Large-scale community echocardiographic screening reveals a major burden of undiagnosed valvular heart disease in older people: the OxVALVE Population Cohort Study. Eur Heart J. 2016;37(47):3515–22.
38. Lopes EL, Beaton AZ, Nascimento BR, Tompsett A, Dos Santos JP, Perlman L, et al. Telehealth solutions to enable global collaboration in rheumatic heart disease screening. J Telemed Telecare. 2018;24(2):101–9.
39. Nascimento BR, Sable C, Nunes MCP, Diamantino AC, Oliveira KK, Oliveira CM, et al. Comparison between different strategies of rheumatic heart disease echocardiographic screening in Brazil: data from the PROVAR (Rheumatic Valve Disease Screening Program) study. J Am Heart Assoc. 2018;7(4):e008039.
40. Nascimento BR, Beaton AZ, Nunes MCP, Diamantino AC, Carmo GA, Oliveira KK, et al. Echocardiographic prevalence of rheumatic heart disease in Brazilian schoolchildren: data from the PROVAR study. Int J Cardiol. 2016;219:439–45.
41. Gensini GF, Alderighi C, Rasoini R, Mazzanti M, Casolo G. Value of telemonitoring and telemedicine in heart failure management. Card Fail Rev. 2017;3(2):116.
42. Bashi N, Karunanithi M, Fatehi F, Ding H, Walters D. Remote monitoring of patients with heart failure: an overview of systematic reviews. J Med Internet Res. 2017;19(1):e18.
43. Yun JE, Park J-E, Park H-Y, Lee H-Y, Park D-A. Comparative effectiveness of telemonitoring versus usual care for heart failure: a systematic review and meta-analysis. J Card Fail. 2018;24(1):19–28.
44. Fraiche AM, Eapen ZJ, McClellan MB. Moving beyond the walls of the clinic: opportunities and challenges to the future of telehealth in heart failure. JACC: Heart Failure. 2017;5(4):297–304.
45. Inglis SC, Clark RA, Dierckx R, Prieto-Merino D, Cleland JG. Structured telephone support or non-invasive telemonitoring for patients with heart failure. Cochrane Database Syst Rev. 2015;103(4) https://doi.org/10.1136/heartjnl-2015-309191.

46. Pekmezaris RTL, Williams M, Patel V, Makaryus A, Zeltser R, et al. Home telemonitoring in heart failure: a systematic review and metaanalysis. Health Affairs (Millwood). 2018;37(12):1983–9.
47. Koehler F, Koehler K, Deckwart O, Prescher S, Wegscheider K, Kirwan BA, et al. Efficacy of telemedical interventional management in patients with heart failure (TIM-HF2): a randomised, controlled, parallel-group, unmasked trial. Lancet. 2018;392(10152):1047–57.
48. Abraham WT, Adamson PB, Bourge RC, Aaron MF, Costanzo MR, Stevenson LW, et al. Wireless pulmonary artery haemodynamic monitoring in chronic heart failure: a randomised controlled trial. Lancet. 2011;377(9766):658–66.
49. Abraham WT, Stevenson LW, Bourge RC, Lindenfeld JA, Bauman JG, Adamson PB. Sustained efficacy of pulmonary artery pressure to guide adjustment of chronic heart failure therapy: complete follow-up results from the CHAMPION randomised trial. Lancet. 2016;387(10017):453–61.
50. Margolis KL, Asche SE, Dehmer SP, Bergdall AR, Green BB, Sperl-Hillen JM, et al. Long-term outcomes of the effects of home blood pressure telemonitoring and pharmacist management on blood pressure among adults with uncontrolled hypertension: follow-up of a cluster randomized clinical trial. JAMA Netw Open. 2018;1(5):e181617.
51. Wald DS, Bestwick JP, Raiman L, Brendell R, Wald NJ. Randomised trial of text messaging on adherence to cardiovascular preventive treatment (INTERACT trial). PLoS One. 2014;9(12):e114268.
52. McManus RJ, Mant J, Franssen M, Nickless A, Schwartz C, Hodgkinson J, et al. Efficacy of self-monitored blood pressure, with or without telemonitoring, for titration of antihypertensive medication (TASMINH4): an unmasked randomised controlled trial. Lancet. 2018;391(10124):949–59.
53. Monahan M, Jowett S, Nickless A, Franssen M, Grant S, Greenfield S, et al. Cost-effectiveness of telemonitoring and self-monitoring of blood pressure for antihypertensive titration in primary care (TASMINH4). Hypertension. 2019;73(6):1231–9.
54. Palmer MJ, Barnard S, Perel P, Free C. Mobile phone-based interventions for improving adherence to medication prescribed for the primary prevention of cardiovascular disease in adults. Cochrane Database Syst Rev. 2018;6:CD012675.
55. Marcolino MS, Maia LM, Oliveira JAQ, Melo LDR, Pereira BLD, Andrade-Junior DF, et al. Impact of telemedicine interventions on mortality in patients with acute myocardial infarction: a systematic review and meta-analysis. Heart. 2019;105(19):1479–86.
56. Oliveira Junior MT, Canesin MF, Marcolino MS, Ribeiro AL, Carvalho AC, Reddy S, et al. Telemedicine guideline in Patient Care with Acute Coronary Syndrome and Other heart Diseases. Arq Bras Cardiol. 2015;104(5 Suppl 1):1–26.
57. DeBusk RF, Miller NH, Raby L. Technical feasibility of an online decision support system for acute coronary syndromes. Circ Cardiovasc Qual Outcomes. 2010;3(6):694–700.
58. Nelson BP, Chason K. Use of ultrasound by emergency medical services: a review. Int J Emerg Med. 2008;1(4):253–9.
59. Wechsler LR, Demaerschalk BM, Schwamm LH, Adeoye OM, Audebert HJ, Fanale CV, et al. Telemedicine quality and outcomes in stroke: a scientific statement for healthcare professionals from the American Heart Association/American Stroke Association. Stroke. 2017;48(1):e3–e25.
60. Nascimento BR, Brant LCC, Marino BCA, Passaglia LG, Ribeiro ALP. Implementing myocardial infarction systems of care in low/middle-income countries. Heart. 2019;105(1):20–6.
61. Filgueiras Filho NM, Feitosa Filho GS, Solla DJF, Argolo FC, Guimaraes PO, Paiva Filho IM, et al. Implementation of a regional network for ST-segment-elevation myocardial infarction (STEMI) care and 30-day mortality in a low- to middle-Income City in Brazil: findings from Salvador's STEMI Registry (RESISST). J Am Heart Assoc. 2018;7(14):e008624.
62. Brasen CL, Madsen JS, Parkner T, Brandslund I. Home management of warfarin treatment through a real-time supervised telemedicine solution: a randomized controlled trial. Telemed J e-Health. 2019;25(2):109–15.

63. Pozzi M, Mitchell J, Henaine AM, Hanna N, Safi O, Henaine R. International normalized ratio self-testing and self-management: improving patient outcomes. Vasc Health Risk Manag. 2016;12:387–92.
64. Heneghan CJ, Garcia-Alamino JM, Spencer EA, Ward AM, Perera R, Bankhead C, et al. Self-monitoring and self-management of oral anticoagulation. Cochrane Database Syst Rev. 2016;7:CD003839.
65. Saia M, Mantoan D, Fonzo M, Bertoncello C, Soattin M, Sperotto M, et al. Impact of the regional network for AMI in the management of STEMI on care processes, outcomes and health inequities in the Veneto region, Italy. Int J Environ Res Public Health. 2018;15(9):1980.
66. Beatty AL, Fukuoka Y, Whooley MA. Using mobile technology for cardiac rehabilitation: a review and framework for development and evaluation. J Am Heart Assoc. 2013;2(6):e000568.
67. Rawstorn JC, Gant N, Direito A, Beckmann C, Maddison R. Telehealth exercise-based cardiac rehabilitation: a systematic review and meta-analysis. Heart. 2016;102(15):1183–92.
68. Frederix I, Hansen D, Coninx K, Vandervoort P, Vandijck D, Hens N, et al. Medium-term effectiveness of a comprehensive internet-based and patient-specific Telerehabilitation program with text messaging support for cardiac patients: randomized controlled trial. J Med Internet Res. 2015;17(7):e185.
69. Peng X, Su Y, Hu Z, Sun X, Li X, Dolansky MA, et al. Home-based telehealth exercise training program in Chinese patients with heart failure: a randomized controlled trial. Medicine. 2018;97(35):e12069.
70. Maddison R, Rawstorn JC, Stewart RAH, Benatar J, Whittaker R, Rolleston A, et al. Effects and costs of real-time cardiac telerehabilitation: randomised controlled non-inferiority trial. Heart. 2019;105(2):122–9.
71. Taylor RS, Dalal H, Jolly K, Moxham T, Zawada A. Home-based versus Centre-based cardiac rehabilitation. Cochrane Database Syst Rev. 2010;(1):CD007130.
72. Frederix I, Hansen D, Coninx K, Vandervoort P, Vandijck D, Hens N, et al. Effect of comprehensive cardiac telerehabilitation on one-year cardiovascular rehospitalization rate, medical costs and quality of life: a cost-effectiveness analysis. Eur J Prev Cardiol. 2016;23(7):674–82.
73. Lopez-Villegas A, Catalan-Matamoros D, Martin-Saborido C, Villegas-Tripiana I, Robles-Musso E. A systematic review of economic evaluations of pacemaker Telemonitoring systems. Rev Esp Cardiol. 2016;69(2):125–33.
74. Bourge RC, Abraham WT, Adamson PB, Aaron MF, Aranda JM Jr, Magalski A, et al. Randomized controlled trial of an implantable continuous hemodynamic monitor in patients with advanced heart failure: the COMPASS-HF study. J Am Coll Cardiol. 2008;51(11):1073–9.
75. Hindricks G, Taborsky M, Glikson M, Heinrich U, Schumacher B, Katz A, et al. Implant-based multiparameter telemonitoring of patients with heart failure (IN-TIME): a randomised controlled trial. Lancet. 2014;384(9943):583–90.
76. De Simone A, Leoni L, Luzi M, Amellone C, Stabile G, La Rocca V, et al. Remote monitoring improves outcome after ICD implantation: the clinical efficacy in the management of heart failure (EFFECT) study. Europace. 2015;17(8):1267–75.
77. Kurek A, Tajstra M, Gadula-Gacek E, Buchta P, Skrzypek M, Pyka L, et al. Impact of remote monitoring on long-term prognosis in heart failure patients in a real-world cohort: results from all-comers COMMIT-HF trial. J Cardiovasc Electrophysiol. 2017;28(4):425–31.
78. Klersy C, Boriani G, De Silvestri A, Mairesse GH, Braunschweig F, Scotti V, et al. Effect of telemonitoring of cardiac implantable electronic devices on healthcare utilization: a meta-analysis of randomized controlled trials in patients with heart failure. Eur J Heart Fail. 2016;18(2):195–204.

Telestroke and Teleneurology

25

Benzion Blech and Bart M. Demaerschalk

Introduction

Stroke is a major cause of disability and mortality in the United States, as well as globally [1]. Over the last few years, tremendous strides have been made in the treatment of acute ischemic stroke, from the US Food and Drug Administration (FDA) approval of intravenous tissue-type plasminogen activator (IV tPA) alteplase to the more recent trials demonstrating the clinical benefits of endovascular thrombectomy interventions up to 24 hours from symptom onset in carefully selected patients [2, 3]. With the rapidly changing pace of stroke care, and expansion of potential intervention windows [4] for patients experiencing an acute ischemic stroke, the idea of telemedicine specifically geared toward acute cerebrovascular disorders came into being, known as *telestroke*, with the main purpose of being able to provide acute stroke care remotely. While current guidelines recommend IV tPA for eligible patients who have symptom onset within 4.5 hours of presentation, the sooner it is given more brain can be potentially saved; this is known as the "time-is-brain" concept [5]. Telestroke can be utilized not only to provide acute stroke care remotely for sites which would otherwise go without expert vascular neurology expertise but also to help improve stroke times, while potentially improving patient outcomes. This chapter discusses the practical definitions of telestroke and teleneurology, as well as the utility, applicability, and network strategies for these models of care.

B. Blech (✉)
Mayo Clinic College of Medicine and Science, Phoenix, AZ, USA
e-mail: blech.benzion@mayo.edu

B. M. Demaerschalk
Medical Director of Center for Connected Care, Cerebrovascular Diseases Division,
Mayo Clinic College of Medicine and Science, Phoenix, AZ, USA

Principles of Telestroke

Telestroke Definitions

The term "telestroke" refers to the use of telemedicine technologies for the care of patients who suffer from ischemic or hemorrhagic cerebrovascular injuries. Telestroke can be considered a subdivision of teleneurology, which encompasses all neurologic care that is performed remotely. As far as teleneurology and telemedicine are concerned, telestroke has been one of the fastest-growing and innovative of the telemedicine fields and has shown promise in all aspects of stroke care, from acute management and prehospital evaluations to chronic management with telerehabilitation. In 2018, the American Heart Association/American Stroke Association (AHA/ASA) released recommendations and guidelines for the use of telestroke in acute ischemic stroke [6].

Telestroke Networks

One of the most crucial elements of utilizing telestroke in the population is defining the idea of *telestroke networks*. A telestroke network is a method of providing telestroke care, and is typically divided into two different network types: the *hub-and-spoke* model and the *distributive* model. The hub-and-spoke model refers to a network that is comprised of a central "hub" site, such as primary or comprehensive stroke center, that then provides telestroke care to other healthcare centers, or "spoke" sites (Fig. 25.1). The hub sites provide not only acute telestroke care but can also participate with training and improvement in telestroke and traditional stroke workflows at spoke sites, as well as expediting transfers for patient who require higher levels of stroke care to the hub site. This model has been shown to be economically favorable and can lead to decreased costs for stroke care across the network [7–9]. Another network that has been described is the *distributive* model. In this setting, there is a central group of telestroke physicians (such as vascular neurologists) who work as part of a group and can be employed across multiple sites or healthcare centers. This group then provides telestroke care to centers contracted in that network (Fig. 25.2). Both models are described by the AHA/ASA as commonly used in telestroke [10].

A major goal of a telestroke network is to provide high-quality vascular neurology expertise with acute stroke management, although certainly the network can be valuable in other areas of stroke care, from inpatient stroke unit management to rehabilitation and beyond. Telestroke participation has been associated with improved stroke care metrics over time for participating hospitals; this could be secondary to improved workflows in stroke management, educational initiatives, and training that can be directed by the hub site [11].

25 Telestroke and Teleneurology

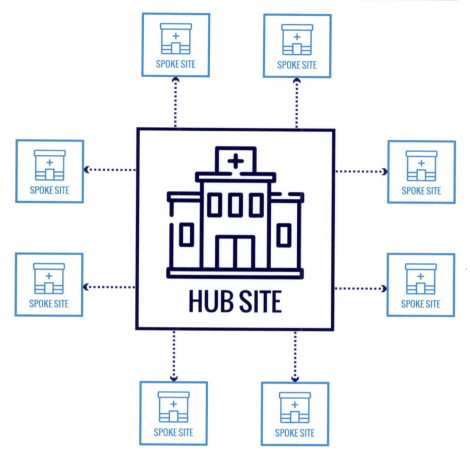

Fig. 25.1 The hub-and-spoke model of telestroke care. In this model, a hospital known as the *hub* – such as a comprehensive stroke center – employs telestroke physicians to provide care to multiple other hospitals or healthcare facilities, which are referred to as *spokes*

Devices

Many devices have been utilized in telemedicine as a whole, including smartphones, telephones, computers, and other mobile devices [12]. While other areas of medicine have been somewhat limited by the technological capabilities of devices used in telemedicine, which can be inferior to in-person examinations [12], teleneurology, and particularly telestroke, has been shown to benefit from telehealth technologies. Mobile devices such as the iPhone, when used in telestroke evaluations, has been shown to have a high inter-method agreement between vascular neurologists, as well as increased physician satisfaction and acceptance [13]. Robotics used in

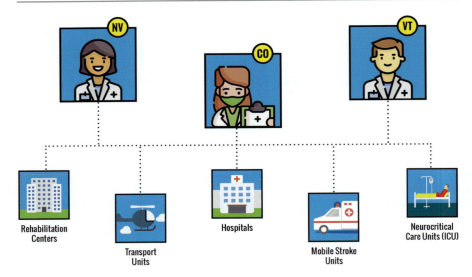

Fig. 25.2 The distributive model of telestroke care. In this model, multiple providers – potentially across multiple healthcare systems – are linked together in the network to provide telestroke services to other sites in need, including hospitals, clinics, mobile stroke units, and others

telestroke assessments has also been well-accepted globally [14], although may be associated with slightly longer assessment times [15]. However, telestroke can be as efficacious as in-person evaluations in terms of outcomes, especially for sites that do not have vascular neurologists available on-site [16].

Telestroke Applications

Prehospital

While telestroke can be utilized during nearly all phases of stroke care, it has traditionally been most commonly been utilized in the Emergency Department (ED) setting. However, prehospital utilization of telestroke devices and workflows can help streamline the acute stroke assessment and expedite care for patients, and possibly reduce morbidity and mortality. It can also provide useful insights for the vascular neurologist regarding the overall clinical status of the patient, as well as help make decisions for correct triaging and routing of patients, such as to a comprehensive stroke center or thrombectomy-capable stroke center for patients suspected of a large vessel occlusion (LVO) and need for endovascular intervention.

Emergency Medical Services

Emergency medical service (EMS) utilization of telemedicine, particularly of telestroke technologies, has been an area of much interest and research in recent years. As EMS personnel are usually the first ones to encounter and examine the patient, performing remote assessments using telestroke methodologies can be a powerful way for other stroke team members to partner with EMS earlier in the course of stroke. EMS hospital prenotification of incoming acute stroke patients has been shown to improve various factors of care, including increasing the number of IV tPA–eligible patients and timelier stroke evaluation [17]. From a technological standpoint, two commonly utilized methods are *telestroke-enabled ambulances* and *mobile stroke units* (MSUs). The telestroke-enabled ambulance is a vehicle that is outfitted with remote audiovisual (AV) capabilities, allowing for instant communication with the telestroke physician [18]. Using these technologies, the treating vascular neurologist can communicate and examine the patient, as well as communicate instantly with EMS personnel. MSUs, on the other hand, have the same capabilities as telestroke-enabled ambulances, but with the added benefit of an on-board computed tomography (CT) scanner, as well as point-of-care laboratory equipment and medications. With the MSU, not only can the assessments be done remotely, but potential interventions can be performed as well, such as the administration of IV tPA in eligible patients, or antihypertensive agents in patients with evidence of intracranial hemorrhage on CT [19]. As MSU care evolves, other pathologies have been identified for intervention as well, such as status epilepticus, cerebral edema from brain tumors, and hypoglycemia, among others [20]. While MSUs have the benefit of acute stroke interventions with the aid of the on-board CT scanner and point-of-care laboratory equipment, telestroke-enabled ambulances can be quicker to deploy, as well as cheaper and more cost-effective, especially in rural areas [21]. More recently, mobile telehealth applications have been developed specifically to facilitate rapid communication between EMS and accepting EDs via chat software, including video and audio communication. This new and rapidly changing area of telehealth has much promise, although research remains to be done to examine patient care and outcomes using such technology.

Early Screening

Prehospital early screening of patients using remote telestroke technologies can be invaluable. Patient screening is important for proper treatment decisions of the patient, and EMS can provide valuable early insights that can potentially change patient management. From an acute stroke perspective, utilization of MSUs or telestroke-enabled ambulances can screen for the presence of an LVO using either the stroke severity with predefined clinical stroke scales (such as the Cincinnati Prehospital Stroke Scale, RACE scale, and others) or the presence of CT angiographic evidence. These screening assessments can affect further treatment and transfer decisions, such as transfer to a thrombectomy-capable stroke centers for patients suspected of an LVO [22, 23].

Emergency Department (ED)

The ED remains the key focus area of telestroke delivery. The responsibility of telestroke in the ED setting is multifaceted, and efficient workflows in this setting are critical for proper management, triage, and decision-making for patients suffering from an acute ischemic or hemorrhagic stroke. When a patient arrives to the ED with suspected stroke, an alert to the consulting telestroke network is activated immediately. Then, the vascular neurologist on call for the network responds and communicates with the ED staff either through traditional methods (such as telephone consultations) or with more advanced telemedicine tools, such as with smartphones or tablets with continuous AV communication, telemedicine platforms, laptop or desktop computers, or robotic telepresence devices. Regardless of the methodology utilized, the key goal of telestroke in the ED setting is the quick evaluation of the patient for possible IV tPA, assistance with management of complications, and potential transfer decisions. Telestroke networks are designed to provide 24/7 accessibility to expert stroke physicians, which allows for continued operation of a stroke center throughout the day and night.

Telestroke consultations can also help identify those with stroke-mimic syndromes using various scoring systems, although a possible stroke mimic syndrome itself is not an absolute contraindication to IV tPA [6, 24–26].

Neurocritical Care and Inpatient

In the hospital setting, telestroke technology can be useful for continued management of stroke patients. Telemonitoring can be performed in the neurocritical care unit, inpatient stroke units, and inpatient rehabilitation centers. Applications in the hospital setting includes monitoring of patients who received IV tPA for complications, including orolingual edema, thrombolysis-related intra- or extracranial hemorrhage, hemorrhagic transformation of stroke, and malignant cerebral edema. Patients identified to have intracranial hemorrhage can be monitored during the inpatient stay for re-bleeding, vasospasm, and cerebral edema. Close monitoring with telestroke modalities can provide critical information on inpatients, regardless of whether IV tPA or endovascular thrombectomy intervention was performed. The telestroke network can also be called upon for acute inpatient stroke alerts for candidacy of treatment eligibility and further cerebrovascular workup and management. In-hospital stroke alerts have been associated with longer treatment times than patients arriving to the ED [27]; telestroke protocols can potentially improve stroke recognition and management. It is vitally important that when implementing a telestroke network, careful attention is directed toward creating inpatient workflows for such inpatient stroke alerts in order to improve patient care.

Telerehabilitation

With regards to posthospital care, telestroke has been studied in rehabilitation settings as well. Telerehabilitation has been shown to be associated with improvements in motor recovery, higher cortical function, and depression [28]. Telehealth evaluations for poststroke dysphagia evaluations and treatment have found to be effective

[29]. While telerehabilitation in the stroke population remains promising, especially in remote and rural areas [30], more research needs to be done to determine the cost-effectiveness utility of such modalities across the broader poststroke population.

Telemedicine to Home

Home telemedicine follow-up appointments or posthospital discharge appointments are feasible for patients with many medical or surgical conditions including cerebrovascular disorders [31]. Telemedicine to a patient's home is particularly feasible when the principle data to be gained is audiovisual, when the principle purposes are dialogue, counseling, and answering questions, when there isn't an indication for a hands-on physical examination, and when the patient resides out of town/state or when there are transportation challenges. In the case of post-discharge telemedicine home visits, there are opportunities to check on recovery and rehabilitation progress, symptoms of recurrent stroke or transient ischemic attack, secondary stroke prevention medication compliance, and side effects, the NIHSS and Modified Rankin Scale, any remaining outpatient diagnostic studies requiring review and communication, and to address patient and family questions. Post-discharge home telemedicine visits may be useful to reduce the risk of early readmissions to hospital.

Secondary Prevention

Remote monitoring of patients for secondary stroke prevention, such as with virtual stroke clinics, has been an area of telestroke with much interest, as many patients in remote and rural areas have difficulty with obtaining continued poststroke care and secondary prevention. However, more research needs to be done in this area before recommendations can be made with regards to telestroke and secondary prevention, and trials are ongoing at this point in time.

Telemedicine for Other Neurologic Conditions (Teleneurology)

While telestroke remains the most actively developed area of teleneurology, many other areas of neurology can benefit from the impacts of telemedicine, especially in hospitals and clinics that do not have constant availability of neurologists to provide specialized neurologic care. Teleneurology has been linked to greater community physician satisfaction and lower rates of patient transfers [32], as well as decreased costs of care and greater patient satisfaction in rural populations [33]. Teleneurology can provide vital services for hospitals and clinics that are unable to provide neurologic care 24/7, and growth of these technological platforms will likely continue to grow in popularity, especially in rural and remote areas.

Inpatient Care

General Inpatient

Teleneurology can be applied to the general inpatient service. Teleneurology networks, unlike telestroke networks, can give a broader range of neuropathology that can be evaluated and treated by network-affiliated remote neurologists. This can allow for many small and rural hospital centers to provide around-the-clock general neurology care. Conditions that have been provided for teleneurological care include epilepsy, malignant cerebral edema associated with brain tumors, delirium and encephalopathy, meningitis, among others. Typically, telestroke and teleneurology remain as separate service lines, although they can be bundled together for network hospitals to provide the widest range of teleneurological services. The same devices utilized in telestroke (such as telephones, smartphones, robots, etc.) can be used in general teleneurology as well. Teleneurology can be especially critical for rural hospitals that are unable to staff the inpatient service with a full-time neurologist and allows for quick and easy access to expert neurologic care at all times of the day or night.

Teleneurocritical Care

In the field of neurocritical care, telemedicine can be a valuable tool in the management of critically ill patients. Intractable epilepsy and status epilepticus patients can be remotely monitored with continuous EEG monitoring, while trained epilepsy specialists can provide alerts and management expertise for hospitals without such care in-house [34]. Management of other acute neurologic conditions, such as malignant cerebral edema and herniation syndromes, can be implemented in a teleneurology network with trained neurologists, neurosurgeons, and radiologist. Coma scales (Glasgow Coma Scale and Mayo Clinic FOUR Score Scale) can be successfully applied to telemedicine examinations of patients in coma in the intensive care unit environment [35]. Brain death evaluations can be performed remotely using teleneurological services as well [36]. Teleneurocritical care can be a useful adjunct for facilities which do not have ready access to neurocritical care physicians and should be designed to work alongside existing critical care physician and workflows.

Outpatient Care

Teleneurology has proven useful to deliver chronic neurologic care to rural patients at community-based outpatient clinics. For instance, veterans living in rural communities of New Mexico, Colorado, Arizona, and Texas receive follow-up teleneurology care at 16 rural outpatient facilities. Parkinson disease (32%), epilepsy (23%), headache (15%), multiple sclerosis (6%), and dementia (5%) were the most common neurological conditions confronted in these outpatient care appointments [37]. Saving time, saving money, or both, was reported by 96% of patient respondents. All the providers expressed that they could deliver excellent care through teleneurology. A similar teleneurology outpatient experience was reported by veterans in California [38].

Remote Patient Monitoring

Teleneurology has been used for the purposes of caring and monitoring outpatient neurological conditions, such as in headache disorders, dementia evaluations, movement disorders, epilepsy, and multiple sclerosis [39]. The idea of remote patient monitoring in teleneurology is a key component of primary and secondary prevention strategies for remote and rural areas that may not have ready access to neurologists. Patients with chronic neurological conditions can face hurdles in mobility and transportation issues, further highlighting the need for cost-efficient methods for proper neurologic care that takes these issues into account, which teleneurology can play a role. Proper outpatient teleneurology care should focus on management of acute and chronic neurologic conditions, as well as triage of patients to correct facilities should the need arise for inpatient management. Some of the main barriers to implementation of teleneurology for management and remote monitoring of patients with chronic neurological conditions include lack of internet access in rural areas, variable familiarity with technology (especially among elderly patients), perceived costs of enrolling in a telehealth practice, disruption of the traditional physician–patient relationship, billing and credentialing issues, among others [40]. As Internet access and telehealth technology become more ubiquitous, expectations are that teleneurology will continue to grow in utilization.

Telerehabilitation

Telerehabilitation has been an area of much interest and research in recent years, especially as telemedicine has become more popular in general. With regards to neurologic disorders, such as stroke, telerehabilitation is designed to manage not only physical activities (such as physical, occupational, and speech therapies), but theoretically improve cognitive function as well. A 2017 Cochrane review examining the utilization of virtual reality (VR) in stroke rehabilitation found that VR did not significantly improve upper limb function when compared to conventional therapies, although can be a useful adjunct to traditional therapy [41]. Although much research remains to be done in this area, it may prove to be a major component of teleneurology and telestroke in the future.

Rural Care

One of the main focuses of telestroke, as well as teleneurology in general, has been to provide high-quality neurovascular care to remote and rural areas that would otherwise go without. Rural areas in the United States are well known to have physician shortages in general when compared to urban centers [42], and access to neurologists can be difficult to come by. The root of this problem is likely multifactorial; costs of recruitment and retention may be too high for a small rural hospital to justify the hiring of full-time vascular neurologist, and smaller facilities may lack the technological capabilities to fully service stroke patients [43]. Telestroke can provide a way for rural areas to benefit from the expertise of stroke neurologists and can be a more cost-effective option as well [7]. As technologic advances continue in the field of telehealth in general, telestroke is predicted to continue to grow and improve, especially in rural areas.

Other Models of Care

Teleneuroradiology

Neuroradiology is vital for teleneurology and telestroke networks. With regards to teleneuroradiology in telestroke, remote CT viewing has been shown to have excellent agreement among teleneurologists and teleradiologists on the presence or absence of radiographic contraindications to IV tPA [44]. More recently, automated methods of LVO detection using artificial intelligence has become utilized in the emergent settings, and have been shown to have high sensitivity and negative predictive value in this regard [45]. Remote multimodal CT evaluations can be performed safely in a rural network [46], which is important for determining possibly thrombectomy candidates in the dawn of the new era of extended windows of up to 24 hours in select patients with LVO and perfusion mismatch on CT perfusion studies [2, 3]. Teleneuroradiology remains a key component for the proper operation of a telestroke network, and continued advances in image acquisition and transmission will further benefit the field.

Teleneurosurgery

Telemedicine in neurosurgery has been an area of interest as well. Remote evaluations of potential neurosurgical candidates with telehealth technologies can decrease transfer rates and lead to better utilization of resources [47]. Neuroendovascular models of teleneurosurgery have shown promise, and perhaps may be utilized in acute stroke care [48, 49]. Other areas of neurosurgery have also shown that telesurgery can be beneficial, including robotic endonasal telesurgery [50]. As remote robotic technology advances, more teleneurosurgical possibilities can be designed and implemented for the benefit of the teleneurology network.

Strategies for Development

Telestroke Network Development

Telestroke network development can be a complex process. Multiple factors need to be weighed before creating a network. First, it is important to define the network type (distributive vs. hub-and-spoke), as well as potential participating hospital centers and clinics. Technological factors, including types of equipment, need to be defined. Appropriate training of both hub and spoke sites needs to be created and implemented efficiently. Guidelines have been published to better guide hospital, healthcare systems, and groups that would like to either create and join an existing telestroke network [51]. These include administrative guidelines (such as management of patient data, workflows, data retrieval policies, quality, and outcome measures) as well as clinical guidelines (such as program goals, staffing models, operational/service hours, and integration strategies) [51]. It may be helpful for health centers with minimal experience with telemedicine communicate with other facilities that have participated with telestroke in the past for guidance on other inherent issues related to telemedicine delivery, such as location, technologic hurdles, and unique patient populations.

Teleneurology Network Development

Similar features that are applicable to telestroke network development apply for teleneurology network development as well, such as network definitions (hub-and-spoke vs. distributive models). However, some factors in teleneurology network development are unique. An important factor in development includes defining the specific diagnoses or concerns that would be handled by the teleneurology service; this can include acute and chronic headache management, epilepsy and status epilepticus, meningitis and encephalitis, movement disorders, and emergencies such as dystonic reactions, and many others. Clear activation guidelines, patient workflows, and transfer criteria need to be developed within the network to maximize efficient patient care. With severe shortages of physicians in general and neurologists in particular, especially in rural and remote areas, teleneurology services can be a vital service for these hospitals and healthcare centers.

Other Important Factors

Equipment utilized by the network should be provided by the organization and should emphasize high-quality AV technology wherever possible. Continued education between the hub and participating sites should be performed on a routine basis, as well as examination of workflows and policies in order to improve patient care through the network. Simulation training between hub and participating sites can be particularly beneficial, and has been linked to improved door-to-needle times for the network [52]. Constant monitoring of the network is important, as is data analytics and examination of factors regarding patient care, such as outcomes and quality measures. While the processes of creating (or joining) a teleneurology/telestroke network may be a daunting task, the focus should always remain on providing and utilizing expert neurologic care for the improvement of patient care.

Future Directions

Telestroke Networks

Telestroke networks should continue to evolve. While much of the focus of telestroke has been delivery of acute stroke care in the prehospital and ED settings, there are many areas for improvement on current telestroke networks. For example, current patient transfer methods may be inadequate for some networks, especially in the setting of recent expanded windows for endovascular therapy; longer transfer times, especially transfers occurring nocturnally, may be associated with decreased likelihood of undergoing endovascular therapy [53]. Future telestroke network directions should focus on continued improvement in all network parameters related to patient care, from prehospital care to discharge from the hospital, and beyond. Efficient patient care workflows need constant refining for optimization in the rapidly changing world of acute cerebrovascular care.

Teleneurology Networks

Teleneurology networks can continue to benefit from growth of the telemedicine world in general. As teleneurological networks continue to grow in popularity, focus should be directed toward optimization of the network in general. Clear workflow guidelines need to be created for physicians, nursing, and other staff on proper utilization of the teleneurology network. Approved indications for activation of the network should be disseminated by the network to participating centers. For neurological emergencies such as meningitis and status epilepticus, it is important for the teleneurology network to focus on ways of rapid activation when needed, and the utilization of high-quality AV methods wherever possible.

Devices

Telemedicine Devices
Technological advances have been and continue to be a major driving force of innovation in telemedicine in general, as well as for teleneurology and telestroke networks. Although traditional methods of communication remain an important means of communication throughout a network (such as with telephone), recommendations are for networks to implement high-quality AV wherever possible, such as with high-speed video conferencing methods [51]. Tablets, in particular, can be a cost-effective method of teleneurology and telemedicine administration compared to traditional telemedicine technologies [32]. With the advent of wearable fitness technologies, such as smartwatches, much research has been focused on possible utilization of these devices with remote patient monitoring for telemedicine care

[54]. Other wearable sensors, such as those that are graphene-based, may be a major component of remote patient monitoring in the future, although scientific and engineering challenges remain [55, 56].

Telestroke Devices

Many devices marketed for telemedicine can be applied for possible telestroke utilization. Some of the features that are particularly important for optimal telestroke usage include high-quality AV capabilities, rapid communication methods for communication between bedside providers and remote telestroke physicians, as well as need for tools to participate with specific acute stroke evaluations, such as the NIH Stroke Scale. As telemedicine technology continues to improve, innovative methods may be uncovered for use in stroke care in the future. Wearable devices, such as Google Glass–based devices, has shown good inter-rater reliability when used for NIH Stroke Scale assessments [57]. Other mobile apps have also been released in recent years focusing particularly on EMS and stroke team intercommunication, which can prove useful for networks that have limited funds or other limitations in installation of traditional telestroke technologies. However, certainly more research needs to be done in this area before widespread recommendations can be made.

Other Devices

Telesonography has been studied in the emergency department settings, and can be comparable when compared to in-person ultrasonography, although more data and studies are needed to evaluate its clinical efficacy [58]. Remote ultrasonography can include carotid duplex and transcranial doppler ultrasounds. While the benefits of such imaging modalities include lower cost and risk to the patient, the inherent limitations of ultrasound may limit its use, such as the fact that it is operator-dependent and difficult to standardize protocols. More research needs to be explored in this area before recommendations for telesonography can be made for use in telestroke assessments. Other devices continue to be developed and tested, such as telehealth-connected patient vital monitors, stethoscopes, otoscopes, retinal scanners, among others. The future landscape for telehealth devices appears promising with continued innovation.

Other Applications

Telestroke networks can also provide the means for acute stroke trial enrollment in a rapid manner, which can lead to more improvements in acute cerebrovascular care in the future [59]. Neurologic education can also be an important function of a network for training, such as for medical students, neurology residents, and cerebrovascular fellows; the American Academy of Neurology (AAN) Telemedicine Work Group has released recommendations on implementation of teleneurology in medical education [60].

Summary

Telestroke is a subspecialty of teleneurology, and one of the most widely studied and innovative areas of telemedicine in general. Telestroke groups, otherwise known as *networks*, are designed to provide care to multiple medical care facilities, which can include prehospital care (such as ground and air ambulances), Emergency Departments, acute stroke units, neurocritical care units, rehabilitation facilities, and clinics. Two types of telestroke networks include the *hub-and-spoke* and the *distributive* models. The hub-and-spoke model refers to a central hub (such as a comprehensive stroke center) that employs telestroke physicians, such as vascular neurologists, radiologists, and neurosurgeons, that provide care to multiple other health facilities, known as *spoke* sites. In the distributive model, a group of telestroke physicians may be employed in multiple locations, that then join to provide network support for other centers and clinics. While telestroke is a popular field, the overall field of teleneurology has been growing as well and can be used to provide expert neurologic care for multiple other indications in both the inpatient and outpatient settings, such as meningitis, epilepsy, multiple sclerosis, and other acute and chronic neurologic conditions. Teleneurology and telestroke continue to gain popularity, but the process of joining and/or creating such as a network can be an arduous task. The first step is to define the type of network, such as the hub-and-spoke or distributive models, the decision of which may depend on specific locale, patient population, and available healthcare resources. While many devices have been developed and utilized for the field of teleneurology and telestroke, the future of device development in this area remains promising with a high level of innovation from the healthcare technology sector. Future directions would include further growth of existing telestroke and teleneurology networks and continued technological advances to make the process of telehealth in neurology as seamless as possible. While the primary focus has been on direct clinical applications such as patient care, it is important to understand the full potential these technologies can offer, such as with rapid stroke trial enrollment, research, and educational opportunities for trainees.

References

1. Katan M, Luft A. Global burden of Stroke. Semin Neurol. 2018;38(2):208–11.
2. Nogueira RG, Jadhav AP, Haussen DC, Bonafe A, Budzik RF, Bhuva P, et al. Thrombectomy 6 to 24 hours after stroke with a mismatch between deficit and infarct. N Engl J Med. 2018;378(1):11–21.
3. Albers GW, Marks MP, Kemp S, Christensen S, Tsai JP, Ortega-Gutierrez S, et al. Thrombectomy for stroke at 6 to 16 hours with selection by perfusion imaging. N Engl J Med. 2018;378(8):708–18.
4. Schellinger PD, Demaerschalk BM. Endovascular stroke therapy in the late time window. Stroke. 2018;49, 2559(10):–2561.
5. Warner JJ, Harrington RA, Sacco RL, Elkind MSV. Guidelines for the early management of patients with acute ischemic stroke: 2019 ypdate to the 2018 guidelines for the early management of acute ischemic stroke. [Internet]. Stroke. 2019. STROKEAHA119027708 p. Available from: http://www.ncbi.nlm.nih.gov/pubmed/31662117.

6. Powers WJ, Rabinstein AA, Ackerson T, Adeoye OM, Bambakidis NC, Becker K, et al. Guidelines for the early management of patients with acute ischemic stroke: a guideline for healthcare professionals from the American Heart Association/American Stroke Association. Vol. 49. Stroke. 2018;2018:46–110.
7. Switzer JA, Demaerschalk BM, Xie J, Fan L, Villa KF, Wu EQ. Cost-effectiveness of hub-and-spoke telestroke networks for the management of acute ischemic Stroke from the hospitals' perspectives. Circ Cardiovasc Qual Outcomes [Internet]. 2013 [cited 2019 Sep 24];6(1):18–26. Available from: https://doi.org/10.1161/circoutcomes.112.967125.
8. Riou-Comte N, Mione G, Humbertjean L, Brunner A, Vezain A, Lavandier K, et al. Implementation and evaluation of an economic model for telestroke: experience from Virtuall, France. Front Neurol. 2017;8(NOV).
9. Al Kasab S, Almallouhi E, Debenham E, Turner N, Simpson KN, Holmstedt CA. Beyond acute stroke: rate of stroke transfers to a tertiary centre following the implementation of a dedicated inpatient teleneurology network. J Telemed Telecare. 2019:1357633X1986809.
10. Wechsler LR, Demaerschalk BM, Schwamm LH, Adeoye OM, Audebert HJ, Fanale C V, et al. Telemedicine quality and outcomes in stroke: a scientific statement for healthcare professionals from the American Heart Association/American Stroke Association. Stroke [Internet]. 2017;48(1). Available from: https://doi.org/10.1161/str.0000000000000114
11. Blech B, O'Carroll CB, Zhang N, Demaerschalk BM. Telestroke program participation and improvement in door-to-needle times. Telemed J E Health [Internet]. 2019 [cited 2019 Oct 2]; Available from: http://www.ncbi.nlm.nih.gov/pubmed/31287782.
12. Ray Dorsey E, Topol EJ. State of telehealth. N Engl J Med [Internet]. 2016 [cited 2019 Sep 24];375(2):154–61. Available from: https://doi.org/10.1056/nejmra1601705
13. Demaerschalk BM, Vegunta S, Vargas BB, Wu Q, Channer DD, Hentz JG. Reliability of real-time video smartphone for assessing national institutes of health stroke scale scores in acute stroke patients. Stroke [Internet] 2012;43(12):3271–7. Available from: https://doi.org/10.1161/strokeaha.112.669150
14. Al-Khathaami AM, Alshahrani SM, Kojan SM, Al-Jumah MA, Alamry AA, El-Metwally AA. Cultural acceptance of robotic telestroke medicine among patients and healthcare providers in Saudi Arabia: results of a pilot study. Neurosciences. 2015;20(1):27–30.
15. O'Carroll CB, Hentz JG, Aguilar MI, Demaerschalk BM. Robotic telepresence versus standardly supervised stroke alert team assessments. Telemed e-Health. 2015;21(3):151–6.
16. Fong WC, Ismail M, Lo JWT, Li JTC, Wong AHY, Ng YW, et al. Telephone and teleradiology-guided thrombolysis can achieve similar outcome as thrombolysis by neurologist on-site. J Stroke Cerebrovasc Dis [Internet]. 2015;24(6):1223–8. Available from: https://doi.org/10.1016/j.jstrokecerebrovasdis.2015.01.022
17. Lin CB, Peterson ED, Smith EE, Saver JL, Liang L, Xian Y, et al. Emergency medical service hospital prenotification is associated with improved evaluation and treatment of acute ischemic stroke. Circ Cardiovasc Qual Outcomes. 2012;5(4):514–22.
18. Barrett KM, Pizzi MA, Kesari V, TerKonda SP, Mauricio EA, Silvers SM, et al. Ambulance-based assessment of NIH Stroke scale with telemedicine: a feasibility pilot study. J Telemed Telecare. 2017;23(4):476–83.
19. Mathur S, Walter S, Grunwald IQ, Helwig SA, Lesmeister M, Fassbender K. Improving prehospital stroke services in rural and underserved settings with mobile stroke units. Front Neurol. 2019;10(March):1–11.
20. Lin E, Calderon V, Goins-Whitmore J, Bansal V, Zaidat O. World's First 24/7 mobile stroke unit: initial 6-month experience at Mercy Health in Toledo, Ohio. Front Neurol. 2018;9(MAY):1–8.
21. Lippman JM, Smith SNC, McMurry TL, Sutton ZG, Gunnell BS, Cote J, et al. Mobile telestroke during ambulance transport is feasible in a rural EMS setting: the iTREAT study. Telemed e-Health [Internet]. 2016;22(6):507–13. Available from: https://doi.org/10.1089/tmj.2015.0155
22. Nehme A, Deschaintre Y, Labrie M, Daneault N, Odier C, Poppe AY, et al. Cincinnati prehospital stroke scale for EMS redirection of large vessel occlusion stroke. Can J Neurol Sci [Internet]. 2019 [cited 2019 Sep 29];1–7. Available from: http://www.ncbi.nlm.nih.gov/pubmed/31303192.

23. Dickson RL, Crowe RP, Patrick C, Crocker K, Aiken M, Adams A, et al. Performance of the RACE score for the prehospital identification of large vessel occlusion Stroke in a suburban/rural EMS Service. Prehospital Emerg Care. 2019;23(5):612–8.
24. Yaghi S, Rayaz S, Bianchi N, Hall-Barrow JC, Hinduja A. Thrombolysis to stroke mimics in telestroke. J Telemed Telecare [Internet]. 2013; Available from: https://doi.org/10.1258/jtt.2012.120510
25. Geisler F, Ali SF, Ebinger M, Kunz A, Rozanski M, Waldschmidt C, et al. Evaluation of a score for the prehospital distinction between cerebrovascular disease and stroke mimic patients. Int J Stroke. 2019;14(4):400–8.
26. Khan NI, Chaku S, Goehl C, Endris L, Mueller-Luckey G, Siddiqui FM. Novel algorithm to help identify stroke mimics. J Stroke Cerebrovasc Dis [Internet]. 2018;27(3):703–8. Available from: https://doi.org/10.1016/j.jstrokecerebrovasdis.2017.09.067.
27. Stecker MM, Michel K, Antaky K, Wolin A, Koyfman F. Characteristics of the stroke alert process in a general Hospital. Surg Neurol Int. 2015;6(1)
28. Sarfo FS, Ulsavets U, Opare-Sem OK, Ovbiagele B. Tele-rehabilitation after stroke: an updated systematic review of the literature. J Stroke Cerebrovasc Dis. 2018;27(9):2306–18.
29. Morrell K, Hyers M, Stuchiner T, Lucas L, Schwartz K, Mako J, et al. Telehealth stroke dysphagia evaluation is safe and effective. Cerebrovasc Dis. 2017;44(3–4):225–31.
30. Tchero H, Tabue Teguo M, Lannuzel A, Rusch E. Telerehabilitation for stroke survivors: systematic review and meta-analysis. J Med Internet Res [Internet]. 2018 [cited 2019 Sep 29];20(10):e10867. Available from: http://www.ncbi.nlm.nih.gov/pubmed/30368437.
31. Lokken TG, Blegen RN, Hoff MD, Demaerschalk BM. Overview for implementation of telemedicine services in a large integrated multispecialty health care system. Telemed e-Health. 2020;26(4):382–7.
32. Harper K, McLeod M, Brown SK, Wilson G, Turchan M, Gittings EM, et al. Teleneurology service provided via tablet technology: 3-year outcomes and physician satisfaction. Rural Remote Health. 2019;19(1)
33. Davis LE, Coleman J, Harnar JA, King MK. Teleneurology: successful delivery of chronic neurologic care to 354 patients living remotely in a rural state. Telemed e-Health. 2014;20(5):473–7.
34. Coates S, Clarke A, Davison G, Patterson V. Tele-EEG in the UK: a report of over 1000 patients. J Telemed Telecare. 2012;18(5):243–6.
35. Adcock AK, Kosiorek H, Parich P, Chauncey A, Wu Q, Demaerschalk BM. Reliability of robotic telemedicine for assessing critically ill patients with the full outline of UnResponsiveness score and Glasgow coma scale. Telemed e-Health. 2017;23(7):555–60.
36. Girkar UM, Palacios R, Gupta A, Schwamm LH, Singla P, May H, et al. Teleneurology consultations for prognostication and brain death diagnosis. Telemed e-Health. 2020;26(4):482–6.
37. Davis LE, Harnar J, Lachey-Barbee LA, Pirio Richardson S, Fraser A, King MK. Using teleneurology to deliver chronic neurologic care to rural veterans: analysis of the first 1,100 patient visits. Telemed e-Health. 2019;25(4):274–8.
38. Schreiber SS. Teleneurology for veterans in a major metropolitan area. Telemed e-Health. 2018;24(9):698–701.
39. Larner AJ. Teleneurology: an overview of current status. Pract Neurol. 2011;11(5):283–8.
40. Wechsler LR, Tsao JW, Levine SR, Swain-Eng RJ, Adams RJ, Demaerschalk BM, et al. Teleneurology applications: report of the telemedicine work group of the American Academy of Neurology. Neurology. 2013;80(7):670–6.
41. Ke L, George S, Thomas S, Je D, Crotty M. Virtual reality for stroke rehabilitation. Virtual Real Stroke Rehabil. 2015;80(2):57–62.
42. Rosenblatt RA, Hart LG. Physicians and rural America. West J Med. 2000;173(5):348–51.
43. Pritt S, Swearingern J, Coustasse A. Telestroke: an approach to the shortage of neurologists in rural areas. 2016; Available from: http://mds.marshall.edu/mgmt_faculty.
44. Demaerschalk BM, Bobrow BJ, Raman R, Ernstrom K, Hoxworth JM, Patel AC, et al. CT interpretation in a telestroke network: agreement among a spoke radiologist, hub vascular neu-

rologist, and hub neuroradiologist. Stroke [Internet]. 2012 [cited 2019 Sep 29];43(11):3095–7. Available from: http://www.ncbi.nlm.nih.gov/pubmed/22984007.
45. Amukotuwa SA, Straka M, Smith H, Chandra RV, Dehkharghani S, Fischbein NJ, et al. Automated detection of intracranial large vessel occlusions on computed tomography angiography. Stroke. 2019;50(10):2790–8.
46. Garcia-Esperon C, Soderhjelm Dinkelspiel F, Miteff F, Gangadharan S, Wellings T, O'Brien B, et al. Implementation of multimodal computed tomography in a telestroke network: five-year experience. CNS Neurosci Ther [Internet]. 2019 [cited 2019 Oct 2];cns.13224. Available from: https://onlinelibrary.wiley.com/doi/abs/10.1111/cns.13224
47. Hassan R, Siregar JA, Azman N. The implementation of teleneurosurgery in the management of referrals to a neurosurgical department in hospital Sultanah Amninah Johor Bahru. Malaysian J Med Sci. 2014;21(2):54–62.
48. Miyachi S, Nagano Y, Hironaka T, Kawaguchi R, Ohshima T, Matsuo N, et al. Novel operation support robot with sensory-motor feedback system for neuroendovascular intervention. World Neurosurg [Internet]. 2019;127:e617–23. Available from: https://doi.org/10.1016/j.wneu.2019.03.221.
49. Bao X, Guo S, Xiao N, Li Y, Shi L. Compensatory force measurement and multimodal force feedback for remote-controlled vascular interventional robot. Biomed Microdevices. 2018;20(3)
50. Wirz R, Torres LG, Swaney PJ, Gilbert H, Alterovitz R, Webster RJ, et al. An experimental feasibility study on robotic endonasal telesurgery. Neurosurgery [Internet]. 2015 [cited 2019 Sep 29];76(4):479–84; discussion 484. Available from: http://www.ncbi.nlm.nih.gov/pubmed/25599203.
51. Demaerschalk BM, Berg J, Chong BW, Gross H, Nystrom K, Adeoye O, et al. American telemedicine association: telestroke guidelines. Telemed e-Health [Internet] 2017;23(5):376–89. Available from: https://doi.org/10.1089/tmj.2017.0006
52. Carvalho VS, Picanço MR, Volschan A, Bezerra DC. Impact of simulation training on a telestroke network. Int J Stroke. 2018;14(5):500–7.
53. Regenhardt RW, Mecca AP, Flavin SA, Boulouis G, Lauer A, Zachrison KS, et al. Delays in the air or ground transfer of patients for endovascular thrombectomy. Stroke. 2018;49(6):1419–25.
54. Wright SP, Hall Brown TS, Collier SR, Sandberg K. How consumer physical activity monitors could transform human physiology research. Am J Physiol Regul Integr Comp Physiol. 2017;312(3):R358–67.
55. Huang H, Su S, Wu N, Wan H, Wan S, Bi H, et al. Graphene-based sensors for human health monitoring. Front Chem. 2019;7(JUN):1–26.
56. Qiao Y, Li X, Hirtz T, Deng G, Wei Y-H, Li M, et al. Graphene-based wearable sensors. Nanoscale. 2019;11(41):18923–45.
57. Noorian AR, Hosseini MB, Avila G, Gerardi R, Andrle AF, Su M, et al. Use of wearable technology in remote evaluation of acute stroke patients: feasibility and reliability of a Google glass-based device. J Stroke Cerebrovasc Dis. 2019;28(10):1–4.
58. Marsh-Feiley G, Eadie L, Wilson P. Telesonography in emergency medicine: a systematic review [Internet]. Vol. 13, PLoS ONE. 2018 [cited 2019 Sep 24]. Available from: https://doi.org/10.1371/journal.pone.0194840.t001.
59. Shoirah H, Wechsler LR, Jovin TG, Jadhav AP. Acute stroke trial enrollment through a telemedicine network: a 12-year experience. J Stroke Cerebrovasc Dis [Internet]. 2019;28(7):1926–9. Available from: https://doi.org/10.1016/j.jstrokecerebrovasdis.2019.03.046.
60. Govindarajan R, Anderson ER, Hesselbrock RR, Madhavan R, Moo LR, Mowzoon N, et al. Developing an outline for teleneurology curriculum. Neurology. 2017;89(9):951–9.

Telemedicine for Prisons and Jail Population: A Solution to Increase Access to Care

26

Rifat Latifi, Kalterina Osmani, Peter Kilcommons, and Ronald S. Weinstein

Introduction

There are more than 10.35 million people held in penal institutions throughout the world [1]. The United States (U.S.) has the largest prison population in the world with almost 2.3 million prisoners; there are more than 1.65 million in China (plus an unknown number in pretrial detention or "administrative detention"); 640,000 in the Russian Federation; 607,000 in Brazil; 418,000 in India; 311,000 in Thailand; 255,000 in Mexico; and, 225,000 in Iran. The countries with the highest prison population rate (the number of prisoners per 100,000 of the national population) are Seychelles (799 per 100,000), followed by the United States (698), St. Kitts & Nevis (607), Turkmenistan (583), U.S. Virgin Islands (542), Cuba (510), El Salvador (492), U.S. Guam (469), Thailand (461), Belize (449), Russian Federation (445), Rwanda (434), and the British Virgin Islands (425) [1]. More than 20,000 people worldwide are detained on death row, where many are living in inhumane conditions and often follow unfair trials [2].

R. Latifi (✉)
Department of Surgery, New York Medical College, School of Medicine and Westchester Medical Center, Valhalla, NY, USA
e-mail: Rifat.Latifi@wmchealth.org

K. Osmani
Department of Medicine, Westchester Medical Center, Valhalla, NY, USA
e-mail: Kalterina.Osmani@wmchealth.org

P. Kilcommons
MedWeb, San Francisco, CA, USA
e-mail: pete@medweb.com

R. S. Weinstein
Arizona Telemedicine Program, The University of Arizona's College of Medicine, Tucson, AZ, USA
e-mail: rweinstein@telemedicine.arizona.edu

© Springer Nature Switzerland AG 2021
R. Latifi et al. (eds.), *Telemedicine, Telehealth and Telepresence*,
https://doi.org/10.1007/978-3-030-56917-4_26

The 2.3 million American prisoners in the criminal justice system are held in 1833 state prisons, 110 federal prisons, 1772 juvenile correctional facilities, 3134 local jails, 218 immigration detention facilities, and 80 Indian country jails, as well as in military prisons, civil commitment centers, state psychiatric hospitals, and prisons in the U.S. territories.

As of 2017, data has demonstrated that six states held at least 20% of those incarcerated under the state prison system's jurisdiction in local jail facilities: Kentucky (29%), Louisiana (55%), Mississippi (27%), Utah (22%), Tennessee (24%), and Virginia (20%). Nationally, according to the U.S. Census, Blacks are incarcerated five times (2306 per 100,000) more than Whites (450 per 100,000), followed by Hispanics (831 per 100,000). Worldwide, marginalized groups, including foreign nationals, minorities, indigenous peoples, people with disabilities, and LGBTQ (lesbian, gay, bisexual, transgender and queer or questioning) people are disproportionately arrested and imprisoned [2]. Almost 11 million people are admitted to local jails annually, and on any given day more than 730,000 people are being held, of whom almost two-thirds are awaiting trial [3]. Yet, according to one report [4], the imprisonment rate for sentenced prisoners under state or federal jurisdiction decreased 2.1% from 2016 to 2017 (from 450 to 440 sentenced prisoners per 100,000 U.S. residents), and 13% from 2007 to 2017 (from 506 to 440 per 100,000). The number of prisoners under state or federal jurisdiction decreased by 18,700 (down 1.2%), from 1,508,100 at year-end in 2016 to 1,489,400 at year-end in 2017. Overall, the federal prison population decreased by 3% from year-end 2016 to year-end 2017. Still, the sheer number of inmates in the U.S. and around the world at any given time is not known because a large number of inmates remain in the process of being sentenced, and thus are not part of the official absolute reported data.

Healthcare in the Prison System

There are a number of issues with the prison population, with the provision of healthcare services as one of the major ones. Healthcare provision to inmates is complex, expensive, it's not uniform, it is often unclear even within the U.S., and the cost is unknown [5]. An overview of government expenditures on prisons across 54 countries shows that it usually amounts to less than 0.3% of their gross domestic product (GDP). The largest expenditure from this goes to staff and infrastructure [2].

The data from the justice department shows that for 2019 the Bureau of Prisoners (BOP) [6] is a complex enterprise with a large budget of over 7 billion, 35,786 FTEs, and 36,016 positions of which 18,674 are correctional officers. This is 1.2% higher than the 2018 Annual Continuing Resolution amount. Only 11% of this budget goes toward medical services and supplies. The provision of healthcare services to an ever-increasing prison population continues to be challenging and the BOP is faced with staffing shortages [6]. Three main factors that contribute to medical staffing challenges are as follows: (1) the majority of medical school graduates do not go to primary care, (2) there is competition in salaries with sister federal agencies (i.e. Veteran Health Administration, Department of Defense, National Institutes of Health, etc.), and (3) it is difficult getting qualified staff to live in the rural locations where prisons are usually located.

Healthcare Problems and Deaths in Prison and Jail Population

Approximately 45% of prison and jail population (average age of 41 years) have multiple chronic conditions. A large number of inmates suffer from chronic diseases, and many who have serious chronic physical illnesses fail to receive appropriate care while incarcerated [7]. Even worse, among the inmates with mental illness, most are not continued on treatments once they are arrested and sentenced. Five clinically based care measures to access to healthcare services has been suggested: access to medical examinations, access to pharmacotherapy, access to prescription medication, access to laboratory tests, and adequacy of acute care [7].

Moreover, worldwide, deaths in custody are common and preventable, with a mortality rate as much as 50% higher than for people outside the prisons. The most common causes are suicide and fatal violent clashes, with other reasons being torture or ill-treatment, infectious diseases, and ill-health [2].

Between 2001 and 2014, there were 50,785 inmate deaths in housed in U.S. state and federal prisons. The number of deaths in state prison was stable between 2013 and 2014, but it increased by 11% in federal prisons. Deaths in state prisons declined in both California (down 13%) and Texas (down 7%) between 2013 and 2014. Yet, these states accounted for 20% of the state prison population and 20% of state prisoner deaths in 2014 [8]. In 2014, the prisoner death rate by state varied from no deaths per 100,000 to 631 deaths per 100,000 state prisoners. The median state-level mortality rate among prisoners was 267 per 100,000 state prisoners [9]. Illness accounted for 87% of deaths in the reported data, although it declined 2%, from 3082 to 3031 deaths, between 2013 and 2014. AIDS-related deaths increased 23% during this period, and respiratory disease deaths increased by 20%. Most concerning, the number of suicides in state prisons increased by 30% from 2013 to 2014, accounting for 7% of all deaths in state prisons in 2014, and it was the largest percentage of deaths due to suicide since 2001. At the same time, heart disease mortality rates among state prisoners continue to increase.

While prison healthcare systems are fascinating and complex, examining of the anatomy of entire prison system and the entire healthcare system intricacies of each clinical disciplines is a science in itself, it out of the scope of this chapter. The author of this chapter has had a long-standing interest in providing healthcare services to inmates, particularly surgical care that started while in training; it has become a major focus while practicing in in Richmond, Virginia, Tucson, Arizona, and Valhalla, New York.

Telemedicine for the Prisoners

Telemedicine can deliver specialty medical services to remote locations in the prison population [6] just as it does in other situations. Currently, the BOP provides health services through dedicated Wide Area Network (WAN) and is performed by large hospital vendors. This is done both to reduce cost, and more importantly, mitigate security risks associated with escorted trips to community facilities. The Federal Medical Center in Lexington contracted with the University of Kentucky Medical Center for 26 specialty telemedicine clinics. The U.S. Medical Center for Federal Prisoners has contracted with Mercy Hospital in Springfield, Missouri, for more than 30 specialty telemedicine services.

The use of telemedicine for prisoners is probably the most common-sense service. It is very costly to transport an inmate to a hospital for a visit, and it is potentially dangerous; moreover, there is no reason to expose the inmate hand-cuffed and in an orange suit to the community of the hospitals. As someone who has personally taken care of many inmates in every location that I have worked, I know firsthand that just about every preoperative and postoperative test and exam, unless we need surgical intervention, can be accomplished via telemedicine. The aim of the chapter is to review the current status, and to explore the possibilities of the use of telemedicine in prisoners, not just in the U.S., but also around the world.

For all the reasons outlined above, telemedicine for prisoners has been suggested and demonstrated to be beneficial, and it is becoming more popular. As early as 1996, there were reports of a major telemedicine program for inmates in Ohio [10]. Other examples have ensued since. But, how often is telemedicine actually used today? Over half of state correctional institutions, and 39% of federal institutions, are using some sort of telehealth or telemedicine application [11]. The most common benefits cited were improved security, personnel safety, costs savings, and access to specialists. The most common barriers cited were costs of technology, resistance from medical personnel, lack of staff technical expertise, and difficulties coordinating services.

On the other hand, in Europe the use of telemedicine is dismal. Telemedicine, as an additional healthcare delivery model, is used only in 11 out of 28 European countries, mostly members of Northern and Western Europe. Only Romania displayed having a pilot project for a nationwide program of telemedicine [12]. The most commonly used service is teleradiology (five countries have it), followed by telepsychiatry and tele-ECG, which are used by four countries. Only two countries use teledermatology, and one has teleassistance for diabetes care. Telecardiology is used in Italy [13] and done in 12 state penitentiaries situated across Apulia, a region in southeastern Italy. Of more than 2015 ECG sent over the phone, 62% showed normal findings that not requiring urgent hospitalization, and 34% showed premature contraction, sinus tachycardia or bradycardia, and permanent atrial fibrillation. Abnormal findings requiring further clinical examination out of prison were found in only 4% (ventricular tachycardia, ischemic ECG anomalies).

Building a telemedicine network only between hospitals and prisons may not be enough as serious operational problems and bureaucratic inflexibility was reported

[14]. These problems include resistance on the part of hospital personnel to the provision of support for telemedicine without additional pay; resistance from the Ministry of Health to the provision of services to prisons, because the prison medical facilities are outside its official jurisdiction; inability of the national health system to interface with the computerized record-keeping system of the Korydallos Prison telemedicine system in Greece; resistance from the prison staff to the implementation of the system (they considered it a threat to their authority, since they could no longer decide whether a particular medical complaint merited transfer of the prisoner to a hospital under guard); and, lack of support from the Ministry of Justice, who permitted lower-ranking officials to erect numerous bureaucratic obstacles to the implementation of the project.

In a study aimed to collate the current evidence related to the use of telemedicine to deliver health services within correctional setting [15], the authors found 36 articles of which 19 (53%) were published during the period of 2010–2018. Most papers were from the U.S. ($n = 23$; 64%), France, and Australia. There were 23 descriptive studies (64%), five costing studies (14%), five experimental studies (14%), two mixed methods (6%), and one qualitative study (3%). The experimental studies were predominantly focused on mental health services ($n = 4$, 80%). The commonest telemedicine intervention used was synchronous videoconferencing ($n = 21$, 58%), while eight articles (22%) described asynchronous interventions. Telemedicine interventions were mainly used for mental health ($n = 13$), and ophthalmology ($n = 4$) disciplines.

Clinical Disciplines Using Telemedicine

While telemedicine can be used for just about every clinical discipline, telepsychiatry has gained popularity [16]. These authors reviewed the literature complemented by a semi-structured interview with a telepsychiatry practitioner, searched five electronic databases, the National Bureau of Justice, the American Psychiatric Association websites, and 49 sources. In addition, they examined the implementation of telepsychiatry in correctional facilities in Arizona, California, Georgia, Kansas, Ohio, Texas, and West Virginia to determine the effect of telepsychiatry on inmate access to mental health. Most telemedicine encounters were completed (92.8%), a treatment plan was established (97.0%), the provider perceived that the technology was adequate to conduct a visit (93.4%), and a follow-up telemedicine appointment was requested (90.8%). Another study was performed in the U.S. Army's European Theater and evaluated the use of telemedicine for inmates [17]. One hundred and seventy-seven ($n = 177$) synchronous telehealth encounters were performed by physician assistant, nurse practitioner, and four physicians. Of these 177 encounters, 114 were Special Housing Unit (SHU) safety checks, and 63 encounters were for physicals, medication management, and a variety of medical complaints including acute infections, abdominal pain, musculoskeletal, and dermatological complaints. The authors found that synchronous telehealth was an effective option for the delivery of high-quality routine medical care for minor illnesses, injuries, and other nonurgent conditions, as well as for general physicals and SHU checks in a correctional facility. Acceptance by providers and clinic staff was found to be high. Inmates were generally satisfied with their telehealth encounters, although a few inmates reported a preference to see providers in-person.

Moreover, telepsychiatry helps with increasing access to mental care [18]. A study from Spain [19] found that the implementation of telemedicine in Spain in the prison settings continued to be scarce and irregular. Others [20] reported that use of psychiatry, neurology, and neurosurgery consultation provided for the two central prisons in South India. In total, 20.7% of them had a severe mental illness, that is, schizophrenia and mood disorders, 20.7% with substance use disorder (alcohol and cannabis), 17% had anxiety disorders, while 17% presented with seizure disorder. Nearly 81.1% of patients (inmates) were advised pharmacotherapy, while 18.9% were suggested further evaluation of illness and inpatient care at the higher center. There are over 80,000 incarcerated high-risk inmates in the U.S. being detained in administrative segregation housing and who may have serious problems and require psychological help. Providing psychologic care to those inmates was reported as an important service, but it has a number of challenges [21]. Telemedicine for correctional facility residents has been reported both for long-term care and for short-term emergencies as well [22]. A total of 530 emergency care records were reviewed with 126 telemedicine consultations performed. Eighty-one of 126 (64%) telemedicine patients did not require transfer to emergency department. The average total time of telemedicine consultation was 30 minutes versus a 2-hour and 45-minute turn-around time for an emergency department evaluation. Live telemedicine interaction has been reported for dermatologic diseases in Korean prisons [23]. Of 406 patients studied, the majority (91.4%) were male, and in 43% infectious disease was the most common type of disease, followed by eczematous disease (29.4%), and diseases of the skin appendages (14.5%). Among the 187 (38.2%) patients who had a follow-up consultation, 162 (86.7%) showed clinical improvement, whereas 21 showed either no change or a worse clinical outcome. The majority (n 1/4254, 62.6%) of patients required a consultation only once, while the remainder (n 1/4152, 37.4%) had two or more consultations.

In another study evaluating the effectiveness, efficiency, and safety of telemedicine for urological care in the male prisoner population [24], the authors found safe and effective methods to provide general urologic care that obviated the initial in-person visits in nearly 90% of patients. The effectiveness of telemedicine was assessed by the following: (1) the concordance of TM and in-person diagnoses; (2) compliance with radiologic and medication orders; and (3) in-person visits saved with telemedicine consultation. Safety, on the other hand, was assessed by analyzing the number of patients in which an emergency department visit was required after a telemedicine visit, and missed or delayed cases of malignancy. Telemedicine has been successfully used in increased testing, diagnosis, and treatment of Hepatis C virus (HCV) in this high-prevalence population [25]. Use of telemedicine to monitor HIV has provided up-to-date, evidence-based human immunodeficiency virus (HIV) management, improved compliance, greater virologic suppression with medication, improved CD4 T-cell counts, fewer adverse drug interactions, and decreased transmission in the community [26]. Furthermore, it has become more demanding, it is efficient (avoids transfers and is decisive), and has a high acceptance among all users [27]. Moreover, telemedicine was used in the HIV population nearing release from an incarcerated state to connect to HIV care post release [28] and was positively received by inmates and case management agencies in the community in Louisiana. Telemedicine has been used for telementoring inmates with, and for, HCV [29] and was reported as an effective method to facilitate eligible prescriber status to medical doctors and upskill other clinicians in correctional facilities to increase the capacity to treat HCV.

Inmate satisfaction with telemedicine was also assessed [30]. Of the 299 inmates surveyed immediately after their teleconsultations, only 9% of 221 who completed questionnaires expressed dissatisfaction with telemedicine. In a study that evaluated provider satisfaction and patient outcomes associated with telemedicine [31], most providers were satisfied with telemedicine for the visit overall (87.0%), they believed that telemedicine improved patient prognosis (88.2%), and perceived that the patient was satisfied (83.0%). In this study, there were 737 patient visits, 92.9% were seen for either infectious disease or mental health (46.2% and 50.2%).

COVID-19 and Prison and Jail System Healthcare

COVID-19 represents the most difficult problem to deal with in prisons and jails that require a major transformation of the system overall, but most importantly ensures timely and proper testing, social distancing, and medical care of this high-risk population [32]. The first case of novel coronavirus 2019 (COVID-19) was diagnosed at Riker's Island, the main jail complex in New York City in mid-March, but within 2 weeks there were 200 more cases. The situation in other jails and prisons is the same; the Cook County jail in Chicago is experiencing the same situation as in early April there were 350 incarcerated persons and staff members that tested positive [33, 34].

On February 20, 2020, there were an estimated 500 new COVID-19 cases in prisons in China, but the data are not available at this time. Due to many factors [35–37], there are significant challenges with the provision of healthcare services even without pandemics like this one. This pandemic, however, adds significant difficulties that have to do with the nature of incarceration, which de facto is the most serious form of quarantine, and potentially social distance. Yet, overcrowded jails and prisons cannot afford such a luxury of social distancing. Chances are that the prison system will continue to fail prisoners now during this pandemic and in the future [38].

Most recently, in an article that outlines the disproportional burden of COVID-19 among immigrants, authors mention the use of virtual visits, but they did not give any further data on frequency, usefulness, or outcomes [39]. Moreover, another paper describing early COVID-19 in jails and prisons of the U.S. does not mention telemedicine at all as one of the methods to mitigate the pandemic [33].

Conclusion

Telemedicine is invaluable for increasing access to the care of prisoners; it can, and should be, implemented worldwide. It is more humane, cost-effective, safer, and can be used for every aspect of clinical care. The current COVID-19 pandemic should further increase the use of telemedicine in the jail and prison population of 2.3 million.

References

1. Walmsley R. World prison population list 11th ed. London: International Center for Prison Studies (ICPS); 2015. https://www.prisonstudies.org/sites/default/files/resources/downloads/world_prison_population_list_11th_edition_0.pdf. Accessed 9 May 2020.
2. Global Prison Trends 2020. London, England; Renal Reform International; 2020. https://cdn.penalreform.org/wp-content/uploads/2020/04/Global-Prison-Trends-2020-Penal-Reform-International.pdf
3. Alston P. Contempt for the poor in US drives cruel policies, says UN expert. OHCHR. https://www.ohchr.org/EN/NewsEvents/Pages/DisplayNews.aspx?NewsID=23172&LangID=E. Accessed 7 May 2020. Published June 4, 2018.
4. Bronson J, Carson AC. Prisoners in 2017. Bureau of Justice Statistics (BJS). https://www.bjs.gov/content/pub/pdf/p17.pdf. Published April 25, 2019. Accessed 6 May 2020.
5. Sridhar S, Cornish R, Fazel S. The costs of healthcare in prison and custody: systematic review of current estimates and proposed guidelines for future reporting. Front Psych. 2018;9:716. https://doi.org/10.3389/fpsyt.2018.00716.
6. FY 2019 Performance budget congressional submission salaries and expenses. The United States Department of Justice Federal Bureau of Prisons. https://www.justice.gov/jmd/page/file/1034421/download. Published 2019.
7. Wilper AP, Woolhandler S, Boyd JW, et al. The health and health car of US prisoners: results of a nationwide survey. Am J Public Health. 2009;99(4):666–72. https://doi.org/10.2105/AJPH.2008.144279.
8. Carson EA, Mulako-Wangato J. Count of total custody population (including private prisons. *Corrections Statistical Analysis Tool- Prisoners.* Bureau of Justice Statistics. Cited by: Noonan ME. Mortality in state prisons, 2001–2014-statistical tables. Bureau of Justice Statistics. https://www.bjs.gov/content/pub/pdf/msp0114st.pdf. Published December 2016.
9. Noonan ME. Mortality in state prisons, 2001–2014-statistical tables. Bureau of Justice Statistics. https://www.bjs.gov/content/pub/pdf/msp0114st.pdf. Published December 2016.
10. Mekhjian H, Warisse J, Gailiun M, et al. An Ohio telemedicine system for prison inmates: a case report. Telemed J. 1996;2(1):17–24. https://doi.org/10.1089/tmj.1.1996.2.17.
11. Larsen D, Stamm BH, Davis K, et al. Prison telemedicine and telehealth utilization in the United States: state and federal perceptions of benefits and barriers. Telemed J E Health. 2004;(10 Suppl):2.
12. Edge C, George J, Black G, et al. Using telemedicine to improve access, cost and quality of secondary care for people in prison in England: a hybrid type 2 implementation effectiveness study. BMJ Open. 2020;10(2):e035837. https://doi.org/10.1136/bmjopen-2019-035837.
13. Brunetti ND, Dellegrottaglie G, Di Giuseppe G, et al. Prison break: remote tele-cardiology support for cardiology emergency in Italian penitentiaries. Int J Cardiol. 2013;168(3):3138–40. https://doi.org/10.1016/j.ijcard.2013.04.022.
14. Anogeianaki A, Anogianakis G, Ilonidis G, et al. The Korydallos, Greece, prisons telemedicine system experience: why technology alone is not a sufficient condition. Stud Health Technol Inform. 2004;98:16–8.

15. Senanayake B, Wickramasinghe SI, Eriksson L, et al. Telemedicine in the correctional setting: a scoping review. J Telemed Telecare. 2018;24(10):669–75. https://doi.org/10.1177/1357633X18800858.
16. Deslich SA, Thistlethwaite T, Coustasse A. Telepsychiatry in correctional facilities: using technology to improve access and decrease costs of mental health care in underserved populations. Perm J. 2013;17(3):80–6. https://doi.org/10.7812/TPP/12-123.
17. Swift C, Cain SM, Needham M. A primary care telehealth experience in a US Army correctional facility in Germany. US Army Med Dep J. 2016:76–80.
18. Kaftarian E. Lessons learned in prison and jail-based telepsychiatry. Curr Psychiatry Rep. 2019;21(3):15. https://doi.org/10.1007/s11920-019-1004-5.
19. Mateo M, Alvarez R, Cobo C, et al. Telemedicine: contributions, difficulties and key factors for implementation in the prison setting. Rev Esp Sanid Penit. 2019;21(2):95–105.
20. Agarwal PP, Manjunatha N, Gowda GS, et al. Collaborative tele-neuropsychiatry consultation services for patients in central prisons. J Neurosci Rural Pract. 2019;10(1):101–5. https://doi.org/10.4103/jnrp.jnrp_215_18.
21. Batastina A, Morgan RD. Connecting the disconnected: preliminary results and lessons learned from a telepsychology initiative with special management inmates. Psychol Serv. 2016;13(3):283–91. https://doi.org/10.1037/ser0000078.
22. Ellis DG, Mayrose J, Jehle DV, et al. A telemedicine model for emergency care in short-term correctional facility. Telemed J E Health. 2001;7(2):87–92. https://doi.org/10.1089/153056201750279584.
23. Seol JE, Park SH, Kim H. Analysis of live interactive teledermatologic consultations for prisoners in Korea for 3 years. J Telemed Telecare. 2018;24(9):623–8. https://doi.org/10.1177/1357633X17732095.
24. Sherwood BG, Han Y, Nepple KG, et al. Evaluating the effectiveness, efficiency and safety of telemedicine for urological care in the male prisoner population. Urol Pract. 2018;5(1):44–51. https://doi.org/10.1016/j.urpr.2017.01.011.
25. Morey S, Hamoodi A, Jones D, et al. Increased diagnosis and treatment of hepatitis C in prison by universal offer of testing and use of telemedicine. J Viral Hepat. 2019;26(1):101–8. https://doi.org/10.1111/jvh.13017.
26. Young JD, Patel M. HIV subspecialty care in correctional facilities using telemedicine. J Correct Health Care. 2015;21(2):177–85. https://doi.org/10.1177/1078345815572863.
27. Blanco Portillo A, Palacios Garcia-Cervigon G, Perez Figueras M, et al. Telemedicina, centros penitenciarios y enfermedad po VIH [Telemedicine, prison and illness associated with HIV]. Rev Esp Quimioter. 2019;32(6):539–44.
28. Brantley AD, Page KM, Zack B, et al. Making the connection: using videoconferencing to increase linkage to care for incarcerated persons living with HIV post-release. AIDS Behav. 2019;23(Suppl 1):32–40. https://doi.org/10.1007/s10461-018-2115-4.
29. Neuhaus M, Langbecker D, Caffery LJ, et al. Telementoring for hepatitis C treatment in correctional facilities. J Telemed Telecare. 2018;24(10):690–6. https://doi.org/10.1177/1357633X18795361.
30. Mekhjian H, Turner JW, Gailiun M, et al. Patient satisfaction with telemedicine in a prison environment. J Telemed Telecare. 1999;5(1):55–61. https://doi.org/10.1258/1357633991932397.
31. Glaser M, Winchell T, Plant P, et al. Provider satisfaction and patient outcomes associated with a statewide prison telemedicine program in Louisiana. Telemed J E Health. 2010;16(4):472–9. https://doi.org/10.1089/tmj.2009.0169.
32. Akiyama MJ, Spaulding AC, Rich JD. Flattening the curve for incarcerated populations-Covid-19 in jails and prisons. N Engl J Med. 2020;382(22):2075–7. https://doi.org/10.1056/NEJMp2005687.
33. Hawks L, Woolhandler S, McCormick D. COVID-19 in prisons and jails in the United States. JAMA Intern Med. 2020;28 https://doi.org/10.1001/jamainternmed.2020.1856.
34. Yang H, Thompson JR. Fighting Covid-19 outbreaks in prisons. BMJ. 2020;369:m1362. https://doi.org/10.1136/bmj.m.1362.

35. Maruschak LM, Berzofsky M, Unangst J. Medical problems of state and federal prisoner and jail inmates, 2011–12. Bureau of Justice Statistics (BJS). https://www.bjs.gov/content/pub/pdf/mpsfpji1112.pdf. Accessed 9 May 2020. Published February 2015.
36. Andrews J. The current state of public and private prison healthcare. Peen Wharton: Public Policy Initiative. https://publicpolicy.wharton.upenn.edu/live/news/1736-the-current-state-of-public-and-private-prison/for-students/blog/news.php#_edn21. Accessed 9 May 2020. Published 2017.
37. Trusts PC. Prison health care: costs and quality. https://www.pewtrusts.org/-/media/assets/2017/10/sfh_prison_health_care_costs_and_quality_final.pdf?la=en&hash=C3120E4248708AB27435866F5EEC12AE24F63DFE. Accessed 9 May 2020. Published 8, 2017.
38. Armstrong S. The prison service is still failing inmates/ healthcare needs. BMJ. 2020;368:m724. https://doi.org/10.1136/bmj.m724.
39. Ross J, Diaz CM, Starrels JL. The disproportionate burden of COVID-19 for immigrants in Bronx, New York. JAMA Intern Med. 2020; https://doi.org/10.1001/jamainternmed.2020.2131.

Part IV

The Next Generation of Telemedicine and Telepresence

Surgical Telementoring and Teleproctoring

27

Rifat Latifi, Xiang Da Dong, Ziad Abouezzi, Ashutosh Kaul, Akia Caine, Roberto Bergamaschi, Aram Rojas, Igor A. Laskowski, Donna C. Koo, Tracey L. Weigel, Kaveh Alizadeh, Nikhil Gopal, Akhil Saji, Ashley Dixon, Bertie Zhang, John Phillips, Jared B. Cooper, and Chirag D. Gandhi

> "Bringing people together by rapid and abridged means is true progress," said Ferdinand Lesseps (1805–1894) of the first successful Transatlantic Telegraphic Cable, "because it allows us to … help each other achieve a better and happier life"
> F Lesseps, Address, 1868. In: *Proceedings at the Banquet Held in Honor of Cyrus W Field*, Metchem & Sons, London, pp. 52–53).

Introduction

Technological advances and surgical ingenuity have made possible to integrate new and innovative surgical intervention. Telementoring and teleproctoring has been evolving over the last decade following the introduction of laparoscopic and robotic

---

R. Latifi (✉) · X. Da Dong · Z. Abouezzi · A. Kaul · A. Caine · R. Bergamaschi · A. Rojas
I. A. Laskowski · D. C. Koo · T. L. Weigel · K. Alizadeh
Department of Surgery, Westchester Medical Center, Valhalla, NY, USA

New York Medical College, School of Medicine, Valhalla, NY, USA
e-mail: Rifat.Latifi@wmchealth.org; xiang.dong@wmchealth.org; Ziad.Abouezzi@wmchealth.org; Ashutosh.Kaul@wmchealth.org; igor.laskowski@wmchealth.org; Tracey.Weigel@wmchealth.org; Kaveh.alizadeh@wmchealth.org

N. Gopal · A. Saji · A. Dixon · B. Zhang · J. Phillips
New York Medical College, School of Medicine, Valhalla, NY, USA

Department of Urology, Westchester Medical Center, Valhalla, NY, USA
e-mail: nikhil.gopal@wmchealth.org; bzhang@student.nymc.edu; phillipsj@wmchealth.org

J. B. Cooper · C. D. Gandhi
New York Medical College, School of Medicine, Valhalla, NY, USA

Department of Neurosurgery, Westchester Medical Center, Valhalla, NY, USA
e-mail: jared.cooper@wmchealth.org; chirag.gandhi@wmchealth.org

© Springer Nature Switzerland AG 2021
R. Latifi et al. (eds.), *Telemedicine, Telehealth and Telepresence*,
https://doi.org/10.1007/978-3-030-56917-4_27

surgery. Early studies have shown it to be a safe addition to traditional methods of teaching and brings surgical expertise to areas of need [1–5]. With wider adaptation of robotic surgery to perform mainstream operations in general surgery, thoracic, urology, gynecological, orthopedic, and other surgical disciplines, the role of telementoring has evolved further. Furthermore, with the widespread of Internet and increased bandwidth allows the mentor and mentee to perform complex cases while having discussion over minute details without disrupting surgical procedures. This has led to the ability to safely perform complex operations over great distances. Previous studies have demonstrated no difference in knowledge and skill acquisition with the use of telementoring compared with onsite traditional mentoring approaches [6, 7].

The Defense Advanced Research Agency (DARPA) and National Aeronautics and Space Administration (NASA) have been at the lead of these processes [8–10]. These efforts have been a key element to the development of telementoring and teleproctoring [10] and integrating telemedicine in the operating room [11–13].

Surgical telementoring and teleproctoring have become acceptable terms, that often are used interchangeably, but they are different. Teleproctoring refers to the supervision of an examination from a distance using telecommunication technology, whereas telementoring is remote guidance or teaching [14].

A remote telemanipulation of any device can be done synchronously (live or real time) or asynchronously (store and forward) based on the application [15, 16]. This type of function is the basis of surgical robotics like the da Vinci system, which is basically a telemanipulation system, a platform for surgical proctoring and mentorship. In September 2001, Professor Jacques Marescaux, who was in New York City, utilized a Zeus robotic system to perform a cholecystectomy on a patient in Strasbourg, France. This event, known as "Operation Lindbergh" was reported widely [16–19]. Mehran Anvari reported a series of surgical procedures between Hamilton and North Bay [20]. Supported by NASA Ronald Merrell explored and develop i-telemedicine testbeds in the jungles of Ecuador and Mt. Everest Base Camp [21, 22]. Others follow suit with research projects that validated the ability to remotely operate a surgical system in an isolated and extreme environment [23–25].

Telementoring and teleproctoring technology can be utilized in many ways. Its most common application being the mentoring of surgeons in new techniques to get them safely past their learning curve. This holds true for new surgeons fresh from residency or fellowship as well as seasoned surgeons introducing new procedures into their armamentarium. For established surgeons looking to incorporate robotic surgery into their practice, most hospitals require a number of proctored cases among a number of other requirements for credentialing. At smaller hospitals this often means a surgeon outside of the physician's specialty is proctoring their cases. Use of telementoring technology would allow for someone with expertise and knowledge of the procedures and diseases being treated to proctor giving an assessment of the surgeon's proficiency, which may ultimately affect patient safety. In the following pages we will examine the utility of telementoring in a number of surgical disciplines.

Telementoring in Oncologic and Hepato-Pancreatico-Biliary (HPB) Surgery

Early adopters of laparoscopy saw the potential for telementoring and started disseminating the knowledge to underserved nations through telementoring. Proof of principle using animal models showed that satisfaction among trainees was high even with a telementoring system [26–33]. Rosser et al. demonstrated the feasibility of telementoring over great distances from the United States to Ecuador for performance of a laparoscopic cholecystectomy in 1999 [21].

Following the development of robotic systems for surgery, a new era in surgical approaches came into being [34, 35]. As mentioned above, remote robotic cholecystectomy, which was first performed in 2001, established the feasibility of robotic telesurgery. Conversely, this also demonstrated the feasibility of robotic teleproctoring without the mentor being physically present onsite. The availability of dual teaching or assisting console, have made possible to have mentors assist mentees with surgical interventions has progressed and is no longer encumbered by inability to provide direct assistance as in laparoscopic mentoring. Therefore, complex surgical oncology cases can also be performed with mentor instructions through remote telementoring and teleproctoring and no longer requires the two surgeons to be in close proximity to perform complex cases.

In addition, during performance of laparo-robotic surgeries, the option of augmented reality can enhance and improve the mentor guidance of the surgical trainees. Vera et al. evaluated an augmented reality platform for assessing its utility in laparoscopic skills [36, 37]. With this technology, trainees learned the skill sets faster than traditional mentoring with similar error rates [36]. However, studies that evaluated telementoring are limited. Typically, they are observational in nature and have low number of cases or mentor–mentees and most all of them are industry supported. In a recent review by Erridge et al., about 74% of the papers reviewed demonstrated only level IV evidence [1]. Similar conclusions were arrived at by the panel convened by Society of American Gastrointestinal Endoscopic Surgeons (SAGES) in 2017 [38]. Comparison of telementoring and onsite training found that the two approaches to offer similar clinical outcomes for the patients, although there are still lingering concerns as evaluations by trainees indicated that even with dual console usage, immediate availability of the mentor can provide demonstrations of hand movements when they are in close proximity [39–41].

Telementoring and Teleproctoring in Bariatric Surgery

Traditionally, metabolic and bariatric surgeons, as in most other surgical disciplines learn of new techniques and technologies either during their training or from peers at national conferences like those sponsored by the Society of American Gastrointestinal and Endoscopic Surgeons (SAGES) and the American Society for Metabolic and Bariatric Surgery (ASMBS), among others. They then return home and attempt to incorporate what they have learned into their practice, at times potentially sacrificing patient safety in the name of innovation [42].

For surgeons traveling to mentor and proctor, there are drawbacks of the costs of travel and time taken away from their own practices. There are also regulatory hoops to jump through to be physically present in the operating room of a different hospital [43].

There is a paucity of published research of telementoring in metabolic and bariatric surgery. However, given the significant improvements and readily available telecommunications technology, remote mentoring has been proposed to mitigate some of the difficulties of performing live, in-person mentoring. SAGES defines telementoring as a "relationship, facilitated by telecommunication technology, in which an expert (Mentor) provides guidance to a less experienced learner (Mentee) from a remote location." [43] Telementoring allows practicing surgeons to receive real-time instruction and feedback without the disadvantages of time spent on travel and to perform a number of complex procedure, [44] but there must be adequate preparation beforehand by both parties engaging in the telementoring experience in order to master established procedures. Fuertes-Guiró et al. reported on a series of 36 patients who underwent laparoscopic bariatric surgery between March 2013 and March 2014, in 20 of which telementoring was utilized [45]. The surgeons at the three hospitals had established relationships with one another through prior joint clinical and operative sessions. The surgeons at the community hospitals had completed less than 50 laparoscopic bariatric cases compared to the university surgeons experience of over 400 cases. Mentored operations took a statistically significant shorter amount of time than non-mentored operations. In this study, patients' postoperative clinical course was also telementored. Patients of telementored cases had a shorter length of stay by 2 hospital days, which was also statistically significant. Three patients from the non-mentored group suffered minor complications compared to none in the mentored group [45].

In 2018, Nguyen et al. published results of collaborative quality improvement project targeted at sleeve gastrectomy [42]. This 4-year project linked mentor bariatric surgeons who have performed at least 75 sleeve gastrectomies with minimally invasive surgery fellow mentees. Participants were affiliated with six hospitals across the United States and South America, although within the US, mentors and mentees from the same state were paired together for medical licensing reasons. None of the hospitals involved required any additional credentialing or malpractice insurance for telementoring activities. Informed consent for telementoring was obtained by the operating surgeon [42].

The Karl Storz VISITOR 1® telementoring platform used mobile technology allowed the mentoring surgeon to view the operating room or the laparoscopic video image, and to telestrate or illustrate on the laparoscopic screen.

In this study, 15 mentees were able to complete the telementoring process. During this process, some logistical and technological limitations were discovered, but there were no reported intraoperative or postoperative complications, and 93% of mentees reported that the experience "exceeded expectations." None of the mentors were dissatisfied with the mentoring experience or the visual or sound quality. The authors concluded that telementoring for laparoscopic sleeve gastrectomy was feasible and valuable to surgeons [42].

The Michigan Bariatric Surgical Collaborative (MBSC), a statewide quality improvement initiative, introduced a peer coaching program in 2015. Coaches were chosen among the top 15 performing surgeons in the state and they were trained to perform coaching sessions based on video review of recorded operative cases of the other less performing surgeons in the state. These sessions took place at quarterly meetings of the MBSC [46].

Another important aspect of telementoring and teleproctoring is to extend autonomy in the operating room to surgical residents and fellows in training. These trainees can have the experience of operating on their own safely while their overseeing attending is watching their every move. Utilizing telementoring in this way can possibly increase trainee satisfaction without sacrificing patient safety. There are more applications in resident education. Altieri et al. utilized the telementoring format to teach residents the SAGES Fundamental Use of Surgical Energy (FUSE) program and directly compared it to in-person mentoring in a multi-institutional randomized controlled trial. Sixty-five surgical trainees from three institutions participated in a FUSE simulation curriculum either with in person ($n = 30$) or remote ($n = 35$) proctoring. They found that both groups had similar and improved examination scores [47].

Rarely addressed in the literature is the role telementoring can play in global health. It can be used to bridge the growing disparities and behavior modification in surgical care in rural areas of the United States and worldwide [48]. Telementoring can now extend to patients and has been shown to result in improved weight loss outcomes and positive behavior change [49, 50].

Low-Tech Examples of Telementoring and Teleproctoring in Plastic Surgery

With increasing access to healthcare even in the most remote areas of the world, there has been a focus to "teach how to fish" which has led to telementoring innovations in surgery. While most plastic surgery, similar to other clinical disciplines, when in a surgical volunteer mission, training of residents and other trainees is done in person, due to safety and security of members of the mission [51]. Training mission was changed telementoring via video conferencing. Various technologies are used such as Skype that allowed us live simultaneous interviews with the doctor and patient [52]. This is effective for semi-elective cases when a didactic dialogue with the local doctors about the best treatment options. With advances in mobile telephony, smartphones have become a primary tool for telementoring in many parts of the world, but studies are still missing. Telepresence via phones during intraoperative consultations can provide live and meaningful guidance and often significantly affect the outcomes of such managements.

Since 2016, we have embraced a new phase in our approach to telementoring which places greater emphasis on broad engagement over broadband. A surgeon network based in sub-Saharan Africa, of over 100 physicians from 15 countries, increasingly relies on WhatsApp as main source of telementoring. This easy application is available to all countries and all on phone formats and is functional with minimal bandwidth. Many doctors have used this platform to ask for recommendation letters, seek information about scholarships, and showcase their successful operations, or ask difficult questions about patient complications and management. Other advantages include message encryption during transmission; allows four-way live video conferencing, and allows topics to be searched on the chat group via a simple function. Just as in the past, telemedicine was used to serve geographically remote areas [53, 54], mobile telephones and other devices can be used to provide both clinical care and telementoring.

Telementoring and Teleproctoring in Colorectal Surgery

The advent of laparoscopic surgery in the 1990s certainly represented a unique opportunity for telementoring. In fact, Rosser et al. published in 1997 a prospective study in telementoring laparoscopic colon resections, which concluded that there was no difference in the performances of the surgeons as well as in the outcomes of the operations when mentoring was carried out with physical presence in the operating room or remotely [7]. Unlike the case of laparoscopic general surgery, the implementation of laparoscopic colorectal surgery has been slow and fought with technical difficulties [55]. A three-phase model for longitudinal mentoring of laparoscopic colon resection for cancer between an academic institution and community hospitals was reported [56]. A 2013 review of clinical outcomes of telementoring identified 33 telementored operations to have been documented in the literature including colorectal surgery among 11 subspecialties [57]. Although on-site mentoring remains the standard, the option of telementoring may address a number of challenges such as the discrepancy between number of experts and number of surgeons requiring mentoring, the time and resources involved in providing on-site mentoring in remote locations, and the current COVID-19 (Coronavirus Disease 2019) pandemic [58].

The feedback from mentees involved in telementored operations at community hospitals has been enthusiastic due to increased understanding of operating room setup, patient positioning, appropriate instrumentation, trocar placement, and chronological sequentiality of surgical steps overall resulting in improved confidence [59]. In addition to increasing access to care in remote areas, telemedicine has also improved the ability to request and provide guidance from colleagues during training and surgical cases [60–63].

Telemedicine in Thoracic Surgery

The development of the da Vinci robotic platform, especially the fourth generation, da Vinci Xi, have allowed many thoracic surgeons to increasingly and rapidly incorporate robotic-assisted surgery into their daily practice as they transition from open to minimally invasive robotic thoracic surgery, often bypassing altogether the technically more challenging video-assisted thoracoscopic (VATS) procedures such as

VATS lobectomy or thymectomy. Robotic-assisted thoracoscopic (RATS) lobectomy has been associated with a decrease in length of stay, blood loss, and conversion to open thoracotomy as compared to VATS lobectomy [64].

In the last decade, with the introduction of the da Vinci Xi four-arm robotic platform, the specialty of thoracic surgery has been one of the fastest adopters of robotics greatly expanding the percentage of thoracic surgeries being performed with minimally invasive laparoscopic and thoracoscopic techniques [65]. Historically, this technology transfer and adoption has predominantly been facilitated through on-site case observation or proctoring, perhaps slowing this adoption of robotics due to the time, issues with individual host hospitals licensing and malpractice requirements, and the cost burden associated with travel of the mentor or mentee. The Society of the American Gastrointestinal and Endoscopic Surgeons (SAGES) has established clear guidelines on teleproctoring [43].

As video-communication technology continued to develop, further advances were also made in the sphere of telementoring. In 2014, Ponsky et al. reported series of video-assisted thoracoscopic lower lobectomy performed by surgeons under the telementoring guidance of pediatric surgeon mentors [66]. Subsequently, usage of the VisitOR1™ robot for telementoring in thoracic cases was reported by Bruns et al. in 2016, in which telementoring allowed two telementors in the US to guide surgical telementees in France to perform a thoracoscopic total thymectomy [67]. Both reports indicate successful completion of the attempted procedures without loss of connection. The telestration and laser pointer features of the VisitOR1™ platform was noted to be especially useful in facilitating telementoring [66, 67].

There has been a rapid increase in the adoption of robotic-assisted thoracoscopic surgery (RATS) by thoracic surgeons due to multiple series and the large body of data now showing improved outcomes such as decrease in postoperative complications and length of stay (LOS) with RATS lobectomies versus VATS or open (thoracotomy) lobectomies for stage I Non-Small Cell Lung Cancer [68]. Questions about the feasibility of robotic telementoring and telesurgery have long interested surgeons [69]. To date, however, a paucity of reports of thoracic robotic telementoring appear in the literature. Pioneers in the field, such as Robert J. Cerfolio, have published their individual nonrandomized case series of anatomic pulmonary lobectomies and segmentectomies in an attempt to share their techniques and help others learn from their experiences [70].

Telementoring and Teleproctoring in Vascular Surgery

Classical telementoring and proctoring can be used in variety of situations [71, 72]. Endovascular surgeries, on the other hand, lends itself especially well to telementoring since these procedures almost always take places with application of live video feeds performed in endovascular suites or hybrid operating rooms that are equipped with sophisticated video feedbacks capabilities. The application of telemedicine mentoring in endovascular interventions for abdominal endovascular aneurysm repair (EVAR) was first described in 1999 by Deaton et al. [73] Another example of great application of teleproctoring in vascular surgery was establishing an EVAR program to serve patients located in a remote Swiss Canton of Ticino and separated by the Alps from specialized medical centers [74]. In addition, the authors conducted a follow-up study prospectively comparing the telementored cohort to the subsequent 86 patients who underwent EVAR from 2003 to 2013 [75].

Analysis of both groups revealed no difference in perioperative mortality and primary technical success rate. In the recent study Lin et al., evaluated hybrid operating room integration using existing hospital network for live streaming of surgical procedur [76] and suggested potential cost savings on top of clear education and expert surgical telementoring advantages.

In 2019, Society for Vascular Surgery established a Mentor Match Program was established to provide resources to medical students, general surgery residents, and younger Society for Vascular Surgery (SVS) members interested in learning more about all aspect of career in vascular surgery [77]. Vascular and Endovascular Surgery Society similarly offers a mentoring program to surgery resident in their last year of training and all members within first 10 years of practice [78]. Although not via telementoring these programs provide potential for easy transition to telemedicine-based applications.

Telementoring in Urology

Ever since Ferdinand Lesseps (1805–1894) said *"Bringing people together by rapid and abridged means is true progress, because it allows us to … help each other achieve a better and happier life"* on the occasion of the first successful Transatlantic Telegraphic Cable [79], humans searched for better way of communicating. The procedure generally regarded as the first true telesurgical experience in urology did not involve a robot but a transrectal ultrasound (TRUS) device in prostate biopsy. TRUS biopsy of the prostate is a cheap, reproducible, and safe bedside procedure but is dependent on the quality and experience of the practitioner. Rovetta et al. envisioned a remote expert controlling and/or training on-site practitioners TRUS biopsy via digital control of the TRUS device itself [80]. In the well-publicized and proof-of-principle 1995 event, a Sankyo SCARA robot (Adept Technology, Inc., Pleasanton, CA) enabled the manual handling of the TRUS device positioned in the patient rectum by the on-site practitioner. There were no complications and biopsies were successfully "guided" demonstrating feasibility despite prohibitive costs and applicability. Credit for the first true telesurgical operation is given to Jacques Marescaux et al. who used a Zeus (Computer Motion Inc., USA)-type marginal manipulator robot to perform a cholecystectomy in Strasbourg, France, from New York, NY. The 2001 procedure, famously dubbed the "Charles Lindbergh operation," required the surgeon to obtain consent from the patient in Europe before flying to New York to perform the surgery on the Zeus device. The mean total delay time was just 155 minutes and a total dissection time of 54 minutes [17]. The following year, surgeons had the opportunity to compare robotic versus manual placement of needles into a $2.5 \times 3 \times 4$ cm silicone renal model of percutaneous stone surgery in 10 possible calyces [81]. That same year, da Vinci telerobotics were used to demonstrate the safe and feasible application of the technique. Surgeons in Cincinnati, Ohio (2400 miles) and Denver, Colorado (1300 miles) performed four nephrectomies in pigs located in Sunnyvale, California. Using only public Internet cable speeds of 2.6–5.3 MB/sec, visibility during the cases was either good or intermittently poor [82]. The development of the da Vinci robot was initially met with skepticism due to its high cost, inability to demonstrate superiority over standard laparoscopic techniques, and lack of benefit for military battlefield use. In the late 1990s, urologic procedures being performed with regularity and increasing interest were laparoscopic donor, partial, and radical nephrectomy, adrenalectomy, pyeloplasty, and lymph node dissection [83–85]. All demonstrated superior short-term outcomes compared to their open counterparts in terms of hospital stay, pain scores, cosmesis, and patient satisfaction. The same was not necessarily true for radical prostatectomy [86]. The small confines of the pelvis, the difficulty of straight laparoscopic suturing, and surgeon posture were among the variables that relegated laparoscopic retropubic prostatectomy to a small handful of surgeons dotting the globe and was never universally accepted [87]. By 1999, Guillineau et al., having acquired expertise with laparoscopic suturing and pelvic reconstruction in gynecologic suspension procedures, re-examined laparoscopic prostatectomy from a posterior and anterior approach [88, 89]. The different technique revolutionized laparoscopic urologic approaches to the prostate but still could not overcome difficulties of surgeon posture and suture placement of a narrow, confined space of the male pelvis. The da Vinci platform, which enables three-dimensional visualization and ease of suture manipulation, was first used for radical prostatectomy by Binder et al., in 2000 [90]. Within a few years, robotic prostatectomy, also referred to as "telepresence" laparoscopic prostatectomy, had gained worldwide appeal because it placed a formerly unfeasible laparoscopic procedure into the hands of mortals. The da Vinci prostatectomy was a paradigm shift in not only prostate cancer surgery but almost all of urology [91–94]. Modern advances in the surgery of the kidney, prostate, and bladder, now envisioned improvements that would not have been feasible during the "open" era. For prostatectomy, great debate exists in the optimization of nonthermal nerve sparing prostatectomy, single-port surgery, and the anatomic nuances that were really appreciated before the visualization of robotics made them easily appreciated [95]. For partial nephrectomy, in which warm ischemia of the cross-clamped kidney may play a role, robotic surgery has increased the awareness and feasibility of nephron sparing surgery as a standard of care for the small renal mass (SRM). For muscle invasive bladder cancers, robotic surgery may play a significant role in minimizing the morbidity of the abdominal wound though still limited by the delays in recovery required of bowel surgery for urinary diversion [96, 97]. Despite the benefit of three-dimensional imaging, range of wrist motion, and surgeon comfort, considerable obstacles remain to da Vinci robotic surgery including cost, economic viability, and learning curve. The majority of large outcome series report that the learning curve to achieve maximal surgical results may be >40 cases for partial nephrectomy and >100 cases for robotic prostatectomy [98, 99]. The combination of telepresence, telestration, and a potentially unlimited distance for digital transmission illustrates the role of robotics in telesurgical education. Telementoring in its simplest form, of supervising and guiding laparoscopic procedures, has been demonstrated since the earliest days of laparoscopic herniorraphy [100]. With deployment of the da Vinci 2000 in the cardiac surgical domain by 1999 and urologic surgery by 2000, educational demands pushed technological developments to improve learning on-site and remotely [101, 102] (Fig. 27.1a, b).

In a recent meta-analysis of all telementoring and telesurgical papers in peer reviewed literature, Hung et al. demonstrated that such educational attempts improve patient safety, better clinical outcomes, and lower costs [103]. Current 2-D telestration, whereby screen annotations drawn by an instructor are perceived elsewhere by the trainee, may be replaced with 3-D images (Fig. 27.2). Jarc et al. developed "ghost tools" that overlay images with perceived depth onto the trainees endoscopic screen including pointers, hands, and "ghost" instruments [104]. Robotic surgery, viewed with skepticism, has moved well into the realm of standards-of-care but still require rigorous evaluation of safety, efficacy, economics, and feasibility [105, 106] Telementoring and telepresence tutoring are already being implemented to allow for experts in the technology to train robotic surgeons at other sites who are initiating those programs [107].

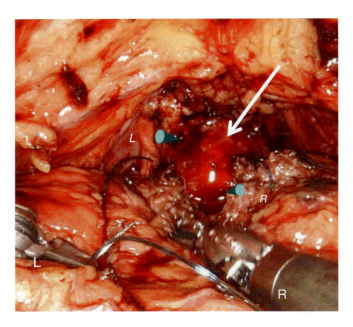

Fig. 27.1 (a) Telestration telementoring during robotic prostatectomy using the da Vinci Xi robotic platform. Contact sensor illustration on a dedicated monitor are transmitted to the visual display of the surgical console via the da Vinci vision cart. (b) Dual robotic da Vinci Xi platform demonstrating the classic telementor–telementee configuration. The dual system allows each surgeon to share the same videoendoscopic image while swapping the control of instruments and using "ghost" telestration to indicate surgical landmarks

Fig. 27.2 Ghost telestration. Da Vinci surgical console image showing (L) and (R) left and right, respectively, robotic needle drivers during bladder neck reconstruction after robotic radical prostatectomy. Also shown are the "ghost" blue cone-shaped icons (small, italicized "L" and "R") which display direct movements from the telementor's left and right hands, respectively, in a second console (see Fig. 27.1b)

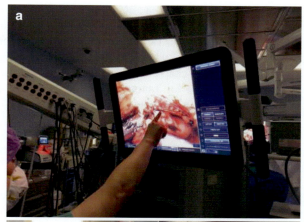

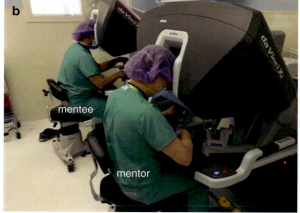

George Campbell (1823–1900), the Eighth Duke of Argyll, in feting Cyrus West Field the year of the completion of the Transatlantic Cable, also remarked that "it is a great comfort to scientific men to be sure that even those discoveries which for year, and even for centuries, remain apparently entirely useless, may at any time and at any moment become serviceable in the highest degree to human family." [108] Thus, as the world continues to become smaller, and travel to distant worlds a reality, telerobotics and its ability to deliver medical care from afar, may have its greatest effects in the centuries to come.

Telepresence and Telementoring in Trauma and Emergency Surgery

Live telementoring in the management of a critically ill trauma patient has been proven lifesaving [109, 110]. In a study by Latifi et al., 59 trauma and general surgery patients were evaluated, wherein 35 (59%) were trauma patients and 24 (41%)

were general surgery patients. For 6 of 35 trauma patients, the telementoring via teletrauma consults were considered potentially lifesaving; 17 patients (29%) were kept in the rural hospitals (8 trauma and 9 general surgery patients).

The best example of telementoring in trauma, emergency, and ICU ae demonstrated in a separate chapter in this book. In this chapter, in order to illustrate the value of telepresence for trauma or teletrauma we will recall a case from Arizona that has been previously reported.

Southern Arizona Teletrauma and Telepresence (SATT) First of Telementoring

The use of telemedicine is long standing, but only in recent years has it been applied to the specialties of trauma, emergency care, and surgery. Despite being relatively new, the concepts of teletrauma, telepresence, and telesurgery are evolving and being integrated into modern care of trauma and surgical patients. The Southern Arizona Telemedicine and Telepresence (SATT) program was an interhospital telemedicine program, while the Tucson eR-link is a link between prehospital and emergency room system, and both are built upon a successful existing award winning Arizona Telemedicine Program and the technical infrastructure of the city of Tucson. These two programs represent examples of integrated and collaborative community approaches to solving the lack of trauma and emergency care issue in the region. These networks will be used by trauma, but also by all other medical disciplines, and as such have become an example of innovation and dedication to trauma care. The first case of trauma managed over the telemedicine trauma program or "teletrauma" was that of an 18-month-old girl who was the only survivor of a car crash with three fatalities (Fig. 27.3). The success of this case and the pilot project of SATT that ensued led to the development of a regional teletrauma program serving close to 1.5 million people.

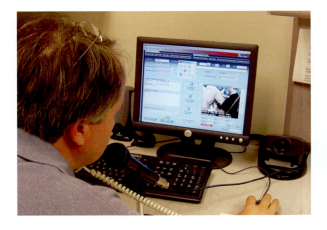

Fig. 27.3 First telementoring for trauma, Tucson, Arizona, 2004. Dr. Latifi assisting a local physician managing an 18-month-old child following severe trauma

An 18-month-old girl was the only survivor of a severe car crash with three fatalities in Agua Prieta, Sonora, Mexico. She was transported to Douglas Hospital in southern Arizona in critical condition 3 hours after the crash. She was hypotensive, oxygen saturation was 70%, Glasgow Coma Scale 7, multiple visible injuries to the head, bilateral lower extremity fractures, and had no intravenous access. The trauma surgeon in Tucson on call that night received a call from the on-duty physician in Douglas, AZ, requesting help and if the patient could be transferred to Trauma Center at the University of Arizona in Tucson. It was her first day on the job, first working day as a physician post family residency, and first day in Arizona! She was scared. A connection was initiated with her through a state-of-the-art telemedicine unit. The trauma surgeon realized why she was visibly shaken; she had a little girl dying in her hands. The patient was hypotensive, hypoxic, in a coma, with multiple visible injuries to her head, and fractures of bilateral lower extremities. Forty-five minutes and a few occasionally nerve-racking exchanges later, the child was resuscitated and stable enough to be placed on the helicopter for a 150 km flight to Tucson. Prior to transfer, the physician in Douglas intubated the patient successfully, but once she was intubated, the saturation was not coming up as expected. Through the telemedicine link, the senior author of this chapter (RL), a trauma surgeon, could see the rising of the lower right chest wall with each manual ventilation. The chest radiography clearly demonstrated that the endotracheal tube was in the right lower lobe. Advising the emergency doctor at the scene, to pull the endotracheal tube back solved the problem of saturation. Grossly dilated stomach was decompressed with a nasogastric tube.

Getting intravenous access in a patient in shock is always difficult, as all the veins are collapsed. The only choice is accessing central veins, such as femoral, jugular, subclavian vein, or osseous access. In a shocked patient, femoral access is the fastest and the safest. However, this was this physician's first femoral stick in child! Using telemedicine, the physician in Douglas was successfully guided through femoral line placement. Once she gained access, the patient could be transfused with packed RBC. Arterial blood gas analysis showed severe acidosis (base deficit 10, from acute blood losses, hemoglobin 5.8 gr/dL). After the patient was placed on the helicopter, the joyful, but exhausted and pale-looking physician turned to the camera, her face filling the screen and said: "Thank you so much for being with us here today. Without you, this child would have died." This image provides perspective in the true value of telemedicine.

During our first teleresuscitation of a severely injured patient, in Arizona, we learned many things about the teletrauma system and what we needed to have in ours teletrauma room, such as dosing medication for kids and adults, headphones for a physician and not a speaker phone, and the angle that we needed to place the camera to see the chest X-ray. Most importantly, and personally, this trauma surgeon reconfirmed that a calm, deliberate voice with clear directions and clear communication is key in handling major trauma and bad situations. During the 45 minutes, teleresuscitation and the long list of intervention that saved this little girl's life were possible only because the trauma surgeon was able to see what was happening 150 km away and how the patient was responding to each intervention, almost each second. The trauma surgeon left the teletrauma room, and went to the trauma bay and waited for the patient. The trauma team saved this child only because it had access to advanced technologies. Without the telemedicine technology (the physician in Douglas was right) this patient undoubtedly would have died. No question about that! She was discharged to home after 14 days in the hospital. Her fractures were fixed, acute respiratory distress syndrome (ARDS) resolved, she was smiling and behaving like any other 18-month-old child. Luckily, her parents were not among the dead in that fatal car crash [109, 110]. Telementoring for trauma and emergency surgery or emergency medicine overall is different than telementoring surgical cases, as we know today. For one, the emergency nature of the injury adds a different dimension. Second, it is rare that the trauma surgeon and the EMS provider or a physician in a remote healthcare institution know each other and work together often enough to be able to coordinate all that is required in saving the life of very sick and or injured patient.

Telemedicine and Telementoring in Neurosurgery

Neurosurgery is considered one of the most cutting-edge and technologically advanced surgical practices, with an ever-growing focus on achieving safer outcomes with increasingly common minimally invasive techniques. Traditionally, neurosurgery is first learned during a 7-year residency with the addition of either an enfolded or postgraduate subspecialty fellowship. Supplemental educational opportunities exist in the form of subspecialty society meetings, national conferences, and departmental skills labs offered by academic institutions. In a more recent effort to keep up with the pace of rapidly evolving neurosurgical practices and techniques, the apprenticeship model has been modified to include virtual simulation models and telementoring. This has been implemented for both residents in training as well as fellows and junior faculty looking to introduce new procedures into their surgical armamentarium.

Unfortunately, within the field of neurosurgery there is still a paucity of published research on telemedicine and telementoring.

Telemedicine within neurosurgery has been most successfully implemented in delivery of acute stroke [112, 113] and trauma care [114]. Trials of tele-stroke, intracranial hemorrhage, and neurotrauma care systems have demonstrated comparable outcomes, as well as reduced costs, in comparison to standard practices [115–117]. A pooled analysis of randomized trials investigating tele-stroke care demonstrated improved decision-making with respect to administration of recombinant tissue plasminogen activator (rt-PA) and no significant differences between the two groups with respect to mortality rates, outcomes, or hemorrhage [112, 113, 118, 119]. Telemedicine has also been utilized in the treatment of chronic neurologic conditions. A study by Davis et al. reported success with providing remote care for chronic neurologic conditions to patients living in rural areas, including patients with movement disorders who had undergone deep brain stimulation [120]. Out of the surveyed patients, 92% reported that the telemedicine service saved them potentially both time and money. The authors estimated that in 354 patients, total savings were more than $48,000, and patient response was overwhelmingly positive, with 95% of patients reporting that they wished to continue their neurological care via telemedicine [119]. The economic impact of telemedicine is from a combination of diminished travel times and reduced lost work time for patients, as well as avoiding unnecessary, expensive transfers to tertiary care centers for subspecialty consultations by physicians [119].

Telementoring has been shown to be comparable to on-site mentorship with respect to knowledge and skill acquisition [121, 122]. The technology used in telementoring and teleproctoring can be used to extend autonomy in the operating room to surgical resident and fellows in training. Importantly, this allows providers in low-resource settings to learn from remote world-class specialists. Mendez et al. utilized robotic long-distance telementoring for six neurosurgical procedures: three craniotomies for brain tumor resection, a craniotomy for arteriovenous malformation resection, a carotid endarterectomy, and a lumbar laminectomy. There were no surgical complications during the procedures, and all patients had uneventful outcomes [123]. Virtual Interactive Presence and Augmented Reality (VIPAR) is a new technology that allows surgeons to deliver real-time virtual assistance and training in remote locations. The technology provides a hybrid perspective of local and remote video feeds, allowing a remote surgeon to digitally survey and comment on the surgical field, highlighting anatomic structures, and providing visual demonstration of operative techniques [124]. VIPAR has been utilized in both neurosurgical and orthopedic procedures for training of resident surgeons in regions in which surgeons skilled in a particular procedure are not readily available [125].

Another novel technology, the CorPath GRX system (Covindus Corp, Waltham, MA), is a proprietary instrument for use in the remote delivery and manipulation of coronary or peripheral guidewires, rapid exchange device, and guide catheters during percutaneous coronary intervention procedures and percutaneous vascular intervention procedures. Given the recent successes of this robotic system in performing percutaneous cardiac interventions [126, 127]. There is a growing enthusiasm about expanding the indications to include the emergent interventional procedures such as stroke thrombectomy and cerebral aneurysm embolization. In addition, for the potential of remote care delivery, the CorPath GRX also provides an exceptionally novel opportunity for telementoring in the future but these applications are still in their infancy.

Telementoring can also be employed in the credentialing process. Optimizing training of practitioners with new technology is critical to minimize the impact of the learning curve on safety. Oftentimes, this means a surgeon outside of the physician's institution has to proctor a predetermined number of early procedures. Use of telementoring allows for an expert with knowledge of the disease process and procedure to remotely proctor and assess the treating surgeon's proficiency. A recent example of this within the neurosurgical arena is well illustrated by the woven endobridge (WEB) device (Microvention, Aliso Viejo, CA); an intrasaccular flow disruptor that is used to treat intracranial wide-necked bifurcation aneurysms. Successful deployment of this device depends on accurate sizing in order to ensure that the device is under compression and presents an adequate barrier to blood inflow at the neck of the aneurysm. Arthur et al. presented a unique simulated training program, which was incorporated into the Web Intrasaccular Therapy (WEB-IT) study to optimize technical performance and patient safety. Surgical rehearsal with the replicator enabled physicians to practice device deployment and communication with proctors. An additional potential benefit was the opportunity to carry out trials of different devices within a given aneurysm. Fluoroscopy and procedure times in the WEB-IT study were not significantly different between those using the simulation model from those under direct proctoring [128].

Challenges of Future of Surgical Telementoring

Despite its opportunities, surgical telementoring has its own challenges, but the most sensitive issue is medical liability and legal aspect and logistics. Prior to experts committing to telementoring community-based surgeons, the legal responsibility of both mentee and mentor are legally documented with detailed accountability for the outcome of the procedure; both mentee and mentor have had documented consultations and/or telemedicine consultations with the patient; both mentee's and mentor's names appear on the patient's informed consent form; the mentor's responsibility to assess the mentee's surgical skills and equipment availability prior to implementation of telementoring program are legally documented; both mentee and mentor have signed agreement regarding the time and the circumstances under which the link could be terminated if disagreement should arise regarding the quality of the surgery; the leadership of both academic institution and community hospital have signed agreement [111].

Because of the above, the introduction of telementoring, surgeons have been asking the pertinent question, "What responsibility does the mentoring physician hold to the patient?" Some believe that the mentor is in a purely advising role and thus is not delivering any care to the patient. Others believe that the mentoring surgeon does indeed have a degree of control over the procedure and is in fact delivering care to the patient. If the latter school of thought is to be accepted as the norm, then it would be a requirement that the mentor hold a medical license in the state where the care is being delivered and proper hospital privileges at the time of the procedure. This can cause difficulty particularly in the United States where licensure in one state does not confer the ability to practice medicine in another state [43]. Credentialing and malpractice liability are other areas of concern. Early precedents have shown that hospitals can accept that a mentor is credentialed and in good standing at their home institution as sufficient for telementoring to occur. The mentoring surgeon may be facing a very low risk of medical liability and thus malpractice coverage is necessary [43]. In published works demonstrating the feasibility of telementoring in bariatric surgery, no additional malpractice coverage was sought after consultation with the insurance carrier [42].

Some surgeons with a desire to teach have expanded the utility of the technology behind one on one telementoring to perform "live surgery" on front of large audiences. These are cases that, with patient consent, are broadcast live in real time. Through this format master surgeon are able to share their technique and decision-making process with fellow surgeons and trainees across various points along the learning curve for a procedure. However, this practice has raised significant concerns. Kallmes et al. documents several ethical issues raised by the practice of live surgical demonstrations. Some of these problems stem from the scheduled nature of these events [129]. There is a fear that patients may be pressured into undergoing procedures to meet the scheduled demands of a live surgery event or have a necessary surgery delayed. In addition, indications for procedures are sometimes observed to be loosened in order to procure patients for these occasions. There is also a potential for an alteration in the normal decision-making processes during live surgery cases. Surgeons may take shortcuts to speed cases along, even subconsciously. These scenarios create conflicts of interest for surgeons who want to care for their patient but also entertain and educate an audience.

There is very limited data to guide the surgical community in the risks and benefits of live surgery. From an educational standpoint the benefits are obvious. How does a patient benefit from this process, if at all? Live surgery events utilizing technology sponsored by industry can have a cost benefit to a patient, which raises more ethical questions than it answers. More importantly, what are the risks to the patient? Studies of live demonstrations of retrograde cholangiopancreatography have shown no difference in complication rates but a trend toward more successful procedures in control groups compared to the live demonstration groups [129].

Despite few challenges, telementoring is an acceptable and important method to advancing the knowledge and surgical procedures. Technological advances will continue, and not be an issue, just as there were not for telemedicine advances overall. Mindset changes of surgeons and leaders of surgical departments will be required. Public education and leadership of surgery resolve to advance surgery will make telementoring more acceptable in the future. Finally, a successful telementoring program will depend on an efficient telementoring system, with the ability to compress video and audio signaling, achieving an adequate transfer rate in the range of 128 Kbps, with an adequate time delay. Time delays of more than 500 minutes carry a higher risk of surgical delay and errors [130]. A virtual private secure network (VPN) is also mandatory between the mentor and mentee facilities, for obvious reasons. Commercial telemonitoring systems are available: Karl Storz OR1 Smartconnect (Karl Storz, Germany), Stryker's Video Network Hub (Stryker, MI USA), etc. [44].

Conclusion

Telementoring and teleproctoring into the operating room have become a reality, but are still a small portion of training new surgeons. The robotics in surgery, once seen with outmost skepticism, has become a standard of care have made possible wider spread of telementoring [131].

References

1. Erridge S, Yeung DKT, Patel HRH, Purkayastha S. Telementoring of surgeons: a systematic review. Surg Innov. 2019;26(1):95–111. https://doi.org/10.1177/1553350618813250.
2. Santok GD, Raheem AA, Kim LHC, et al. Proctorship and mentoring: Its backbone and application in robotic surgery. Investig Clin Urol. 2016;57Suppl 2:S114–20. https://doi.org/10.4111/icu.2016.57.S2.S114.
3. Bruschi M, Micali S, Porpiglia F, et al. Laparoscopic telementored adrenalectomy: the Italian experience. Surg Endosc. 2005;19:836–40.
4. Julien JS, Perrier ND. Video telementoring to accelerate learning of new surgical techniques. JAMA Surg. 2016;151:671–3.
5. El-Sabawi B, Magee W III. The evolution of surgical telementoring: current applications and future directions. Ann Transl Med. 2016;4:391. https://doi.org/10.21037/atm.2016.10.04.
6. Moore RG, Adam JB, Partin AW, et al. Telementoring of laparoscopic procedures: initial clinical experience. Surg Endosc. 1996;10:107–10.
7. Rosser JC, Wood M, Payne JH, et al. Telementoring. A practical option in surgical training. Surg Endosc. 1997;11:852–5.
8. Lendvay TS, Hannaford B, Satava RM. Future of robotic surgery. Cancer J. 2013;19(2):109–19.
9. Takács A, Nagy DA, Rudas IJ, Haidegger T. Origins of surgical robotics: from space to the operating room. Acta Polytechnica Hungarica. 2016;13(1):13–30.
10. Doarn CR, Nicogossian AE, Merrell RC. Applications of telemedicine in the United States space program. Telemed J. 1998;4(1):19–30.
11. Doarn CR. Telemedicine in tomorrow's operating room: a natural fit. Surg Innov. 2003;10(3):121–6.
12. Bharathan R, Aggarwal R, Darzi A. Operating room of the future. Best Pract Res Clin Obstet Gynaecol. 2013;27(3):311–22.
13. Merrell RC, Jarrell BE, Schenkman NS, Schoener B, McCullough K. Telemedicine for the operating room of the future. Surg Innov. 2003;10(2):91–4.
14. https://www.sages.org/wiki/teleproctoring/
15. Lii NY, Leidner D, Schiele A, Birkenkampf P, Pleintinger B, Bayer R. Command robots from orbit with supervised autonomy: an introduction to the meteron supvis-justin experiment. In: Proceedings of the Tenth Annual ACM/IEEE International Conference on Human-Robot Interaction Extended Abstracts: ACM; 2015. p. 53–4.
16. Diana M, Marescaux J. Robotic surgery. BJS. 2015;102(2):e15–28.
17. Marescaux J, Leroy J, Gagner M, et al. Transatlantic robot-assisted telesurgery. Nature. 2001;413(6854):379–80. Erratum 2001; 414(6865):710.
18. Anvari M, McKinley C, Stein H. Establishment of the world's first telerobotic remote surgical service: for provision of advanced laparoscopic surgery in a rural community. Ann Surg. 2005;241(3):460–4.
19. Marescaux J, Rubino F. Telesurgery, telementoring, virtual surgery, and telerobotics. Curr Urol Rep. 2003;4(2):109–13.
20. Anvari M. Robot-assisted remote telepresence surgery. Semin Laparosc Surg. 2004;11(2):123–8.
21. Rosser JC Jr, Bell RL, Harnett B, Rodas E, Murayama M, Merrell R. Use of mobile low-bandwidth telemedical techniques for extreme telemedicine applications. J Am Coll Surg. 1999;189(4):397–404.17.
22. Angood PB, Satava R, Doarn C, Merrell R, E3 Group. Telemedicine at the top of the world: the 1998 and 1999 Everest extreme expeditions. Telemed J E Health. 2000;6(3):315–25.
23. Sterbis JR, Hanly EJ, Herman BC, et al. Transcontinental telesurgical nephrectomy using the da Vinci robot in a porcine model. Urology. 2008;71(5):971–3.19.
24. Doarn CR, Anvari M, Low T, Broderick TJ. Evaluation of teleoperated surgical robots in an enclosed undersea environment. Telemed J E Health. 2009;15(4):325–35.

25. Harnett BM, Doarn CR, Rosen J, Hannaford B, Broderick TJ. Evaluation of unmanned airborne vehicles and mobile robotic telesurgery in an extreme environment. Telemed J E Health. 2008;14(6):539–44.
26. Sereno S, Mutter D, Dallemagne B, Smith CD, Marescaux J. Telementoring for minimally invasive surgical training by wireless robot. Surg Innov. 2007;14(3):184–91. https://doi.org/10.1177/1553350607308369.
27. Marescaux J, Leroy J, Rubino F, et al. Transcontinental robot-assisted remote Telesurgery: feasibility and potential applications. Ann Surg. 2002;235:487–92.
28. Ereso AQ, Garcia P, Tseng E, Dua MM, Victorino GP, Guy LTS. Usability of robotic platforms for remote surgical teleproctoring. Telemed J E Health. 2009;15(5):445–53.
29. Fleet R, Tounkara FK, Ouimet M, Dupuis G, Poitras J, et al. Portrait of trauma care in Quebec's rural emergency departments and identification of priority intervention needs to improve the quality of care: a study protocol. BMJ. 2016;6(4):e010900.
30. Liss MA, McDougall EM. Robotic surgical simulation. Cancer J. 2013;19(2):124–9.
31. Ereso AQ, Garcia P, Tseng E, Gauger G, Kim H, Dua MM, et al. Live transference of surgical subspecialty skills using telerobotic proctoring to remote general surgeons. J Am Coll Surg. 2010;211(3):400–11.
32. Latifi R. Telemedicine for trauma and intensive care: changing the paradigm of telepresence. In: Technological advances in surgery, trauma and critical care. New York: Springer; 2015. p. 51–7.
33. Rolston DM, Meltzer JS. Telemedicine in the intensive care unit: its role in emergencies and disaster management. Crit Care Clinics. 2015;31(2):239–55.
34. Smith AL, Scott EM, Krivak TC, Olawaiye AB, Chu T, Richard SD. Dual-console robotic surgery: a new teaching paradigm. J Robot Surg. 2013;7:113–8.
35. Jarc AM, Shah SH, Adebar T, et al. Beyond 2D telestration: an evaluation of novel proctoring tools for robot-assisted minimally invasive surgery. J Robot Surg. 2016;10:103–9.
36. Vera AM, Russo M, Mohsin A, et al. Augmented reality telementoring (ART) platform: a randomized controlled trial to assess the efficacy of a new surgical education technology. Surg Endosc. 2014;28:3467–72.
37. Andersen D, Popescu V, Cabrera ME, et al. Medical telementoring using an augmented reality transparent display. Surgery. 2016;159:1646–53.
38. Augestad M, Han H, Paige J, et al. Educational implications for surgical telementoring: a current review with recommendations for future practice, policy, and research. SAGES. 2017;
39. Miller JA, Kwon DS, Dkeidek A, et al. Safe introduction of a new surgical technique: remote telementoring for posterior retroperitoneoscopic adrenalectomy. ANZ J Surg. 2012;82:813–6.
40. Mirheydar H, Jones M, Koeneman KS, Sweet RM. Robotic surgical education: a collaborative approach to training postgraduate urologists and endourology fellows. JSLS. 2009;13:287–92.
41. Santomauro M, Reina GA, Stroup SP, L'Esperance JO. Telementoring in robotic surgery. Curr Opin Urol. 2013;23:141–5.
42. Nguyen NT, Okrainec A, Anvari M, et al. Sleeve gastrectomy telementoring: a SAGES multi-institutional quality improvement initiative. Surg Endosc. 2018;32(2):682–7. https://doi.org/10.1007/s00464-017-5721-8.
43. Schlachta CM, Nguyen NT, Ponsky T, Dunkin B. Project 6 Summit: SAGES telementoring initiative. Surg Endosc. 2016;30(9):3665–72. https://doi.org/10.1007/s00464-016-4988-5.
44. Antoniou SA, Antoniou GA, Franzen J, et al. A comprehensive review of telementoring applications in laparoscopic general surgery. Surg Endosc. 2012;26(8):2111–6. https://doi.org/10.1007/s00464-012-2175-x.
45. Fuertes-Guiró F, Vitali-Erion E, Rodriguez-Franco A. A program of telementoring in laparoscopic bariatric surgery. Minim Invasive Ther Allied Technol. 2016;25(1):8–14. https://doi.org/10.3109/13645706.2015.1083446.
46. Shubeck SP, Kanters AE, Sandhu G, Greenberg CC, Dimick JB. Dynamics within peer-to-peer surgical coaching relationships: early evidence from the Michigan Bariatric Surgical Collaborative. Surgery. 2018;164(2):185–8. https://doi.org/10.1016/j.surg.2018.03.009.

47. Altieri MS, Carmichael H, Jones E, Robinson T, Pryor A, Madani A. Educational value of telementoring for a simulation-based fundamental use of surgical energy™ (FUSE) curriculum: a randomized controlled trial in surgical trainees [published online ahead of print, 2020 May 4]. Surg Endosc. 2020; https://doi.org/10.1007/s00464-020-07609-1.
48. Huang EY, Knight S, Guetter CR, et al. Telemedicine and telementoring in the surgical specialties: a narrative review. Am J Surg. 2019;218(4):760–6. https://doi.org/10.1016/j.amjsurg.2019.07.018.
49. Messiah SE, Sacher PM, Yudkin J, et al. Application and effectiveness of eHealth strategies for metabolic and bariatric surgery patients: a systematic review. Digit Health. 2020;6:2055207619898987. https://doi.org/10.1177/2055207619898987.
50. Coldebella B, Armfield NR, Bambling M, Hansen J, Edirippulige S. The use of telemedicine for delivering healthcare to bariatric surgery patients: a literature review. J Telemed Telecare. 2018;24(10):651–60. https://doi.org/10.1177/1357633X18795356.
51. https://missionrestore.org/missionrestores-east-african-regional-training-2018-begins/. Last accessed 24 May 2020.
52. Alizadeh K. Commentary on: complications after global surgery tourism. Aesthet Surg J. 2019;39(7):972–3.
53. Benschoter RA. Multipurpose television. Ann, NY: Academy Sciences; 1967. p. 471–8.
54. Wittson CL, Benschoter RA. Two-way television: helping the medical center reach out. Amer J Psychiat. 1972;129(5):624–7.
55. Sebajang H, Trudeau P, Dougall A, et al. The role of telementoring and tele- robotic assistance in the provision of laparoscopic colorectal surgery in rural areas. Surg Endosc. 2006;20:1389–93.
56. Schlachta CM, et al. A model for longitudinal mentoring and telementoring of laparoscopic colon surgery. Surg Endosc. 2009;23:1634–8.
57. Augestad KM, Bellika JG, Budrionis A, et al. Surgical telementoring in knowledge translation–clinical outcomes and educational benefits: a comprehensive review. Surg Innov. 2013;20(3):273–81.
58. Angelos G, Dockter AG, Gachabayov M, Latifi R, Bergamaschi R. Emergency colorectal surgery in a COVID-19 pandemic epicenter. Surg Tecnol Int. 2020;14:36:sti36/1297.
59. Anvari M. Telesurgery: remote knowledge translation in clinical surgery. World J Surg. 2007;31:1545e1550.
60. Latifi R, Peck K, Satava R, Anvari M. Telepresence and telementoring in surgery. Stud Health Technol Inform. 2004;104:200–6.
61. Doarn CR, Latifi R. Telementoring and teleproctoring in trauma and emergency care. Cur Trauma Rep. 2016;2:138–43.
62. Latifi R, Doarn CR. Perspective on COVID-190: finally, telemedicine at center stage [published online ahead of print, 2020 May 14]. Telemed J E Health. 2020;https://doi.org/10.1089/tmj.2020.132.
63. Leung T, Vyas D. Robotic surgery: applications. Am J Robot Surg. 2014;1(1):1–64.
64. Liang H, Liang W, Zhao L, Chen D, Zhang J, Zhang Y, et al. Robotic versus video-assisted lobectomy/segmentectomy for lung cancer: a meta-analysis. Ann Surg. 2018;268(2):254–9.
65. Cerfolio RJ, Bryant AS, Skylizard L, Miniich DJ. Initial consecutive experience of completely portal robotic pulmonary resection with 4 arms. J Thorac Cardiovasc Surg. 2011;142(4):740–6.
66. Ponsky TA, Bobanga ID, Schwachter M, Stathos TH, Rosen M, Parry R, et al. Transcontinental telmentoring with pediatric surgeons: proof of concept and technical considerations. J Laparoendosc Adv Surg Tech A. 2014;24(12):892–6.
67. Bruns NE, Irtan S, Rothenberg SS, Bogen EM, Kotobi H, Ponsky TA. Trans-Atlantic telemonitoring with pediatric surgeons: technical considerations and lessons learned. J Laparoendosc Adv Surg Tech A. 2016;26(1):75–8.
68. Yang H, Woo KM, Sima CS, et al. Long-term survival based on the surgical approach to lobectomy for clinical stage I non-small cell lung cancer: comparison of robotic, video-assisted thoracic surgery, and thoracotomy lobectomy. Ann Surg. 2017;264(2):431–7.

69. Dewey TM, Mak MJ. Lung cancer. Surgical approaches and incisions. Chest Surg Clin N Am. 2000;10(4):803–20.
70. Cerfolio RJ, Bess KM, Wei B, Minnich DJ. Incidence, results, and our current intraoperative technique to control major vascular injuries during minimally invasive robotic thoracic surgery. Ann Thorac Surg. 2016;102(2):394–9.
71. Proctoring versus precepting Medical Staff Leader Insider, Credentialing Resource Center Digest – Volume 7, Issue 43 October 25, 2006.
72. Schneider A, Wilhelm D, Bohn U, Wichert A, Feussner HJ. An evaluation of a surgical telepresence system for an intrahospital local area network. Telemed Telecare. 2005;11:408–13.
73. Deaton DH, Balch D, Kesler C, Bogey WM, Powell CS. Telemedicine and endovascular aortic grafting. Am J Surg. 1999;177(1):75–7. https://doi.org/10.1016/s0002-9610(98)00309-2.
74. Di Valentino M, Alerci M, Bogen M, et al. Telementoring during endovascular treatment of abdominal aortic aneurysms: a prospective study. J Endovasc Ther. 2005;12:200–5.
75. Porretta AP, Alerci M, Wyttenbach R, et al. Long-term outcomes of a telementoring program for distant teaching of endovascular aneurysm repair. J Endovasc Ther. 2017;24(6):852–8.
76. Lin CC, Chen YP, Chiang CC, Chang MC, Lee OK. Real-time streaming of surgery performance and intraoperative imaging data in the hybrid operating room: development and usability study. JMIR Med Inform. 2020;8(4):e18094. Published 2020 Apr 22. doi:https://doi.org/10.2196/18094.
77. https://www.mdedge.com/vascularspecialistonline/article/209996/society-news/enroll-mentor-match-program-svsconnect
78. Jacobs BN, Boniakowski AE, Osborne NH, Coleman DM. Effect of mentoring on match rank of integrated vascular surgery residents. Ann Vasc Surg. 2020;64:285–29.
79. Lesseps F. Address. In: proceedings at the Banquet held in honor of Cyrus W Field. London: Metchem & Sons; 1868. p. 52–3.
80. Rovetta A, Sala R. Execution of robot-assisted biopsies within the clinical context. J Image Guid Surg. 1995;1(5):280–7.
81. Challacombe B, Patriciu A, Glass J, et al. A randomized controlled trial of human versus robotic and telerobotic access to the kidney as the first step in percutaneous nephrolithotomy. Comput Aided Surg. 2005;10(3):165–71.
82. Sterbis JR, Hanly EJ, Herman BC, et al. Transcontinental telesurgical nephrectomy using the da Vinci robot in a porcine model. Urology. 2008;71(5):971–3.
83. Winfield HN, et al. Laparoscopic adrenalectomy: the preferred choice? A comparison to open adrenalectomy. J Urol. 1998;160(2):325–9.
84. Clayman RV, et al. Laparoscopic nephrectomy: initial case report. J Urol. 1991;146(2):278–82.
85. Ratner LE, et al. Laparoscopic live donor nephrectomy. Transplantation. 1995;60(9):1047–9.
86. Schuessler WW, et al. Laparoscopic radical prostatectomy: initial short-term experience. Urology. 1997;50:854.
87. Schuessler WW, Schulam PC, Clayman RV, Vancaille TH. Laparoscopic radical prostatectomy: initial case report. J Urol. 1992;147(1):246–8.
88. Guillonneau B, Cathelineau X, Barret E, Rozet F, Vallancien G. Radical laparoscopic prostatectomy: early results in 28 cases. Presse Med. 1998;27(31):1570–4.
89. Guillonneau B, et al. Laparoscopic radical prostatectomy: the Montsouris experience. J Urol. 2000;163(2):418–22.
90. Binder J, Kramer W. Robotically-assisted laparoscopic radical prostatectomy. BJU Int. 2001;87(4):408–41.
91. Skarecky D et al. Robotic-assisted radical prostatectomy after the first decade: surgical evolution or new paradigm, ISRN Urology. 2013; PMID: 23691367, pp 1–22.
92. Menon M, Tewari A, Baize B, Guillonneau B, Vallancien G. Prospective comparison of radical retropubic prostatectomy and robot-assisted anatomic prostatectomy: the Vattikuti Urology Institute experience. Urology. 2002;60(5):864–8.
93. Ficarra V, Novara G, Rosen RC, et al. Systematic review and meta-analysis of studies reporting urinary continence recovery after robot-assisted radical prostatectomy. Eur Urol. 2012;62(3):405–41.

94. Patel VR, Palmer KJ, Coughlin G, Samavedi S. Robot-assisted laparoscopic radical prostatectomy: perioperative outcomes of 1500 cases. J Endourol. 2008;22(10):2299–305.
95. Agarwal D. Initial experience with da Vinci single-port robot-assisted radical prostatectomies. Eur Urol. 2020;77(3):373–9.
96. Hussein AA, et al. A comparative propensity score-matched analysis of perioperative outcomes of intracorporeal vs extracorporeal urinary diversion after robot-assisted radical cystectomy: results from the International Robotic Cystectomy Consortium. BJU Int. 2020;126(2):265–72.
97. Bochner BH, Dalbagni G, Marzouk KH, et al. Randomized trial comparing open radical cystectomy and robot-assisted laparoscopic radical cystectomy: oncologic outcomes. Eur Urol. 2018;74(4):465.
98. Sivaram A, et al. Learning curve of minimally invasive radical prostatectomy: comprehensive evaluation and cumulative summation analysis of oncological outcomes. Urol Oncol. 2017;35(4):149.
99. Bravi C, et al. The impact of experience on the risk of surgical margins and biochemical recurrence after robot-assisted radical prostatectomy: a learning curve study. J Urol. 2019;202:108–13.
100. Cubano M, et al. Long distance telementoring. A novel tool for laparoscopy aboard the USS Abraham Lincoln. Surg Endosc. 1999;13:673–8.
101. Rassweiler JJ, et al. Future of robotic surgery in urology. BJU Int. 2017;120:822–41.
102. Fernandes E, et al. The role of the dual console in robotic surgical training. Surgery. 2013;155:1–4.
103. Hung AJ, et al. Telementoring and telesurgery for minimally invasive procedures. J Urol. 2018;199:355–69.
104. Jarc AM, et al. Beyond 2D telestration: an evaluation of novel proctoring tools for robot-assisted minimally invasive surgery. J Robot Surg. 2016;35:957–62.
105. Checcucci E, et al. Single-port robot-assisted radical prostatectomy: a systematic review and pooled analysis of the preliminary experiences. BJU Int. 2020;126(2):265–72.
106. Chang Y, et al. Robotic perineal radical prostatectomy: initial experience with the da Vinci Si robotic system. Urol Int. 2020:1–6.
107. Veneziano D, Is remote live urologic surgery a reality? Evidences from a systematic review of the literature. World J Urol. 2019.
108. Duke of Argyll. Address. In: Proceedings at the Banquet held in honor of Cyrus W Field. London: Metchem & Sons; 1868. p. 20.
109. Latifi R, Hadeed GJ, Rhee P, O'Keeffe T, Friese RS, Wynne JL, et al. Initial experiences and outcomes of telepresence in the management of trauma and emergency surgical patients. Am J Surg. 2009;198(6):905–10. https://doi.org/10.1016/j.amjsurg.2009.08.011.
110. Latifi R, Weinstein RS, Porter JM, Ziemba M, Judkins D, Ridings D, et al. Telemedicine and telepresence for trauma and emergency care management. Rev Scand J Surg. 2007;96:281–9.
111. Francis N, Fingerhut A, Bergamaschi R, Motson R, editors. Training in minimal access surgery manual: Springer-Verlag; 2014.
112. Demaerschalk BM, Bobrow BJ, Raman R, et al. Stroke team remote evaluation using a digital observation camera in Arizona: the initial mayo clinic experience trial. Stroke. 2010;41:1251–8.
113. Demaerschalk BM, Raman R, Ernstrom K, Meyer BC. Efficacy of telemedicine for stroke: pooled analysis of the Stroke Team Remote Evaluation Using a Digital Observation Camera (STRokE DOC) and STRokE DOC Arizona telestroke trials. Telemed J E Health. 2012;18:230–7.
114. Latifi R, Olldashi F, Dogjani A, Dasho E, Boci A, El-Menyar A. Telemedicine for Neurotrauma in Albania: initial results from case series of 146 patients. World Neurosurg. 2018;112:e747–53. https://doi.org/10.1016/j.wneu.2018.01.146.
115. Bailes JE, Poole CC, Hutchison W, Maroon JC, Fukushima T. Utilization and cost savings of a wide-area computer network for neurosurgical consultation. Telemed J. 1997;3:135–9.

116. Duchesne JC, Kyle A, Simmons J, et al. Impact of telemedicine upon rural trauma care. J Trauma. 2008;64:92–7.
117. Moya M, Valdez J, Yonas H, Alverson DC. The impact of a telehealth web-based solution on neurosurgery triage and consultation. Telemed J E Health. 2010;16:945–9.
118. Meyer BC, Raman R, Hemmen T, et al. Efficacy of site-independent telemedicine in the STRokE DOC trial: a randomised, blinded, prospective study. Lancet Neurol. 2008;7:787–95.
119. Kahn EN, La Marca F, Mazzola CA. Neurosurgery and telemedicine in the United States of America: assessment of the risks and opportunities. World Neurosurg. 2016;89:133–8. https://doi.org/10.1016/j.wneu.2016.01.075.
120. Davis LE, Coleman J, Harnar J, King MK. Teleneurology: successful delivery of chronic neurologic care to 354 patients living remotely in a rural state. Telemed J E Health. 2014;20:473–7.
121. Sebajang H, Trudeau P, Dougall A, et al. The role of telementoring and telerobotic assistance in the provision of laparoscopic colorectal surgery in rural areas. Surg Endosc. 2006;20:1389e1393.
122. Ereso AQ, Garcia P, Tseng E, et al. Live transference of surgical subspecialty skills using telerobotic proctoring to remote general surgeons. J Am Coll Surg. 2010;211(3):400e411.
123. Mendez I, Hill R, Clarke D, et al. Robotic long-distance telementoring in neurosurgery. Neurosurgery. 2005;56:434–40.
124. Akhigbe T, Zolnourian A, Bulters D. Mentoring models in neurosurgical training: review of literature. J Clin Neurosci. 2017;45:40–3. https://doi.org/10.1016/j.jocn.2017.07.025.
125. Huang EY, Knight S, Guetter CR, et al. Telemedicine and telementoring in surgical specialties: a narrative review. Am J Surg. 2019;218:760–6.
126. Mahmud E, Schmid F, Kalmar P, et al. Feasibility and safety of robotic peripheral vascular interventions: results of the RAPID trial. JACC Cardiovasc Interv. 2016;9(19):2058–64.
127. Weisz G, Metzger DC, Caputo RP, et al. Safety and feasibility of robotic percutaneous coronary intervention: PRECISE (percutaneous robotically-enhanced coronary intervention) study. J Am Coll Cardiol. 2013;61(15):1596–600.
128. Arthur A, Hoit D, Coon A, et al. Physician training protocol within the WEB intrasaccular therapy (WEB-IT) study. J Neuro Intervent Surg. 2018;10(5):500–4.
129. Kallmes DF, Cloft HJ, Molyneux A, Burger I, Brinjikji W, Murphy KP. Live case demonstrations: patient safety, ethics, consent, and conflicts. Lancet. 2011;377(9776):1539–41. https://doi.org/10.1016/S0140-6736(11)60357-7.
130. Anvari M. The impact of latency on surgical precision and task completion during robotic-assisted remote telepresence surgery. Comput Aided Surg. 2005;10:93–9.
131. George EI, Brand TC, LaPorta A, Marescaux J, Satava RM. Origins of robotic surgery: from skepticism to standard of care. JSLS. 2018;22(4):e2018.00039. https://doi.org/10.4293/JSLS.2018.00039.

The Promise and Hurdles of Telemedicine in Diabetes Foot Care Delivery

Bijan Najafi, Mark Swerdlow, Grant A. Murphy, and David G. Armstrong

Background: Public Health Significance of Diabetic Foot Ulcers (DFUs)

More individuals are dying of chronic noncommunicable diseases (NCD) than acute diseases associated with disasters, trauma, or infection. Diabetes is the quintessential NCD, and the prevalent and long-neglected diabetic foot ulcer (DFU) and accompanying lower extremity complications rank among the most debilitating and costly sequelae of this syndrome in both the developed and developing world [1].

Foot ulcers in people with diabetes constitute a silent, sinister syndrome. Approximately ten million people with diabetes mellitus (34%) will develop a DFU in their lifetime in the USA alone [2]. These wounds often become chronic (70% remain unhealed after 3 months of usual care) and can lead to amputation. Every 1.2 seconds someone in the world develops an ulcer, and every 20 seconds someone loses a lower limb due to diabetes [2]. Direct healthcare costs are substantial, ranging from US$3096 for a superficial ulcer to US$107,900 for an ulcer resulting in amputation [3].

Perhaps no complication of DFU is more significant than amputation, which occurs at a rate of 10% per DFU. At least 70% of amputations are potentially preventable [4]. Additionally, Hispanics and African Americans appear to be at

---

B. Najafi (✉)
Interdisciplinary Consortium for Advanced Motion Performance (iCAMP), Division of Vascular Surgery and Endovascular Therapy, Michael E. DeBakey Department of Surgery, Baylor College of Medicine, Houston, USA
e-mail: Bijan.Najafi@bcm.edu

M. Swerdlow · G. A. Murphy · D. G. Armstrong
Southwestern Academic Limb Salvage Alliance (SALSA), Department of Surgery, Keck School of Medicine of University of Southern California, Los Angeles, CA, USA
e-mail: mswerdlo@usc.edu; gamurphy@usc.edu

© Springer Nature Switzerland AG 2021
R. Latifi et al. (eds.), *Telemedicine, Telehealth and Telepresence*,
https://doi.org/10.1007/978-3-030-56917-4_28

increased risk for lower extremity amputation (LEA) compared to other ethnic groups and may also be less likely to undergo advanced care to prevent limb loss. In low-income populations, the risk of major LEA is estimated to be 38% higher than the highest-income regions ($p < 0.05$) [5]. These data suggest an important gap in effectively managing diabetic foot ulcers, particularly among lower-income individuals, and is most important for those living in remote areas with limited access to interdisciplinary care.

Promises of Telemedicine for Diabetic Foot Management

Telemedicine (also referred as telehealth, telecare, remote care, or virtual care) has been defined as "medicine practiced at a distance" and is mainly used for remote management of chronic diseases [6]. Telemedicine interactions take place either in real time (e.g., videoconferencing or telephone) or asynchronously (e.g., store-and-forward transmission of data using email). Monitoring applications have been either automatic (e.g., passive monitoring of activity using room sensors) or have required a patient action (e.g., transmit plantar wound pictures using the buttons on a tablet or smartphone). Educational applications have either employed specially designed devices or depended on web access from PCs or smartphones [6].

In recent years, thanks to advances in telecommunication systems, telemedicine has emerged as one the most economic and patient-friendly methods for delivering follow-up care to patients with DFUs [7]. Considering that some wounds take many months to heal and are at significant risk for infection and amputation, replacing regular clinic visits with a better way to remotely track healthy wound healing is desperately needed. This need, along with the paucity of wound care specialists (it is estimated that less than 0.2% of all nurses are wound care specialists [8]), has promoted the application of telemedicine in remote and rural areas.

Furthermore, it is often reported that the collaboration between primary healthcare and wound specialist is not sufficient, leading to referral delays and severe consequences such as emergency and hospital admission [5, 9]. Telemedicine may address these gaps and assist in improving communication with wound care specialists, increasing access to care, optimizing patient referral, reducing the need for transportation to outpatient clinics, and potentially reducing healthcare costs while improving patient satisfaction and quality of care. Increased connectivity among people via smart devices has made it possible to develop and implement telecare programs for people with diabetes-related foot problems from wound monitoring to DFU-prevention consultations. In particular, as health care providers searching for alternatives to deliver timely care to patients with diabetic foot syndrome during current COVID-19 pandemic, it is tempting to imagine a post-COVID future may lead to some positive changes in healthcare for managing diabetic foot syndrome, particularly in promoting the use of preventive and personalized care via tele-medicine care delivery model.

Key Barriers to Telemedicine Adoption for Diabetic Foot Management

The use of telemedicine to manage chronic conditions is sharply increasing worldwide thanks to its cost-effectiveness and decreased utilization of resources, while providing timely, patient-centered care. Although the promise of telemedicine for managing chronic conditions such as asthma, heart failure, COPD, diabetes, and hypertension is well established, high-quality studies on the effectiveness of telemedicine in diabetic foot disease and wound care management are scarce, limiting the generalizability of most findings.

Several barriers may give healthcare executives pause when it comes to the adoption of telemedicine for diabetic foot management. These include: (1) patient acceptability, awareness, and trust in virtual care offerings; (2) effectiveness; (3) quality of care delivery for remote wound management; (4) reliability compared to in person clinic visits; and (5) concerns around the cost to implement. These challenges and recommendations to successfully navigate them are discussed in the following sections.

Patient Acceptability, Awareness, and Trust in Virtual Care Offerings

There are few studies that examine how the incorporation of telemedicine impacts the experiences of patients receiving DFU care. In-depth knowledge of patients' experiences and their perception of the care provided can help evaluate whether use of telemedicine is an appropriate way to improve DFU care.

In 2015, Rasmussen et al. [10] explored key organizational factors in the implementation of telemedicine in wound care. They conducted eight semi-structured interviews, including individual interviews with leaders and an IT specialist and focus group interviews with the clinical staff. A qualitative data analysis of the interviews was performed to analyze the healthcare professionals' and leaders' perception of the organizational changes caused by the implementation of the intervention. They reported that telemedical setup enhanced confidence among collaborators and improved the wound care skills of visiting nurses from the municipality. Focus on the visiting nurses' training was highlighted as a key factor in the success to securing implementation. Several concerns were also identified, such as lack of multidisciplinary wound care teams, patient responsibility, and lack of patient interaction with the physician. Finally, they concluded that telemedicine could provide an additional option to offer patients after an individual assessment of their health condition.

In 2016, Strom et al. used individual semi-structured interviews to study patients' experiences with telemedicine wound care follow-up as compared to traditional care. Twenty-four patients were recruited and randomized in the intervention group (use of telemedicine, $n = 13$) and control group (use of traditional care, $n = 11$). The results show that competent wound management from health professionals was of great importance to patients' feelings of security during wound care irrespective of their type of follow-up care. They concluded that telemedicine can be an important supplement in the wound care process, but its efficacy will depend on whether it is used as intended and if continuity of care is present. They also recommended that education and practical training in the use of telemedicine should be given to all primary healthcare professionals.

In 2017, Kolltveit et al. [11] conducted a qualitative study in 10 focus groups across different working settings to identify what various healthcare professionals perceived as facilitating engagement and participation with telemedicine. They identified four key conditions for the successful implementation of telemedicine for wound care: technology and training that were user-friendly, the presence of a telemedicine champion in the work setting, the support of committed and responsible leaders, and effective communication channels at the organizational level. They concluded that attention to the distinct needs of each staff group is an essential condition for effective implementation of telemedicine for wound care.

Effectiveness of Telemedicine to Manage Diabetic Foot Care Compared to Traditional Care

There are few studies that have examined the effectiveness of telemedicine to improve diabetic foot care and wound outcomes. Thus, convincing evidence to support the clinical efficacy of telemedicine in wound management compared to traditional care is still lacking.

In 2015, Zarchi et al. [12] used a prospective cluster randomized controlled study to examine whether the delivery of wound management advice from a team of wound-care specialists using telemedicine significantly improved the likelihood of wound healing compared with the best available conventional practice. A total of 90 chronic wound patients in home care were recruited and split into intervention (use of telemedicine, $n = 50$) and control (use of traditional care, $n = 40$) groups. During the 1-year follow-up, complete wound healing was achieved in 35 patients (70%) in the telemedicine group compared with 18 patients (45%) in the conventional group. After adjusting for several covariates, the difference between groups was statistically significant with an adjusted hazard ratio of 2.19. They concluded that using telemedicine is an effective method to connect home-care nurses to wound experts in order to improve the management of chronic wounds.

In 2009, Terry et al. [13] compared wound outcomes in 103 subjects with 160 pressure ulcers or non-healing surgical wounds, who were randomly assigned into three groups: Group A ($n = 40$) received weekly visits via telemedicine consulting with a wound-care specialist, group B ($n = 28$) had weekly visits in person with a wound specialist, and group C ($n = 35$) received usual and customary care. Their results suggest that group A had increased time to heal, length of stay, costs, and visits compared with groups B and C despite similar distribution of subject characteristics (e.g., age, Braden score, total activity of daily living (ADL) score, and race). But group A had disproportionally larger and more numerous pressure ulcers and larger non-healing surgical wounds. They concluded that telemedicine is a useful communication tool in wound management with its efficacy dependent on wound size and type. They also recognized several limitations in their study including insufficient power and large distribution in wound severity in their recruited subjects.

In 2013, Vowden et al. [14] proposed the use of digital pen-and-paper technology and a modified smartphone to remotely monitor and support the effectiveness of wound management in nursing home residents. To demonstrate the effectiveness of this program, they conducted a randomized controlled pilot study in 16 nursing homes, recruiting a total of 39 patients with wounds. They reported that the proposed telemedicine care delivery system provided improved patient outcomes and that it may offer cost savings by improving dressing selection, decreasing inappropriate referral, and decreasing healing time. They also reported that despite initial anxiety related to the technology, most nursing home staff found the system valuable and many were keen to see the trial continue as part of routine patient management.

A 2015 RCT study by Ramussen et al. [15] compared telemedical and standard outpatient monitoring in diabetic foot ulcer patients. Patients were randomized to telemedical monitoring ($n = 193$) or standard outpatient monitoring ($n = 181$). Telemedical monitoring protocol consisted of two consultations in the patient's home and one consultation at the outpatient clinic. Standard practice consisted of three outpatient clinic visits. The three-visit cycle was repeated until study end point, defined as complete ulcer healing, amputation, or death, for up to 1 year. While a trend in increasing wound healing ratio (hazard ratio = 1.11) and reducing foot amputation (hazard ratio = 0.87) were found through telemedicine monitoring, these trend were not statistically significant ($p > 0.40$). However, a significant mortality incidence was observed in the telemedicine group (hazard ratio = 8.68, $p < 0.001$). They recommended further study to better identify these patient subgroups that may have a poorer outcome through telemedicine monitoring. In a critique to the Ramussen et al. study, Muller et al. [16] shared their experience implementing telemedicine with home nurses in France. They claimed that they stopped their trial prematurely after realizing that many of the nurses involved in their study were not trained to deal with chronic wounds; this specialized training is essential for the success of telemedical wound care. Furthermore, they claimed that the quality of data and wound pictures were not sufficiently standardized in Ramussen et al., which may explain part of the negative outcomes from the telemedicine group. They further concluded that adequate initial training and ongoing support are essential for the successful implementation of wound-care telemedicine.

In 2018, Smith-Strøm et al. [17] examined the effectiveness of telemedicine follow-up for diabetic foot ulcer care compared to standard of care using a RCT design. They randomized 182 adults with DFU between the telemedicine ($n = 94$) and standard of care ($n = 88$) groups. Participants were recruited from three clinical sites in western Norway (2012–2016). The intervention group received telemedicine follow-up care in the community; the control group received standard of care. The primary end point was healing time, and the secondary end points were amputation, death, number of consultations per month, and patient satisfaction. Their results suggest that telemedicine was not inferior to standard of care regarding healing time (mean difference −0.43 months, 95% CI −1.50, 0.65). When comparing risk from death and amputation were taken into account, there was no significant difference in healing time between the groups (sub-hazard ratio 1.16, 95% CI 0.85, 1.59). The telemedicine group had a significantly lower proportion of amputations (mean difference −8.3%, 95% CI −16.3%, −0.5%), and there were no significant differences in the proportion of deaths, number of consultations, or patient satisfaction between groups; however, the direction of the effect estimates for these clinical outcomes favored the telemedicine group. They concluded that the use of telemedicine technology can be a relevant alternative and supplement to usual care, at least for patients with more superficial ulcers.

From above studies, we speculate that efficacy of telemedicine for wound management is dependent on DFU severity, size, and adequate initial training. In particular, when wounds are superficial, telemedicine could have better outcomes and lower costs than conventional care. On the other hand, for complex wounds, telemedicine could be served as a supplement to conventional care to improve communication and management plan. Irrespective of type of wound, adequate initial training and ongoing support are essential for the successful and cost-effective implementation of wound-care telemedicine.

Efficiencies of Telemedicine for Delivery of Care for Foot Disease in Remote Area

Inefficiencies and communication gaps continue to hamper both effective care delivery and a reduction in costs while improving the quality of healthcare and overall population health [18]. With the rapid evolution of the healthcare industry, healthcare delivery organizations are leveraging innovative solutions to meet these challenges. Several studies have suggested that telemedicine is an effective tool to improve access to patients in need of diabetic foot care and facilitate the communication between wound care specialists and patients.

In 2016, Kolltveit et al. [19] explored healthcare professionals' experience in the initial phase of introducing telemedicine technology in 10 different wound care groups, including home-based care, primary care, and outpatient hospital clinics. The participants reported experiencing meaningful changes to their practice arising from telemedicine, especially associated with improved wound assessment knowledge, skills, and documentation quality. Kolltveit et al. concluded that using telemedicine intervention enabled the participating healthcare professionals to approach their DFU patients with increased knowledge, better wound assessment skills, and heightened confidence.

In 2017, Turnin et al. [20] examined whether telemedicine could improve healthcare access in rural areas for management of DFUs. A vehicle was equipped with a satellite dish and medical equipment for screening ophthalmological, renal, vascular, and neuropathic damage as well as assessing the level of diabetic foot ulceration risk. Onboard, a nurse performed some or all of the tests on patients who had no diabetes review for over a year. The data were entered into a computer and transmitted by satellite for interpretation by designated specialists. The results were sent to patients, general practitioners (GPs), and diabetologists. Over approximately 3 years, 228 screening days were held in six rural departments; in total, 1545 patients were screened and 93.4% were diagnosed with type 2 diabetes. Of these, 17–32% of tests detected pathologies including 18.7% diabetic retinopathy, 31.9% microalbuminuria, 17.2% lower limb arteriopathy, 28.3% peripheral neuropathy, and 28.2% high risk of foot ulceration (grade 2: 20.6% and grade 3: 7.6%). They concluded that telemonitoring-enabled screening a larger number of patients in need of urgent care and thus helped to improve healthcare access through its innovative organization and use of satellite technology.

Reliability of Telemedicine Compared to In-person Visit

Very few studies compared head-to-head telemedicine care and in-person care. Telemedicine for wound care is mainly dependent on the quality of wound pictures. For instance, even with high-quality images, assessing the need for debridement and detecting infection may be limited.

In 2007, Binder et al. [21] conducted a case series study including 16 patients with 45 leg ulcers of different origins. After an initial outpatient visit when the leg ulcers were assessed and classified, teledermatological follow-up was done by home care nurses. Relevant clinical information and one to four digital images of the wound and surrounding skin were transmitted weekly via a secure website to an expert at the wound-care center who assessed the wound and made therapeutic recommendations. They claimed that 89% of transmitted images (644 out of 707) had excellent or sufficient quality for giving confident therapeutic recommendations. They concluded that the acceptance of telemedicine for wound care treatment recommendations from wound experts is very high, and thus, telemedicine offers great potential for long-term wound care.

In 2011, Bowling et al. [22] compared the ability of wound inspection from images with in-person inspection. They requested two clinicians to document clinically relevant features from 20 different wound images captured using a novel imaging system that provided three-dimensional wound images, including wound area and depth. Next, the wounds were inspected in person, and the results were compared with the documented notes. They reported an overall agreement for remote versus in-person assessments but noticed lower agreement on subjective clinical assessments, such as value of debridement to improve healing. This was linked to a limitation of the imaging technique to capture certain characteristics such as moistness and exudation. However, they reported that clinicians gave positive feedback on visual fidelity and concluded that the three-dimensional wound images could accurately measure and assess a diabetic foot wound remotely.

Cost-Effectiveness of Telemedicine for Diabetic Foot Care

The ideal goal of telemedicine is to facilitate a productive interaction between patient and healthcare provider in order to achieve improved treatment results at lower treatment costs. Although several studies have examined the benefits of telemedicine in both improving outcomes and facilitating interactions between patients and specialists, few studies examined whether telemedicine could also reduce the cost of care compared to conventional face-to-face patient consultation.

In 2007, Litzinger et al. [23] examined the potential benefit of telemedicine in reducing the need for wound ostomy continence (WOC) nurse visits with a 2-year prospective study design. In their study, home health aides trained in telehealth technology assisted with the evaluations of severe wounds using video teleconferencing equipment that enabled the WOC nurse to evaluate wounds from a remote location. This decreased the travel time for the WOC nurse increased the frequency of specialized wound consultations, and facilitated the development of comprehensive treatment plans for multiple patients. They recruited 35 patients receiving multiple wound care evaluations, averaging 7 visits in the first year and 11.3 visits in the second year, for a total of 470 virtual visits. In their estimates of savings from telemedicine, they reported 421.2 hours of saved nursing visits, a cost reduction of US$9449, miles not traveled totaling 30,500 (reducing costs by an additional US$11,875.87 for mileage reimbursement), and travel time saved totaling 916.8 hours (reducing costs still further by US$20,850). After deducting the administrative cost, they claimed that the net program savings were US$25,208. However, this did not factor in the costs of teleconferencing equipment.

In 2008, Dobke et al. [24] evaluated the impact of telemedicine consults on patients with chronic wounds by recruiting 30 patients from long-term care skilled nursing facilities who were referred to the ambulatory wound-care program for wound assessment and preparation of management plans. To facilitate communication with a surgical wound care specialist, telemedicine feedback was provided prior to face-to-face consultation to 15 randomly selected patients. The telemedicine consult included virtual consultation with a field wound nurse who provided remote wound assessment, described rationale for the suggested wound management with emphasis on wound risk projections, and explained the prevention and benefits of surgical intervention. The telemedicine impact was measured by assessing the duration of the subsequent face-to-face consultation and patient satisfaction with further care decisions as well as by validation of a decisional conflict scale. Their results suggested a significant reduction in duration of face-to-face direct consultation by an average of 70% and an average of 46% improvement in patient satisfaction rate. They concluded that telemedicine consults preceding face-to-face evaluation improved patient satisfaction and understanding of their care as well as increased the perception of shared decision making regarding wound care.

In 2013, Sparsa et al. [25] proposed the use of telemedicine to manage chronic wounds (leg ulcers, pressure ulcers, and diabetic ulcers) in older adults living in retirement homes. Specifically, they explored whether telemedicine intervention for wound care could reduce the number of ambulance transports; 10 establishments were provided with a digital camera and their own secure e-mail address in order to allow photographs to be sent anonymously. They documented the number of tele-expertise consultations given, the chronic wound type, the number of hospitalizations or medical consultations, and the number of ambulance trips avoided over 2 years. During this period, photographs of 34 patients presenting with 26 chronic wounds (10 pressure ulcers, 2 diabetic foot ulcers and 14 leg ulcers) received telemedicine consultations. They concluded that this program helped avoid 20 trips for patients, enable rapid hospitalization of nine patients, and provide timely wound management for patients residing in establishments for the elderly.

In 2016, Fasterholdt et al. [26] conducted the first randomized controlled trial study to compare cost-effectiveness of telemedicine versus standard monitoring in patients with diabetic foot ulcers in southern Denmark. A total of 374 patients were randomized to either telemonitoring or standard monitoring. Telemonitoring consisted of two tele-consultations in the patient's own home and one consultation at the outpatient clinic; standard monitoring consisted of three outpatient clinic consultations. The two groups did not present significant differences in terms of demographic and clinical characteristics. Although the amputation rate was similar in the two groups, a reduction in cost was observed thanks to telemonitoring care on average by €2039 per patient over a 6-month period. The difference in cost was related to total staff time used on outpatient consultation, amounting to 156 minutes for the telemonitoring group versus 266 minutes in standard group. However, the observed reduction in cost wasn't statistically significant, and thus they concluded that a telemonitoring service of this form had similar costs and effects as standard monitoring.

Future Directions

Telemedicine is getting "smarter" thanks to artificial intelligence (AI) and connected in-home devices including smart wearables, voice-enabled technologies, and smartphones [27–29]. With the help of AI, patients can be prompted to check their feet, glucose levels, or weight, and enter the results into mobile patient portals. Even better, they can transmit the results to their physicians in real time. These fast-growing, low-cost, and widely available resources can help predict one's risk for foot ulcers, infections, peripheral arterial disease, frailty, and other diabetes-associated complications, ultimately saving limbs and lives [29, 30].

One of the fast-developing infrastructures promising to revolutionize the diabetic foot care industry is the Internet of Things (IoT) [31]. It is expected that 50% of healthcare over the next few years will be delivered via virtual platforms. This has accelerated the development of a new market named "digital wellness," which combines digital technology and healthcare [31]. Digital technology–based healthcare is regarded as a natural choice for remote, home-based, and long-term care of patients with chronic conditions due to its low cost, high accuracy, and continuous monitoring and tracking capabilities.

IoT involves a system of devices, machines, or anything with the ability to transfer data without the need for a human to implement the communication [32]. Fueled by the recent adaptation of a variety of enabling wireless technologies such as radio-frequency identification (RFID) tags, wearable sensors, and actuator nodes, the IoT has stepped out of its infancy to become the next revolutionary technology in transforming the Internet into a fully integrated "Future Internet" [32]. As we move from World Wide Web (www; static pages web) to Web2 (social networking web) to Web3 (ubiquitous computing web), the need for data-on-demand using sophisticated intuitive queries increases significantly. What has made IoT the next big thing is not just its machine-to-machine component, but the potential of sensor-to-machine interaction. With the increasing development of health sensors, there is a growing opportunity to utilize IoT for medical data collection and analysis. It is expected that integration of these tools into the healthcare model has the potential of lowering annual costs of chronic disease management by close to one-third [33]. While the use of IoT for medical applications is still in its infancy, significant business decisions have recently been taken by major information and communication technology companies like Google, Apple, Cisco, and Amazon to position themselves in the IoT landscape. For example, in 2014, Novartis partnered with Google to develop sensor-technologies like a smart lens and a wearable device to measure blood glucose levels [34]. In 2017, Amazon partnered with Merck and Luminary Labs on the Alexa Diabetes Challenge with the goal of improving the experience of people living with diabetes using Alexa (cloud-based voice service) devices [29, 35]. As the IoT continues to develop, further potential exists to develop and facilitate management of chronic conditions at home, including effective strategies for both the prevention and healing of diabetic foot disease.

Recently, a few technologies adopted the concept of IoT to provide preventive care for diabetic foot disease and reduce the need for regular clinic visits [27, 30]. In 2017, Frykberg et al. [36] proposed a smart mat based on the telehealth concept that could address the limitations of previous thermography tools. They studied a novel in-home connected foot mat (Podimetrics Mat™, Somerville, MA, USA; Fig. 28.1) for remote monitoring of plantar temperature that may be used to predict DFU risk and better stratify those in need of urgent foot care. This simple-to-use system was designed to require no configuration or setup by the user who simply had to step on the mat with both feet for 20 seconds daily. Using an embedded cellular component, the collected data are streamed to a cloud. Using an image processing tool, an integrated program compares the temperature profile between feet. In their study, they demonstrated that a threshold difference of ≥ 2.22 °C between corresponding sites on opposite feet correctly predicts 97% of DFU with an average lead time of 37 days. Adherence to the mat was high with 86% of participants using the mat at least three times per week with an average use of five times per week. While this accuracy and lead time could be sufficient to better target those who need urgent care, the technology suffers from an important limitation: While the 2.22 °C threshold provided 97% sensitivity, it yielded just 43% specificity [36]. Increasing the threshold value increases specificity but decreases sensitivity. However, the observed high sensitivity and sufficient lead time (37 days) seem to be promising for both effective triaging and coaching the user to alter their behavior to reduce DFU risk.

There are other digital health developments that could supplement telemedicine technology with practical information to detect feet at risk of DFU and extend

28 The Promise and Hurdles of Telemedicine in Diabetes Foot Care Delivery

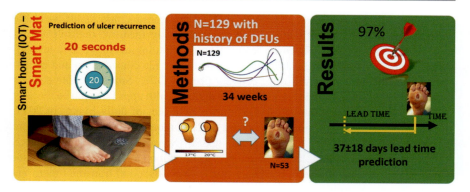

Fig. 28.1 Summary of Frykberg et al. [36] study: In a prospective cohort observational study of patients in foot ulcer remission, Frykberg et al. [36] demonstrated that 20 s of daily monitoring plantar temperature using a smart mat (Podimetrics LLC, MA, USA) and an asymmetry temperature of greater than 2.22 °C enables predicting incidence of ulcer recurrence with 97% accuracy and an average lead time of 37 ± 18 days (mean ± standard deviation). In this study, 129 eligible subjects were recruited and followed for up to 34 weeks, leading to 53 incidents of DFU. Then, using machine learning, an optimum threshold of 2.22 °C was identified to yield a trade-off between longest lead time and detection with highest accuracy. This technology could be used as an add-on to telemedicine, as collected data could provide practical information to health professionals to provide personalized consultation to prevent incident of DFU or schedule clinic visits for a detailed examination. (This figure was created based on the Frykberg et al. study [36])

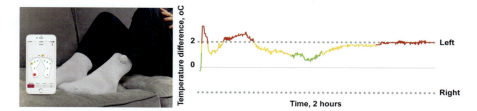

Fig. 28.2 Siren Socks enable continuous and remote plantar temperature monitoring, which may be used as an early warning system for DFU. This data could be used by healthcare professionals to provide personalized recommendations for daily physical activities or preventative actions to perform before a foot ulcer develops. (This figure was created based on Reyzelman et al. study [37])

ulcer-free days. Siren Care (Siren Diabetic Socks, Neurofabric, Siren Care Inc., San Francisco, CA; Fig. 28.2) [37] is an example of such recent developments; they use smart textiles to continuously monitor plantar temperature and then engage patients to reduce risk. However, the acceptability of these technologies and their advantage compared to a daily single point assessment like the Podimetrics Mat remain to be studied. Similarly, new technologies enable temperature measurements of shoe insoles and simultaneous assessment of plantar pressure, temperature, and lower extremities joint angles [38]. These technologies may 1 day improve the triaging of those at a high DFU risk and eventually assist with personalized prevention recommendations via telemedicine.

Thanks to advances in smartphones, mobile applications, and smart wearable sensors, the ability to continuously and simultaneously measure multiple values associated with DFUs has become a reality. These technologies enable remote monitoring that can be used by health professionals to provide consultation and education via telemedicine in order to effectively prevent DFU. Smart flexible sensors implanted in socks or insoles combined with digital health apps have paved the way for monitoring plantar tissue stress [39] during activities of daily living. In 2017, Raviglione et al. [40] proposed the concept of daily monitoring of plantar pressure in people at risk of DFU using a smart textile (Sensoria socks, Sensoria Inc., Redmond, WA, USA; Fig. 28.3a). Their system contained a textile pressure sensor attached to a stretchable band, hardware that collects data and transmits them via Bluetooth to a smartphone, a cloud-enabled data collection-and-storage app, and a clinician-facing web dashboard that displays the collected data. They concluded that this technology could determine optimal offloading in the community setting and assist with DFU prevention. This concept may also be a useful add-on to telemedicine as this remotely collected data would be easily accessible by health professionals and could be used to make personalized recommendations for DFU education and prevention. Recently, Sensoria and Optima (Optima Molliter, Civitanova, Italy, Fig. 28.3b), an Italian offloading company, collaborated to design the MOTUS Smart Boot, which facilitates real-time offloading efficacy assessment and weight-bearing physical activity dosage management. The technology could be transformative for effective management of DFU as practical information to manage plantar wounds – including offloading adherence and level of weight-bearing activities taken with and without offloading – can be remotely collected and accessed

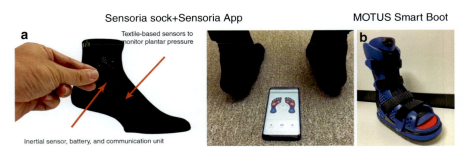

Fig. 28.3 (**a**) Sensoria socks (Sensoria Fitness Inc., Redmond, WA, USA) monitor plantar pressure under three plantar regions of interest including the heel, first metatarsal head, and fifth metatarsal head. They include an anklet that snap to socks' sensors for transmitting data. (**b**) Optima and Sensoria teamed up to design a smart offloading boot named MOTUS Smart Boot that facilitates the real-time monitoring of offloading efficacy and daily dosage of weight-bearing activities .Both technologies could be adopted for telemedicine consultations as they allow remote monitoring of mechanical risk factors such as plantar pressure and level of weight-bearing activities. These remote measurements could serve as digital biomarkers of DFUs and can be utilized by healthcare professionals to provide personalized consultation to prevent or mange DFU. (Images provided from Sensoria with permission to publish)

via a secure cloud. The collected information could be shared with healthcare professionals for effective consultation via telemedicine, which in turn may improve adherence to offloading or dosage management for harmful weight-bearing physical activities; this could ultimately contribute to decreased wound healing times [29, 41]. While the clinical validity of this offloading is unclear at the time of drafting this chapter, the added value it may provide should be confirmed in future clinical trials.

Conclusions

We live in a world where technology is increasingly integrated into every aspect of our lives. With the miniaturization of processors, advancements in sensor technologies, consistent availability of electrical power, ubiquitous Internet access, and significant strides in machine learning and artificial intelligence, emergent solutions are being developed to improve healthcare delivery, patient satisfaction, and population health across different disciplines while reducing the cost of care.

While still in its infancy, recent studies have suggested that delivery of care via telemedicine is acceptable, reliable, and comparably effective to an in-person visit but its efficacy depends on type and severity of wounds as well as adequate initial training. It may also promote patient involvement, care coordination, and effective communications between patients and caregivers. In particular, the combination of telemedicine, wearables, mobile health, and IoT enables reducing in-person visits and allows physicians to remotely monitor patients, track patient adherence, detect the early stages of medical conditions, and triage those who need immediate supervised care. In addition, the use of supplementary information via remote monitoring of DFU risk factors and digital biomarkers could empower healthcare professionals to provide personalized consultations via telemedicine; this may improve acceptability, efficacy, and ultimately adoption of these technologies for delivery of care to patients with or at-risk of DFU.

Telemedicine can be also used to supplement diabetic foot care by providing both educational and motivational support. While this application of the technology for diabetic foot care is still in its infancy, and its cost-effectiveness is debated, with the exponential speed of technological development and increase in technology investment for healthcare applications it is anticipated that healthcare and care delivery for chronic conditions such as diabetic foot disease will undergo dramatic changes in the near future.

In particular, the COVID-19 pandemic exposes our health care system's weaknesses for timely care delivery for patients with diabetic foot disease. For instance, this outbreak shows that traditional healthcare delivery models for managing chronic illness like diabetes are not at scale to handle situations like the global COVID-19 crisis. Because people with diabetes represents a fragile population, it is recommended to avoid unnecessary diabetes-related hospital admissions to reduce the risk of COVID-19 exposure in the hospital. This is disrupting the best practices for preventing diabetes-related complications including diabetic foot ulcer. As health care providers searching for alternatives to deliver timely care to patients with diabetic foot syndrome, it is tempting to imagine a post-COVID future may lead to increased acceptability and at scale adaptation of telemedicine to improve preventive care, smartly triage those who need to be seen in outpatient or inpatient clinic, and supporting acute and subacute care at home [42]

Effective adoption of telemedicine for diabetic foot care, will require (1) user-friendly technology; (2) sufficient training for healthcare professionals, especially during its initial phase; (3) ongoing healthcare professional telemedicine training; (4) enthusiasm for using telemedicine by healthcare professionals, patients, and caregivers; and (5) improved robustness of the intervention plan for remote managing of diabetic foot disease. An important first step in accomplishing all of these will be to increase the awareness of the value-added telemedicine offers; we hope this chapter will mark another important step in doing so.

References

1. Barshes NR, Sigireddi M, Wrobel JS, Mahankali A, Robbins JM, Kougias P, et al. The system of care for the diabetic foot: objectives, outcomes, and opportunities. Diabet Foot Ankle. 2013;4
2. Armstrong DG, Boulton AJM, Bus SA. Diabetic foot ulcers and their recurrence. N Engl J Med. 2017;376:2367–75.
3. Hunt NA, Liu GT, Lavery LA. The economics of limb salvage in diabetes. Plast Reconstr Surg. 2011;127 Suppl 1:289S–95S.
4. Rogers LC, Andros G, Caporusso J, Harkless LB, Mills JL Sr, Armstrong DG. Toe and flow: essential components and structure of the amputation prevention team. J Am Podiatr Med Assoc. 2010;100:342–8.
5. Skrepnek GH, Mills JL Sr, Armstrong DG. A diabetic emergency one million feet long: disparities and burdens of illness among diabetic foot ulcer cases within emergency departments in the United States, 2006–2010. PLoS One. 2015;10:e0134914.
6. Wootton R. Twenty years of telemedicine in chronic disease management–an evidence synthesis. J Telemed Telecare. 2012;18:211–20.
7. Tchero H, Noubou L, Becsangele B, Mukisi-Mukaza M, Retali GR, Rusch E. Telemedicine in diabetic foot care: a systematic literature review of interventions and meta-analysis of controlled trials. Int J Low Extrem Wounds. 2017;16:274–83.
8. Rees RS, Bashshur N. The effects of TeleWound management on use of service and financial outcomes. Telemed J E Health. 2007;13:663–74.
9. Lazzarini PA, Clark D, Mann RD, Perry VL, Thomas CJ, Kuys SS. Does the use of store-and-forward telehealth systems improve outcomes for clinicians managing diabetic foot ulcers?: a pilot study. Wound Pract Res. 2010;18:164.
10. Rasmussen BS, Jensen LK, Froekjaer J, Kidholm K, Kensing F, Yderstraede KB. A qualitative study of the key factors in implementing telemedical monitoring of diabetic foot ulcer patients. Int J Med Inform. 2015;84:799–807.
11. Kolltveit BH, Gjengedal E, Graue M, Iversen MM, Thorne S, Kirkevold M. Conditions for success in introducing telemedicine in diabetes foot care: a qualitative inquiry. BMC Nurs. 2017;16:2.
12. Zarchi K, Haugaard VB, Dufour DN, Jemec GBE. Expert advice provided through telemedicine improves healing of chronic wounds: prospective cluster controlled study. J Invest Dermatol. 2015;135:895–900.
13. Terry M, Halstead LS, O'Hare P, Gaskill C, Ho PS, Obecny J, et al. Feasibility study of home care wound management using telemedicine. Adv Skin Wound Care. 2009;22:358–64.

14. Vowden K, Vowden P. A pilot study on the potential of remote support to enhance wound care for nursing-home patients. J Wound Care. 2013;22:481–8.
15. Rasmussen BS, Froekjaer J, Bjerregaard MR, Lauritsen J, Hangaard J, Henriksen CW, et al. A randomized controlled trial comparing telemedical and standard outpatient monitoring of diabetic foot ulcers. Diabetes Care. 2015;38:1723–9.
16. Muller M, David-Tchouda S, Margier J, Oreglia M, Benhamou PY. Comment on Rasmussen et al. A randomized controlled trial comparing telemedical and standard outpatient monitoring of diabetic foot ulcers. Diabetes Care. 2015;38:1723–9. Diabetes Care. 2016;39:e9–10.
17. Smith-Strom H, Igland J, Ostbye T, Tell GS, Hausken MF, Graue M, et al. The effect of telemedicine follow-up care on diabetes-related foot ulcers: a cluster-randomized controlled non-inferiority trial. Diabetes Care. 2018;41:96–103.
18. Clarke JL, Bourn S, Skoufalos A, Beck EH, Castillo DJ. An innovative approach to health care delivery for patients with chronic conditions. Popul Health Manag. 2017;20:23–30.
19. Kolltveit BC, Gjengedal E, Graue M, Iversen MM, Thorne S, Kirkevold M. Telemedicine in diabetes foot care delivery: health care professionals' experience. BMC Health Serv Res. 2016;16:134.
20. Turnin MC, Schirr-Bonnans S, Chauchard MC, Deglise P, Journot C, Lapeyre Y, et al. DIABSAT telemedicine itinerant screening of chronic complications of diabetes using a satellite. Telemed J E Health. 2017;23:397–403.
21. Binder B, Hofmann-Wellenhof R, Salmhofer W, Okcu A, Kerl H, Soyer HP. Teledermatological monitoring of leg ulcers in cooperation with home care nurses. Arch Dermatol. 2007;143:1511–4.
22. Bowling FL, King L, Paterson JA, Hu J, Lipsky BA, Matthews DR, et al. Remote assessment of diabetic foot ulcers using a novel wound imaging system. Wound Repair Regen. 2011;19:25–30.
23. Litzinger G, Rossman T, Demuth B, Roberts J. In-home wound care management utilizing information technology. Home Healthc Nurse. 2007;25:119–30.
24. Dobke MK, Bhavsar D, Gosman A, De Neve J, De Neve B. Pilot trial of telemedicine as a decision aid for patients with chronic wounds. Telemed J E Health. 2008;14:245–9.
25. Sparsa A, Doffoel-Hantz V, Bonnetblanc JM. Assessment of tele-expertise among elderly subjects in retirement homes. Ann Dermatol Venereol. 2013;140:165–9.
26. Fasterholdt I, Gerstrom M, Rasmussen BS, Yderstraede KB, Kidholm K, Pedersen KM. Cost-effectiveness of telemonitoring of diabetic foot ulcer patients. Health Informatics J. 2018;24(3):245–58.
27. Najafi B. Digital health for monitoring and managing hard-to-heal wounds. In: Smartphone based medical diagnostics: Academic Press; 2020. p. 129–58.
28. Piaggesi A, Lâuchli S, Bassetto F, Biedermann T, Marques A, Najafi B, et al. Advanced therapies in wound management: cell and tissue based therapies, physical and bio-physical therapies smart and IT based technologies. J Wound Care. 2018;27:S1–S137.
29. Basatneh R, Najafi B, Armstrong DG. Health sensors, smart home devices, and the internet of medical things: an opportunity for dramatic improvement in care for the lower extremity complications of diabetes. J Diabetes Sci Technol. 2018;12:577–86.
30. Najaf B, Reeves ND, Armstrong DG. Leveraging smart technologies to improve the management of diabetic foot ulcers and extend ulcer-free days in remission. Diabetes Metab Res Rev. 2020;6 Suppl 1:e3239.
31. Murthy DN, Kumar BV. Internet of Things (IoT): is IoT a disruptive technology or a disruptive business model? Indian J Market. 2015;45:18–27.
32. Gubbi J, Buyya R, Marusic S, Palaniswami M. Internet of Things (IoT): a vision, architectural elements, and future directions. Futur Gener Comput Syst. 2013;29:1645–60.
33. J. Haughom, "Is the health sensor revolution about to dramatically change healthcare," Healthcare Transformation, 2017: https://www.healthcatalyst.com/health-sensors-revolution-change-healthcare. Accessed 31 Sep 2020.
34. Senior M. Novartis signs up for Google smart lens. Nat Biotechnol. 2014;32:856.

35. Coombs B. How Alexa's best skill could be as a home health-care assistant. In: Health care: CNBC; 2017.
36. Frykberg RG, Gordon IL, Reyzelman AM, Cazzell SM, Fitzgerald RH, Rothenberg GM, et al. Feasibility and efficacy of a smart mat technology to predict development of diabetic plantar ulcers. Diabetes Care. 2017;40:973–80.
37. Reyzelman AM, Koelewyn K, Murphy M, Shen X, Yu E, Pillai R, et al. Continuous temperature-monitoring socks for home use in patients with diabetes: observational study. J Med Internet Res. 2018;20:e12460.
38. Najafi B, Mohseni H, Grewal GS, Talal TK, Menzies RA, Armstrong DG. An optical-fiber-based smart textile (smart socks) to manage biomechanical risk factors associated with diabetic foot amputation. J Diabetes Sci Technol. 2017;11:668–77.
39. Lazzarini PA, Crews RT, van Netten JJ, Bus SA, Fernando ME, Chadwick PJ, et al. Measuring plantar tissue stress in people with diabetic peripheral neuropathy: a critical concept in diabetic foot management. J Diabetes Sci Technol. 2019;13:869–80.
40. Raviglione A, Reif R, Macagno M, Vigano D, Schram J, Armstrong D. Real-time smart textile-based system to monitor pressure offloading of diabetic foot ulcers. J Diabetes Sci Technol. 2017;11:894–8.
41. Najafi B, Grewal GS, Bharara M, Menzies R, Talal TK, Armstrong DG. Can't stand the pressure: the association between unprotected standing, walking, and wound healing in people with diabetes. J Diabetes Sci Technol. 2017;11:657–67.
42. Najaii B. "Post the pandemic: how will COVID-19 transform diabetic foot disease management?,' J Diabetes Sci Technol, 2020;14:764–766.

Telemedicine in Austere Conditions

Charles R. Doarn

Introduction

Each of you may have a specific idea of what an austere or extreme environment is. A place with limited resources – electrical power, transportation, knowledge, telecommunication, basic medial capabilities, etc. Perhaps a health condition or the resultant impact of a disaster, a pandemic, or even danger. There are many places around the world (and even above it) that are austere and, in many cases, extreme.

Over the past several decades and even into antiquity, humans have found themselves in geographical places where there is very little to support survivability. With the advent of telecommunications in the late nineteenth century and the seemingly unabated growth in information technology, the world appears to be more connected than ever. Information, regardless of subject, can be available at our fingertips. Yet access to and availability of healthcare services may still be a challenge for many, regardless of their location.

The integration of telecommunications and information systems has provided a platform for healthcare services, including remote monitoring, guidance, effective clinical management, and education by eliminating the barriers of distance, time, and geography [1–3]. While many of these locations are considered austere, telemedicine and telehealth have been integrated and utilized to support individuals in those environments. Some efforts are mission critical, some support research initiatives, and some focus on providing healthcare to areas that are devoid of basic services or much-needed clinical expertise.

Each of the examples presented here are illustrative of how telemedicine and telehealth have been and continue to be deployed in austere and often extreme environments [4–6].

C. R. Doarn (✉)
Department of Environmental and Public Health Sciences, University of Cincinnati College of Medicine, Cincinnati, OH, USA
e-mail: charles.doarn@uc.edu

© Springer Nature Switzerland AG 2021
R. Latifi et al. (eds.), *Telemedicine, Telehealth and Telepresence*,
https://doi.org/10.1007/978-3-030-56917-4_29

Fig. 29.1 Laika in the contaiment unit on an SS20 Intercontintental Ballistic Missile. (Courtesy of Roscosmos)

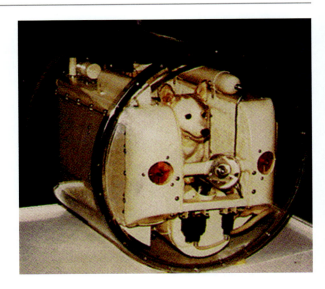

Space

The most extreme and austere environment is human spaceflight. Aside from the United States (U.S.), the Union of Soviet Socialist Republics (USSR), and the Peoples Republic of China, no other nation has yet launched humans to low Earth orbit. Only the U.S. has sent humans to the moon, and that was more than 50 years ago. From the earliest days of space exploration, men and women who have flown in space have been linked to medical personnel on the ground. In fact, the very first application of telemedicine in space was with a dog named Laika, who was sent aloft by the USSR on *Sputnik 2* in 1957 (Fig. 29.1) [5, 8]. Laika's vital signs were monitored from the ground during her flight at a perigee of 131 miles and apogee of 1031 miles (an elliptical orbit). This early development and application of telemetry provided the framework for monitoring astronauts and cosmonauts during spaceflight and in the case of the American program, monitoring the astronauts on the surface of the moon during the Apollo missions from 1969 to 1972 (See Fig. 29.2).

Over the past six decades, space exploration has involved hundreds of individuals who have lived and worked in space. Space stations and spacecraft are several hundred miles above the Earth, and the environment is considered both extreme and austere. While there has been an increase in onboard medical capability from the early 1960s, there is critical link to medical personnel and authority on the ground. Telemedicine is a key component of human spaceflight and has been used effectively since the very early 1960s [8–10].

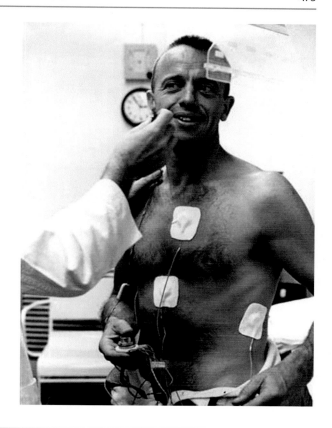

Fig. 29.2 Alan Shepherd with medical watches for wireless telemetry to ground controllers. (Courtesy of NASA)

Battlefield

In the early 1990s, the U.S. military had not fully embraced the concept of integrating telemedicine into battlefield medicine [11]. The U.S. Army began to explore the use of telemedicine in faraway places like Somalia [12]. The U.S. Navy began to integrate teleradiology in the mid-1990s [13]. This early work lead to the development of a multimillion dollar–funded effort known as the U.S. Army's Telemedicine and Advance Technology Research Center (TATRC) [14]. This multiyear effort, mostly through Congressional earmarks, helped usher in changes in protocols and new technologies, deployed at various echelons of care across the world.

In the mid-1990s, Dr. Richard Satava, a program manager at the Defense Advanced Research Projects Agency (DARPA), began discussing virtual reality and telepresence to support military medicine [15]. His work at DARPA was also instrumental in the development of robotic surgery with Stanford Research Institute and the eventual commercialization of da Vinci robotic surgical system [16]. Similar work with other robotics systems, funded in part by National Aeronautics and Space Administration (NASA), also resulted in a competing platform in the late 1990s – Computer Motion's Zeus platform [16].

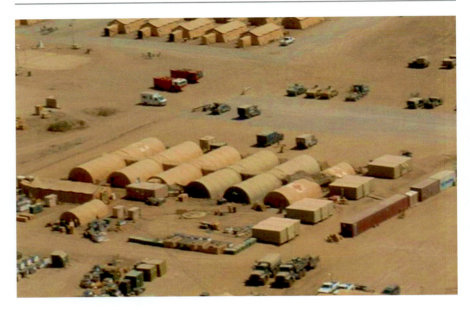

Fig. 29.3 US military field hospital

With each successful military engagement, regardless of the theater, telemedicine and telehealth have become fully integrated in military medicine. No matter where a warfighter may find themselves, there is some form of capability to reach back from the extreme and austere environment they may be deployed to [17]. This might have included war zones like Iraq or Afghanistan or ships at sea or even humanitarian missions (Fig. 29.3).

If a warfighter is injured and cannot return to their assigned post or they become a veteran, the Department of Veteran's Affairs provides a plethora of telemedicine and telehealth capabilities to support care such as posttraumatic stress disorder (PTSD) across 19 geographically dispersed Veterans Integrated Service Networks (VISNs) [18].

While militaries around the world may have been late adopters and integrators of telemedicine and telehealth, they now fully embrace it and, in many cases, especially in the U.S., have been pioneers in developing new technologies and approaches [14].

Alpine

Ever since Sir Edmund Hillary and Sherpa Tenzing Norgay summited Mt. Everest in 1953, there has been a steady increase in climbing expeditions to achieve what only a few can. Every climber must start their mission from Everest Base Camp (south side in Nepal at 17,589 ft or north side in Tibet at 16,900 ft). The majority of teams approach the summit from Nepal (Fig. 29.4). Supplies, including medical

Fig. 29.4 Climbers ascending Everest

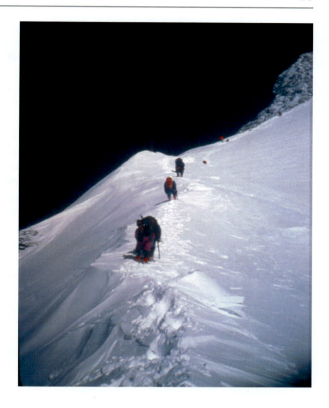

supplies, are carried overland and up to Base Camp by Sherpas and yaks (domesticate bovines). Base camps are both extreme and austere. A medical rescue is pretty challenging and very expensive.

In 1996, a group of climbers perished on the mountain. One of the team members, Jon Krakauer wrote a book about this alpine disaster – *Into Thin Air* [19]. Krakauer was on Rob Hall's climbing team. Those that perished were impacted by weather, schedule, and supply problems, notably oxygen. In 1998 and 1999, a research collaboration, involving the NASA Commercial Space Center at Yale University and The Explorer's Club, explored the possibility of integrating telemedicine to determine if it might serve as a significant tool in preventing morbidity and mortality on the world's highest mountain. The research group conducted real-time physiological monitoring of select climbers [7, 20, 21]. The team even reviewed an emergency ophthalmological case of a Sherpa via a real-time, low-bandwidth video conference [22].

Other research on Everest, including ultrasound [23] and some teleradiology [24] has been conducted. While much of this research has focused on climbers, the population of the Himalayas also require healthcare. Telemedicine has been deployed and studied in Nepal for acute and chronic care as well as emergency care [25, 26].

Today's telemedicine and telehealth technology can be easily deployed in mountainous terrain that is characterized by austerity and isolation. However, it must be well thought out as there remains many geographical and weather challenges.

Jungle

Many individuals, indeed entire populations who live in remote jungles of Central and South America, Africa, and other equatorial regions of the world, must have access to healthcare. While many may see the shaman or medicine man for natural healing, modern medicine has found its way into these remote and austere environments [27]. Over the past century or so, teams of medical personnel (doctors and nurses) travel to various countries around the world to support primary care in a variety of clinical disciplines and surgery.

In the late 1990s and early 2000s, our research team, led by Ronald Merrell and funded by NASA, embarked on a variety of research initiatives designed to explore telemedicine in low resource settings. While the Everest work was mentioned above, the focus here is on surgical care in Ecuador. A research team made episodic trips in concert with the Cinterandes Foundation. The villages visited were characterized by remoteness with austere conditions: one with limited electrical power, telecommunications, reliable medical supply chain, and adequately trained healthcare personnel. Surgical care was conducted in a mobile facility (Fig. 29.5). During

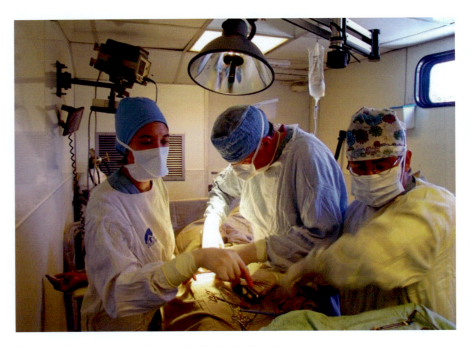

Fig. 29.5 Surgeons at work in a mobile facility in Ecuador

a variety of surgical cases, the local surgical team (remote) was in communication with individuals back at the university in the US. Cases involved remote anesthesia [28], telementoring [29], and intermittent surgical services in primary care [30].

While the utility and efficacy of telemedicine in jungle regions of Ecuador has been well documented, work in Panama, Brazil, and central Africa also showcases the successful application of telemedicine in austere environments. In Latin America, countries may very well require a health systems approach to further expand and integrate telemedicine across all of Central and South America [31]. Developing a top-down strategy may be key in establishing telemedicine in Panama [32].

Brazil, a key emerging player on the world stage has begun to really embrace telemedicine and telehealth [33]. While challenges remain, research has shown that there are no barriers to monitoring health along the Amazon or in the Amazon. In 2008, an individual swam the entire Amazon River from high in the mountains at Atalaya, Peru to the Atlantic Ocean at Belém, Brazil. Over 66 days, the medical research team used telemedicine to provide medical support his swim [34]. Furthermore, telemedicine has been applied for tuberculosis and leprosy in several austere and inhospitable locals [35, 36].

Surgical care in remote regions of Kenya using Internet-based technology demonstrated cost-efficiency for prescreening patients [37]. Figure 29.6 illustrates

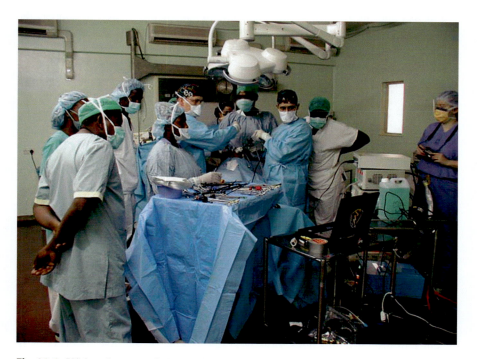

Fig. 29.6 US-based surgeons in Kenya linked to the US via telemedicine

surgeons in an operating theater in Kenya linked to consultants in Richmond, Virginia.

A significant amount of research has been conducted worldwide in austere environments. The results continue to push healthcare forward. Healthcare tools that would not have been common is austere and remote environments are now more readily available, including ultrasound [38] and other digital solutions.

Ships at Sea/Oil Rigs

In early 2020, at the beginning of the COVID-19 pandemic, there were several cruise ships that were impacted by both death and severe illness brought on by the virus [39, 40]. Passenger ships and naval vessels may very well be stocked with medical personnel and a variety of medical capabilities, but they still depend on telemedicine for access to definitive care or at least guidance. In some cases, cruise ships may not have a physician on board [41]. The U.S. Navy utilizes telemedicine from its ships at sea, especially for injuries and infectious diseases [13, 42, 43].

While maritime telemedicine is provided to ships at sea and the medical care capability may not necessarily be austere, emergency evacuation is not an easy task due to many factors, including location, hostile forces, weather, etc. This same thought applies to oil rigs. Much has been published on health care issues in the North Sea and the Gulf of Mexico and how telemedicine is used to support the crews who live and work in these very remote locations [44–46].

While naval vessels are under the authority of the flag and nation for which they sail, other vessels must be aware of legal and medico-legal issues that may arise. This involves the ship's captain contacting Telemedical Maritime Assistance Service when there is a medical need [47]. While telemedicine may be challenging, both the captain and the consulting physician have responsibilities with legal implications.

Disasters and Pandemics

When a disaster strikes, most of the world is not prepared [48]. Infrastructure is damaged or destroyed, including buildings, telecommunications, medical support, transportation, etc. (see Fig. 29.7). Basic resources are no longer readily available, thus, the austere nature of the environment. Morbidity and mortality rise sharply, and the survivors are left to deal with what might be unimaginable conditions, which fosters posttraumatic stress disorder [49]. Disasters are impactful immediately, but it is the aftermath and its toll on public health and life itself where the need lies [50].

Over the past several decades, telemedicine has been applied in the aftermath of earthquakes, hurricanes, tsunamis, humanitarian response to refugees, and most recently to a highly infectious virus COVID-19. One of the first applications of significant size was the Soviet Armenia earthquake in 1988. Telemedicine was deployed and was shown to be highly effective [8, 51, 52]. This system, once it was up and operating post disaster, was easily adapted to respond to a second disaster in

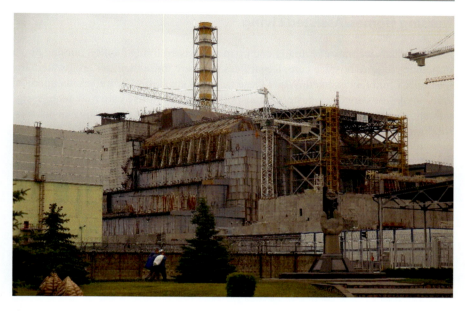

Fig. 29.7 Encasement of Chernobyl nuclear power station, Ukraine

Ufa, Russia. Telemedicine in disaster management plays a significant role [53–55]. Médecins Sans Frontières has used telemedicine effectively through many of its various deployments of physicians and medical teams [56] and field hospitals in disaster regions also incorporate telemedicine [57].

While there is a plethora of work in the field of deploying telemedicine, the commonality is that each catastrophic event, regardless of destruction, morbidity, and mortality, is extreme and austere. Medical personnel and the supply chain are destroyed, delayed, or not working at all. Telemedicine provides a level of comfort to those on the frontline by those who are remote. They provide guidance, expertise, and a virtual helping hand when there is no other alternative.

Often disasters are related to some natural or manmade occurrence. It is not often that a virus or bacterium can bring an entire world to the throws of chaos and economic calamity. Highly infectious diseases like the coronavirus (COVID-19) run through populations quickly bringing mortality and despair. Up to this point, widescale adoption and integration of telemedicine in a normal healthcare system was challenging regardless of the location of the patient and providers. Telemedicine basically went from 0 to 60 in a matter of seconds. Whole health systems increase their utilization by thousands of percentages. Telemedicine has been widely adopted across the world in an effort to alleviate the pressure on the health care system [58]. A quick search on PubMed (on May 27) indicates over 16,490 manuscripts on COVID-19 have been published in 2020. Before 2020, there were none. The pandemic may very well linger for some time, affecting the entire populations of the world, and it will be the effective use of telemedicine that will be significant adjunct to our healthcare workers and all of us as well.

Nursing Homes/Assisted Living

As individuals we may eventually end up in an assisted living facility, nursing home or perhaps require hospice care. Regardless of where these facilities are located, the residence often feel isolated. While these facilities are staffed by nurses, the medical care capabilities are often austere. Transportation to definitive care may require significant coordination and may not be timely. This is where technology in sensors, robotics, and telemedicine come into play [59]. Geriatricians can utilize telemedicine to monitor and manage the elderly population effectively [60]. Gillespie et al. reported on standards for evaluation and management of telemedicine in nursing facilities [61]. In addition, a variety of robotic systems and sensors have been deployed and studied as part of the ecosystem for the elderly [62, 63].

While independent living is encouraged, challenges for individuals remain. Telemedicine offers capabilities that can enhance and enable us to remain in our homes or facilities that permit monitoring of physical and mental state. Even in a large metropolitan area, a person's home may in fact be austere and challenging for that individual to obtain the necessary care needed and expected.

Conclusions

In 1968, as the *Apollo* spacecraft came around the dark side of the moon, the Earth, that blue dot in the starlit blackness of space, was home to billions of people. The Earth looked small juxtaposed to space. While Earth appears large to us, it is indeed smaller today, not in size but in the interconnectedness we experience. Information and communications technologies have lessened the austereness of our world, by enabling us to communicate in real time. This chapter provided a very informative review of how telemedicine has been applied in austere conditions. From space and the battlefields to elder care, telemedicine has been applied successful. Over the past century or so, telemedicine and telehealth have evolved in stature and capability. While there have been barriers placed in front of its path, including technological, political, or economical, they seem to have been removed during the COVID-19 pandemic. Whether they return and hamper consumerism remains an unknown. Sometimes telemedicine is the only way to get medical attention.

References

1. Penninga L, Lorentzen AK, Davis C. A telemedicine case series for acute medical emergencies in Greenland: a model for austere environments. Telemed J E Health. 2020;26(8):1066–70; [Epub ahead of print].
2. Kirkpatrick AW, McKee JL, McBeth PB, Ball CG, LaPorta A, Broderick T, Leslie T, King D, Wright Beatty HE, Keillor J, Tien H. The Damage Control Surgery in Austere Environments Research Group (DCSAERG): a dynamic program to facilitate real-time telementoring/telediagnosis to address exsanguination in extreme and austere environments. J Trauma Acute Care Surg. 2017;83(1 Suppl 1):S156–63.

3. Pamplin JC, Davis KL, Mbuthia J, Cain S, Hipp SJ, Yourk DJ, Colombo CJ, Poropatich R. Military Telehealth: a model for delivering expertise to the point of need in austere and operational environments. Health Aff (Millwood). 2019;38(8):1386–92.
4. Szawarski P, Hillebrandt D. Doctor won't see you now: changing paradigms in mountain medicine. Postgrad Med J. 2018;94(1109):182–4.
5. Doarn CR. Telemedicine in extreme environments: analogs for space flight. Stud Health Technol Inform. 2003;97:35–41.
6. Merrell RC, Cone SW, Rafiq A. Telemedicine in extreme conditions: disasters, war, remote sites. Stud Health Technol Inform. 2008;131:99–116.
7. Satava R, Angood PB, Harnett B, Macedonia C, Merrell R. The physiologic cipher at altitude: telemedicine and real-time monitoring of climbers on Mount Everest. Telemed J E Health. 2000;6(3):303–13.
8. Doarn CR, Nicogossian AE, Merrell RC. Applications of telemedicine in the United States space program. Telemed J. 1998;4(1):19–30.
9. Ushakov IB, Orlov OI, Baevskiĭ RM, Bersen'ev EI, Chernikova AG. Conception of health: space-earth. Fiziol Cheloveka. 2013;39(2):5–9. (In Russian).
10. Doarn CR, Lavrentyev VA, Orlov OI, Nicogossian AE, Grigoriev AI, Ferguson EW, Merrell RC. Evolution of telemedicine in Russia: the influence of the space program on modern telemedicine programs. Telemed J E Health. 2003;9(1):103–9.
11. Rayman RB. Telemedicine: military applications. Aviat Space Environ Med. 1992;63(2):135–7.
12. Crowther JB, Poropatich R. Telemedicine in the U.S. Army: case reports from Somalia and Croatia. Telemed J. 1995;1(1):73–80.
13. Bakalar RS. From ship to shore: "telemedicine at the deckplates" the telemedicine multimedia integrated distribute network (MIDN) project. J Digit Imaging. 1997;10(3 Suppl 1):142.
14. Blanchet KD. The U.S. Army Telemedicine and Advanced Technology Research Center (TATRC). Telemed J E Health. 2006;12(4):390–5.
15. Satava RM. Virtual reality and telepresence for military medicine. Comput Biol Med. 1995;25(2):229–36.
16. Satava RM. Robotic surgery: from past to future—a personal journey. Surg Clin North Am. 2003;83(6):1491–500.
17. McNicholas JE. TeleHealth in the modern era of military medical consultation. Mil Med. 2018;183(5-6):110–2.
18. Kruse CS, Atkins JM, Baker TD, Gonzales EN, Paul JL, Brooks M. Factors influencing the adoption of telemedicine for treatment of military veterans with post-traumatic stress disorder. J Rehabil Med. 2018;50(5):385–92.
19. Krakuaer J. Into thin air: a personal account of the Mt. Everest disaster. New York: Anchor Books/Doubleday; 1999.
20. Harnett BM, Satava R, Angood P, Merriam NR, Doarn CR, Merrell RC. The benefits of integrating Internet technology with standard communications for telemedicine in extreme environments. Aviat Space Environ Med. 2001;72(12):1132–7.
21. Angood PB, Satava R, Doarn C, Merrell R, E3 Group. Telemedicine at the top of the world: the 1998 and 1999 Everest extreme expeditions. Telemed J E Health. 2000;6(3):315–25.
22. Kreshak J. Technical and cultural challenges of remote health care on Everest. Yale J Biol Med. 1999;72(1):29–31.
23. Otto C, Hamilton DR, Levine BD, Hare C, Sargsyan AE, Altshuler P, Dulchavsky SA. Into thin air: extreme ultrasound on Mt Everest. Wilderness Environ Med. 2009;20(3):283–9.
24. Bicakci K, Baykal N. EVEREST: an efficient method for verification of digital signatures in real-time teleradiology. Stud Health Technol Inform. 2004;107(Pt 2):1241–5.
25. Ganapathy K, Chawdhry V, Premanand S, Sarma A, Chandralekha J, Kumar KY, Kumar S, Guleri R. Telemedicine in the Himalayas: operational challenges-a preliminary report. Telemed J E Health. 2016;22(10):821–35.
26. Ganapathy K, Alagappan D, Rajakumar H, Dhanapal B, Rama Subbu G, Nukala L, Premanand S, Veerla KM, Kumar S, Thaploo V. Tele-emergency services in the Himalayas. Telemed J E Health. 2019;25(5):380–90.

27. Hultkrantz A. The Shaman and the medicine-man. Soc Sci Med. 1985;20(5):511–5.
28. Cone SW, Gehr L, Hummel R, Rafiq A, Doarn CR, Merrell RC. Case report of remote anesthetic monitoring using telemedicine. Anesth Analg. 2004;98(2):386–8.
29. Rosser JC Jr, Bell RL, Harnett B, Rodas E, Murayama M, Merrell R. Use of mobile low-bandwidth telemedical techniques for extreme telemedicine applications. J Am Coll Surg. 1999;189(4):397–404.
30. Doarn CR, Fitzgerald S, Rodas E, Harnett B, Prabe-Egge A, Merrell RC. Telemedicine to integrate intermittent surgical services into primary care. Telemed J E Health. 2002;8(1):131–7.
31. LeRouge CM, Gupta M, Corpart G, Arrieta A. Health system approaches are needed to expand telemedicine use across nine Latin American nations. Health Aff (Millwood). 2019;38(2):212–21.
32. Vega S, Marciscano I, Holcomb M, Erps KA, Major J, Lopez AM, Barker GP, Weinstein RS. Testing a top-down strategy for establishing a sustainable telemedicine program in a developing country: the Arizona telemedicine program-US Army-Republic of Panama initiative. Telemed J E Health. 2013;19(10):746–53.
33. Maldonado JM, Marques AB, Cruz A. Telemedicine: challenges to dissemination in Brazil. Cad Saude Publica. 2016;32(Suppl 2):e00155615. [Article in English, Portuguese].
34. Latifi R, Stanonik Mde L, Merrell RC, Weinstein RS. Telemedicine in extreme conditions: supporting the Martin Strel Amazon Swim Expedition. Telemed J E Health. 2009;15(1):93–100.
35. Angel DI, Alfonso R, Faizal M, Ricaurte O, Baez JA, Rojas A, Barato P, Patarroyo ME, Patarroyo MA. Cutaneous tuberculosis diagnosis in an inhospitable Amazonian region by means of telemedicine and molecular biology. J Am Acad Dermatol. 2005;52(5 Suppl 1):S65–8.
36. Paixão MP, Miot HA, de Souza PE, Haddad AE, Wen CL. A university extension course in leprosy: telemedicine in the Amazon for primary healthcare. J Telemed Telecare. 2009;15(2):64–7.
37. Lee S, Broderick TJ, Haynes J, Bagwell C, Doarn CR, Merrell RC. The role of low-bandwidth telemedicine in surgical prescreening. J Pediatr Surg. 2003;38(9):1281–3.
38. Ogedegbe C, Morchel H, Hazelwood V, Hassler C, Feldman J. Demonstration of novel, secure, real-time, portable ultrasound transmission from an austere international location. Conf Proc IEEE Eng Med Biol Soc. 2012;2012:5794–7.
39. Dahl E. Coronavirus (Covid-19) outbreak on the cruise ship Diamond Princess. Int Marit Health. 2020;71(1):5–8.
40. Mouchtouri VA, Dirksen-Fischer M, Hadjichristodoulou C. Health measures to travelers and cruise ships in response to COVID-19. J Travel Med. 2020;27(3):taaa043. Epub ahead of print.
41. Holt TE, Tveten A, Dahl E. Medical emergencies on large passenger ships without doctors: the Oslo-Kiel-Oslo ferry experience. Int Marit Health. 2017;68(3):153–8.
42. Davis K, Perry-Moseanko A, Tadlock MD, Henry N, Pamplin J. Successful implementation of low-cost tele-critical care solution by the U.S. Navy: initial experience and recommendations. Mil Med. 2017;182(5):e1702–7.
43. Schallhorn CS, Richmond CJ, Schallhorn JM. Military teleconsultation services facilitate prompt recognition and treatment of a case of syphilitic uveitis aboard a United States navy aircraft carrier at sea during combat operations without evacuation capability. Telemed J E Health. 2020;26(6):821–26; Epub ahead of print.
44. Ponsonby W, Mika F, Irons G. Offshore industry: medical emergency response in the offshore oil and gas industry. Occup Med (Lond). 2009;59(5):298–303.
45. Webster K, Fraser S, Mair F, Ferguson J. A low-cost decision support network for electrocardiograph transmission from oil rigs in the North Sea. J Telemed Telecare. 2008;14(3):162–4.
46. Mair F, Fraser S, Ferguson J, Webster K. Telemedicine via satellite to support offshore oil platforms. J Telemed Telecare. 2008;14(3):129–31.
47. Ricci G, Pirillo I, Rinuncini C, Amenta F. Medical assistance at the sea: legal and medico-legal problems. Occup Med (Lond). 2009;59(5):298–303.
48. Doarn CR, Latifi R, Poropatich RK, Sokolovich N, Kosiak D, Hostiuc F, Zoicas C, Buciu A, Arafat R. Development and validation of telemedicine for disaster response: the North Atlantic Treaty Organization Multinational System. Telemed J E Health. 2018;24(9):657–68.

49. Naushad VA, Bierens JJ, Nishan KP, Firjeeth CP, Mohammad OH, Maliyakkal AM, ChaliHadan S, Schreiber MD. A systematic review of the impact of disaster on the mental health of medical responders. Prehosp Disaster Med. 2019;34(6):632–43.
50. Randolph R, Chacko S, Morsch G. Disaster medicine: public health threats associated with disasters. FP Essent. 2019;487:11–6.
51. Houtchens BA, Clemmer TP, Holloway HC, Kiselev AA, Logan JS, Merrell RC, Nicogossian AE, Nikogossian HA, Rayman RB, Sarkisian AE, Siegel JH. Telemedicine and international disaster response: medical consultation to Armenia and Russia via a telemedicine spacebridge. Prehosp Disaster Med. 1993;8(1):57–66.
52. Nicogossian AE, Doarn CR. Armenia 1988 earthquake and telemedicine: lessons learned and forgotten. Telemed J E Health. 2011;17(9):741–5.
53. Latifi R, Tilley EH. Telemedicine for disaster management: can it transform chaos into an organized, structured care from the distance? Am J Disaster Med. 2014;9(1):25–37.
54. Lurie N, Carr BG. The role of Telehealth in the medical response to disasters. JAMA Intern Med. 2018;178(6):745–6.
55. Simmons S, Alverson D, Poropatich R, D'Iorio J, DeVany M, Doarn CR. Applying telehealth in natural and anthropogenic disasters. Telemed J E Health. 2008;14(9):968–71.
56. Delaigue S, Bonnardot L, Steichen O, Garcia DM, Venugopal R, Saint-Sauveur JF, Wootton R. Seven years of telemedicine in Médecins Sans Frontières demonstrate that offering direct specialist expertise in the frontline brings clinical and educational value. J Glob Health. 2018;8(2):020414.
57. Naor M, Heyman SN, Bader T, Merin O. Deployment of field hospitals to disaster regions: insights from ten medical relief operations spanning three decades. Am J Disaster Med. 2017;12(4):243–56.
58. Rockwell KL, Gilroy AS. Incorporating telemedicine as part of COVID-19 outbreak response systems. Am J Manag Care. 2020;26(4):147–8.
59. Troudet P, Mignen F, Boureau AS, Berrut G, Georgeton E. Impact of geriatric teleconsultations on hospitalization of elderly living in nursing homes. Geriatr Psychol Neuropsychiatr Vieil. 2019;17(3):261–70.
60. Morley JE. Telemedicine: coming to nursing homes in the near future. J Am Med Dir Assoc. 2016;17(1):1–3.
61. Gillespie SM, Moser AL, Gokula M, Edmondson T, Rees J, Nelson D, Handler SM. Standards for the use of telemedicine for evaluation and management of resident change of condition in the nursing home. J Am Med Dir Assoc. 2019;20(2):115–22.
62. Marcelino I, Laza R, Domingues P, Gómez-Meire S, Fdez-Riverola F, Pereira A. Active and assisted living ecosystem for the elderly. Sensors (Basel). 2018;18(4):pii:E1246.
63. Koceska N, Koceski S, Beomonte Zobel P, Trajkovik V, Garcia N. A telemedicine robot system for assisted and independent living. Sensors (Basel). 2019;19(4):pii:E834.

Correction to: Telemedicine, Telehealth and Telepresence

Rifat Latifi, Charles R. Doarn, and Ronald C. Merrell

Correction to:

R.Latifi at al. (eds.), Telemedicine, Telehealth and Telepresence, https://doi.org/10.1007/978-3-030-56917-4

Chapters 1, 6, 12 and 17 were originally published non-open access. They have been converted to open access under a CC BY 4.0 license and the Copyright is now with "The Author(s)". The book has also been updated with this change.

The updated version of the book can be found at https://doi.org/10.1007/978-3-030-56917-4

© The Author(s) 2021
R. Latifi et al. (eds.), *Telemedicine, Telehealth and Telepresence*,
https://doi.org/10.1007/978-3-030-56917-4_30

Index

A

Access
 disparities in, 333
 neonatologists, 338
 to pediatric dermatologic services, 335
 and utilization, 335
Accountable care models (ACO), 149
Accountable care organizations (ACO), 116, 150
Activity-based costing, 145, 146
Acute myocardial infarction (AMI), 391
Admission, discharge, and transfer (ADT), 65
Advanced Research Projects Agency (ARPA), 266
Agency for health research quality (AHRQ), 79, 141
Albania telemedicine network, 32
Albanian diabetes association, 36
Alpine environment, 475
Alteplase, 401
Ambulatory telehealth consultations, 334
American academy of dermatology, 107
American academy of family medicine, 157
American academy of family practice, 107
American college of surgeons (ACS), 98
American health information management association (AHIMA), 134
American hospital association (AHA), 129
American medical association, 107, 157
American national standards institute, 68
American psychiatry association's (APA) practice guideline, 104
American recovery and reinvestment act of 2009, 69
American t elemedicine association's (ATA) standards and guidelines committee, 102
American Telemedicine Association (ATA), 107, 157, 235, 367
American speech-language-hearing association, 107
Andhra Pradesh, 217–218
Anxiety, 375
Apollo Telehealth Services (ATHS), 208
Applied behavior analysis (ABA), 347, 356, 359
Arizona elemedicine council (ATC), 182
Arizona rural telecommunications network (ARTN), 172
Arizona telemedicine council (ATC), 172, 173, 176
 analysis of, 177
 Burns–Weinstein partnership, 183–186
 challenges, 186
 government attendees, 177, 179
 industry classifications, 177
 legislation, 183
 longitudinal analysis of, attendance, 181, 182
 meeting, 179, 181
 members, of past and present, 182
 membership, 176
Arizona telemedicine program (ATP), 5, 172, 173
Army trauma training center (ATTC), 58
ARPA net (ARPANET), 266
Artificial intelligence (AI), 11, 259, 266–267, 463
Assistant secretary for planning and evaluation (ASPE), 80
Association of american medical colleges (AAMC), 16
Asynchronous interpretation, 63
Asynchronous systems, 241
ATA ocular telehealth special interest group's (SIG) guidelines, 102

Audit cycle, 382
Austere conditions
  alpine, 474–476
  battlefield, 473–474
  disasters and pandemics, 478–479
  jungle, 476–477
  nursing homes/assisted living, 480
  ships at sea/oil rigs, 478–479
  space, 472–473

B
Bariatric surgery, 433–435
Bipartisan budget act of 2018 (BBA), 116
Brief communication technology-based service, 119
Broadband global area network (BGAN), 46
Bundled payments for care improvement advanced program (BPCI), 121
Burn
  assessment, 307
  billing and documentation, 317–318
  global efforts, 315–316
  intubation, 312
  mortality and morbidity worldwide, 307
  opportunities for telemedicine, 308–309
  outpatient telemedicine, 315
  over and under triage, 311
  over-usage, aeromedical transport, 313–314
  pediatric care, 314
  policies and protocols/agreement required, 316
  size and severity assessment, 308–310 (*see also* Teleburn)
  teleconsultation, 317
  virtual examination, 311–312
Business Associate Agreement (BAA), 136
Business planning, telemedicine, 141–143

C
Cabo verde telemedicine network, 33
Cabo verde, telemedicine program, 37–39
California's licensing law, 130
CardioMEMS, 388
Cellular/mobile broadband technology, 46
Center for connected health olicy (CCHP), 175
Center for medicaid and medicare services, 44, 80, 117, 141, 162
Centre for research on the epidemiology of disasters (CRED) programs, 58
Child Ready program, 239
Chiranjeevi Yojana (CY), 207
Clinical child therapy, 348–352

Clinical decision support systems (CDSS), 323
Clinical effectiveness research (CER), 78
Clinical telemedicine, 43
  guidelines, 43, 45
  policies and protocols, 45
  remote monitoring, 43
  technical requirements, 45, 46
    data reporting, 47
    data security and accessibility, 46
    teleconsultations, 46
  telemedicine modalities, 44, 45
Colorectal surgery, 436
Communicable disease outbreaks, 236
Communication network options, 246
Communication technology-based services, 119
  brief communication technology-based service, 119
  interprofessional internet consultation, 119
  remote evaluation of pre-recorded patient information, 119
Comprehensive joint replacement (CJR), 121
Computed tomography (CT) scanners, 15
Computerized cognitive behavioral therapy (cCBT), 375
Confederation of Indian Industry (CII), 205
Consolidated-clinical document architecture (C-CDA), 65
Continued quality improvement (CQI) plan, 244, 249
Continuing medical education (CME), 29, 131
Continuity of care document (CCD), 65
Conventional healthcare providers, 246
Core HIE data sets, 66
2019 Coronavirus (COVID-19), 129
  prison and jail system healthcare, 425
  related DTC telehealth surge, 280
  pandemic, 478, 480
  telemedicine, 478
Corporate memory, 176
Cost effectiveness, 213–214
Crichton, michael, 3
Crichton, Michael, 4, 5, 8, 10
Critical Care Medicine Society (CCMS) website data, 321

D
da Vinci platform, 265
Data communication networks, 46
Decision support systems (DSS), 380
Defense Advanced Research Agency (DARPA), 432
Depression, 375
Diabetic foot ulcers (DFUs)

Index

foot care delivery
   barriers to telemedicine adoption, 457
   cost-effectiveness, 462–463
   delivery in remote area, 460–461
   vs. in-person visit, reliability, 461
   patient acceptability, 457–458
   telemedine vs. traditional care, 458–460
   public health significance of, 455–456
   telemedicine for, 456
Digital health, 464, 466
Digital health interventions (DHIs), 375
Digital technology-based health care, 463
Direct secure messaging (DSM), 70
Direct to consumer telehealth, 340–341
Direct-to-consumer (DTC)
   messaging, 143
   telehealth, 278, 280–282, 289
   telemedicine, 150, 151, 153, 154
      business planning, 152
      cost of, 153
      revenue analysis, 154
Direct-to-enrollee (employee) (DTE), 150
Direct-to-hospital (DTH) telehealth, 276, 278
Direct-to-patient (DTP), 150
Disaster management, 51
   administrative requirements, 59
   disaster classifications, 53
   four phases of, 53
   incorporation, of telemedicine
      during COVID-19, 57
      during disaster, 56, 57
      post-disaster, 57
      pre-disaster, 56
      training and simulation, 58
   incorporation, of telemedicine during COVID-19, 57
   24/7 mass casualty center, 53, 54
Disaster, healthcare in, 478–479
Dissemination and intervention science
   origin of, 79
   in United States, 78, 79
Distance education, 283, 289
Distance learning and telementoring, 268
Division for cancer prevention and control, 79
Drones, 261
Drug enforcement administration (DEA), 44

E
Educational videoconferencing system, 29
e-Health, 259
eHealth Exchange, 69
Electronic health record (EHR), 64, 67, 248, 267

Electronic medical record (EMR), 267, 367
Electronic patient records (EPRs), 267
Emergency and disaster response, phases of, 55
Emergency departments (EDs), 369
Emergency events database (EM-DAT), 53
Emergency triage, treatment and transport model (ET3), 121
End-stage-renal disease (ESRD), 115
Evidence-based medicine (EBM), 97
Extension for Community Health Outcomes (ECHO) model, 237
Extension for Community Healthcare Outcomes (ECHO) project, 268
Extreme environment, *see* Austere conditions

F
Face-to-face consent, 132
Face-to-face interactions, 162
Fast healthcare interoperability resources (FHIR), 68
Federal and state privacy and security regulations, 73
Federal communications commission (FCC), 142
Federal office of rural health policy (ORHP), 160
Federation of state medical boards (FSMB), 131
Fee-for-service (FFS), 149
Five patients. the hospital explained, 10–12
Foot ulcer remission, 465
Forward surgical team (FST), 58
Frantic networking, 187
Full time equivalents (FTEs), 142, 151

G
Geospatial analysis, 281–282
Geospatial information systems (GIS), 67
Glasgow Coma Scale (GCS), 295
Global health, 235
Global positioning system (GPS), 56
Gross domestic product (GDP), 54

H
Hageseth v. superior court of california, 130, 131
Harvard medical school (HMS), 3, 15, 16
Head injuries, 298, 299
Healers, 246
Health and human services (HHS), 142

Health care financing administration (HCFA), 141
Health information exchange (HIE), 65, 67
　creating standards, 65–68
　and telemedicine, 63, 64
Health information exchanges (HIEs), 69, 248
Health information technology (HIT), 160
Health information technology for economic and clinical health act (HITECH Act), 69
Health insurance portability and accountability act (HIPAA), 29, 134, 136
Health internetwork access to research initiative (HINARI), 29
Health level seven international (HL7), 68
Health system capabilities, 245
Heart failure (HF), 386
HIE and telemedicine integration, 64
Himalayas, 216–217
Hospital Dr. Agostinho Neto (HAN), 38
Hub-and-spoke model, 403

I
"Improving healthcare systems" (IHS), 84
India, telehealth
　challenges, 197
　public private partnerships, health care, 203–207
　service providers/supporters, 198
Indo-UK Institute of Health (IUIH), 203
Infant mortality rate, 37
Informal transmissions, 134
Informed consent, telemedicine, 132, 133
Initiate-build-operate-transfer (IBOT), 20, 26
　building phase, of robust infrastructure, 28–30
　implementation
　　albania telemedicine program, 34–36
　　clinical results, 36, 37
　initiating phase, 27, 28
　operating phase, 30
　transferring phase, 30, 31
Innovation, study of telemedicine, 14, 15
Insecure transmissions, 134
Institute for clinical systems improvement (ICSI), 99
Institute of medicine (IOM), 84
Integrated Telemedicine and e-Health program, 34
Intensive care units (ICUs), *see* Tele-ICU
Intensivists, 322
International Telecommunication Union (ITU), 316

International virtual e-hospital, 22
Internet of Medical Things, 242
Internet of Things (IoT), 463
Internet Protocol (IP) networks, 366
Interprofessional internet consultation, 119
Interstate medical license compact (IMLC), 131, 290
Intravenous alteplase (IV tPA), 401

J
Jail system healthcare, COVID-19 and, 425
Jharkhand Digital Dispensaries programme, 219–220
Joint legislative budget committee (JLBC), 172
Jungles, healthcare in, 477

K
Kaiser permanente medical group (KPMG), 99
Karnataka Integrated Telemedicine and Tele-health Project (KITTH), 205
Kidney care choices (KCC) model, 121
Knowles, John H., 3–6
Kosova telemedicine network, 31
Kosova telemedicine program, 20–26

L
Labor and delivery and newborn settings, 338–339
Land mines, 53
Licensing, 130
　Hageseth v. superior court of california, 130, 131
　IMLC, 131
Local area networks (LAN), 46
Logan International airport MGH medical station multi-specialty telemedicine program (LIA-MGH-TP), 3
Logan international airport MGH medical station telemedicine program, 6–8
LOINC, 66
Low- income countries (LIC), 28
Lower extremity amputation, 456

M
Machine learning (ML) algorithms, 323
Man-made disasters, 53
Marine biology laboratory (MBL), 8
Mass casualty centers (MCC), 54
Massachusetts general hospital (MGH), 3

Index   489

Massachusetts institute of technology (MIT), 11
Master patient index (MPI), 70
Maternal mortality rate, 37
Medicaid fee for service, 122, 123
Medicaid managed care, 125
Medi-Cal, 123
Medical records, telemedicine, 134
Medicare access and CHIP reauthorization act of 2015 (MACRA), 150
Medicare advantage (MA) plans, 121
Medicare advantage plans (MA), 116
Medicare payment categories, 117
Medicare reimbursement policies, 115, 116
Medicare telehealth reimbursement, fee-for-service, 118
Medicare telehealth services, 117, 119
Medication-assisted treatment (MAT), 83
Merit-based incentive payment system (MIPS), 150
Metropolitan area network (MAN), 46
MGH medical station telemedicine program, 6, 7
MGH telemedicine trainees, 4, 5
M-health, 242, 259
Middle- income countries (MICC), 28
Military, 261
Millennium Development Goals (MDG), 236
Ministry of health and social affairs (MOHSA), 34
Mobile health (mHealth), 262, 283
Model Concessionaire agreements (MCA), 206
Moutainous terrain, 476
Multinational telemedicine system (MnTS), 58
Myocardial infarction systems, 391

N

National cancer institute (NCI), 79
National center of biomedical engineering (NCBE), 36
National committee on quality assurance (NCQA), 99
National consortium of telehealth resource centers (NCTRC), 134
National Health Policy (NHP), 203
National institute of health (NIH), 6, 78, 141
National Quality Forum (NQF), 249
National Rural Telemedicine Network (NRTN), 205
National thermal power corporation (NTPC), 223–225
Nation-wide HIE, 69

NATO science for peace and security (SPS) program, 58
Natural disaster, 51, 53
Neurology, *see* Teleneurology
Neurology/telestroke program, 39
Neurosurgery, 444–446
Neurotrauma, 37
New mexico health information collaborative (NMHIC) model, 71, 72
New York Heart Association (NYHA) functional classification, 388
NMHIC consent model, 71
Non-communicable disease (NCD)
    quintessential, diabetes, 455
    screening, 225
Non-governmental organizations (NGOs), 20
Non-reimbursement state policy issues, 125
Novel coronavirus 2019 (COVID-19), *see* 2019 Coronavirus (COVID-19)

O

Office for the advancement of telehealth (OAT), 101, 142
Office of rural health policy, 141
Office of the national coordinator (ONC), 69, 160
Oral anticoagulant users, 392
Organization for safety and cooperation, 20

P

Pandemics, 478–479
Parent-child interaction therapy (PCIT), 348
Patient centered outcomes research institute (PCORI), 78–80
    extramural funding, 81
    funding opportunities, 81
    telehealth, defined, 80
    telehealth-related content analysis
        funding, levels of, 86
        health conditions, 84
        intervention strategies, 87
        location and organization, 89
        patient populations, 85
        publications, 90
        research study designs, 86, 87
    telehealth-related research portfolio analysis, 82, 83
    telehealth-related research project, 81, 82
    telemedicine, defined, 80, 81
Patient monitoring, 283, 287
Patient protection and affordable care act, 79
Patient trust assessment tool (PATAT), 162

Patient-centered care, 77
Patient-centered data home (PCDH), 69
Patient-centered medical home (PCMH)
    approach, 147
Patient-centered outcomes research (PCOR)
    trust fund, 80
Patient-powered research networks
    (PPRN), 83
PCORI funding announcements (PFAs), 81
PCORI telehealth-related research
    projects, 90
Pediatric ambulatory care, 334–335
Pediatric behavioral and mental health,
    336
Pediatric cardiology, 37
Pediatric emergency telehealth
    services, 339–340
Pediatric psychology
    interventions, 348, 352–356
    issues in, 347
Peripheral neuropathy, 461
Physician liability, 137
    Frazier v. University of Mississippi
        Medical Center, 137, 138
    malpractice, 137
Physician-patient relationship, 135
Plain old telephone service (POTS), 46
Plastic surgery, 435–436
Podimetrics Mat, 465
Point-of-care limited ultrasound (PLUS), 56
Policy statements, 100
Portable satellite applications, 46
Position statements, 100
Prehospital care, 412, 414
Prehospital telemedicine, 296–297
Prison system
    COVID-19 and, 425
    healthcare in, 420–421
    rate by countries, 419
Prisoners
    clinical disciplines using
        telemedicine, 423–425
    telemedicine for, 422–423
Privacy, risks to, 136
Private payer laws, 124, 125
Project ECHO, 335
Protected health information (PHI),
    64, 70, 136
Public private partnerships, health care
    global perspective, 200–203
    Indian scenario, 203–207
    specific state government
        initiatives, 206–207
    standard, 198–200

Q
Qualified healthcare professional (QHP), 120
Quality of care
    in children, 339
    telehealth pediatric emergency
        consultations, 339
    telehealth services, 341

R
Radio corporation of america (RCA), 8
Rashtriya Swasthya Bima Yojana, 205
Real time teleconsultation, 241
Real-time video, 240
Real-time videoconferencing, 241
Regional HIE collaboration, 70
Regional telemedicine centers (RTCs), 28
Remote evaluation of pre-recorded patient
    information, 119
Remote monitoring, 407, 409, 464, 466, 471
    See also Austere conditions
Remote patient monitoring (RPM), 149,
    243, 333
    cost of, 147
    financial impact, 148
    PCMH approach, 147
    planning, 147
    reducing complications, risk
        population, 147
    revenue of, 148
    shared savings calculation, 149
Remote physiologic monitoring (RPM), 120
Return on investment (ROI), 249
Revenue model, 146
Risk-sharing payment models, 121
Robotic telepathology, 5
Robotics, 259, 263–265
Rural America
    future applications in, 163, 164
    healthcare cost, 161, 162
    level of complexity, 163
    patient's trust, in telemedicine, 162
    transportation, 163
Rural health policy, 159–161
Rural telemedicine, 276, 278–280
RxNORM, 66

S
Scholastic aptitude test (SAT), 185
School-based health centers, 337–338
Selfie telemedicine, 133, 134
Sensoria socks, 466
Sensors, 263

Index

Service Provider Directory (SPD), 276, 279–280
Service Provider Summit (SPS), 276, 277
Shared savings program, 149
Siren socks, 465
Small business association, 143
Small office home office networks (SOHO), 46
Smartphone apps in medicine, 262
SNOMED, 66
Social determinants of health (SDOH), 73
Social security act, 79
Southern Arizona teletrauma and telepresence (SATT), 442–444
Space, 260
Space, telemedicine application in, 473
Specialty consultations via telemedicine, 243
State plan amendment (SPA), 123
State telehealth reimbursement policies
 medicaid fee for service, 122, 123
 medicaid managed care, 125
 private payer laws, 124, 125
Store-and-forward telehealth ambulatory, 335
Strategic health information exchange collaborative (SHIEC), 69
Stroke
 acute ischemic, 401
 care, 401
 in United States, 401 (*see also* Telestroke)
Substance use disorders (SUDs), 116
Sustainable Development Goals (SDG), 236, 237, 249
Swinfen Charitable Trust Expert Consultation Web site, 242
Synchronous telepsychiatry (STP), 365
Synchronous videoconferencing, 63

T

Technology enabled remote health care (TeRHC), 197
 in Andhra Pradesh, 217–218
 barriers to adoption, 215–216
 challenges in communication, 214
 conceptualisation, 208–209
 contact with community, 212–213
 cost effectiveness, 213–214
 in Himalayas, 216–217
 Jharkhand Digital Dispensaries programme, 219–220
 performance assessment, 214–215
 societal influences, 215
 strategy and planning, 209–210
 training and re-training, 211–212

TUVER, 223–226
Uttar Pradesh Telemedicine programme, 220–223
Telebehavioral studies
 in child health services, 348
 diagnostic accuracy, 348
 group-based interventions, 359
 intervention group, 352
 literature, 352
 outreach setting, 359
Teleburn
 guidelines, 317
 unit, 316
Telecardiology, 39
 cardiac rehabilitation, 392
 decision support systems, 380
 emergency services, 390–392
 health promotion and prevention, 380
 high-level KPIs, 395
 hypertension, 388–390
 monitoring and management, 394–396
 myocardial infarction systems, 391
 oral anticoagulants, 392
 pacemaker telemonitoring, 393
 patients with heart failure, 386
 in primary care, 379–386
 remote monitoring using implantable devices, 393–394
 REMOTE-CR, 393
 tele ECG service, 394
 teleconsultation, 381–385
 telediagnosis, 385–386
 tele-education, 386
 Telehab III study, 392
 telemonitoring, 387, 388
 tele-regulation, 385
Telecommunications connectivity, 24
Telecommunications technology, 80
Teleconsultation, 227, 381–385
 audits, 383–384
 service, 381
Tele-dermatology, 39, 335
Telediagnosis service, 385
TeleECHO Session, 238
Tele-endocrinology, 39
Telehealth, 97
 certification, 108
 EBM, 97, 98
 history of, 100–103
 in India (*see* India, telehealth)
 position statements, 100
 standard of care, 108, 109
 standards and guidelines, 99, 100, 104, 105

TeleHealth network grant program
(TNGP), 142
Telehealth patient portal, 190–194
defined, 189
electronic health record, 189
medical information, 189
outcome, 191
patient-centered care, 190
protection, of privacy, 194
records management, 190
Telehealth Resource Center (TRC), 175
Telehealth technology assessment center
(TTAC), 175
Tele-ICU
challenges and barriers, 325–327
mortality and morbidity, 324–325
prevalence, 323–324
protocols and patients (setting)
selection, 327–328
specialists and intensivists, 323
Telemedicine center of kosova (TCK), 23
Telemedicine program of kosova (TMPK), 29
Telemedicine standards and guidelines, 105
Telemedicine visits vs. in-person care,
financial impact, 146
Telemedicine vs. in-person visits, cost of, 145
Telementoring
in bariatric surgery, 433–435
challenges, 446–447
in colorectal surgery, 436
in geriatrics, 268
in hepato-pancreatico-biliary surgery, 433
Karl Storz VISITOR 1®, 434
in neurosurgery, 444–446
in oncologic surgery, 433
in plastic surgery, 435–436
remote, 433
vs. teleproctoring, 432
and tele-supervision, 239
in trauma and emergency surgery, 441–442
in urology, 438–441
in vascular surgery, 437–438
SAGES Fundamental Use of Surgical
Energy (FUSE) program, 435
use of, 432
utility of, 432
Teleneonatology, 108
Teleneurology, 39
applications, 413
benefit of, 410
devices, 403–404, 412–413
network development, 411
networks, 408, 412
outpatient care, 409

rural care, 409–410
Teleneuroradiology, 410
Teleneurotrauma, 39, 300, 301
Tele-ophthalmology (MeEK), 218–221
Teleorthopedics, 39
Teleotolaryngology, 39
Telepathology, 5
Telepresence
in trauma and emergency surgery, 441–442
of trauma surgeon, 298
robotic devices, 406
Teleproctoring
in bariatric surgery, 433–435
characteristics, 432
in colorectal surgery, 436
in plastic surgery, 435–436
remote, 433
robotic, 433
in vascular surgery, 437–438
vs. telementoring, 432
Telepsychiatry, 101
clinical, 366
consultation-liaison, 368–369
correctional systems, 370
definition, 365
digital health interventions, 375
effectiveness, 371
emergency departments, 369
home-based, 370
legal and regulatory issues, 374
metrics and populations, 371
models and settings, 367–371
nursing home, 371
outpatient model, 367
practice guidelines and training, 372–374
remote camera control, 366
residency program, 373
in schools, 370
stepped care systems, 368
in United States, 366
Teleradiology, 39, 475
services, 205
software, 36
Tele-regulation, 385
Telerehabilitation, 406–407
Telesonography, 413
Telestroke
applications, 404–406
definitions, 401, 402
distributive model of, 404
emergency department, 405–406
hub-and-spoke model of, 403
neurocritical care and inpatient, 406
prehospital, 404–405

principles of, 402–404
rural care, 409–410
teleneuroradiology, 410
Telestroke software, 36
Tele-supervision, 239
Tele-surgery, 39, 433, 437
Teletrauma care (TCC)
    acceptance of, 293
    advanced trauma program, 295
    clinical accuracy of, 298
    consultation, 297
    experiences with, 293
    fly and with no data, 295
    in rural hospitals, 299
    in rural settings, 298
    sustainability programs, 301–303
Teleurology, 39
Television microscopy, 11
Texas law, 133
The joint commission, 107
Thoracic surgery, 436–437
Traditional healers, 246
Traditional telemedicine business plan, 144
Transfers to trauma centers, 295, 297, 298, 300
Transmission Control Protocol and Internet Protocol (TCP/IP), 266
Tufts medical school (TMS), 6
Tuver Health & Wellness Centre (THWC) project, 225

U
U.S. agency for international development (USAID), 20
U.S. Census Bureau, 159
U.S. department of health and human services (HHS), 69, 134, 160
Ulcer recurrence, 465
United Nations Economic Commission for Europe (UNECE) Standard, 200
United nations high commissioner for refugees (UN-HCR), 20
United nations interim administration mission in kosova (UNMIK), 20
United states core data set for interoperability (USCDI), 65

University clinical center of kosova (UCCK), 20
University of arizona, 34
Urban telemedicine, 278
Urology, 440
US department of health and human services, 134
US department of veterans affairs (VA), 78
Utah health information network (UHIN), 69
Utilization review accreditation committee (URAC), 99
Uttar Pradesh Telemedicine programme, 220–223

V
Value-based insurance design (VBID) model, 121
Value-based payment model, 121
Vascular surgery, 437–438
Veteran's Affairs (VA) telepsychiatry system, 365
Video microscopy, 8
Videoconferencing
    clinical child interventions using, 348
    interventions using, 347
    PCIT over, 348
    systems, 240
    techniques, 367
Virtual reality, 240
Virtual reality environments, 239

W
War and conflict related disasters, 53
Wearable sensors, 463, 464, 466
Web-based educational programs, 26
Web-based second opinions, 241
Weinstein, Ronald S., 3, 5, 8, 9, 186
Workflow integration, 247
World health organization (WHO), 19, 53, 129
World Wide Web, 266
Wound healing, 456, 458, 459, 467

Z
Zeus platform, 265

Printed in the United States
by Baker & Taylor Publisher Services